HEPATOBILIARY AND PANCREATIC SURGERY

HEPATOBILIARY AND PANCREATIC SURGERY

Imaging Strategies and Surgical Decision Making

Edited by

Stephen R. T. Evans, M.D.

George Washington University Medical Center
Washington, DC

Susan M. Ascher, M.D.

Georgetown University Medical Center
Washington, DC

WILEY-LISS

A JOHN WILEY & SONS, INC., PUBLICATION

New York / Chichester / Weinheim / Brisbane / Singapore / Toronto

This book is printed on acid-free paper. ♾

Published simultaneously in Canada.

While the authors, editors, and publisher believe that drug selection and dosage and the specification and usage of equipment and devices, as set forth in this book, are in accord with current recommendations and practice at the time of publication, they accept no legal responsibility for any errors or omissions, and make no warranty, express or implied, with respect to material contained herein. In view of ongoing research, equipment modifications, changes in governmental regulations and the constant flow of information relating to drug therapy, drug reactions, and the use of equipment and devices, the reader is urged to review and evaluate the information provided in the package insert or instructions for each drug, piece of equipment, or device for, among other things, any changes in the instructions or indication of dosage or usage and for added warnings and precautions.

Library of Congress Cataloging-in-Publication Data:

Hepatobiliary and pancreatic surgery : imaging strategies and surgical decision making / Stephen R. T. Evans, Susan M. Ascher.
p. cm.
Includes bibliographical references and index.
ISBN 0-471-14755-9 (cloth : alk. paper)
1. Liver—Imaging. 2. Biliary tract—Imaging. 3. Pancreas—Imaging. 4. Surgery—Decision making. I. Evans, Stephen R. T. II. Ascher, Susan.
[DNLM: 1. Biliary Tract Surgery. 2. Liver—surgery. 3. Pancreas—surgery. 4. Liver Diseases—diagnosis. 5. Pancreatic Diseases—diagnosis. 6. Diagnostic Imaging. WI 770 H5299 1998]
RC847.5.I42H48 1998
617.5′56—dc21
DNLM/DLC
for Library of Congress 97-37513
CIP

Printed in the United States of America.

10 9 8 7 6 5 4 3 2 1

To all my students and residents,
whose inquisitiveness and intellectual curiosity
have been the source that stimulates my passion for teaching.

Stephen R. T. Evans, M.D.

To Robert K. Zeman, M.D.,
Mentor and Friend.

Susan M. Ascher, M.D.

CONTENTS

PREFACE

In the 1960s and 1970s it was not unusual for a patient with pancreatic or hepatobiliary disease to undergo initially an ultrasound of the right upper quadrant or epigastrium followed by a computed tomographic scan, upon which an angiogram would be performed, and lastly a magnetic resonance imaging to clarify the disease process. In the midst of all these studies a nuclear medicine consultation may or may not have been obtained, again in hopes of elucidating the problem.

This scenario is soon to become a thing of the past given the tremendous time and cost associated with multiple and duplicate radiographic studies. It is therefore imperative for the radiologist and surgeon to understand the inherent advantages and disadvantages of each imaging study for any given disease process involving the gallbladder, biliary tree, liver, or pancreas. Not only will selecting the proper imaging study improve cost effectiveness, but it will also expedite the evaluation of the patient, leading to a more timely and accurate diagnosis.

This is a first attempt to develop a hybrid medical text between two complementary specialties that focuses on the clear-cut advantages and disadvantages of each imaging modality, with overviews for each anatomic section, and attempts to clarify which study should be done first, second, third, and so on. Obviously there will be considerable controversy, even among surgeons, as to which study should be done, and certainly among radiologists and surgeons. But on the whole there is probably far more agreement than disagreement as to where to begin with imaging and where to finish. We feel the unique structure of this text will lend itself to filling a very necessary niche as a textbook of direct clinical application, useful not just at the practicing clinician level, but also at the medical student, resident, and junior practitioner levels. The extensive reviews on each imaging modality for the four separate anatomic sections, coupled with the large number of imaging studies with parallel illustrations, allows for a much easier understanding of the strengths and weaknesses of each study. Additionally, the surgical summaries at the end of each anatomic section with flow diagrams directing the practitioner in a methodical fashion for work-up of the specific disease process being evaluated make this book quite user-friendly with direct clinical application. We hope this serves the surgical community and ultimately enhances the care of patients with pancreatic and hepatobiliary disease.

Stephen R. T. Evans, M.D.
Susan M. Ascher, M.D.

Washington, DC
February, 1997

CONTRIBUTORS

Firas H. Al-Kawas, M.D., Department of Medicine, Division of Gastroenterology, Georgetown University Medical Center, Washington, DC

Susan M. Ascher, M.D., Department of Radiology, Georgetown University Medical Center, Washington, DC

David C. Brooks, M.D., Department of Surgery, Harvard University Medical School, Boston, MA

Ravi S. Chari, M.D., Department of Surgery, The University of Toronto, Toronto, Ontario, Canada

Cirrelda Cooper, M.D., Department of Radiology, Georgetown University Medical Center, Washington, DC

Donald F. Denny, Jr., M.D., Department of Radiology, The Medical Center at Princeton, Princeton, NJ

Mark D. Duncan, M.D., Department of Surgery, Johns Hopkins Bayview Medical Center, Baltimore, MD

Stephen R. T. Evans, M.D., Department of Surgery, George Washington University Medical Center, Washington, DC

Stephen W. Fry, M.D., Department of Medicine, Division of Gastroenterology, Georgetown University Medical Center, Washington, DC

Brian Garra, M.D., Department of Radiology, Georgetown University Medical Center, Washington, DC

Gregory G. Ginsberg, M.D., Department of Medicine, Division of Gastroenterology, University of Pennsylvania Health Systems, Philadelphia, PA

Stephen C. Horii, M.D., Department of Radiology, University of Pennsylvania Medical Center, Philadelphia, PA

Nikolaos L. Kelekis, M.D., Department of Radiology, University of North Carolina at Chapel Hill, Chapel Hill, NC

Keith D. Lillemoe, M.D., Department of Surgery, The Johns Hopkins Medical Institutions, Baltimore, MD

Steven V. Lossef, M.D., Department of Radiology, Georgetown University Medical Center, Washington, DC

Sean M. Mahan, M.D., Department of Radiology, Georgetown University Medical Center, Washington, DC

Russell J. Nauta, M.D., Department of Surgery, Division of General Surgery, Georgetown University Medical Center, Washington, DC

Jeffrey D. Neitlich, M.D., Department of Radiology, Yale University School of Medicine, New Haven, CT

Cuong C. Nguyen, M.D., Department of Gastroenterology, Mayo Clinic Scottsdale, Scottsdale, AZ

Eric K. Outwater, M.D., Department of Radiology, Thomas Jefferson University Hospital, Philadelphia, PA

Theodore N. Pappas, M.D., Department of Surgery, Duke University Medical Center, Durham, NC

Leslie M. Scoutt, M.D., Department of Radiology, Yale University School of Medicine, New Haven, CT

Richard C. Semelka, M.D., Department of Radiology, University of North Carolina at Chapel Hill, Chapel Hill, NC

Mohsen Shabahang, M.D., Department of Surgery, Georgetown University Medical Center, Washington, DC

Paul M. Silverman, M.D., Department of Radiology, Georgetown University Medical Center, Washington, DC

Robert K. Zeman, M.D., Department of Radiology, University of Vermont College of Medicine, Burlington, VT

Harvey A. Ziessman, M.D., Department of Radiology, Georgetown University Medical Center, Washington, DC

HEPATOBILIARY AND PANCREATIC SURGERY

I

GALLBLADDER

1

ULTRASOUND OF THE GALLBLADDER

Brian Garra, M.D.
Georgetown University Medical Center
Washington, DC

Despite the availability of several imaging modalities capable of evaluating the right upper quadrant, ultrasound remains the initial procedure of choice for evaluation of right upper quadrant symptoms and possible gallbladder disease. Ultrasonic examination of the gallbladder and right upper quadrant has the advantage of being highly sensitive to gallbladder pathology while requiring no injection of intravenous contrast material. Ultrasound scanners are also portable, making them usable in intensive care units on critically ill patients where the scan can be performed quickly. Moreover, a comprehensive exam is possible; ultrasound may detect abnormalities other than of the gallbladder that may be responsible for a patient's symptoms. Finally, unlike radionuclide biliary tree scanning, gallbladder ultrasound does not depend on proper hepatic function to achieve adequate visualization.

ULTRASONIC EXAMINATION TECHNIQUES

For proper visualization of gallstones and other pathology the gallbladder must be adequately distended. This is usually ensured by an overnight fast of 8–12 hr, although a 4-hr fast may be used in situations where the study must be performed quickly. Occasionally adequate distension can be achieved only after a second day of fasting. In this situation the patient should be instructed to take only clear liquids after the first day and not to drink coffee, which may cause gallbladder contraction. Also, no barium procedures should be performed on a patient for 2 days prior to the examination.

Scanning ordinarily should be performed with the highest-frequency transducer that can satisfactorily image the posterior portion of the gallbladder. One should usually start with a 5 MHz transducer and move to a 3.5 MHz transducer if the 5 MHz transducer is not able to penetrate sufficiently deep into the patient to visualize the gallbladder.

The patient is usually scanned in a supine or in oblique left lateral decubitus position. Scanning is usually performed in deep inspiration from a subcostal approach or during tidal respiration via an intercostal approach. Occasionally a semiprone or erect position is necessary to demonstrate movement of gallstones within the gallbladder. As noted above, examination after a second day of fasting may be necessary if the gallbladder is not clearly seen or if the gallbladder is only partially distended. When the gallbladder is examined, both longitudinal and transverse images are obtained. Images evaluating the cystic duct are also obtained if possible, and images of the common hepatic duct near the gallbladder are obtained to check for extrahepatic biliary duct dilatation. For contractility studies it may be necessary to measure the length, width, and thickness of the gallbladder for calculation of gallbladder volumes.

ANATOMY

The gallbladder is located in the right upper quadrant with the neck of the gallbladder in close proximity to the right portal vein near the porta hepatis. Gallbladders vary widely in size and shape but typically the gallbladder is roughly pear-shaped with a maximum transverse diameter of approximately 5 cm when distended. The length of the gallbladder may be up to 12–14 cm when distended. The contracted gallbladder generally has a diameter of between 10 and 15 mm and exhibits a somewhat thickened wall. The normal wall of a distended gallbladder is less than 3 mm thick and appears as a single echogenic line. The lumen of the gallbladder is usually anechoic. The cystic duct that connects the gallbladder with the remainder of the biliary tree is often difficult to visualize. This structure may be several centimeters in length and may connect with the common bile duct at some distance from the gallbladder itself. The valves in the neck of the gallbladder and cystic duct are moderately echogenic structures, which often exhibit refractive acoustic edge shadowing and may on occasion simulate gallstones.

GALLBLADDER ABNORMALITIES

Gallstones

Gallstones are the commonest abnormality of the gallbladder and are also the commonest cause of right upper quadrant symptomatology. Gallstones are typically composed of a mixture of three components: cholesterol, calcium bilirubinate, and calcium carbonate. In fact less then 10% of gallstones are pure, containing only one of the components. Sonographically a gallstone appears as an echogenic focus lying within the gallbladder that exhibits acoustic shadowing and movement when the patient's position is changed (Fig. 1). The shadow usually appears sharp and well defined, unlike the ill-defined "dirty" shadow associated with bowel gas. The shadow appears to arise from the center of the echogenic focus, not from the edges as do refractive acoustic shadows. For shadowing to occur, the stone generally must be at the focus of the transducer, especially for small gallstones. For this reason adjustable focus transducers are better suited to gallbladder examination because the focus can be set to the depth of the dependent proportion of the gallbladder where stones usually lie. Calculi that are either very small or not very dense may not produce a significant acoustic shadow (1). If small stones are present, it may be possible to position the patient so that several stones lie on top of one another to enhance the acoustic shadow visibility (2). If the gallstones are multiple, they may form a layer with posterior acoustic shadowing in the dependent portion of the gallbladder. Gallstones are generally denser than bile and thus sink to the dependent portion of the gallbladder. If oral cholecystographic contrast has been given, however, the bile becomes more dense relative to the gallstones and the gallstones may float in the midportion of the gallbladder (3). Gallstones may completely fill a contracted gallbladder, making the gallbladder hard to find or causing it to simulate bowel. A contracted gallbladder, however, produces a better-defined acoustic shadow than does gas-filled bowel and does not change over time. Also one may see the wall of the gallbladder anterior to the gallstones (Fig. 2). This appearance has been called the wall-echo-shadow triad (WES sign) or the double-arc shadow sign (4, 5).

Other structures may simulate gallstones. Valves in the cystic duct and neck of the gallbladder may be echogenic and may produce refractive acoustic shadows, making them difficult to distinguish from gallstones. Of course these structures do not change their position when the patient is repositioned. An impacted stone in the neck of the gallbladder, however, may be hard to identify as a separate structure. Although gallstones generally change their position in the gallbladder when the patient position is changed from supine to decubitus or from supine to erect, gallstones may be adherent to the gallbladder wall (owing to inflammation) and thus may not move. In this situation shadowing is the only criterion that can be used to identify them.

Several maneuvers may be used to increase gallstone visibility. Placing the patient in the erect position may move a gallstone from the neck of the gallbladder to the fundus, where it becomes more readily visible. A 360° roll of the patient and reexamination of the gallbladder may dislodge stones in the region of the neck of the gallbladder and make them easier to visualize. Gallstones must be distinguished from tumefacient sludge and polyps. These lesions do not exhibit acoustic shadowing.

Sludge

Sludge is particulate matter within bile. Typically it is composed of cholesterol crystals and/or calcium bilirubinate. It appears usually as low- to mid-level echoes within the gallbladder, often layering posteriorly. However, sludge may appear as rounded masses (tumefacient sludge or sludge balls) of low- to mid-level echogenicity that do not exhibit acoustic shadowing but that move when the patient's position is changed (Fig. 3). Sludge is usually seen in association with biliary stasis and may be seen in up to 31% of patients 10 days after surgery (6). Sludge balls may gradually develop into gallstones. When this happens one sees gradually increasing echogenicity of the sludge, coupled with a gradual decrease in size of the sludge balls, followed eventually by the development of acoustic shadowing (7).

Polyps

Gallbladder polyps appear as moderately echogenic foci lying adjacent to the gallbladder wall. These foci produce no acoustic shadowing and, because they are

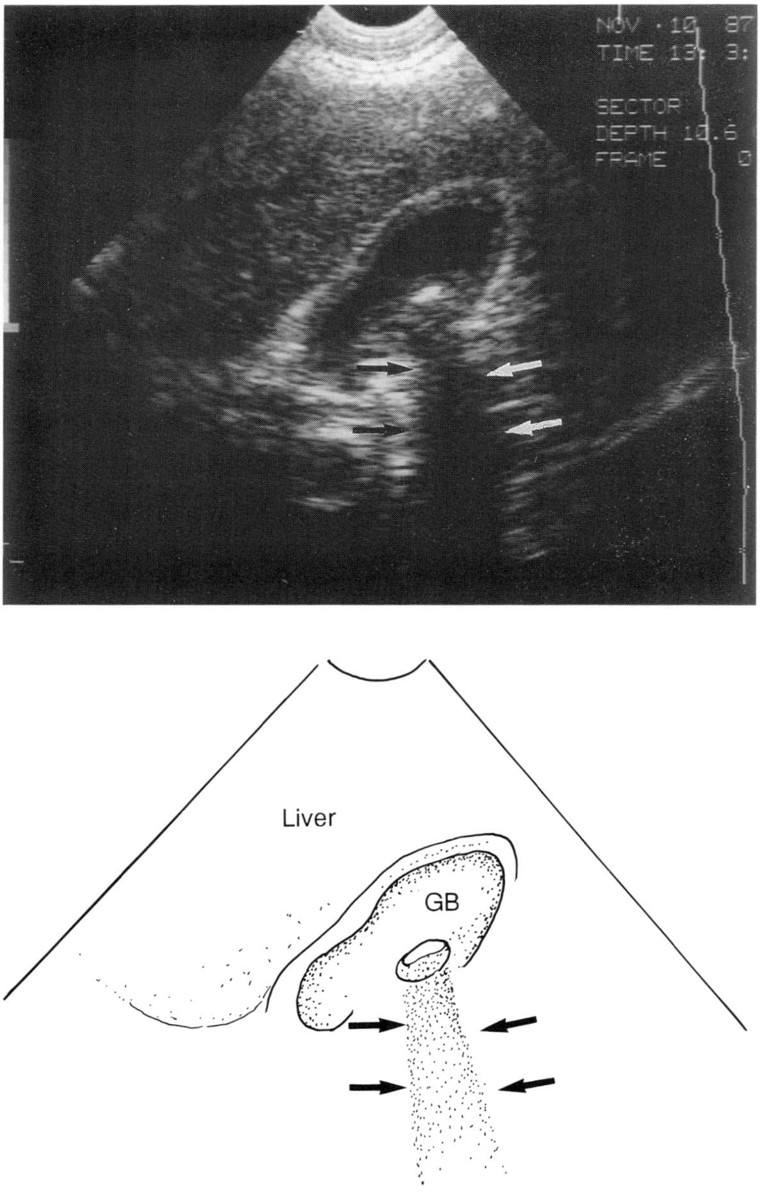

(A)

Figure 1. Gallbladder in a supine patient (figure and drawing A) containing an echogenic stone with acoustic shadowing (arrows, A). The stone is surrounded by moderately echogenic sludge. When the patient is placed in the erect position, the stone and sludge (arrows, B) move from the center of the gallbladder to the dependent part of the fundus (B, next page).

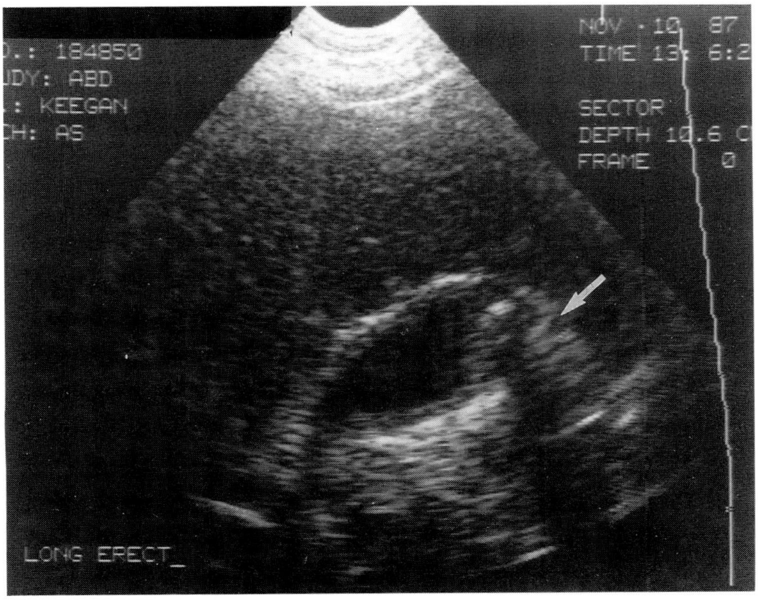

(B)

Figure 1 *(Continued)*

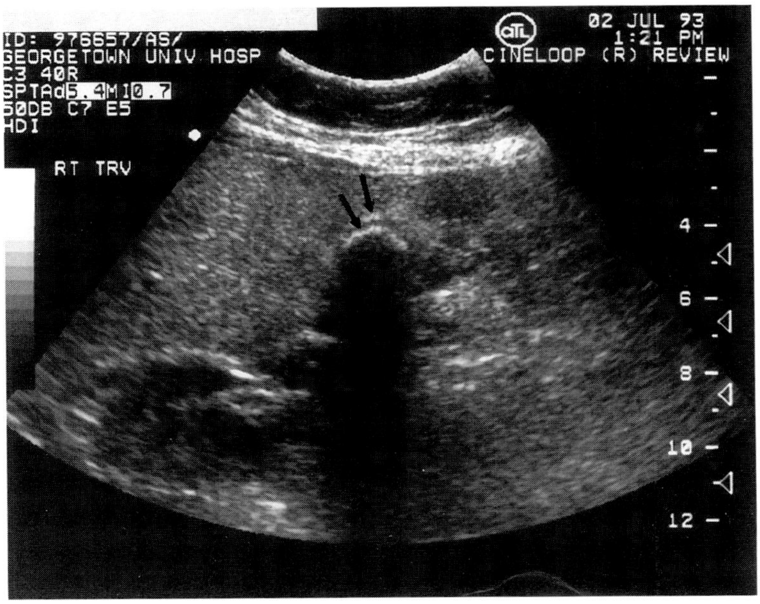

Figure 2. A contracted gallbladder filled with stones appears as an double echogenic line (arrows) with a sharp acoustic shadow. This is known as the wall-echo-shadow complex or the double-arc shadow sign.

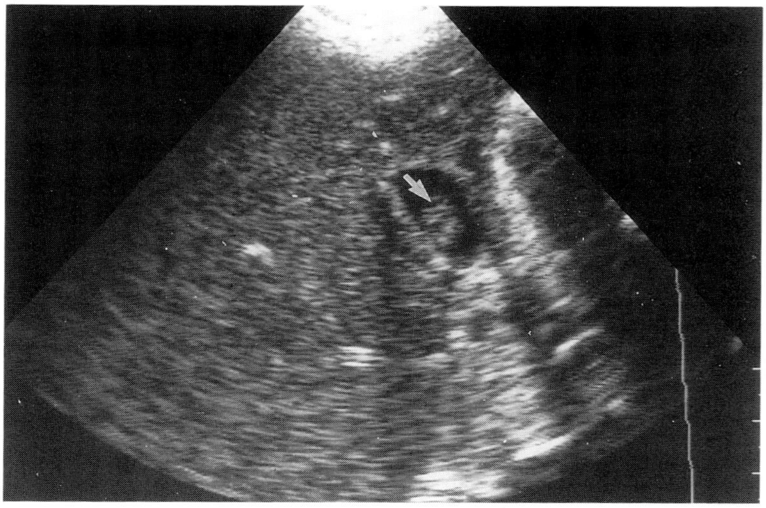

Figure 3. A sludge ball in the gallbladder appears as a moderately echogenic mass (arrow) that moves with changes in position.

attached to the gallbladder wall, exhibit no movement with repositioning of the patient. Usually a gallbladder polyp represents a cholesterol polyp or, much less commonly, an adenomatous polyp. Polyps are benign tumors but other tumors most be considered in the differential diagnosis. Gallbladder carcinoma and metastatic disease to the gallbladder wall should both be considered, but these lesions are usually larger and associated with focal gallbladder wall thickening. Polyps are not usually associated with gallbladder wall thickening.

ACUTE CHOLECYSTITIS

Acute cholecystitis is usually caused by obstruction of the neck of the gallbladder or cystic duct by a stone. This obstruction eventually causes inflammation of the gallbladder wall and possibly even infection of the gallbladder. Acute cholecystitis therefore is associated with stones in 90–95% of patients, with the remainder of acute cholecystitis patients having the diagnosis of acalculous cholecystitis. Sonography is useful both for suggesting the diagnosis of acute cholecystitis (8–10) and for evaluating other possible causes of right upper quadrant pain (Table 1). Sonography can also distinguish acute from chronic cholecystitis with relatively high accuracy (11, 12).

The sonographic findings of acute cholecystitis are gallstones, tenderness over the gallbladder, and wall thickening. Gallstones and tenderness over the gallbladder are the two primary signs of acute cholecystitis. It is important to remember that impacted stones in the cystic duct may not be seen owing to confusion with adjacent gallbladder polyps or the valves of Heister. Tenderness over the gallbladder is a reliable sign but may also be seen in marked distension of the gallbladder in patients

Table 1. Sonography and acute cholecystitis

Study	Sensitivity (%)	Specificity (%)	Reference
Worthen et al., 1981	100	96	8
Freitas et al., 1982	81	60	11
Samuels et al., 1983	97	64	12
Gill et al., 1985	91	92	13
Van Weelde et al., 1986	89	98	14
Shea et al., 1994 (composite results)	94	78	15

without cystic duct obstruction. The evaluation of gallbladder tenderness is more accurate with sonography than with physical examination because of the ability of sonography to identify precisely the location of the gallbladder. In a study of Ralls and colleagues (13) the positive predictive value of tenderness over the gallbladder was 92%. The wall thickening seen in acute cholecystitis typically appears as moderately echogenic wall thickening, often with striated lucencies in the wall representing areas of edema and fluid accumulation (14) (Fig. 4). A fluid-fluid level noted in a gallbladder involved with acute cholecystitis suggests the presence of empyema, though sludge may occasionally mimic this appearance.

Radionuclide scanning of the gallbladder is a very sensitive method for detecting obstruction of the cystic duct and may be used to confirm cholecystitis if the sonographic findings are equivocal (8, 10). Complications of acute cholecystitis include gangrenous cholecystitis and perforation of the gallbladder. Gangrenous cholecystitis is characterized by markedly irregular gallbladder wall thickening. In these patients right upper quadrant pain may actually be decreased because of denervation of the gallbladder wall. Perforation of the gallbladder frequently occurs near the fundus of the gallbladder. It results in a fluid collection adjacent to the gallbladder, and a localized fluid collection adjacent to the gallbladder fundus should suggest the possibility of perforation in the proper clinical setting. Other causes of pericholecystic fluid include pancreatitis and peptic ulcer disease (15).

EMPHYSEMATOUS CHOLECYSTITIS

Emphysematous cholecystitis is a variant of cholecystitis caused by infection of the gallbladder due to gas-forming bacteria. Stones are often not visualized in this entity. A significant percentage of these patients have diabetes mellitus. The sonographic findings suggesting emphysematous cholecystitis include an echogenic focus within the gallbladder lumen or in the gallbladder wall with posterior ring down or a comet-tail appearance. Gas within the gallbladder wall may also appear as an echogenic arc (16).

ACALCULOUS CHOLECYSTITIS

Acalculous cholecystitis is a difficult sonographic diagnosis because the patients by definition do not have gallstones, which is the easiest gallbladder abnormality to

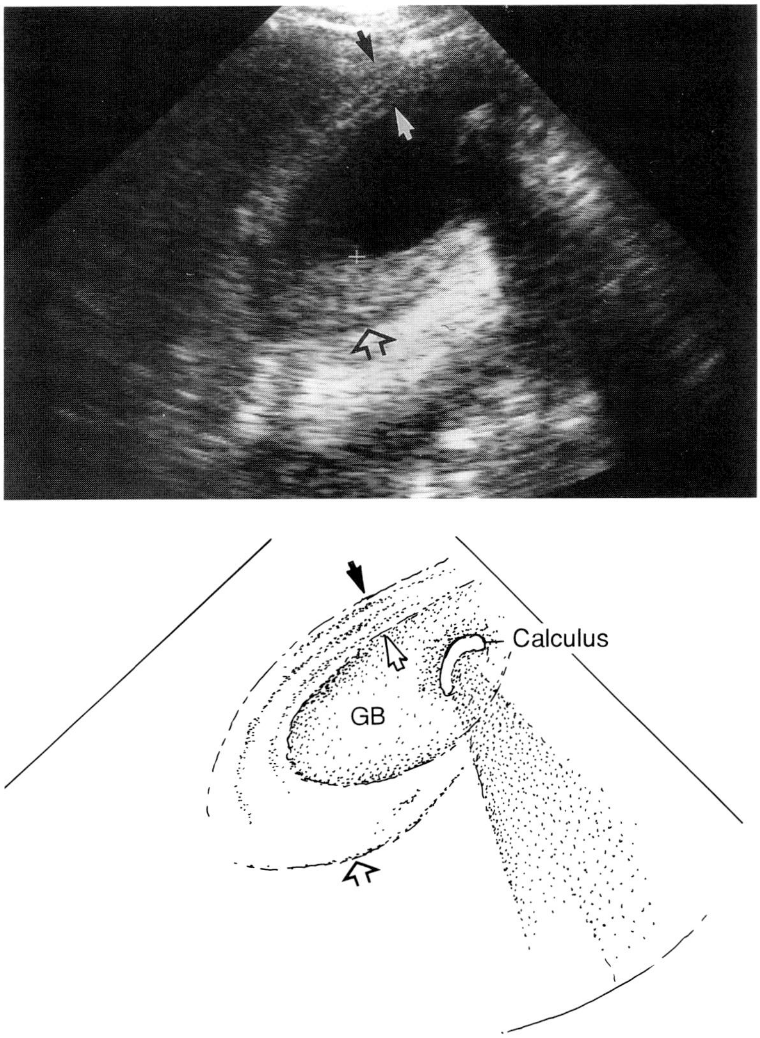

Figure 4. Acute inflamed gallbladder showing layered wall thickening anteriorly (solid arrow), focal thickening posteriorly (open arrow), and a shadowing gallstone in the fundus.

identify. The sonographic Murphy sign is also relatively unreliable because patients with a distended gallbladder without inflammation may also have some tenderness, and patients with acalculous cholecystitis are usually hospitalized for other serious illness and have many other potential sources of right upper quadrant pain. The diagnosis is usually suggested when gallbladder wall thickening is identified without other apparent causes. Radionuclide scanning is reported to be sensitive but not very specific. Lack of contraction of the gallbladder after cholecystokinin stimulation has been reported to be a useful diagnostic test (17). In an ill patient with right upper quadrant pain where acalculous cholecystitis is considered, ultrasound guided

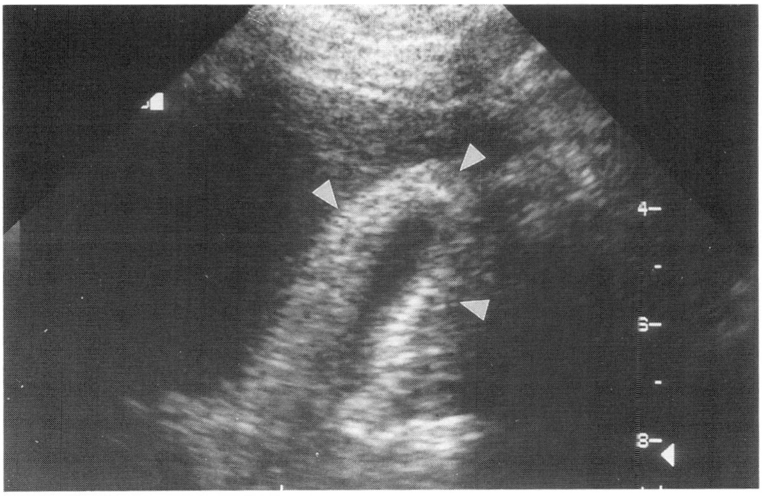

Figure 5. Chronic cholecystitis with a thickened, markedly echogenic gallbladder wall (arrowheads).

biliary aspiration and culture may be useful. This is readily accomplished if the gallbladder is distended. This can be accomplished using an 18-gauge Chiba needle with a roughened outer sheath or roughened stylet to aid in sonographic visualization. A route of access should be chosen that passes through a portion of the liver so that intraperitoneal biliary leakage from the gallbladder is not a problem. After the gallbladder is punctured, as much bile as possible should be aspirated from the gallbladder to lessen the chances of bile leakage.

CHRONIC CHOLECYSTITIS

Chronic cholecystitis may be a sequel to acute cholecystitis but more often develops in the absence of apparent attacks of acute inflammation. Typically these patients have chronic symptoms of right upper quadrant pain and almost invariably gallstones. It occurs most often in middle-aged and older obese females. Sonographically the gallbladder may appear small and contracted or may be normal sized. Gallbladder wall thickening (usually echogenic) is a useful diagnostic feature but is present in only about 25% of the patients with the diagnosis (9, 18) (Fig. 5). Gallstones are present in virtually all cases but the gallstones may be difficult to identify in a contracted gallbladder. Calcification of the gallbladder (porcelain gallbladder) may be present and Rokitansky–Aschoff sinuses may also be visible.

HYPERPLASTIC CHOLECYSTOSES (ADENOMYOMATOSES)

Hyperplastic cholecystosis is an entity characterized by noninflammatory hyperplasia of one or more elements of the gallbladder wall. The commonest form of this entity is called adenomyomatosis, in which there is thickening of the epithelial and

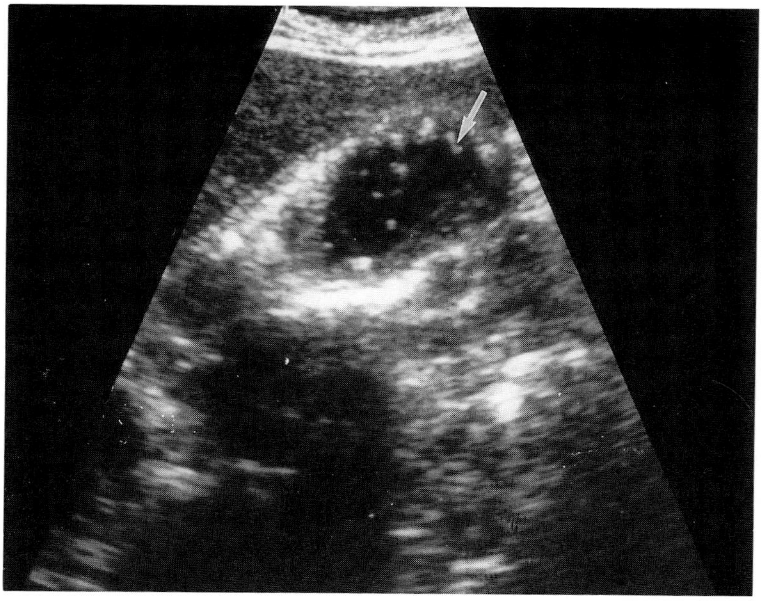

Figure 6. Gallbladder involved with adenomyomatosis showing thickening of the wall and multiple echogenic foci in the lumen, some having a comet-tail appearance (arrow). The echogenic foci represent cholesterol crystals, Rokitansky–Aschoff sinuses, or both.

muscularis layers. This process may produce either diffuse or focal gallbladder wall thickening. When the process is focal the lesion may be called an adenomyoma pathologically. One may also see septation or focal luminal narrowing of the gallbladder. The septation must be distinguished from the Phrygian cap, which is a normal variant. In adenomyomatosis, one may see small anechoic cavities in the gallbladder wall. These represent Rokitansky–Aschoff sinuses, which are small herniations of lining epithelium into the gallbladder wall (19, 20). One may see a comet-tail artifact from a Rokitansky–Aschoff sinus or from small cholesterol crystals within the lumen of the gallbladder or within the gallbladder wall (21, 22) (Fig. 6). The comet-tail artifacts look very similar to those produced by small gas collections in the gallbladder but the patient is relatively asymptomatic. Some investigators believe that hyperplastic cholecystoses are a variant of chronic cholecystitis.

GALLBLADDER CARCINOMA

Carcinoma of the gallbladder is the commonest tumor of the gallbladder wall and is considerably more common than the benign tumors of the gallbladder (23). It is thought to be associated with chronic cholecystitis and cholelithiasis and is significantly more frequent in calcified (porcelain) gallbladders (24). The most common sites of gallbladder carcinoma are in the fundus or the neck of the gallbladder. Sonographically carcinoma of the gallbladder appears as a focal echogenic thick-

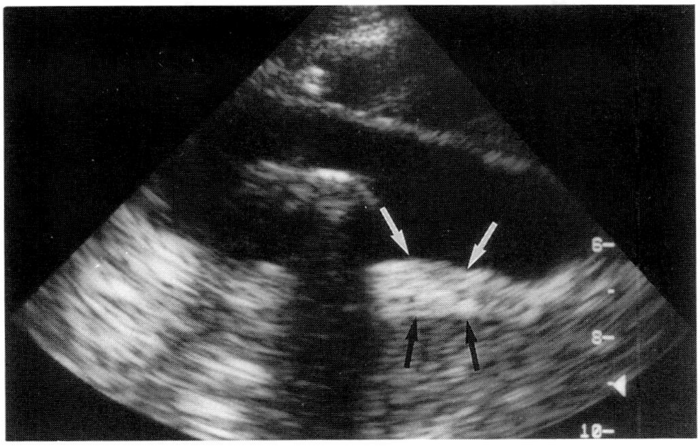

Figure 7. Focal thickening of the posterior gallbladder wall (arrows) and a gallstone. The thickening proved to be carcinoma of the gallbladder.

ening of the gallbladder wall, often nearly obliterating the lumen (Fig. 7). In fact in many cases one may see only an ill-defined mass in the gallbladder fossa. Gallstones are present in 80–90% of the cases. Gallbladder wall calcifications, biliary duct dilatation, periportal lymph nodes, and liver metastases may also be seen.

Numerous other causes of gallbladder wall thickening have been reported (Table 2). Hepatitis may produce gallbladder wall thickening particularly along the side of the gallbladder facing the liver. Hypoalbuminemia typically produces gallbladder wall thickening that has a characteristic appearance of two echogenic lines with a central hypoechoic region (Fig. 8) Congestive heart failure also produces a similar appearance. Ascites may also produce gallbladder wall thickening, which usually has an appearance similar to that of congestive heart failure or hypoalbuminemia but may also have a more echogenic uniform appearance. Renal disease, AIDS, and sepsis also have been reported to produce gallbladder wall thickening. An adjacent inflammatory process such as regional enteritis involving the duodenum

Table 2. Causes of gallbladder wall thickening

Underdistension
Acute or chronic inflammation
Ascites
Hypoalbuminemia
Gallbladder carcinoma
Renal disease
AIDS
Sepsis
Graft versus host disease
Adjacent inflammatory process
Varices

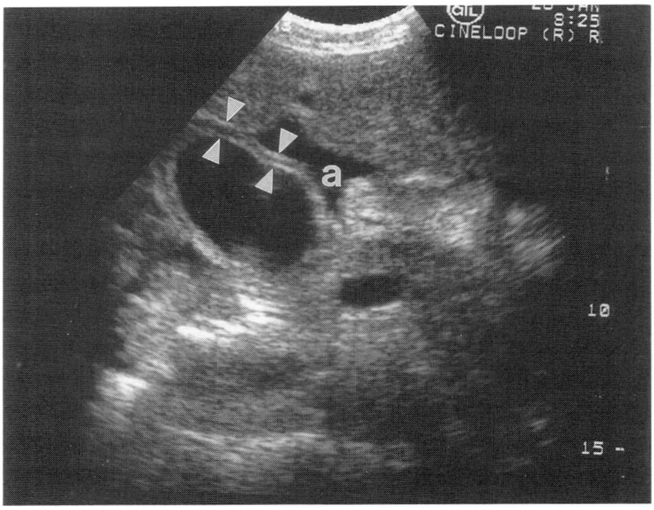

Figure 8. Thickening of the gallbladder wall due to hypoalbuminemia and ascites (a). The gallbladder wall thickening appears as two thin echogenic lines with a hypoechoic center (arrowheads).

can produce gallbladder wall thickening as well. Graft versus host disease has more recently been reported to produce gallbladder wall thickening. The gallbladder wall thickening in this entity is typically hyperechoic. Also, a poorly distended gallbladder wall normally has a somewhat thickened wall. If the gallbladder is distended to a maximum diameter of less than 2 cm and mild gallbladder wall thickening is present it may be assumed that the thickening is due to underdistension. Finally, varices of the gallbladder wall in patients with portal hypertension may produce an unusual form of thickening of the gallbladder wall with hypoechoic regions at the edge of the gallbladder wall representing the enlarged vessels (Fig. 9). Color Doppler ultrasound can readily identify the vascular nature of these structures.

Although sonography has demonstrated high accuracy in the detection of acute cholecystitis, strategies to improve its sensitivity and specificity further are being investigated. Color Doppler imaging has been investigated, with both increased flow (28) and decreased flow (29) being reported. So far, color Doppler seems to be limited by lack of sensitivity to flow in small arteries and arterioles. In the future, this situation may be remedied by the use of sonographic contrast agents or by the application of power Doppler instrumentation, which is much more sensitive than traditional color Doppler.

Both Doppler sensitivity and resolution of small structures in the gallbladder and biliary tree may be improved by moving the transducer closer to the organ and using a higher ultrasound frequency. In the future, high-resolution, high-frequency probes mounted on catheters or on endoscopes may be used to visualize the gallbladder and its blood supply. These techniques are invasive, however, and will probably never replace imaging through the abdominal wall.

In summary, the utility of sonographic evaluation of the gallbladder has been well established. Although many of the findings are somewhat nonspecific, when

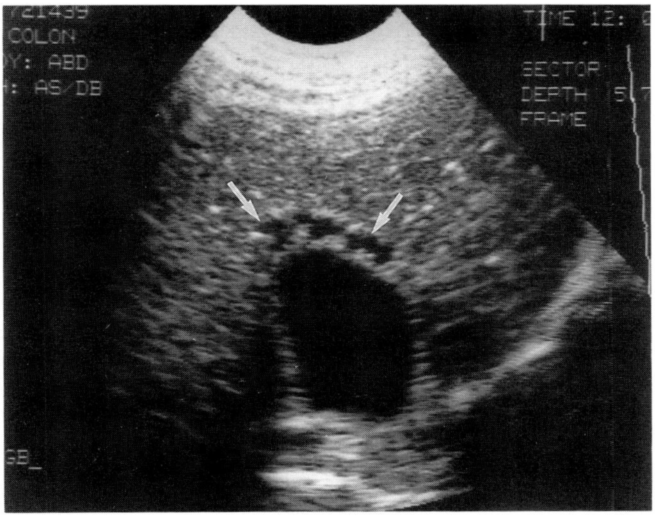

Figure 9. Gallbladder wall varices may appear as irregular lucencies in the wall (arrows) that may simulate wall thickening.

used in conjunction with appropriate clinical history and other laboratory tests, sonography enables one to diagnose many gallbladder disorders accurately and assists one in ruling out other types of pathology in the right upper quadrant.

REFERENCES

1. Crade M, Taylor KJW, Rosenfield AT, et al. Surgical and pathologic correlation of cholecystonosonography and cholecystography. *AJR.* 1978;131:227–229.
2. Laing FC. The gallbladder and bile ducts. In: Rumack CM, Wilson SR, Charboneau JW, eds. *Diagnostic Ultrasound.* St. Louis: Mosby-Year Book Inc.; 1991:106–144.
3. Scheske GA, Cooperberg PL, Cohen MM. Floating gallstones: the role of contrast material. *J Clin Ultrasound.* 1980;8:227–231.
4. MacDonald FR, Cooperberg PL, Cohen MM. The WES triad: a specific sonographic sign of gallstones in the contracted gallbladder. *Gastrointest Radiol.* 1981;6:39–41.
5. Raptopoulos V, D'Orsi C, Smith E, et al. Dynamic cholecystosonography of the contracted gallbladder: the double-arc-shadow sign. *AJR.* 1982;138:275–278.
6. Bolondi L, Gaiani S, Testa S, et al. Gallbladder sludge formation during prolonged fasting after gastrointestinal tract surgery. *Gut.* 1985;26:734–738.
7. Britten JS, Golding RH, Cooperberg PL. Sludge balls to gallstones. *J Ultrasound Med.* 1984;3:81–84.
8. Worthen NJ, Uzler JM, Funamara JL. Cholecystitis: prospective evaluation of sonography and 99 mTc-HIDA cholescintigraphy. *AJR.* 1981;137:973–978.
9. Laing FC, Federle MP, Jeffrey RB, et al. Ultrasonic evaluation of patients with acute right upper quadrant pain. *Radiology.* 1981;140:449–455.

10. Shuman WP, Mack LA, Rudd TG, et al. Evaluation of acute right upper quadrant pain: sonography and 99mTc-PIPIDA cholescintigraphy. *AJR*. 1982;139:61–64.
11. Cooperberg PL, Burhenne HJ. Real-time ultrasonography. Diagnostic technique of choice in calculous gallbladder disease. *New Engl J Med*. 1980;302:1277–1279.
12. McIntosh DMF, Penney HF: Gray scale ultrasonography as a screening procedure in the detection of gallbladder disease. *Radiology*. 1980;136:725–727.
13. Ralls PW, Colletti PM, Lapin SA, et al. Real-time sonography in suspected acute cholecystitis. *Radiology*. 1985;155:767–771.
14. Cohan RH, Mahony BS, Bowie JD, et al. Striated intramural gallbladder lucencies on ultrasound studies: predictors of acute cholecystitis. *Radiology*. 1987;164:31–35.
15. Nyberg DA, Laing FC. Ultrasonographic findings in peptic ulcer disease and pancreatitis that simulate primary gallbladder disease. *J Ultrasound Med*. 1983;2:303–307.
16. Bloom RA, Libson E, Lebensart PD, et al. The ultrasound spectrum of emphysematous cholecystitis. *J Clin Ultrasound*. 1989;17:251–256.
17. Mirvis SE, Vainright JR, Nelson AW, et al. The diagnosis of acute acalculous cholecystitis: a comparison of sonography, scintigraphy, and computed tomography. *AJR*. 1986;147:1171–1175.
18. Sanders RC. The significance of sonographic gallbladder wall thickening. *J Clin Ultrasound*. 1980;8:143–146.
19. Robbins SL, Cotran RS, Kumar V. *Pathologic Basis of Disease*. 3rd ed. Philadelphia: W. B. Saunders; 1984:949.
20. Jutras JA. Hyperplastic cholecystoses. *AJR*. 1960;83:795.
21. Raghavendra BN, Subramanyam BR, Balthazer EJ, et al. Sonography of adenomyomatosis of the gallbladder: radiologic-pathologic correlation. *Radiology*. 1983;146: 747–752.
22. Lafortune M, Gariepy G, Dumont A, et al. The V-shaped artifact of the gallbladder. *AJR*. 1986;147:505–508.
23. Ilingworth CFW. Carcinoma of the gallbladder. *Br J Surg*. 1936;23:4.
24. Polk HC. Carcinoma in the calcified gallbladder. *Gastroenterology*. 1966;50:582.

2

COMPUTED TOMOGRAPHY OF THE GALLBLADDER

Robert K. Zeman, M.D.
University of Vermont College of Medicine
Burlington, VT

Computed tomography (CT) is generally not used as a screening technique in the patient with suspected gallbladder disease. Ultrasonography and cholescintigraphy with iminodiacetic acid derivatives are the real workhorses in this setting. Computed tomography may be useful, however, as a problem solver in patients with complicated cholecystitis or in staging gallbladder carcinoma.

CHOLELITHIASIS AND CHOLECYSTITIS

Computed tomography is not as sensitive as ultrasound in the detection of gallstones, but did detect 79% of stones present on ultrasound in one retrospective study (1). 70% of stones are of high attenuation whereas the remainder are either of soft-tissue density or radiolucent compared to bile. Those stones that are radiolucent can be expected to have the highest cholesterol content. Gas-containing fissures in stones give rise to the so-called Mercedes-Benz sign on CT similar to that observed on plain radiographs.

Acute cholecystitis gives rise to a broad range of findings on CT (2–4). Although many of the findings are nonspecific, the presence of multiple findings usually allows an accurate diagnosis to be made. On contrast-enhanced scans, intramural edema is frequently present in acute cholecystitis. It is manifest as a low-attenuation band or multiple bands separating the gallbladder mucosa from submucosal layers analogous to that reported on ultrasound (5, 6) (Fig. 1). Areas of low-attenuation edema or hyperemia in the adjacent liver may also be present. Stranding within the pericholecystic fat indicates extension of inflammation into the surrounding structures. Similar findings have been described in both calculous and acalculous cholecystitis

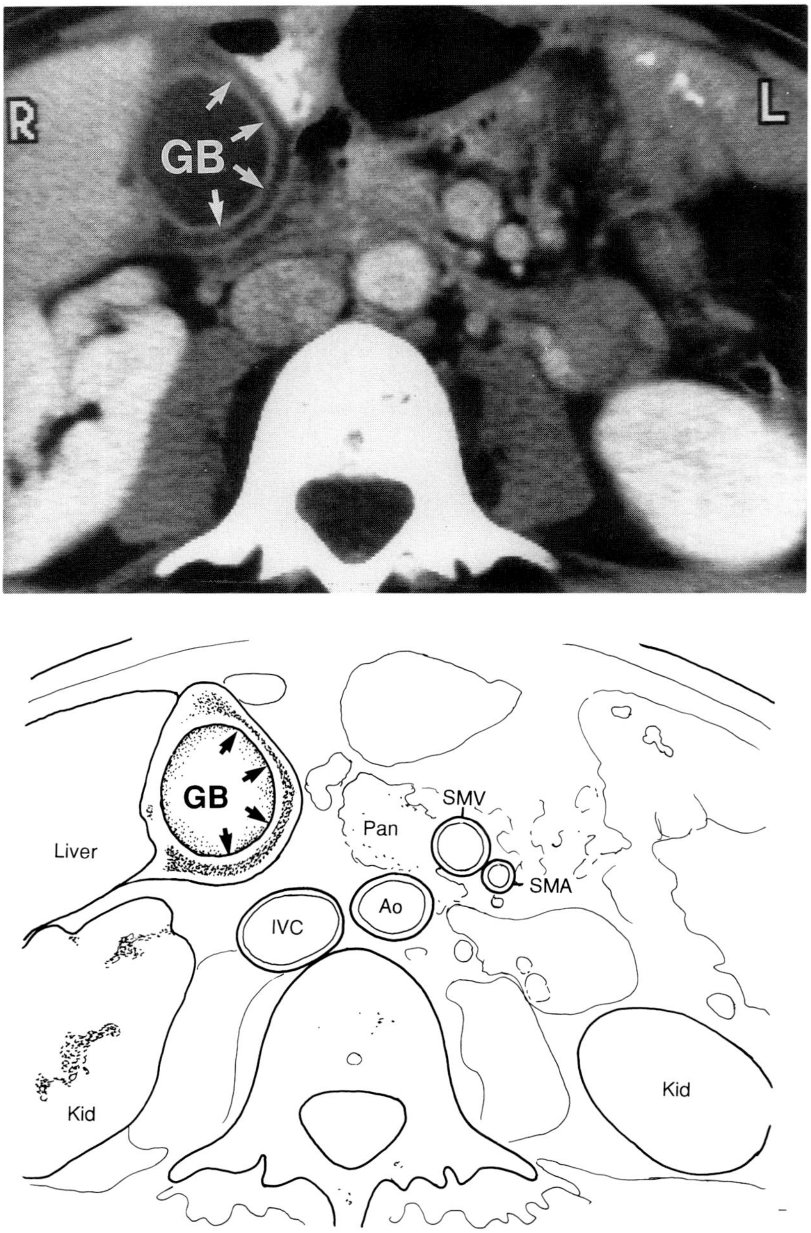

Figure 1. CT of acute cholecystitis. Contrast-enhanced CT reveals a uniform band of low-attenuation edema (arrows) within the gallbladder (GB) wall. The finding of wall edema, when coupled with pericholecystic inflammatory stranding, is very suggestive of acute cholecystitis. (Copyright Robert Zeman, M.D.; used by permission.)

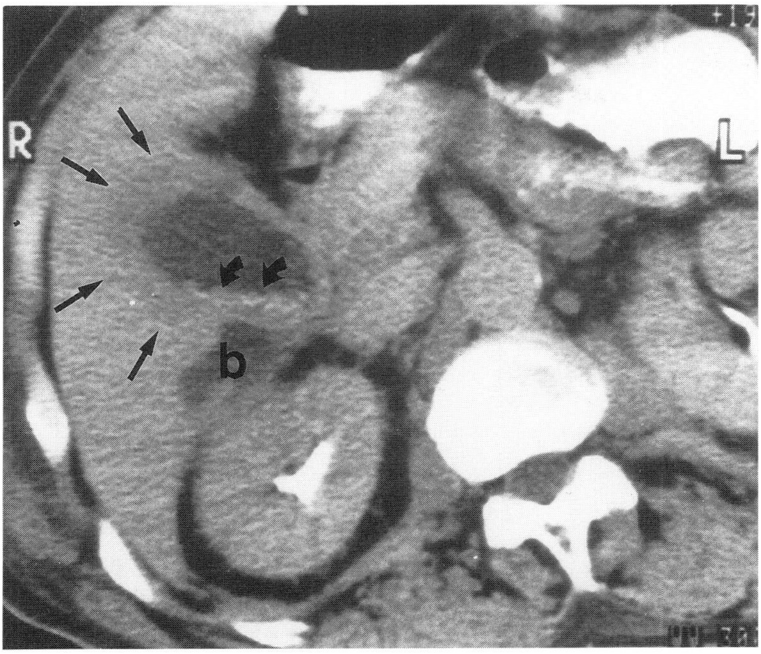

Figure 2. CT of acute cholecystitis with perforation. Contrast-enhanced CT demonstrates a thick-walled gallbladder with a rim of inflammation extending into the adjacent liver (arrows). A small biloma (b) has formed in Morrison's pouch with hepatic subcapsular extension due to perforation. Multiple small gallstones are present (curved arrows). (Copyright Robert Zeman, M.D.; used by permission.)

(7). Small collections of pericholecystic fluid may also be identified. Gallbladder wall thickening, gallbladder distension, and gallstones are at best nonspecific findings in acute cholecystitis.

Computed tomography is usually not necessary in the evaluation of uncomplicated cholecystitis. In cases where complications such as gallbladder perforation, pericholecystic abscess, or emphysematous cholecystitis are being considered, CT can offer valuable information prior to surgery. Perforation of the gallbladder and pericholecystic abscess may look quite similar. Perforation occurs in patients with severe inflammation or gangrenous cholecystitis. A mortality of 19–24% has been reported (8). Both perforation and pericholecystic abscess show evidence on CT of a fluid collection adjacent to the gallbladder, and severe inflammatory stranding in the pericholecystic fat (Fig. 2). Abscesses tend to loculate early, whereas bilomas tend to be associated with more free fluid prior to developing a well-defined wall. Computed tomography attenuation numbers do not allow distinction of a biloma from abscess. The presence of gas bubbles, however, does indicate abscess formation. The only specific test to confirm bile leakage is nuclear cholescintigraphy. When severe inflammation is present, and the gallbladder is collapsed owing to perforation, it may be impossible to distinguish complicated cholecystitis from a perforated carcinoma.

Emphysematous cholecystitis is suggested on sonography when indistinct, "dirty" shadowing with reverberation artifact is seen arising from the gallbladder wall or lumen. When this finding is present, a plain film should first be used to look for

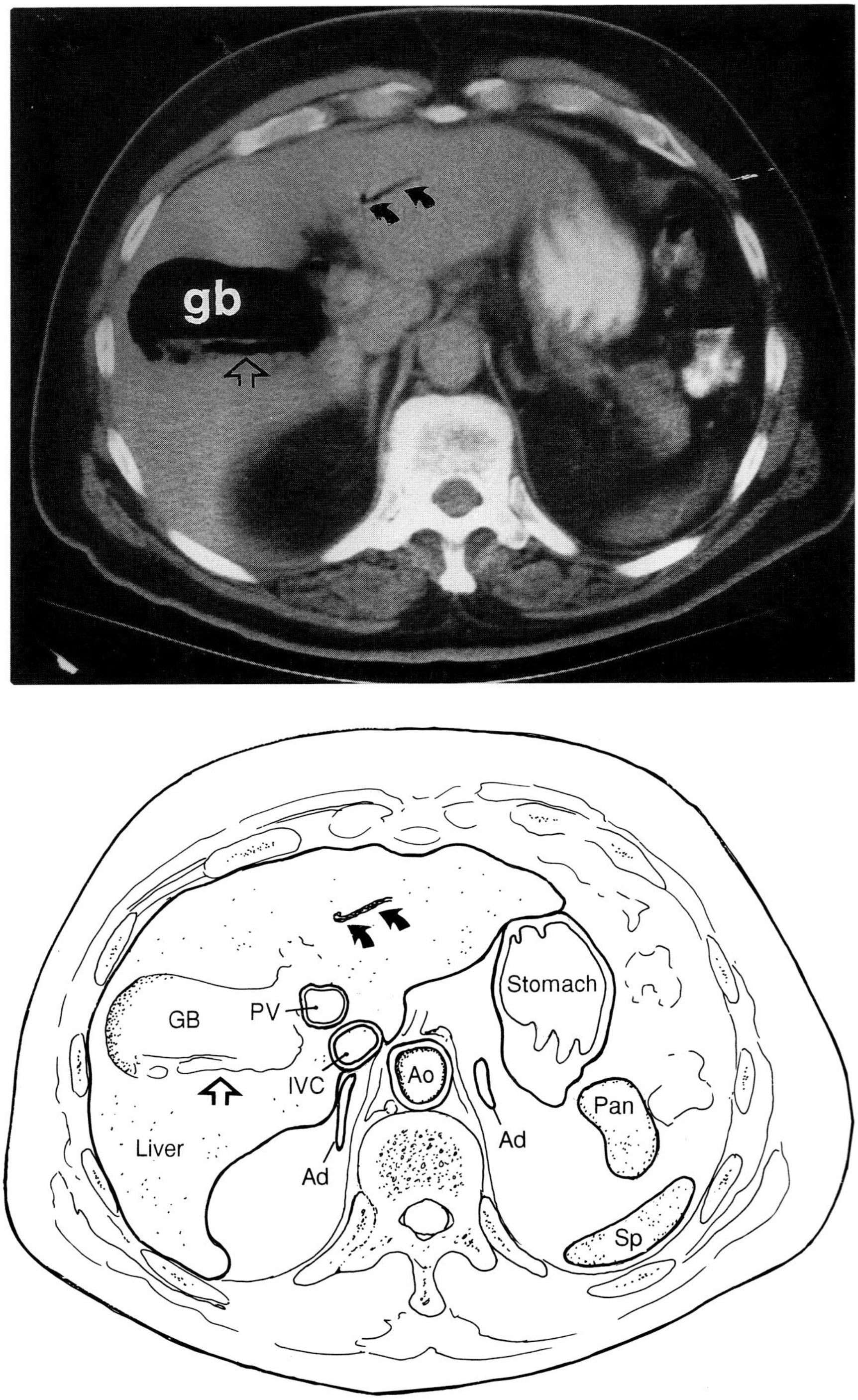

Figure 3. CT of emphysematous cholecystitis revealing a gas-filled gallbladder (GB) containing sludge and debris (open arrow). Gas and infection have extended into the left hepatic duct (curved arrows) because the inflammatory occlusion of the cystic duct was partial. This is unusual, but can occur. (Copyright Robert Zeman, M.D.; used by permission.)

gallbladder gas suggestive of the diagnosis of emphysematous cholecystitis. If the plain film is equivocal, which may occur due to dilatation of adjacent bowel loops and duodenal ileus, CT can usually resolve the confusion (Fig. 3). Computed tomography can be used to gauge the extent of inflammation, and in severe cases, gas may be seen tracking into the hepatoduodenal ligament, adjacent liver, and surrounding mesentery. Emphysematous cholecystitis is especially common in elderly diabetics, and increases the risk of perforation fivefold over nonemphysematous cholecystitis. In the acutely ill patient, gas in the gallbladder suggests the need for relatively expeditious cholecystectomy.

Mirizzi syndrome (acute cholecystitis with erosion of a cystic duct stone directly into the common hepatic duct) results in simultaneous acute cholecystitis and biliary obstruction (9). Computed tomography will demonstrate biliary dilatation, thickening and/or low-attenuation edema in the gallbladder wall, and pericholecystic inflammatory changes suggestive of acute cholecystitis (Fig. 4). The inflammatory mass that results may actually protrude into the common hepatic duct and mimic a polypoid tumor on cholangiography. In severe cases, the entire right upper quadrant may become engulfed in inflammation, distorting the surgical biliary anatomy.

GALLBLADDER NEOPLASMS

Small protuberances arising from the gallbladder wall are commonly the result of adenomas, adenomyomas, and cholesterol polyps. Only adenoma is truly a neoplastic lesion; the latter entities are more appropriately classified as hyperplastic cholecystopathies, and are often associated with chronic inflammatory disease of the gallbladder. Adenomyomas usually occur in the fundus, eccentrically compress the gallbladder, and may be up to several centimeters in diameter despite their benign nature. Some fundal adenomyomas may demonstrate opacification of a central Rokitansky–Aschoff sinus on oral cholecystography, but more often than not the diagnosis rests on surgical exploration.

Carcinoma of the gallbladder results in greater than 7000 deaths per year in the United States. Survival statistics are comparable to that of pancreatic carcinoma. There is a clear association with porcelain gallbladder. Gallbladder carcinoma exhibits three common morphological patterns (10, 11). These are a large polypoid mass, focal or diffuse gallbladder wall thickening, and a large infiltrative mass engulfing the gallbladder and invading the surrounding liver. A large polypoid mass is the most common form, occurring in 42% of patients studied by Weiner et al. (12).

Once carcinoma is suspected, CT may be used to stage the lesion preoperatively. Resection is not precluded by involvement of adjacent organs, but it is common to see extension into the hepatoduodenal ligament, adjacent liver, common hepatic duct, and pericholecystic fat (Fig. 5). Because resection of the adjacent liver may be necessary, it is important to use CT to map the segmental anatomy and determine if the tumor has extended superiorly to involve the right portal vein. Porta hepatis or celiac adenopathy may occur. The tumor may invade and even obstruct the duodenum or hepatic flexure. Although resection is possible in many cases, recurrence is also very common.

Other tumors of the gallbladder are rare. We have seen gallbladder sarcomas present as bulky masses with polypoid extension into the bile duct mimicking Mirizzi

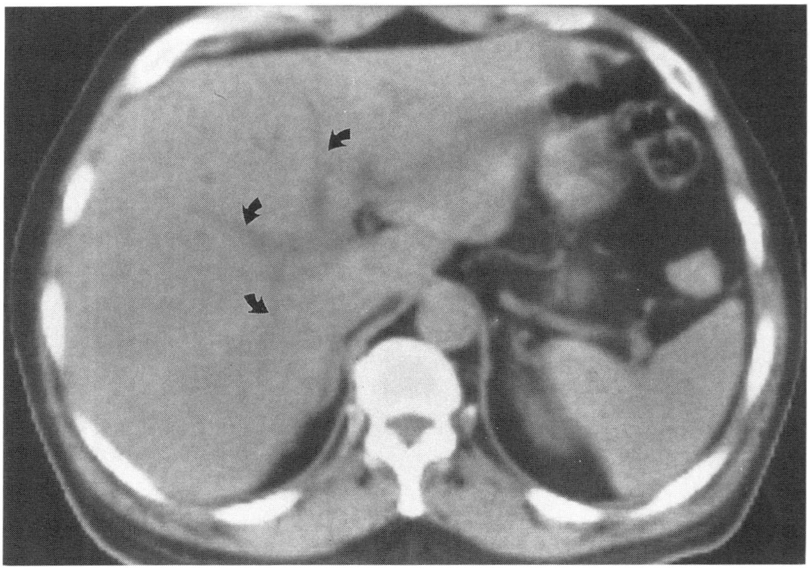

(A)

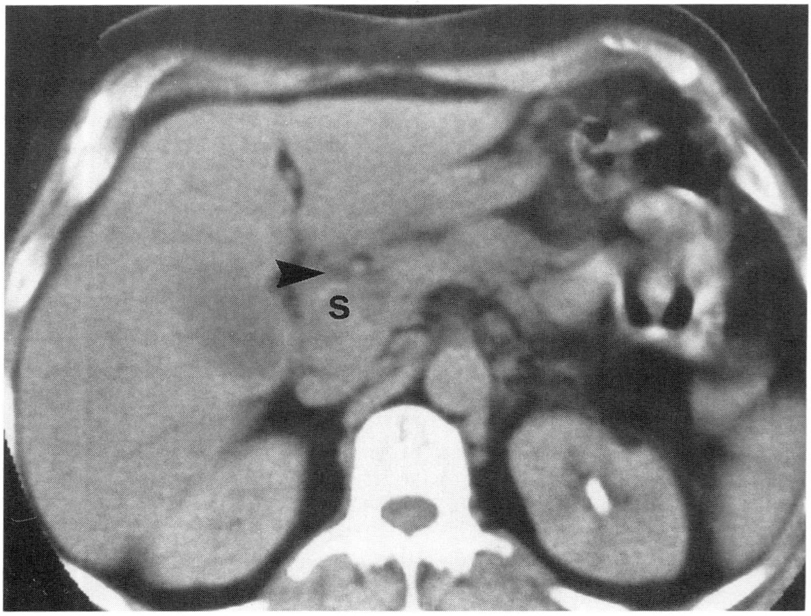

(B)

Figure 4. Mirizzi syndrome. (A) CT scan shows presence of multiple dilated ducts (curved arrows). (B) CT scan several centimeters caudad shows a stone (S) which is displacing the common hepatic duct (arrowhead) anteriorly. Unlike choledocholithiasis, the stone is not clearly centered within the common hepatic duct. (C, next page) Further caudad, the dilated gallbladder (gb) is seen. A band of intramural low-attenuation edema is present (arrows). (D, next page) Cholangiogram shows the cystic duct stone (S) protruding into the bile duct (arrows) and producing obstruction of the common hepatic duct characteristic of Mirizzi syndrome. Courtesy of Churchill Livingstone (13).

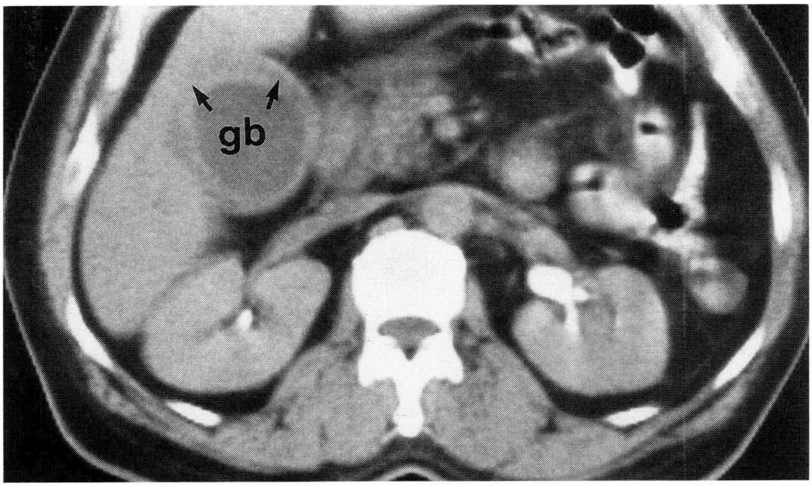

(C)

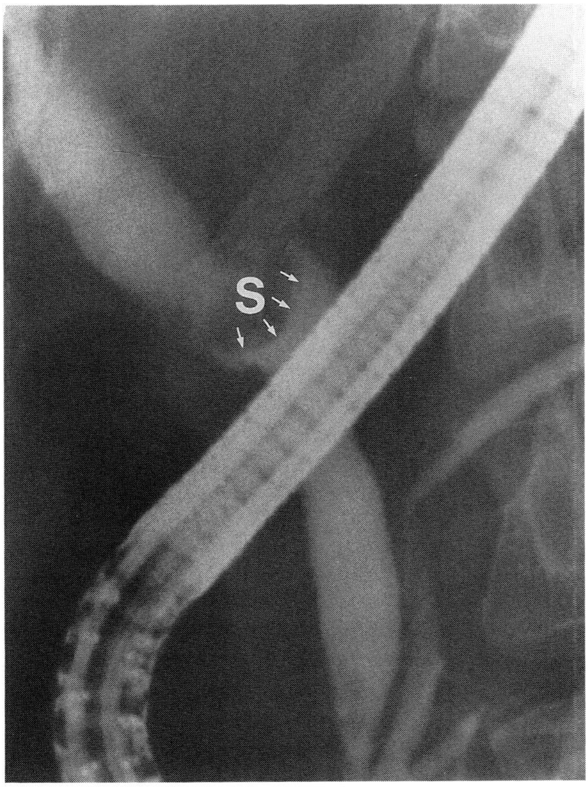

(D)

Figure 4 (*Continued*)

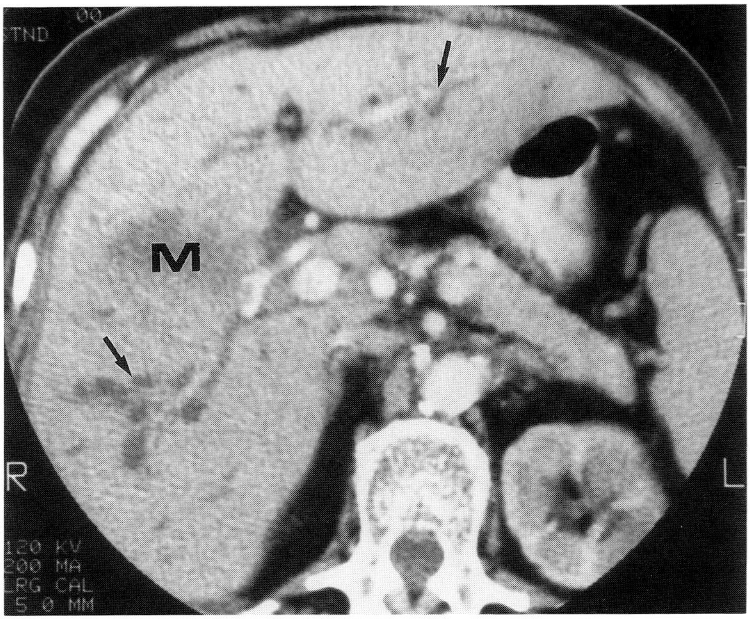

(A)

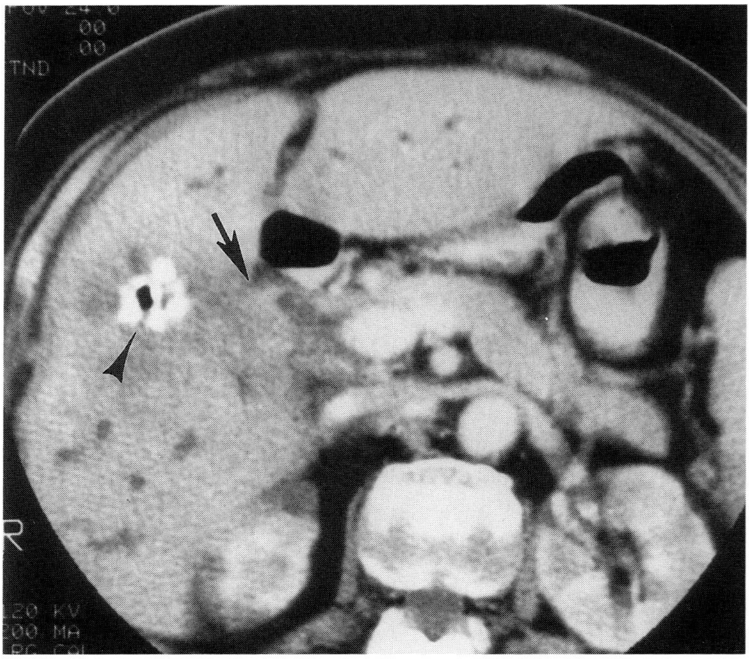

(B)

Figure 5. CT of invasive carcinoma of the gallbladder. (A) Enhanced CT section reveals a large mass (M) arising from the gallbladder and extending into the hepatic parenchyma. The intrahepatic bile ducts are dilated (arrows). (B) 2 cm caudad to A, the mass is seen projecting into the pancreatoduodenal space, and involving the duodenum (arrow). The cause of gas within the cluster of gallstones (arrowhead) most likely was due to the presence of a malignant fistulous tract. Courtesy of Churchill Livingstone (13).

syndrome. They are rapidly aggressive with frequent spread into the surrounding structures. Metastatic melanoma is the most common metastasis to involve the gallbladder. It may be evident as a polypoid or infiltrative mass.

REFERENCES

1. Barakos JA, Ralls PW, Lapin SA, Johnson MB, Radin DR, Colletti PM, Boswell WD, Halls JM. Cholelithiasis: evaluation with CT. *Radiology.* 1987;162:415–418.
2. Kane RA, Costello P, Duszlak E. Computed tomography in acute cholecystitis: new observations. *AJR.* 1983;141:697–701.
3. Terrier F, Becker CD, Stoller C, Triller JK. Computed tomography in complicated cholecystitis. *J Comput Assist Tomogr.* 1984;8:58–62.
4. Smathers RL, Lee JKT, Heiken JP. Differentiation of complicated cholecystitis from gallbladder carcinoma by computed tomography. *AJR.* 1984;143:255–259.
5. Teefey SA, Baron RL, Bigler SA. Sonography of the gallbladder. Significance of striated (layered) thickening of the gallbladder wall. *AJR.* 1991;156:945–947.
6. Cohan RH, Mahony BS, Bowie JD, Cooper C, Baker ME, Illescas FF. Striated intramural gallbladder lucencies on US studies. Predictors of acute cholecystitis. *Radiology.* 1987;64:31–35.
7. Mirvis SE, Vainright JR, Nelson AW, et al. The diagnosis of acute acalculous cholecystitis. A comparison of sonography, scintigraphy and CT. *AJR.* 1986;147:1171–1175.
8. Strohl EL, Diffenbaugh WG, Baker JH, et al. Collective reviews: gangrene and perforation of the gallbladder. *Int Obstet Surg.* 1962;114:1–7.
9. Clemmet AR, Lowman RM. The roentgen features of the Mirizzi syndrome. *AJR.* 1965;4:480–483.
10. Lane J, Buck JL, Zeman RK. Primary carcinoma of the gallbladder: a pictorial essay. *Radiographics.* 1989;9:209–228.
11. Yeh HC. Ultrasonography and computed tomography of carcinoma of the gallbladder. *Radiology.* 1979;133:167–173.
12. Weiner SN, Koenigsberg M, Morehouse H, Hoffman J. Sonography and computed tomography in the diagnosis of carcinoma of the gallbladder. *AJR.* 1984;142:735–739.
13. Zeman RK, Burrell MI. *Gallbladder and Bile Duct Imaging. A Clinical Radiologic Approach.* New York: Churchill Livingstone; 1987.

3

NUCLEAR MEDICINE

Harvey A. Ziessman, M.D.
Georgetown University Medical Center
Washington, DC

Cholescintigraphy can be very useful in the evaluation of patients with gallbladder disease because it provides information on physiology (bile flow through the cystic duct) and function (gallbladder contraction) in contrast to anatomy alone.

ACUTE CHOLECYSTITIS

Pathophysiology

Obstruction of the cystic duct is the usual precipitating event in acute cholecystitis. This is most commonly caused by a calculus, much less commonly by mucus plugging or functional obstruction from inflammation and edema. Cystic duct obstruction produces increased intraluminal pressure. Bile flow through the cystic duct is impeded and blood flow impaired. The gallbladder becomes distended and edematous, inflammatory cell infiltration ensues, and mucosal hemorrhage and infarction follow. When obstruction persists, complications such as infection, gangrene, or perforation can result.

Functional versus Anatomic Imaging

Cholescintigraphy can confirm the clinical diagnosis of acute cholecystitis by detecting the primary underlying pathophysiology, that is, obstruction of the cystic duct, manifested by nonfilling of the gallbladder. In contrast, ultrasonography attempts to make the diagnosis by detecting stones, gallbladder distension, wall thickening or edema, and pericholecystic fluid, all anatomic findings and secondary changes.

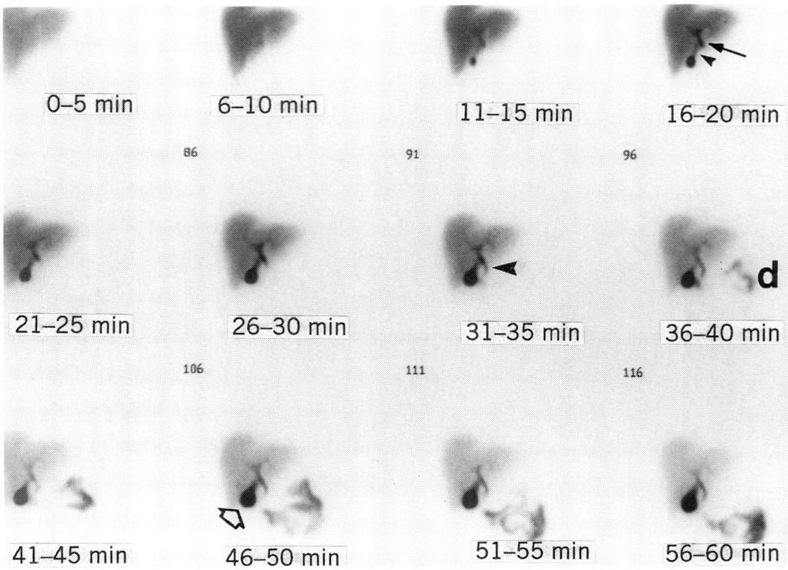

Figure 1. Normal Tc 99m IDA study. On these 5-min summed images, the common hepatic duct is seen at 11–16 min (arrow), the cystic duct by 16 min (small closed arrowhead), and the common duct at 31 min (larger closed arrowhead), and the gallbladder progressively fills from 11 to 46 min (open arrowhead). There is normal biliary-to-duodenum (d) transit first seen at about 36 min.

METHODOLOGY

Patient Preparation

The patient should be fasting for 3–4 hr prior to beginning the study. More than 60% of normal subjects do not show gallbladder visualization in the nonfasted state. Digestion and emptying of a large meal often takes several hours. Fat and protein entering the small bowel stimulate duodenal release of cholecystokinin, causing gallbladder contraction, which can prevent radiolabeled bile entry. Not eating for 3–4 hr prior to the study ensures that a false positive study (nonfilling of the gallbladder in a patient without cholecystitis) will not result.

When a patient has been fasting for longer than 24–48 hr, the gallbladder may not visualize because it is full of viscous concentrated bile due to the lack of stimulation to contract. This, too, can prevent bile entry. Cholecystokinin, or 0.02 μg/kg of Sincalide®, the physiologically active C-terminal octapeptide, can be administered intravenously in an attempt to empty the gallbladder. After allowing time for relaxation of the gallbladder, imaging can begin 30 min later.

Radiopharmaceuticals

Although a number of different radiopharmaceuticals (radioactive drugs) have been investigated over the years, two are presently used in the United States for cholescintigraphy, Tc 99m DISIDA or disofenin (Hepatolite®) and Tc 99m BIDA or mebrofenin (Choletec®). Technetium Tc 99m is the radioactive label (radiotracer) and HIDA (hepatic IDA) is the generic term for the iminodiacetic acid derivative drugs. Both are extracted with high efficiency by hepatocytes by the same mechanism as bilirubin, then rapidly secreted into the bile unconjugated, where they follow biliary flow. The two radiopharmaceuticals are quite similar. The biliary tree can be visualized by both agents with bilirubin levels as high as 20–30 mg %. Mebrofenin has slightly better hepatic extraction (98 versus 88%) and more rapid hepatobiliary clearance ($T_{1/2}$ of 17 versus 19 min) than disofenin. This moderate advantage may have clinical importance in patients with severe hepatic insufficiency.

Imaging

After intravenous injection of the technetium-labeled IDA, the patient lies supine for 60 min while images are made with a gamma camera. Images are acquired frequently on computer (1 frame/min) and formatted on hard-copy radiographic film every 2–5 min. The resulting images show the dynamic uptake and clearance of the radiopharmaceutical by the liver, filling of the gallbladder, and passage into the small bowel (Fig. 1). Review of the study on computer in cinematic mode can sometimes be helpful diagnostically.

Diagnostic Criteria

In a normal study, the gallbladder fills within 60 min and the Tc 99m IDA transits from the biliary ducts to the small intestine (Fig. 1). Gallbladder visualization rules out acute cholecystitis with a high degree of certainty. Acute cholecystitis is diagnosed if there is no gallbladder filling, but normal biliary-to-bowel transit (Fig. 2). Patients with no filling of the gallbladder within 1 hr require delayed imaging. The diagnosis of acute cholecystitis can be made if the gallbladder has not visualized within 4 hr. Most patients with delayed gallbladder filling (between 1 and 4 hr) have chronic cholecystitis (Fig. 3). However, they represent a small subgroup because the gallbladder is visualized in most patients with chronic cholecystitis in the first hour (>95%). Delayed filling is probably due to a partial cystic obstruction caused by previous inflammation. Morphine sulfate can be used as an alternative to delayed imaging with a total study time of only 60–90 min (Fig. 4).

Morphine Sulfate-augmented Cholescintigraphy

Morphine sulfate increases intraductal pressure at the sphincter of Oddi. This produces a functional partial common duct obstruction. The increased common duct pressure causes preferential bile flow through the cystic duct, if it is patent.

The dose of morphine sulfate used, 0.04 μg/kg (approximately 2 mg) is considerably lower than the dose usually used for analgesia. Side effects are rare. The most common method is to infuse it over 1 min intravenously if the gallbladder has not filled by 1 hr and there has been normal biliary-to-bowel transit with no suggestion of common duct obstruction. The reason for the latter requirement is that once morphine is administered, one can no longer differentiate common duct obstruction from drug effect. The study is completed 30 min after morphine administration. In

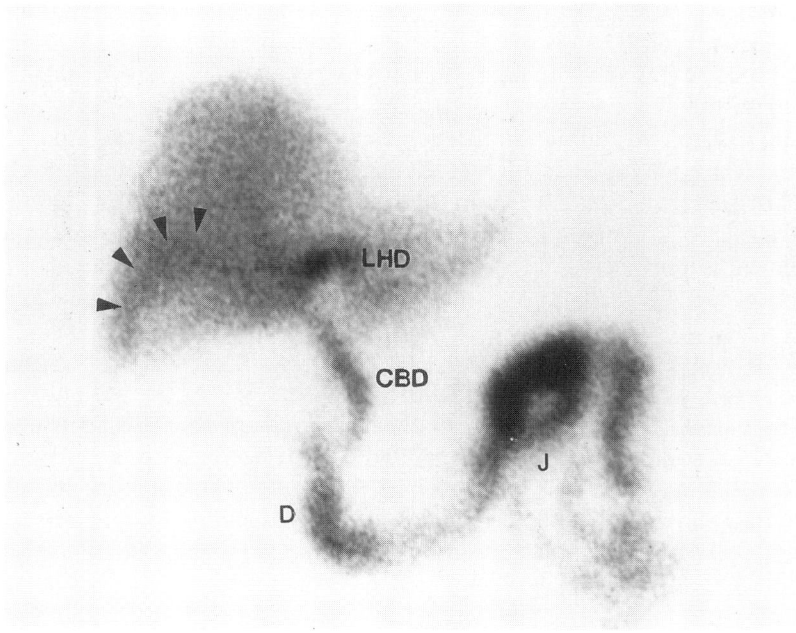

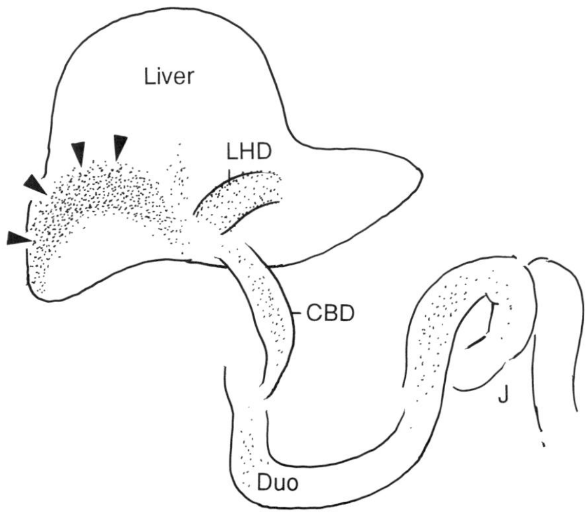

Figure 2. Acute cholecystitis with the "rim sign." This 60-min image shows the common duct, duodenal, and more distal small bowel. No gallbladder visualization is seen and there is a rim of increased activity adjacent to the gallbladder fossa (arrowheads), the rim sign. The rim sign is diagnostic of acute cholecystitis and delayed imaging or morphine is not required to make the diagnosis. The left hepatic duct (LHD) is prominent but not abnormal. The common bile duct (CBD), duodenum (Duo), and jejunal (J) activity are noted.

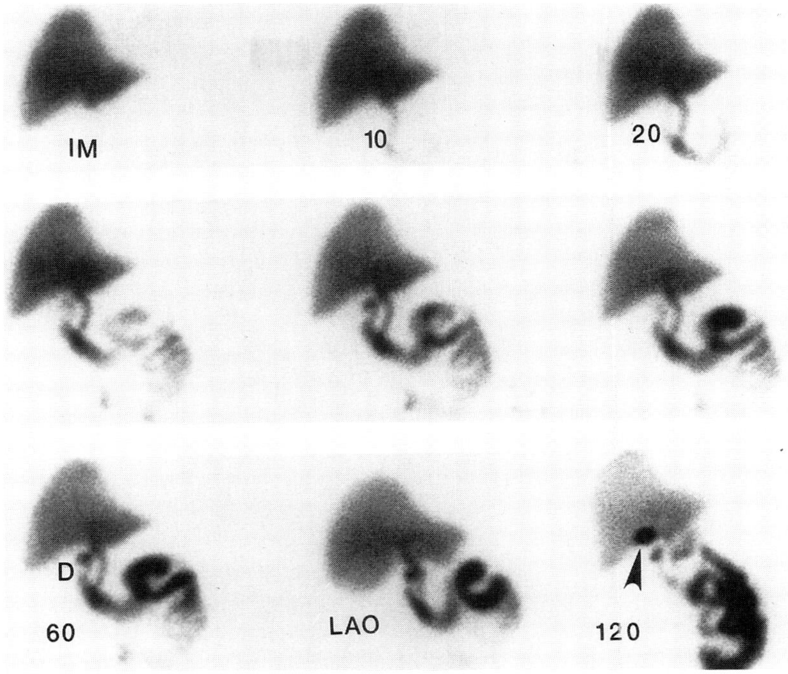

Figure 3. Delayed gallbladder filling. There is normal biliary-to-bowel transit but no definite gallbladder filling by 60 min. Two images show focal activity that raise the question of a gallbladder, but this is duodenal (D) activity, as demonstrated by its spontaneous clearance and posterior position on the left anterior oblique (LAO) view. The ultimate filling of the gallbladder (arrowhead) is in the expected but different position at 120 min.

patients without cystic duct obstruction, the gallbladder begins to fill promptly after infusion, often within 5–10 min (Fig. 5). If there is no filling by 30 min, the study is consistent with the diagnosis of acute cholecystitis. Morphine can be given as early as 30 min, completing the entire study by 60 min (1).

Rim Sign

In addition to nonfilling of the gallbladder, 25–35% of patients with acute cholecystitis have the additional imaging finding of increased hepatic uptake adjacent to the gallbladder fossa, called the "rim sign" (Fig. 2). The rim sign is due to focally increased Tc 99m IDA hepatic extraction. At surgery, the gallbladder is sometimes noted to be adherent to the liver capsule. Pathologically, the inflammatory process in the gallbladder wall can be seen to penetrate into the adjacent liver (2). As a result of the inflammation, the liver parenchyma receives increased blood flow, which delivers more radiotracer to that region of the liver, which extracts it with a very high efficiency. Regional hepatic clearance may also be delayed owing to obstruction of the biliary canaliculi by the inflammatory edema.

Detecting a rim sign has clinical importance because this finding has been associated with an increased incidence of gallbladder perforation and gangrene (3–5).

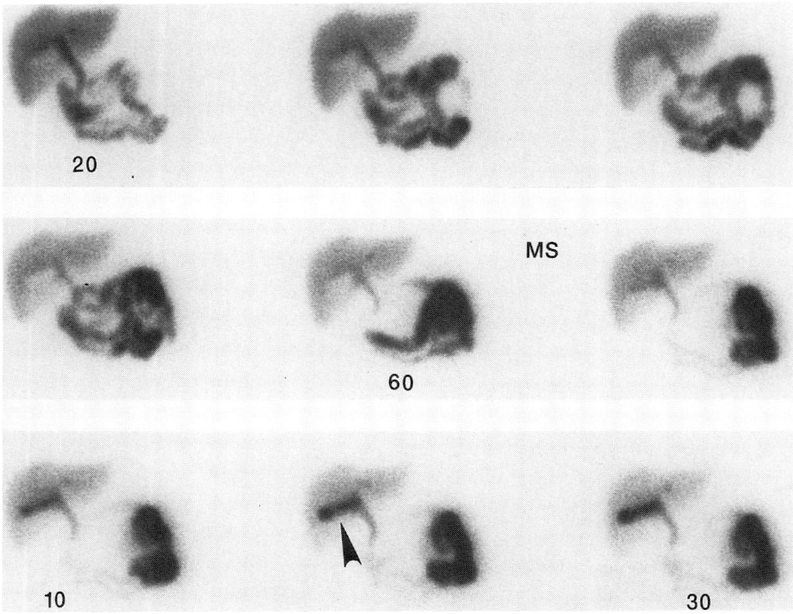

Figure 4. Morphine-augmented cholescintigraphy. No gallbladder filling is noted through 60 min. Morphine sulfate, 2 mg, is then given intravenously and prompt gallbladder (arrowhead) filling occurs. This study rules out acute cholecystitis.

There is evidence that even patients who do not have perforation and/or gangrene have a more severe cholecystitis and are at risk for developing complications. Hemorrhage and necrosis, late findings in the pathological spectrum of acute cholecystitis, are common, compared to edema and white cell infiltration, seen in the earlier stages of acute cholecystitis (2). The rim sign is very specific for the diagnosis of acute cholecystitis. Therefore it can be a valuable finding in patients who have an increased likelihood of a false positive study, for example, after prolonged fasting or hyperalimentation or in patients with a severe intercurrent illness (see section on accuracy of cholescintigraphy below). If the rim sign is present, one can be sure that the study is a true positive and not a false positive (5, 6). Because the rim sign is so specific for acute cholecystitis, the study can be discontinued at 1 hr rather than obtaining delayed imaging or using morphine.

Acute Acalculous Cholecystitis

Acute *acalculous* cholecystitis is a serious life-threatening illness that occurs in hospitalized patients who have had extensive burns, trauma, shock, or sepsis, for example. It is seen in less than 5% of patients requiring cholecystectomy. The disease often presents atypically, leading to a delay in diagnosis and associated high morbidity (55%) and mortality (30%) (7). As the name suggests, it is not caused by a stone. Although the cystic duct may be obstructed by inflammatory debris, edema, or inspissated bile, in many patients it is patent, but the gallbladder wall is inflamed as a result of infection, ischemia, or toxins. Because the cystic duct may not be obstructed, concern has been expressed regarding the potential for false negative cholescintigraphy, either by dislodging the stone or forcing tracer around an obstruction. However, most studies have shown a high sensitivity for detecting this disease (>90%). If the gallbladder visualizes in a patient with clinically suspected acute acalculous cholecystitis, cholecystokinin can be administered to determine if the gallbladder contracts normally (abnormal is less than 35% emptying). If it does, cholecystitis can be ruled out. If the gallbladder does not contract, it is consistent with a diseased gallbladder; however, this does not differentiate acute from chronic disease. In this situation, a radiolabeled white blood cell study (In 111 or Tc 99m HMPAO) can confirm or exclude the diagnosis (8, 9).

Accuracy of Cholescintigraphy

Over the years many investigations have reported a high accuracy of cholescintigraphy for confirming the clinical diagnosis of acute cholecystitis. In an early, large series of 296 patients, Weissmann et al. reported a sensitivity of 95% and a specificity of 98% (10). Numerous other investigations have found similar excellent results with sensitivities ranging from 95 to 100% and specificities of 94–100% (11–15) (Table 1).

Although there is general consensus that cholescintigraphy is highly sensitive for detection of acute cholecystitis, the reported specificity has varied considerably, with a false positive rate ranging from 0.6 to 27% (10, 17, 18). To a large degree the poor results are due to the use of different methodologies, populations, and diagnostic criteria (16). For example, a patient population with a high prevalence of severe intercurrent illness, prolonged fasting, and/or hyperalimentation would be expected to have a lower test specificity than a more general referral population. In addition, sensitivity and specificity can change dramatically in the same patient population by varying the criteria and technique (19). Use of different standards for final diagnosis can result in very different sensitivity and specificity. Using liberal pathological criteria (edema and inflammatory cell infiltration) as the standard, in contrast to more strict criteria (hemorrhagic necrosis) will improve sensitivity and decrease specificity and vice versa. The percent of the study population with chronic

Table 1. Accuracy of cholescintigraphy for diagnosis of acute calculous cholecystitis

		Cholescintigraphy		Ultrasonography	
Study	Reference	Sensitivity (%)	Specificity (%)	Sensitivity (%)	Specificity (%)
Cheng et al. (1979)	11		100		77
Freitas et al. (1980)	13	100	90		
Szlabick et al. (1980)	12	100	98	78	
Weissmann et al. (1981)	10	95	99		
Zeman et al. (1981)	14	98	81	67	82
Mauro et al. (1982)	15	100	94		
Samuels et al. (1983)	48	97	93	97	64

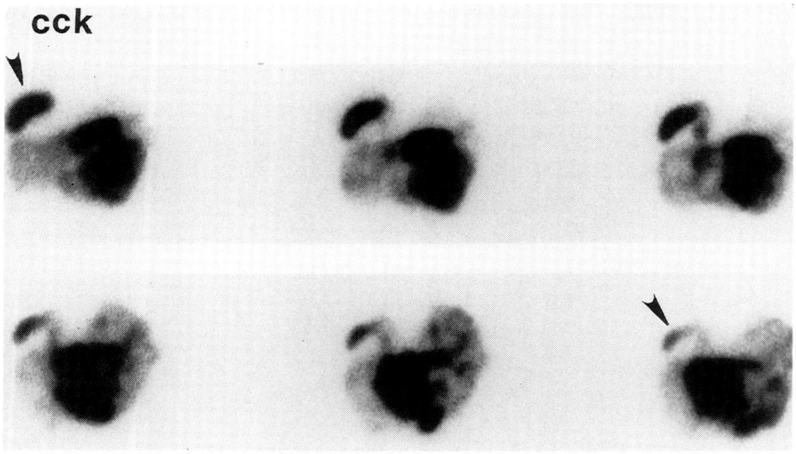

(A)

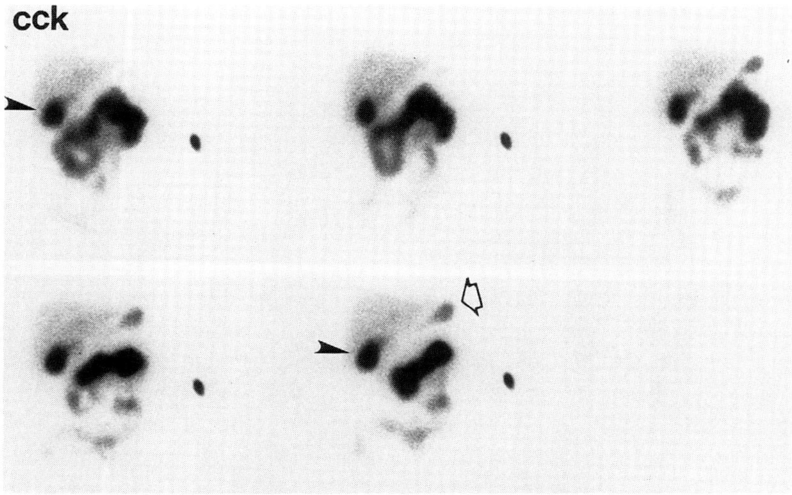

(B)

Figure 5. CCK-stimulated cholescintigraphy. (A) After the initial normal 60-min study, the liver has completely washed out. The gallbladder (arrowheads) shows excellent contraction in response to CCK. (B) In another patient the gallbladder (closed arrowheads) shows almost no response to CCK. Note some enterogastric reflux (open arrowhead). (C, next page) Regions of interest are drawn around the gallbladder and adjacent liver, and a background-subtracted gallbladder time–activity curve is generated, from which 40% gallbladder emptying is determined.

cholecystitis can also influence the overall reported results. Some reports with poorer accuracy used nonfilling of the gallbladder at 1 hr to make the diagnosis of acute cholecystitis. It is now well appreciated that imaging for up to 4 hr is required to minimize the false positive rate (20).

In summary, cholescintigraphy has a very good specificity as well as sensitivity if proper technique and appropriate diagnostic imaging criteria are used. The pre-

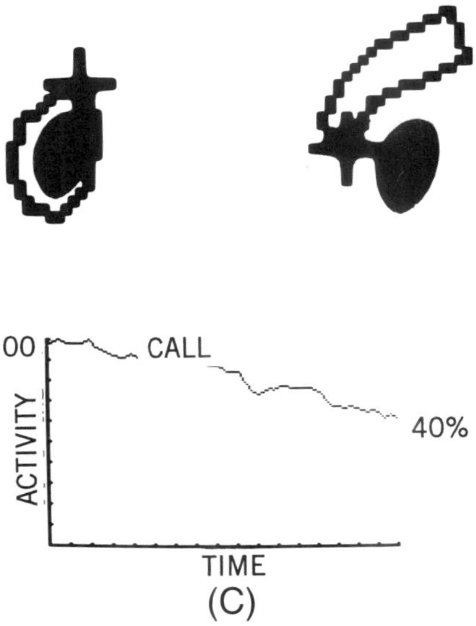

Figure 5. *(Continued)*

dictive value of a positive test (persistent nonvisualization) for acute cholecystitis is greater than 90%, whereas normal or delayed gallbladder visualization has a negative predictive value of 99% (16).

Numerous studies have now confirmed that morphine-augmented cholescintigraphy gives results comparable to delayed imaging (1, 21–27) (Table 2). Some investigators have found it to be superior to delayed imaging, with a higher specificity and positive predictive value (28).

Sick hospitalized patients have an increased rate of false positive studies due to prolonged fasting, hyperalimentation (29–32), and the presence of serious intercurrent illness (33–35). Patients with hepatic insufficiency have delayed hepatic uptake and excretion of bile; therefore, the gallbladder may not fill in the usual time course. Delayed images of 12–24 hr may be required to detect gallbladder filling. Although most patients with chronic cholecystitis have normal studies, a rare patient will have cystic duct obstruction due to chronic inflammation, and less than 5% will

Table 2. Accuracy of morphine-augmented cholescintigraphy

Study	Reference	Sensitivity [No. Patients (%)]	Specificity [No. Patients (%)]
Choy et al.	21	23/24 (96)	35/35 (100)
Kim et al.	22	11/11 (100)	18/18 (100)
Keslar and Turbiner	24	19/19 (100)	10/12 (83)
Vasquez et al.	25	10/10 (100)	22/26 (85)
Fig et al.	27	15/16 (94)	22/32 (69)
Flanebaum and Aldens	23	28/29 (97)	38/49 (95)
Fink-Bennett et al.	26	35/37 (95)	23/24 (96)
Kistler et al.	1	13/14 (93)	14/18 (78)

Table 3. Accuracy of cholescintigraphy for diagnosis of acute acalculous cholecystitis

Study	Reference	Sensitivity [No. Patients (%)]
Shuman et al.	36	13/19 (68)
Weissmann et al.	38	14/15 (93)
Mirvis et al.	35	18/19 (95)
Swayne	39	37/49 (93)
Frazee et al.	7	10/10 (100)
Ramanna et al.	37	11/11 (100)

have delayed gallbladder filling by 4 hr (20). Being aware of these clinical situations, using proper methodology and, when indicated, intervening with cholecystokinin or morphine sulfate as discussed above, one can minimize false positives, with an overall specificity of about 95% (16).

Cholescintigraphy is reported to have a slightly lower sensitivity for acute acalculous cholecystitis than for the calculous form (Table 3). One study has reported a sensitivity of 68%. In that study ultrasonography showed similar results (67%) (36). However, numerous other series have shown a good sensitivity for its detection by cholescintigraphy (93–100%) (36–38).

Cholescintigraphy versus Ultrasonography

Because many findings have been reported as useful in the sonographic detection of acute cholecystitis, but few are specific, major and minor criteria have been put forth. Major criteria include demonstration of gallstones, intramural lucencies, and a positive sonographic Murphy's sign. Although most patients with acute cholecystitis have gallstones, gallstones do not necessarily indicate acute inflammation. In one study of patients seen in the emergency room with suspected acute cholecystitis and imaging evidence of gallstones, 40% did not have acute cholecystitis (39). Detection of a calculous lodged in the cystic duct is specific, but very rarely seen. Intramural lucencies represent subserosal edema, a fairly specific finding, but this is seen in only 70% of patients with acute cholecystitis (40, 41). The findings of diffuse gallbladder thickening and pericholecystic fluid are neither sensitive nor specific. The sonographic Murphy's sign has been reported to have a predictive value for acute cholecystitis of 88% (42); however, others have not found such good results (16). The technique is subjective and has many pitfalls. Its sensitivity is reported to be low in gangrenous gallbladders and acute acalculous cholecystitis (44).

Most studies comparing the techniques have shown the superiority of cholescintigraphy over ultrasonography (42, 43, 47) (Table 1). One prospective study that directly compared real-time ultrasonography with cholescintigraphy showed similar sensitivities for making the diagnosis of acute cholecystitis (97%), but scintigraphy showed significantly better specificity (93 versus 64%, $p < .001$) (48).

Cholescintigraphy has numerous other advantages. It can detect bile leaks, biliary obstruction, and importantly, early and low-grade obstruction in the absence of dilated ducts (49), which can mimic or coexist with acute cholecystitis. Cholescintigraphy is objective and not operator-dependent. The radiation dose to the patient is very low, similar to that received from a chest X-ray and considerably less than from a kidney, ureter, and bladder roentgenographic series. Allergic reactions are rare.

When the clinical index of suspicion for acute cholecystitis is high, scintigraphy should be used as the primary method of evaluation. When the referring physician is less certain of the diagnosis, scintigraphy can rule it out with a high degree of certainty. Ultrasonography in conjunction with cholescintigraphy may be useful in patients who have an increased likelihood of a false positive cholescintigraphic study. Ultrasonography is most useful for detection of chronic cholecystitis, biliary duct disease, or nonbiliary disease.

CHRONIC CHOLECYSTITIS

Chronic Calculous Cholecystitis

Most patients with chronic cholecystitis have normal conventional radionuclide cholescintigraphy. Less than 5% have delayed gallbladder visualization and a few have nonvisualization of the gallbladder. Ultrasonography, and less often these days oral cholecystography, are the methods of choice for making the diagnosis of chronic cholecystitis. The presence of gallstones is consistent with the diagnosis. However, cholescintigraphy can sometimes play a role in selected patients, for example, those with cholelithiasis, but atypical abdominal pain. Here the surgeon may want to be certain that the patient's pain is indeed related to chronic cholecystitis and not to some other disease process. In these patients, cholecystokinin can be given to evaluate gallbladder function. Although about half of patients with cholelithiasis have a low gallbladder ejection fraction, most patients with *symptomatic* chronic cholecystitis have a poorly functioning or nonfunctioning gallbladder as manifested by gallbladder ejection fraction of less than 35% (50–52). A normal ejection fraction would suggest that the patient's pain is more likely caused by some other disease, for example, irritable bowel syndrome.

Chronic Acalculous Cholecystitis

Cholescintigraphy now plays an important role in the diagnosis of *chronic acalculous cholecystitis.* Although less than 10% of patients with chronic cholecystitis have the acalculous form, these patients present with identical symptoms and gallbladder histopathology, except for the absence of stones. Other names used for this entity have included gallbladder spasm, gallbladder dyskinesia, and cystic duct syndrome. In the past, this was a very difficult clinical diagnosis to confirm objectively. Ultrasonography and oral cholecystography are usually normal. Surgeons understandably hesitate to operate on clinical suspicion alone because other causes of abdominal pain may mimic biliary colic. In the past, patients with less typical symptoms were sometimes diagnosed incorrectly. However, if the patient found a bold surgeon who was willing to operate, the diagnosis could be confirmed pathologically and the patient cured. Understandably, a noninvasive method for confirming the diagnosis has long been sought.

There has been evidence over the years to suggest that a chronically diseased gallbladder does not contract normally and that this information could be used diagnostically. In the 1950s and 1960s fatty meal or cholecystokinin-stimulated oral cholecystography was investigated with the hope of making the diagnosis of chronic acalculous cholecystitis. However, mixed results were reported regarding its clinical diagnostic accuracy (53–60), perhaps owing to the various different techniques used and the subjective methods for estimating gallbladder contraction.

With the advent of cholescintigraphy, several preliminary investigations reported the radionuclide method to be useful in confirming the clinical diagnosis of chronic acalculous cholecystitis (61–65). However, because two studies reported less encouraging results (66, 67), some skepticism and controversy remained regarding the diagnostic utility of cholecystokinin (CCK) cholescintigraphy (68). The publication of two recent excellent investigations (69, 70) as well as many other confirmatory studies (71–78) have now convincingly shown that CCK-augmented cholescintigraphy is very accurate for confirming the clinical diagnosis of chronic acalculous cholecystitis and predicting response to cholecystectomy.

Enthusiasm for the role of CCK cholescintigraphy for confirming this diagnosis was generated by a large retrospective study of 374 patients with clinically suspected chronic acalculous cholecystitis and a low gallbladder ejection fraction as determined by CCK cholescintigraphy (69). In this study, surgery and histopathological examination confirmed a diseased gallbladder in 94% of the patients with a low gallbladder ejection fraction. Symptoms resolved in 105/108 patients following cholecystectomy. The negative predictive value of a normal gallbladder ejection fraction was 91%.

A particularly convincing prospective study (70) randomized all patients who had low gallbladder ejection fractions into two groups, cholecystectomy or no operation. Of those having cholecystectomy, 91% had symptom resolution and all showed histopathological evidence of chronic cholecystitis. Patients who did not have surgery continued to be symptomatic.

Today CCK-stimulated cholescintigraphy has become the accepted method for evaluating gallbladder function and for confirming the diagnosis of chronic acalculous cholecystitis. However, it should be pointed out that the above investigations were performed in patients who had been thoroughly worked up for other diseases and followed for a period of time; that is, they represent a population of patients with a high likelihood of disease. This test should not be performed when the patient is acutely ill or as an alternative to a complete work-up and adequate follow-up time before surgery is contemplated. Other diseases should be excluded and the patient followed for a time so that other disease processes become manifest. Patients less thoroughly evaluated or followed for a brief period may have an increased false positive rate (80) because numerous other diseases and drugs are also known to cause a low gallbladder ejection fraction. Some of these are listed in Table 4.

Fatty Meal versus Cholecystokinin Infusion

Intravenously administered cholecystokinin (CCK, Sincalide) has advantages over fatty meal stimulation of the gallbladder because the former does not depend on gastric emptying and intestinal absorption. Cholecystokinin-augmented cholescintigraphy is a more rapid and reproducible test. Changes in gallbladder volume in

Table 4. Diseases and drugs known to affect gallbladder emptying[a]

Diseases	Drugs
Obesity	Morphine
Diabetes mellitus	Atropine
Sickle cell disease	Calcium blockers
Irritable bowel syndrome	Histamine two-receptor stimulating drugs
Truncal vagotomy	Progesterone and birth control pills
Pancreatic insufficiency	Octreotide
Sprue	Excess calcium
Achalasia	

[a]This is not an all-inclusive list.

response to fatty meals or CCK have been measured with real-time ultrasonography. One small retrospective study reported that ultrasonography predicted histological changes of chronic cholecystitis in 62% of patients with chronic acalculous cholecystitis, similar to oral cholecystography, but considerably less than cholescintigraphy, 89% (63). Cholecystokinin-stimulated cholescintigraphy has the additional advantages that continuous imaging can be performed, it is not operator-dependent, and the test is inherently quantitative.

Methodology for Cholecystokinin Cholescintigraphy

Approximately 1 hr after injection when the gallbladder has completely filled, Sincalide is infused intravenously. In the past and still at many institutions, 0.02 μg/kg Sincalide is infused over 3 min (shorter infusions are not given because it is well known that they can result in spasm of the gallbladder neck) and imaging is performed for 20 min. However, there are a number of advantages to infusing the Sincalide at a lower dose rate, for example, the same 0.02 μg/kg but over 30 min (80). This slower method of CCK infusion is more physiological (81), results in better emptying, and more clearly separates normal from abnormal (80, 82). The more rapid infusion method sometimes results in false positives (low ejection fractions) in normal volunteers (80, 82). The slower infusion method does not produce adverse side effects of nausea and abdominal cramping. Although it has been believed by some that the patient's pain response to CCK could predict the disease (53, 56, 58), in fact, this has not proved to be the case because it has been demonstrated that a large number of normal subjects and patients with other diseases, for example, irritable bowel syndrome, can have pain with CCK infusion (80–84).

After complete filling of the gallbladder, the CCK study is acquired on computer (1-min frames × 30 min). Cholecystokinin is infused for 30 min during this acquisition period, 0.02 μg/kg over 30 min. Although hard-copy images can demonstrate poor or good contraction (Fig. 5A–C), a strong point of the radionuclide study is that accurate quantitation can be performed. On computer, a region of interest is drawn for the gallbladder and for liver background adjacent to the gallbladder, from which a time–activity curve is generated. The gallbladder ejection fraction is calculated by dividing the peak gallbladder counts minus the minimum counts by the peak counts, after correcting for background. An ejection fraction of less than 35% emptying is abnormal.

REFERENCES

1. Kistler AM, Ziessman HA, Gooch D, Bitterman P. Morphine-augmented cholescintigraphy in acute cholecystitis: a satisfactory alternative to delayed imaging. *Clin Nucl Med.* 1991;16:404–406.
2. Meekin GK, Ziessman HA, Klappenbach RS. Prognostic value and pathophysiologic significance of the rim sign in cholescintigraphy. *J Nucl Med.* 1987;28:1679–1682.
3. Brachman MB, Tanasescu DE, Ramanna L, et al. Acute gangrenous cholecystitis: radionuclide diagnosis. *Radiology.* 1984;158:63–66.
4. Smith R, Rosen JM, Alderson PO. Gallbladder perforation: diagnostic utility of cholescintigraphy in suggested subacute or chronic cases. *Radiology.* 1986;158:63–66.
5. Bushnell DL, Perlman SB, Wilson MA, Polcyn RE. The rim sign: association with acute cholecystitis. *J Nucl Med.* 1986;27:353–356.
6. Swayne LC, Ginsberg HN. Diagnosis of acute cholecystitis by cholescintigraphy: significance of pericholecystic hepatic uptake. *AJR.* 1989;152:1211–1213.
7. Frazee RC, Nagorney DM, Mucha P. Acute acalculous cholecystitis. *Mayo Clinic Proc.* 1989;64:163–167.
8. Datz FL. Utility of indium-111 labeled leucocyte imaging in acute acalculous cholecystitis. *AJR.* 1986;147:813–814.
9. Fink-Bennett D, Clarke K, Tsai D, et al. Indium-111-leukocyte imaging in acute cholecystitis. *J Nucl Med.* 1991;323:803–804.
10. Weissmann HS, Badia J, Sugarman LA, et al. Spectrum of cholescintigraphic patterns in acute cholecystitis. *Radiology.* 1981;138:167–175.
11. Cheng TH, Davis MA, Seltzer SC, et al. Evaluation of hepatobiliary imaging by radionuclide scintigraphy, ultrasonography, and contrast cholangiography. *Radiology.* 1979; 133:761–767.
12. Szlabick RE, Catto JA, Fink-Bennett D, et al. Hepatobiliary scanning in the diagnosis of cystic duct obstruction. *Ann Surg.* 1980;115:540–544.
13. Freitas JE, Fink-Bennett D, Thrall DM, et al. Efficacy of hepatobiliary imaging in acute abdominal pain. *J Nucl Med.* 1980;21:919–924.
14. Zeman RK, Burrell MI, Cahow CE, et al. Diagnostic utility of cholescintigraphy and ultrasonography in acute cholecystitis. *Am J Surg.* 1981;141:446–451.
15. Mauro MA, McCartney WH, Melmed JR. Hepatobiliary scanning with 99mTc-PIPIDA in acute cholecystitis. *Radiology.* 1982;142:193–197.
16. Freitas JE. Cholescintigraphy. In: Murray IPC, Ell PJ, eds. *Nuclear Medicine in Clinical Diagnosis and Treatment.* Edinburgh: Churchill Livingstone; 1994:77–86.
17. Shuman WP, Mack LA, Rudd TG, et al. Evaluation of acute right upper quadrant pain: Sonography and Tc-99m PIPIDA cholescintigraphy. *AJR.* 1982;139:61–63.
18. Worthen NJ, Uszler JM, Funamura JL. Cholecystitis: Prospective evaluation of sonography and 99m Tc-HIDA cholescintigraphy. *AJR.* 1981;137:973–978.
19. Freitas JE, Coleman RE, Nagle CE, et al. Influence of scan and pathologic criteria on the specificity of cholescintigraphy: concise communication. *J Nucl Med.* 1983;24: 876–879.

20. Weissmann HS, Sugarman LA, Badia JD, et al. Improving the specificity and accuracy of Tc-99m IDA cholescintigraphy with delayed views. *J Nucl Med.* 1980;21:17.
21. Choy D, Shi EC, McLean RG, et al. Cholescintigraphy in acute cholecystitis: use of intravenous morphine. *Radiology.* 1984;151:203–207.
22. Kim EE, Pjura G, Lowry P, et al. Morphine-augmented cholescintigraphy in the diagnosis of acute cholecystitis. *AJR.* 1986;147:1177–1179.
23. Flanebaum L, Aldens SM. Morphine cholescintigraphy. *Surg Gynecol Obstet.* 1990; 171:227–232.
24. Keslar PJ, Turbiner ELT. Hepatatobiliary imaging and the use of intravenous morphine. *Clin Nucl Med.* 1987;12:592–596.
25. Vasquez TE, Rimkus DS, Pretorius HT, Greenspan G. Intravenous administration of morphine sulfate in hepatobiliary imaging of acute cholecystitis: a review of clinical efficacy. *Nucl Med Commun.* 1988;9:217–222.
26. Fink-Bennett D, Balon H, Robbins T, Tsai D. Morphine-augmented cholescintigraphy: its efficacy in detection of acute cholecysitis. *J Nucl Med.* 1991;32:1231–1233.
27. Fig LM, Wahl RL, Stewart RE, Shapiro B. Morphine-augmented hepatobiliary scintigraphy in the severely ill: caution is in order. *Radiology.* 1990;175:473–476.
28. Kim CK, Tse KMK, Juweid M, et al. Cholescintigraphy in the diagnosis of acute cholecystitis: morphine augmentation is superior to delayed imaging. *J Nucl Med.* 1993; 34:1866–1870.
29. Larsen MJ, Klingensmith III WC, Kuni CC. Radionuclide hepatobiliary imaging: nonvisualization of the gallbladder secondary to prolonged fasting. *J Nucl Med.* 1982;23:1003–1005.
30. Sippo WC, Moreno AJ, Cabellon S, Turnbull GL. The effect of prolonged fasting and total parenteral nutrition on hepatobiliary imaging with technetium-99m DISIDA. *Clin Nucl Med.* 1987;12:169–172.
31. Warner BW, Hamilton FN, Silberstein EB, et al. The value of hepatobiliary scans in fasted patients receiving total parenteral nutrition. *Surgery* 1987;102:595–601.
32. Shuman WP, Gibbs P, Rudd TG, Mack LA. PIPIDA scintigraphy for cholecystitis: false positives in alcoholism and total parenteral nutrition. *AJR.* 1982;138:1–5.
33. Garner WL, Marx MV, Fabri PJ. Cholescintigraphy in the critically ill. *Am J Surg.* 1988;155:727–729.
34. Kalff V, Froelich JW, Lloyd R, Thrall JH: Predictive value of an abnormal hepatobiliary scan in patients with severe intercurrent illness. *Radiology.* 1983;146:191–194.
35. Mirvis SE, Vainright JR, Nelson AW, et al. The diagnosis of acute alcalculous cholecystitis: a comparison of sonography, scintigraphy, and CT. *AJR.* 1986;147:1171–1175.
36. Shuman WP, Rogers JV, Rudd TG, et al. Low sensitivity of sonography and cholescintigraphy in acalculous cholecystitis. *AJR.* 1984;142:531–534.
37. Rammana L, Brachman MB, Tanasescu DE, et al. Cholescintigraphy in acute acalculous cholecystitis. *Am J Gastroenterol.* 1984;79:650–653.
38. Weissmann HA, Berkowitz D, Fox MS, et al. The role of technetium 99m iminodiacetic acid cholescintigraphy in acute acalculous cholecystitis. *Radiology.* 1983;146:177–200.
39. Swayne LC. Acute acalculous cholecystitis: sensitivity in detection using technetium-99m iminodiacetic acid cholescintigraphy. *Radiology.* 1986;160:33–38.
40. Weissmann HS, Freeman LM. The biliary tract. In: *Freeman and Johnson's Clinical Radionuclide Imaging.* 3rd ed. Philadelphia: W. B. Saunders Company; 1984:879–1050.
41. Cohan RH, Mahony BS, Bowie, et al. Striated intramural gallbladder lucencies on US studies. Predictors of acute cholecystitis. *Radiology.* 1987;164:31–35.

42. Teefey SA, Baron RL, Bigler SA. Sonography of the gallbladder. Significance of striated (layered) thickening of the gallbladder wall. *AJR.* 1991;156:945–948.
43. Laing FC, Federlye MP, Jeffery RB, Brown TW. Ultrasonic evaluation of patients with acute right upper quadrant pain. *Radiology* 1981;140:449–455.
44. Ralls PW, Colletti PM, Lapin SA, et al. Real time sonography in suspected acute cholecystitis. *Radiology* 1985;155:767–771.
45. Simeone JF, Brink JA, Mueller PR, et al. The sonographic diagnosis of acute gangrenous cholecystitis: importance of the Murphy sign. *AJR.* 1989;152:289–290.
46. Zeman RK, Burrell MI, Cahow CE, et al. Diagnostic utility of cholescintigraphy and ultrasonography in acute cholecystitis. *Am J Surg.* 1981;141:446–451.
47. Freitas JE, Mirkas SH, Fink-Bennett DM, et al. Suspected acute cholecystitis: comparison of hepatobiliary imaging versus ultrasonography. *Clin Nucl Med.* 1982;7:364–367.
48. Samuels BI, Freitas JE, Bree RL, et al. A comparison of radionuclide hepatobiliary imaging and real-time ultrasonography for the detection of acute cholecystitis. *Radiology.* 1983;147:207–210.
49. Zeman RK, Lee C, Jaffe MH, Burrell MI. Hepatobiliary scintigraphy and sonography in early biliary obstruction. *Radiology.* 1984;153:793–798.
50. Fisher RS, Stelzer F, Rock E, Malmud LS. Abnormal gallbladder emptying in patients with gallstones. *Dig Dis Sci.* 1992;27:1019–1024.
51. Thompson JC, Fried GM, Ogden WD, et al. Correlation between release of cholecystokinin and contraction of the gallbladder in patients with gallstones. *Ann Surg.* 1982; 195:670–676.
52. Shaffer EA, McOrmond P, Duggan H. Quantitative cholescintigraphy: Assessment of gallbladder filling and emptying and duodenogastric reflux. *Gastroenterology.* 1980; 79:899–906.
53. Valberg LS, Jabbari M, Kerr JW, et al. Biliary pain in young women in the absence of gallstones. *Gastroenterology.* 1971;60:1020–1026.
54. Goldstein F, Grunt R, Margulies M. Cholecystokinin cholecystography in the differential diagnosis of acalculus gallbladder disease. *Am J Dig Dis.* 1974;19:835–849.
55. Nora PF, McCarthy W, Sanez N. Cholecystokinin cholecystography in acalculus gallbladder disease. *Arch Surg.* 1974;108:507–511.
56. Nechis M, King MC, Murphy RA. Cholecystokinin cholecystography in the diagnosis of acalculous extrahepatic biliary tract disorders. *Am J Gastroenterol.* 1978;70:593–599.
57. Griffin WO, Bivins BA, Rogers EL. Cholescystokinin cholecystography in the diagnosis of gallbladder disease. *Ann Surg.* 1980;191:636–641.
58. Lennard TWJ, Farndon JR, Taylor RMR. Acalculous biliary pain: diagnosis and selection for cholecystectomy using cholecystokinin test for pain reproduction. *Br J Surg.* 1984;71:368–370.
59. Dunn FH, Christen EC, Reynolds J, et al. Cholecystokinin cholecystography. *JAMA.* 1974;228:997–1003.
60. Nathan MH, Newman A, McFarland J, et al. Cholecystokinin cholecystography. *Radiology.* 1969;93:1–8.
61. Topper TE, Ryerson TW, Nora PF. Quantitative gallbladder imaging following cholecystokin. *J Nucl Med.* 1980;21:694–696.
62. Pickleman J, Peiss RL, Henkin R, et al. The role of sincalide cholescintigraphy in the evaluation of patients with acalculous gallbladder disease. *Arch Surg.* 1985;120:693–697.
63. Brugge WR, Brand DL, Atkins, et al. Gallbladder dyskinesia in chronic acalculous cholecystitis. *Dig Dis Sci.* 1986;31:461–467.

64. Fink-Bennett D, DeRidder P, Kolozsi W, et al. Cholecystokinin cholescintigraphic findings in the cystic duct syndrome. *J Nucl Med.* 1985;26:1123–1128.

65. Raptopouloos V, Compton CC, Doherty P, et al. Chronic acalculous gallbladder disease: multiimaging evaluation with clinical-pathologic correlation. *AJR.* 1986;147:721–724.

66. Westlake PJ, Hersfield NB, Kelly JK, et al. Chronic right upper quadrant pain without gallstones: Does HIDA scan predict outcome after cholecystectomy? *Am J Gastroenterol.* 1990;85:986–990.

67. Davis GB, Berk RN, Scheible FW, et al. Cholecystokinin cholecystography, sonography, an scintigraphy: detection of chronic acalculous cholecystitis. *AJR.* 1982;139:1117–1121.

68. Ruffolo TA. The value of HIDA imaging in acalculus right upper quadrant pain: "Spin the wheel, Vanna!" *Am J Gastroenterol.* 1991;86:375–376.

69. Fink-Bennett D, DeRidder P, Kolozsi WZ, et al. Cholecystokinin cholescintigraphy: detection of abnormal gallbladder motor function in patients with chronic acalculous gallbladder disease. *J Nucl Med.* 1991;32:1695–1699.

70. Yap L, Wycherley AG, Morphett AD, et al. Acalculous biliary pain: cholecystectomy alleviates symptoms in patients with abnormal cholescintigraphy. *Gastroenterology.* 1991;101:786–793.

71. Middleton GW, Williams JH. Is gallbladder ejection fraction a reliable predictor of acalculous gallbladder disease. *Nucl Med Commun.* 1992;13:894–896.

72. Halverson JD, Garner BA, Siegel BA, et al. The use of hepatobiliary scintigraphy in patients with acalculous biliary colic. *Arch Intern Med.* 1992;152:1305–1307.

73. Misra DC, Blossom GB, Fink-Bennett D, Glover JL. Results of surgical therapy for biliary dyskinesia. *Arch Surg.* 1991;126:957–960.

74. Zech ER, Simmons LB, Soballe PW, et al. Cholecystokinin enhanced hepatobiliary scanning with ejection fraction calculation as an indicator of diseases of the gallbladder. *Surg Gynecol Obstet.* 1991;172:21–24.

75. Reed DN, Fernandez M, Hicks RD. Kinevac-assisted cholescintigraphy as an accurate predictor of chronic acalculus gallbladder disease and the likelihood of symptom relief with cholecystectomy. *Am Surgeon.* 1993;59:273–277.

78. Sorenson MK, Fancher S, Lang NP, et al. Abnormal gallbladder nuclear ejection fraction predicts success of cholecystectomy in patients with biliary dyskinesia. *Am J Surg.* 1993;166:672–675.

79. Harvey RF, Read AE. Effect of cholecystokinin on colonic motility and symptoms in patients with the irritable-bowel syndrome. *Lancet.* 1973;1:1–3.

80. Ziessman HA, Fahey FH, Hixson DJ. Calculation of a gallbladder ejection fraction: advantage of continuous sincalide infusion over the three minute infusion method. *J Nucl Med.* 1992;33:537–541.

81. Krishnamurthy S, Krishnamurthy GT. Cholecystokinin and morphine pharmacological intervention during 99mTc-HIDA cholescintigraphy: a rational approach. *Semin Nucl Med.* 1996;26:16–24.

82. Sarva RP, Shreiner DP, Van Thiel D, Yingvorapant N. Gallbladder function: methods for measuring filling and emptying. *J Nucl Med.* 1985;26:140–144.

83. Sykes D. The use of cholecystokinin in diagnosing biliary pain. *Ann Royal Coll Surgeons.* 1982;64:114–116.

84. Harvey RF, Read AE. Effect of cholecystokinin on colonic motility and symptoms in patients with the irritable bowel-syndrome. *Lancet.* 1973;1:1–3.

4

MAGNETIC RESONANCE IMAGING OF THE GALLBLADDER

Nikolaos L. Kelekis, M.D., and Richard C. Semelka, M.D.
University of North Carolina at Chapel Hill
Chapel Hill, North Carolina

The role of magnetic resonance imaging (MRI) in investigating gallbladder disease is currently expanding. Fat-suppressed spoiled gradient echo images and dynamic administration of gadolinium contrast agents are effective at demonstrating diseases of the gallbladder. The recent implementation of MR cholangiographic techniques in combination with the tissue imaging sequences (spoiled gradient echo, SGE, and fat-suppressed SGE) has resulted in comprehensive evaluation of gallbladder and biliary tract disease.

MAGNETIC RESONANCE TECHNIQUES

Magnetic resonance techniques for imaging the gallbladder may employ either black signal bile or bright signal bile techniques.

Pre- and postcontrast T1-weighted sequences are generally referred to as dark bile techniques in the investigation of the biliary system. Normal bile is not concentrated in the biliary tree and is low in signal intensity on T1-weighted images. Dilute bile in the gallbladder is low in signal intensity on T1-weighted images. Concentrated bile in the gallbladder may have high signal intensity on T1-weighted images due to its high protein and/or cholesterol concentration. A gradual transition from dark bile to bright bile in the dependent part of the gallbladder may be observed. Bile is high in signal on T2-weighted images.

Techniques that generate bright signal biliary fluid are referred to as MR cholangiopancreatography (MRCP). These techniques are based on heavily T2-weighted pulse sequences. As a result, stationary fluids, including bile and pancreatic ducts,

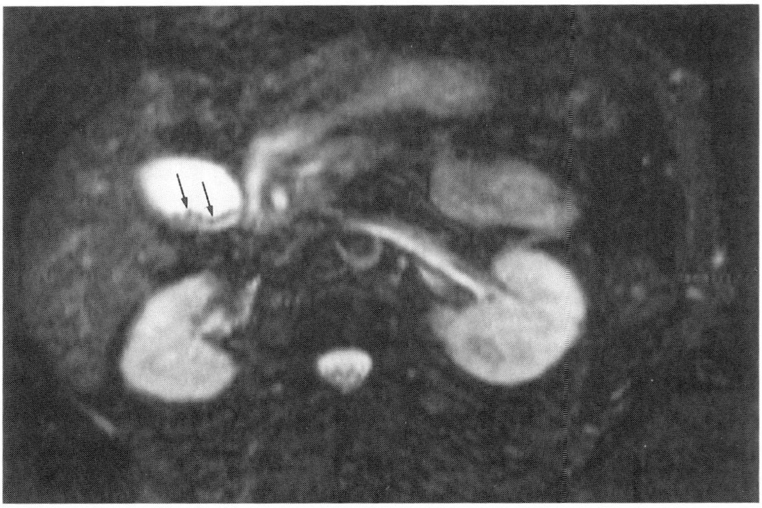

Figure 1. Gallstones. T2FS image. Multiple gallstones (arrows) are readily identified as signal-void filling defects in a background of bright bile.

have a high signal intensity, whereas solid organs and flowing blood have a low signal intensity. This combination of imaging characteristics results in high contrast between the high signal of bile and the low signal of background tissue on MRCP images. Sequences may be performed in a breath-hold period lasting from 1 to 20 sec. Half Fourier snapshot turbo spin echo (HASTE) is a thin-section single shot technique that appears to have considerable clinical utility because it is inherently independent of breathing, does not suffer substantially from magnetic susceptibility artifacts, and provides good resolution imaging of all the abdominal viscera.

Sequences useful for the demonstration of the gallbladder wall include T1-weighted fat suppressed images with and without gadolinium chelates (1). Gadolinium-enhanced T1-weighted fat-suppressed imaging is particularly well suited for the demonstration of abnormal ductal/periductal superficial spreading tissue as seen in ascending cholangitis and cholangiocarcinoma. Fat-suppressed images are better performed as breath-hold techniques such as fat-suppressed SGE because they avoid respiratory artifacts (2).

BENIGN DISEASES

Calculous Disease

Calculi are generally signal void on MR images because of lack of mobile protons. Occasionally they may contain sufficient water or lipid components to render them high in signal on T1-weighted SGE images. Calculi are well shown on MR images in which bile is high in signal (Figs. 1, 2). Breathing-independent MRCP sequences are particularly effective owing to high contrast between high-signal bile and low-signal calculi and lack of motion artifacts. Small calculi are routinely identified on

MR images, and MR exceeds CT in their detection owing to the inherent high contrast on bright biliary fluid techniques between low-signal calculi and high-signal bile.

Acute Cholecystitis

The high sensitivity of gadolinium-enhanced fat-suppressed images to inflammatory changes make this an optimal MR technique to assess patients in whom a diagnosis of acute cholecystitis is entertained, but findings of traditional imaging techniques such as sonography are equivocal (1). The gallbladder wall and adjacent tissues demonstrate increased enhancement on these images (Fig. 3), and the degree of enhancement has been shown to be more accurate than wall thickness measurements in the distinction of acute cholecystitis from other entities (3). The increased enhancement of the gallbladder wall may be accompanied by transient enhancement of the pericholecystic hepatic parenchyma on the immediate post-gadolinium SGE images, observed in 70% of patients with acute cholecystitis (Fig. 2) (3). Periportal high-signal intensity on T2-weighted images may be observed in the setting of acute cholecystitis. This is, however, a nonspecific appearance observed in a variety of biliary, liver, and pancreatic diseases (4).

In cases of acute hemorrhagic cholecystitis MRI can detect the presence of blood degradation products in the thickened gallbladder wall and help differentiate this condition from a gallbladder carcinoma (Fig. 4).

Chronic Cholecystitis

In chronic cholecystitis the gallbladder appears small and irregularly shaped, with a thickened, mildly enhanced wall on gadolinium-enhanced fat-suppressed images (Fig. 5). A distinguishing feature between acute and chronic cholecystitis on MR images is the degree of mural enhancement and enhancement of pericholecystic tissues. Late enhancement in cases of chronic cholecystitis may reflect the fibrotic changes of the gallbladder wall. The degree and extent of enhancement reflects the severity of the inflammatory process.

MALIGNANT DISEASES

Gallbladder Cancer

Gallbladder cancer is characterized on imaging studies by a mass filling or replacing the gallbladder or by a mass protruding into the gallbladder lumen (5, 6). Focal or diffuse thickening of the gallbladder wall >1 cm is highly suggestive of the diagnosis (Fig. 6) (5). Extension of tumor into liver is shown well on T2-weighted images and gadolinium-enhanced images, whereas extension into pancreas and adjacent tissue is shown well on T1-weighted fat-suppressed images prior to and following gadolinium administration. Associated biliary calculi are well shown on most imaging sequences (Fig. 7).

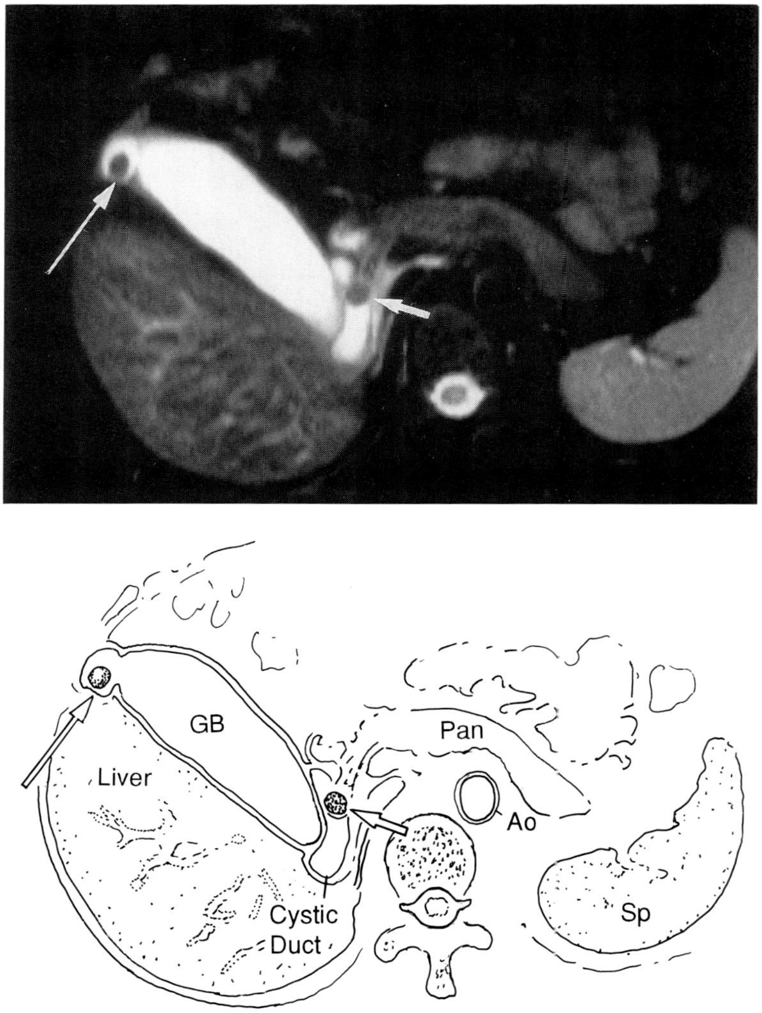

(A)

Figure 2 (Legend, next page).

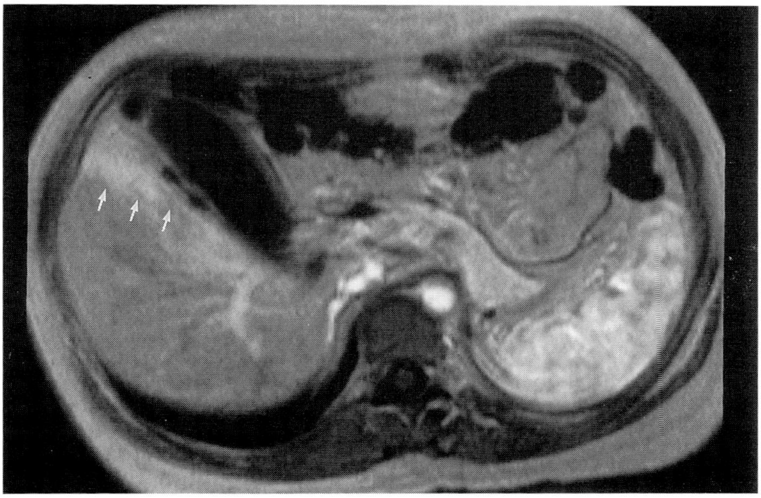

(B)

Figure 2. Cholelithiasis with acute cholecystitis. T2FS image and drawing (A), and immediate post-gadolinium SGE (B) images. The T2FS image shows a gallstone in the fundus of the gallbladder (long arrow, A, preceding page) as a rounded dark filling defect in a background of high-signal intensity bile. A second gallstone (short arrow, A, preceding page) is impacted in the cystic duct. The immediate post-gadolinium SGE image shows thickened gallbladder wall with mild enhancement. Pericholecystic fluid is identified as a dark zone immediately adjacent to the gallbladder wall. Transient increased enhancement of the liver parenchyma adjacent to the gallbladder is noted (arrows, B), which reflects hyperemic inflammatory changes due to the close proximity to the inflamed gallbladder wall.

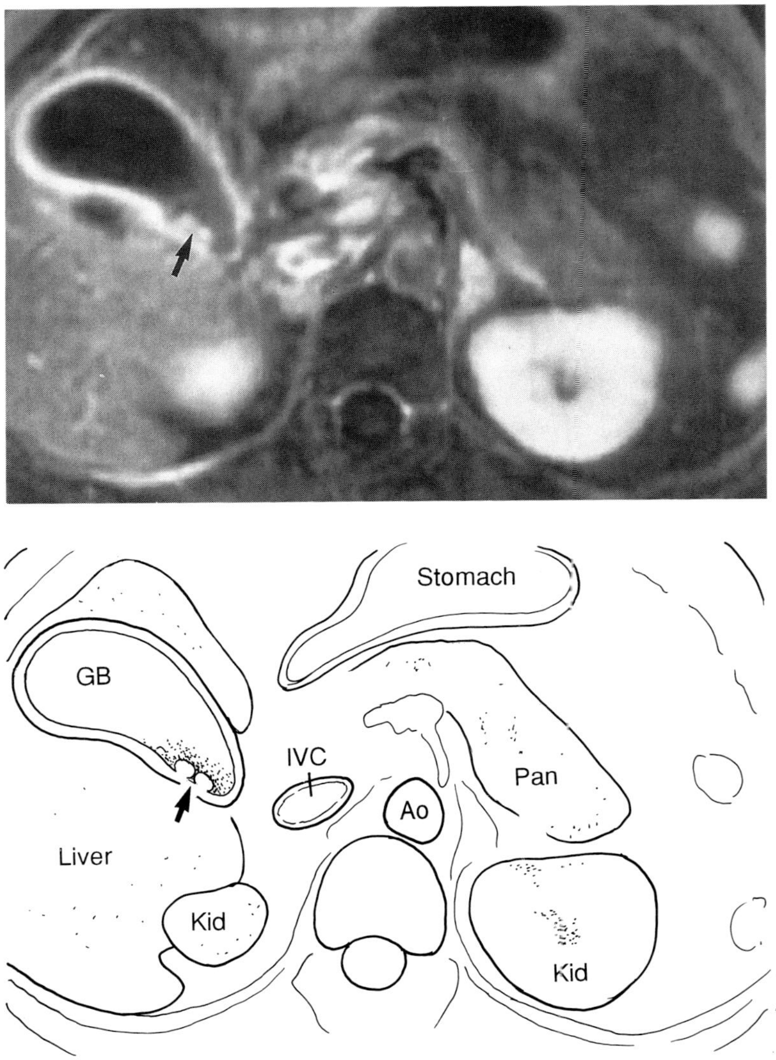

Figure 3. Acute cholecystitis. Post-gadolinium T1-weighted fat-suppressed spin echo image. The gallbladder wall is thickened (5 mm), and demonstrates substantial enhancement, a feature consistent with acute cholecystitis. Two small enhancing polyps are also depicted (arrow). Reproduced with permission from Reference 1.

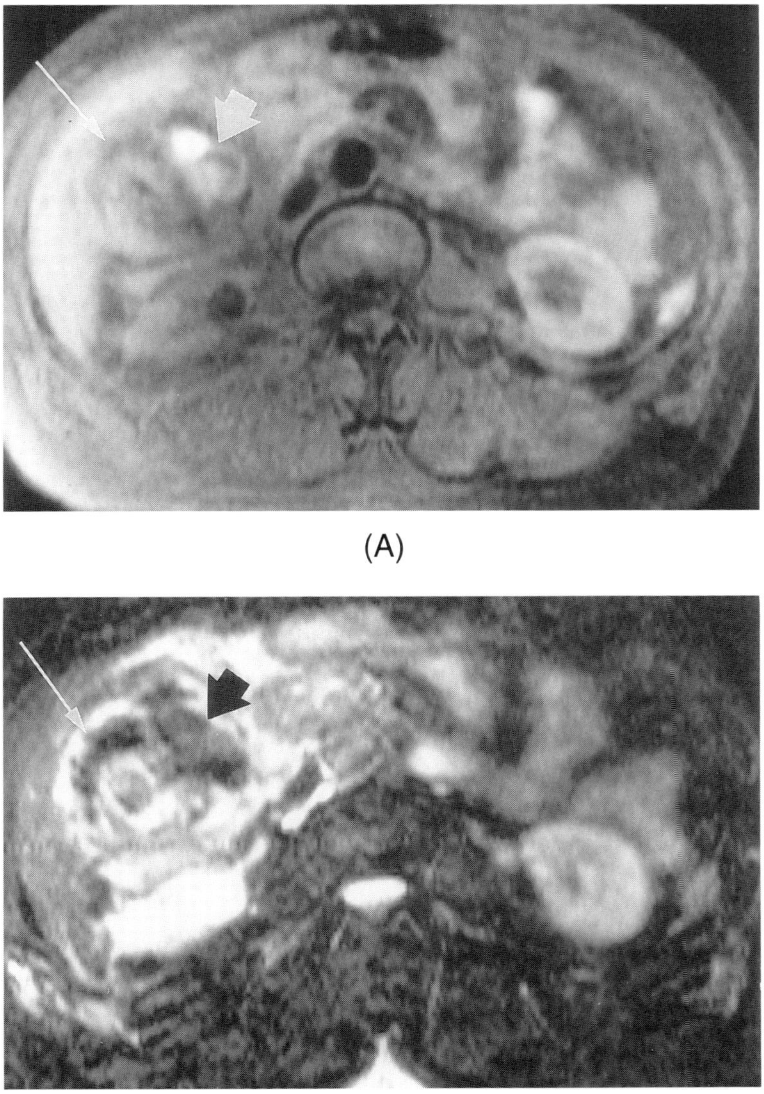

(A)

(B)

Figure 4. Hemorrhagic cholecystitis. Precontrast T1-weighted fat-suppressed spin echo (A) and T2FS (B) images. The gallbladder wall is thickened and is mixed low and high in signal intensity on both images (long arrows, A, B), reflecting the presence of blood products. The gallbladder contains a gallstone and pericholecystic fluid also contains blood products in different stages of degradation (large arrow, A, B).

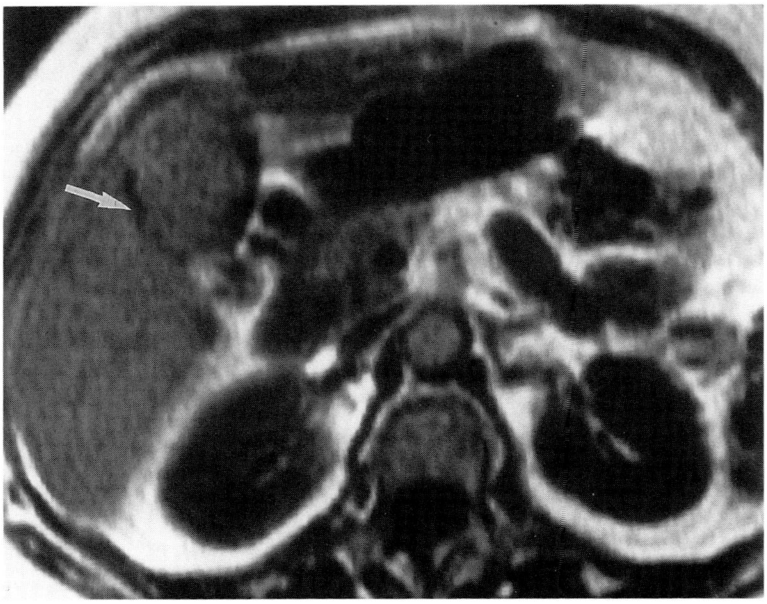

(A)

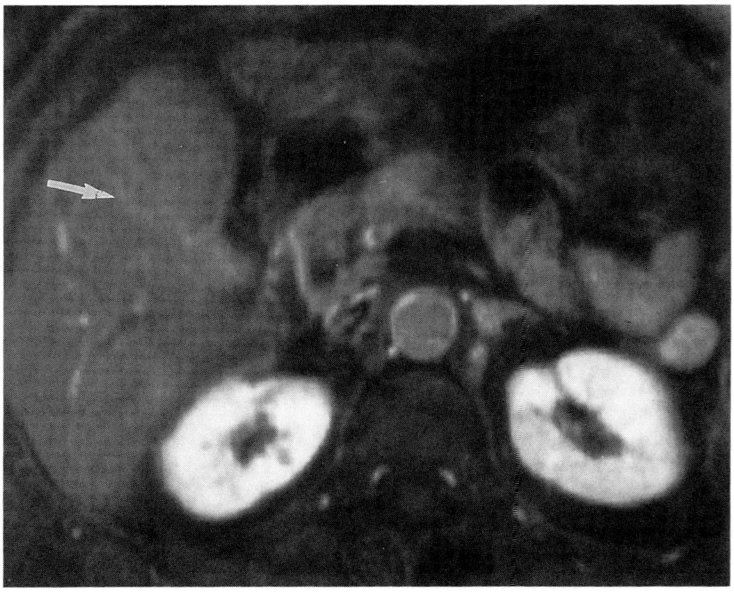

(B)

Figure 5. Chronic cholecystitis. Precontrast SGE (A) and post-gadolinium T1-weighted fat-suppressed spin echo (B) images. The gallbladder wall is thickened, is low in signal intensity on the precontrast SGE image (arrow, A), and demonstrates mild enhancement on the delayed post-gadolinium image (arrow, B), reflecting fibrotic changes. Reproduced with permission from Reference 1.

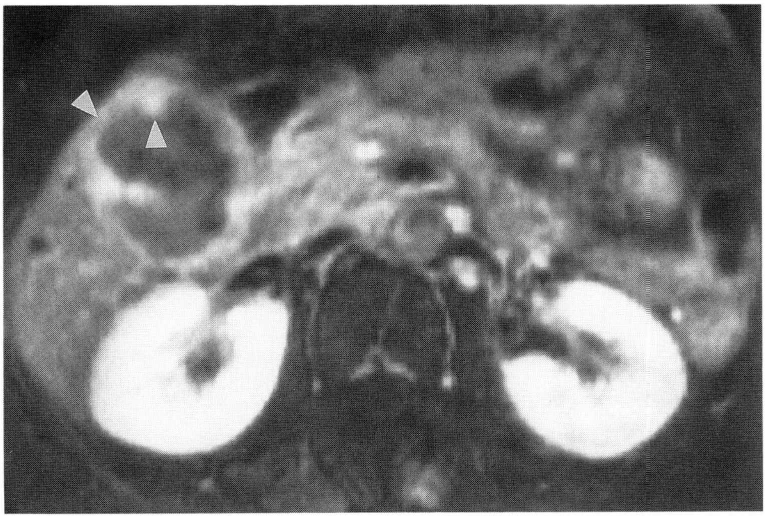

Figure 6. Carcinoma of the gallbladder. Post-gadolinium T1-weighted fat-suppressed spin echo image shows irregular nodular thickening of the gallbladder wall with moderate enhancement (arrowheads). Reproduced with permission from Reference 1.

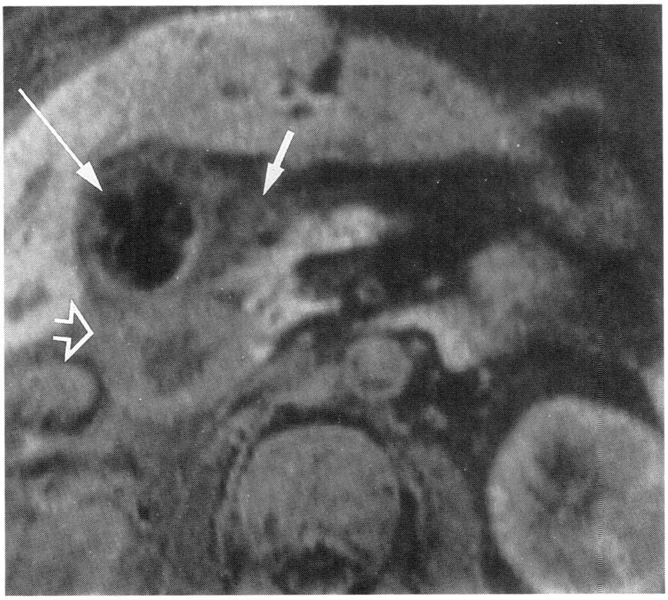

Figure 7. Gallbladder cancer. Precontrast T1-weighted fat-suppressed spin echo image. The gallbladder wall is substantially thickened and contains signal-void gallstones (long arrow). The presence of a scalloped margin of the high-signal pancreas confirms invasion by tumor (small arrow). The mass is invading the duodenum, which possesses a thick wall (open arrow). Reproduced with permission from Reference 1.

REFERENCES

1. Semelka RC, Shoenut JP, Mickflickier AB. The gallbladder and biliary tree. In: Semelka RC, Shoenut JP, eds. *MRI of the Abdomen with CT Correlation.* New York: Raven Press; 1993:43–52.
2. Low RN, Sigeti JS, Francis IR, et al. Evaluation of malignant biliary obstruction: efficacy of fast multiplanar spoiled gradient-recalled MR imaging vs spin-echo MR imaging, CT, and cholangiography. *AJR.* 1994;162:315–323.
3. Loud AP, Semelka RC, Kettritz U, Brown JJ, Reinhold C. MRI of acute cholecystitis: comparison with the normal gallbladder and other entities. *Magn Reson Imaging.* 1996;14:349–355.
4. Matsui O, Kadoya M, Takashima T, Kameyama T, Yoshikawa J, Tamura S. Intrahepatic periportal abnormal intensity on MR images: an indication of various hepatobiliary diseases. *Radiology.* 1989;171:335–338.
5. Rooholamini SA, Tehrani NS, Razavi MK, et al. Imaging of gallbladder carcinoma. *Radiographics* 1994;14:291–306.
6. Sagoh T, Itoh K, Togashi K, et al. Gallbladder carcinoma: evaluation with MR imaging. *Radiology* 1990;174:131–136.

5

ORAL CHOLECYSTOGRAPHY, ENDOSCOPIC RETROGRADE CHOLANGIO-PANCREATOGRAPHY, OTHER IMAGING TECHNIQUES

Mark D. Duncan, M.D.
Johns Hopkins Bayview Medical Center
Baltimore, Maryland

ORAL CHOLECYSTOGRAPHY

For half a century following its introduction by surgeons Graham, Cole, and Copher in 1924, oral cholecystography (OCG) provided the only avenue for radiographic imaging of the gallbladder (1). Relying on biliary physiology, this test provided functional as well as anatomic information in gallbladder disease. With the introduction of high-resolution real-time ultrasonography, biliary scintigraphy, computerized tomography, and more recently magnetic resonance imaging, OCG was relegated to a secondary if not antiquated status. The recent enthusiasm for nonsurgical management of calculous disease has seen a reemergence of OCG as perhaps a more accurate tool in selecting and following patients for either chemolitholysis or extracorporeal shock wave lithotripsy. Oral cholecystography has also proved useful in the diagnosis of chronic cholecystitis, in evaluating right upper quadrant symptoms in sonogram-negative patients, and in evaluating noncalculous disease of the gallbladder.

Technical Considerations

Iodine-containing compounds replaced phenolphthalein derivatives used in pioneering cholecystography to allow for oral administration (2). Agents in current use

Table 1. Nonopacification of the gallbladder following oral cholecystogram

Failure of Absorption
Poor patient compliance
Fasting
Gastrointestinal diverticula
Gastrointestinal obstruction
Malabsorption
Peritonitis
Pancreatitis
Crohn's disease
Cholestyramine therapy
Hepatocellular Dysfunction
Hepatitis
Cirrhosis
Obstructive jaundice
Biliary Obstruction
Gallbladder agenesis
Surgically absent gallbladder
Impacted common duct stone
Malignant obstruction
Cholecystitis
Acute cholecystitis
Chronic cholecystitis

Data adapted in part from Gore RM, Levine MS, Laufer I. *Textbook of Gastrointestinal Radiology.* Philadelphia: W. B. Saunders Company; 1994.

include iopanoic acid (Telepaque, Winthrop Pharmaceuticals, New York, NY), sodium tyropanoate (Bilopaque, Winthrop Pharmaceuticals, New York, NY), calcium ipodate (Oragrafin), and iocetamic acid (Cholebrine). The recommended dose of each is 3 g. After oral ingestion, the cholecystographic agent is absorbed in the ileum, from which it is transported to the liver via lymphatics and the portal venous system. Once in the liver, it is conjugated to glucuronide by the hepatocyte and then excreted into the bile. In the presence of a patent ductal system and normally functioning gallbladder, the contrast is taken up in the gallbladder and concentrated. Interruption at any point in this pathway may lead to poor or no opacification of the gallbladder (Table 1). Mechanical problems such as bowel obstruction and diverticula or functional malabsorption as in pancreatitis may prohibit absorption of the cholecystographic agent. Fasting or impaired bile salts prohibit absorption in the intestine. Hepatic dysfunction can prevent glucuronide conjugation. A patent cystic duct and proximal biliary tree are of course required for gallbladder visualization. The contrast agent will not be concentrated if the gallbladder fails to reabsorb water. The reabsorptive capacity of the gallbladder also permits reabsorption of the iodinated contrast, although seldom to a degree that would prohibit visualization.

Iopanoic acid (Telepaque) is most commonly used; it is lipid soluble and thus requires the presence of bile salts in the small bowel to facilitate absorption. Its biliary peak concentration is reached 14–17 hr following ingestion, and radiographic examination is scheduled for the morning following evening administration of a 3-g dose. The other agents are more water soluble and have a shorter time to opacification. Sodium tyropanoate (or ipodate) may be more appropriate for patients unable to eat or with disruption of the enterohepatic circulation. Its peak concentration is 10 hr after administration and it is taken at bedtime prior to morning radiography. Ipodate may be used for same-day studies or on inpatients with gallbladder visualization beginning as early as 5 hr. The gallbladder is visualized in 75% of patients following a single oral dose. In the remaining 25%, a second dose of 3 g is administered and the radiographs are repeated the following day. Two-thirds of these patients demonstrate gallbladder filling on this second dose, often termed the double dose method. Provided the remaining patients lack the nonbiliary causes of failure to visualize listed above and in Table 1, they can be conclusively stated to have gallbladder disease. Nonopacification of the gallbladder with absorbed and excreted contrast material in the bowel implies impaired gallbladder water absorption or contrast diffusion through an inflamed gallbladder wall, diagnostic of cholecystitis.

On the day of examination, a preliminary kidney, ureter, bladder roentgenographic series is obtained. Multiple views, including upright, supine, and oblique views, are important to evaluate the full anatomy of the gallbladder by opacifying fundus, Hartmann's pouch, and a Phrygian cap if present, as well as to assess the motility of any intraluminal filling defects (Figs. 1, 2). The upright view may demonstrate buoyancy of stones. The supine view importantly provides less magnification with shorter table to gallbladder distance, and further delineates the infundibulum and neck. Multiple views further allow distinction of multiple stones for more accurate assessment of number and size. A 70-kV peak is typically used with 100-mm photospot exposures, with adjustments for patient size and physique.

Side effects of OCG are diarrhea, dysuria, nausea, and vomiting. Oral cholecystography is relatively contraindicated in patients with gout owing to the uricosuric effect of the contrast agents, and in patients with reactions to iodine. In rare situations, rectal administration of the cholegraphic agent may be considered. Oral cholecystographic agents may also be used in conjunction with other imaging modalities such as spiral computerized tomography.

Cholecystokinin Stimulation and Fatty Meal Stimulation

Gallbladder contraction may be stimulated following a fatty meal or administration of cholecystokinin (CCK) (Fig. 3). Not all centers routinely perform stimulation studies. In CCK stimulation, cholecystokinin (Sincalide, Squibb Diagnostic, Princeton, NJ), 0.02 μg/kg, is given intravenously over 30 min. Side effects include nausea, vomiting, and abdominal discomfort. The fatty meal may be a commercial preparation (Neocholex, Lafayette Pharmaceuticals, Lafayette, IN) or a standard liquid or solid preparation. Stimulation by CCK or a fatty meal may allow opacification of the hepatic ducts and common bile duct, which may not be seen on routine OCG. Stones in the neck of the gallbladder that are missed by conventional OCG

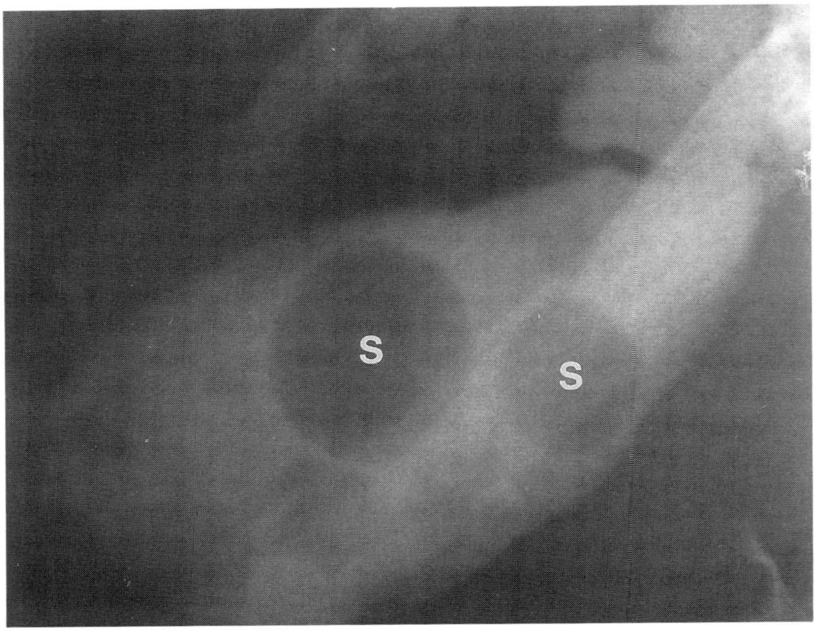

Figure 1. Opacification of the gallbladder on OCG demonstrating several large stones (S). (Copyright Robert Zeman, M.D.; used by permission.)

may be discerned following stimulation. Although concentration of contrast and contraction of the gallbladder are evident following stimulation by either method, OCG is unreliable for evaluating gallbladder ejection fraction, which is best left to scintigraphy. The significance of lack of contraction in an opacified gallbladder is uncertain. Finally, stimulation with gallbladder contraction forces contrast into the common bile duct. Demonstration of a patent, nondilated common duct prior to laparoscopic cholecystectomy may obviate consideration of or need for cholangiography or endoscopic retrograde cholangiopancreatography (ERCP).

Utilization in Calculous Disease and Acute Cholecystitis

Sonography and biliary scintigraphy are unarguably the mainstays of imaging in calculous disease and acute cholecystitis (3). Some stones, however, are missed on ultrasound. Oral cholecystography remains a good study for demonstrating gallbladder calculi (Figs. 1, 2, 4). Obtaining an OCG on patients with suspected calculous disease with normal or equivocal sonographic findings is prudent (4, 5).

Utilization in Chronic Cholecystitis

The oral cholecystogram can be a useful tool in evaluating chronic cholecystitis. Although sonography is routinely performed and generally supported in the literature, reports of specificity based on pathological criteria of chronic cholecystitis must be viewed with suspicion because few true-negative results exist. Surgically

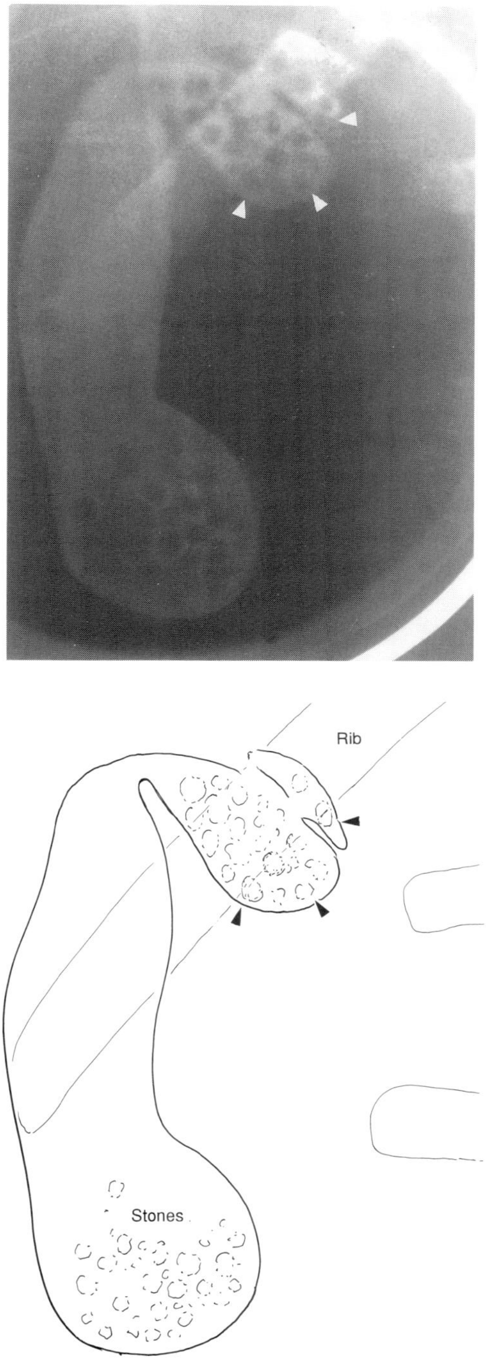

Figure 2. OCG demonstrating the Phrygian cap (arrowheads), with delineation of multiple calculi (copyright Robert Zeman, M.D.; used by permission). Phrygian cap connotes resemblance to the headgear traditionally worn in Phrygia, central Asia minor (now Turkey); it is due to accentuation of the normal second fold near the neck of the gallbladder.

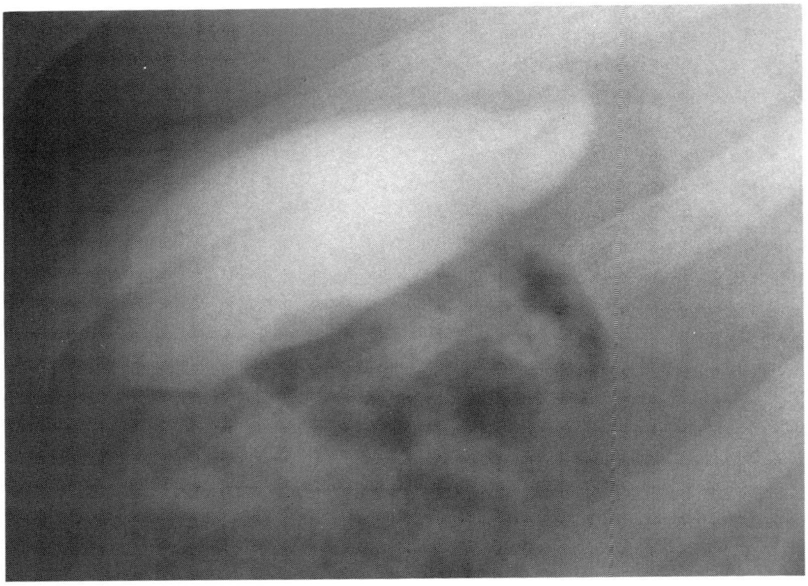

(A)

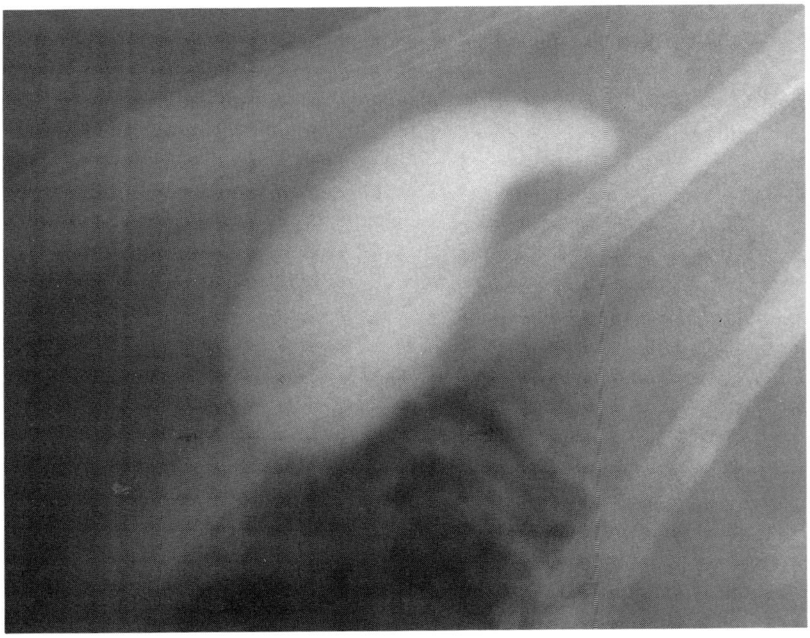

(B)

Figure 3. Normal OCG (A) pre- and (B) post-fatty meal stimulation. (Copyright Robert Zeman, M.D.; used by permission.)

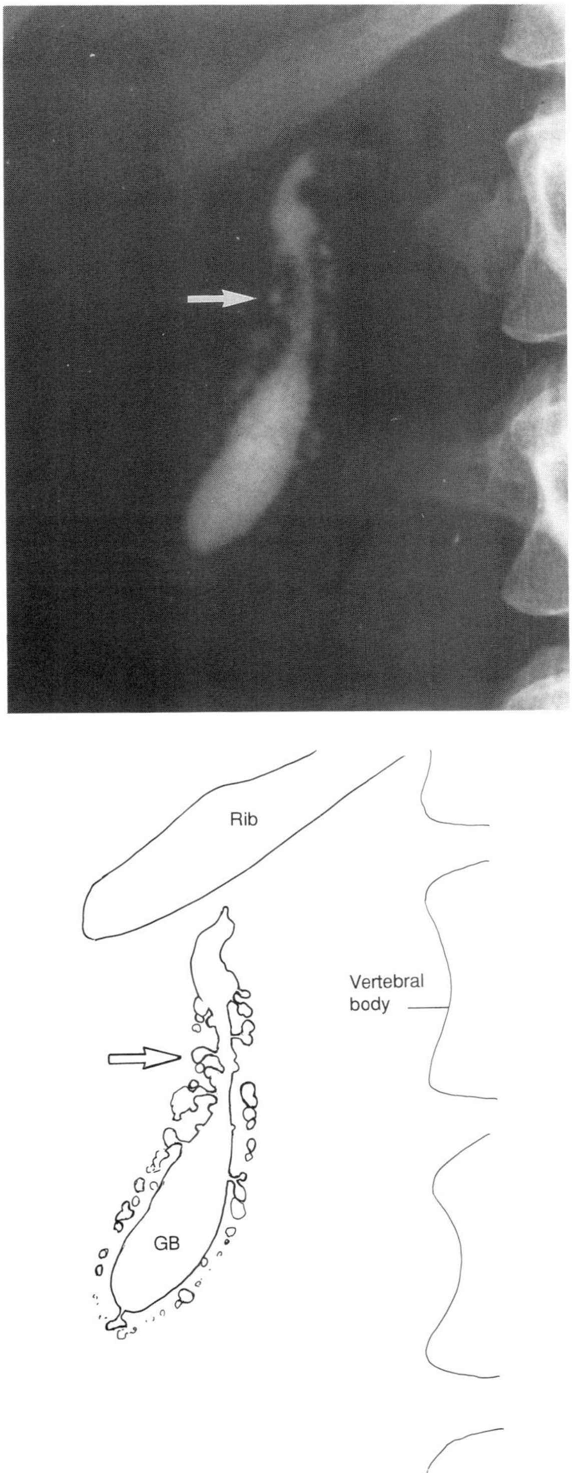

Figure 4. Rokitansky–Aschoff sinuses (arrow) in a case of adenomyomatosis of the gallbladder. (Copyright Robert Zeman, M.D.; used by permission.)

excised gallbladders are rarely called normal; only 0.5% of gallbladders from a combined series of 384 were called normal (6). The diagnosis of chronic cholecystitis pathologically is far from rigid. In a retrospective review utilizing patient outcome data to answer the question of superiority of ultrasound versus OCG, the two techniques were comparable in evaluating chronic cholecystitis. Oral cholecystography was 83% sensitive and 97% specific; ultrasound was 86% sensitive and 90% specific (6). This study excluded patients with acute cholecystitis, in whom it is generally agreed that ultrasound should be performed and OCG would be inappropriate. Several authors recently have reappraised OCG and ultrasound in evaluating cholecystitis in both prospective and retrospective studies (5–8). Although few, if any, would recommend returning to cholecystography as the primary imaging modality, the data support the accuracy of OCG when appropriately performed and interpreted. The use of OCG is highly appropriate in evaluating sonogram-negative or equivalent patients with right upper quadrant or biliary type symptoms (4, 5). Similarly, OCG should be used in such patients for whom other studies, including hepatic iminodiacetic acid or computed tomography (CT) scan are nonrevealing. Oral cholecystography can additionally aid in the related but somewhat ambiguous diagnosis of gallbladder dysmotility (9, 10).

Utilization in Noncalculous Disease

Noncalculous disease of the gallbladder is well visualized by OCG. Hypertrophy, polyps, and tumors are delineated by contrast. Adenomyomatosis of the gallbladder, characterized by mucosal and muscular hypertrophy of the gallbladder wall of unknown etiology, may be focal or diffuse. Cholecystography is the best method to image adenomyomatosis. Opacification of Rokitansky–Aschoff sinuses during gallbladder contraction is pathognomonic of diffuse adenomyomatosis (Fig. 4). Stimulation with a fatty meal or CCK contracts the gallbladder and emphasizes the Rokitansky–Aschoff sinuses; this is also helpful when mass effect narrows the lumen. Cholesterolosis refers to subepithelial accumulation of cholesterol-laden histiocytes and may form polyps up to 1 cm in size. Adenomatous polyps may also occur. Gallbladder carcinoma, the fifth most common gastrointestinal malignancy, is rarely diagnosed at a curative stage (11). Oral cholecystography should be considered to rule out carcinoma in any mass lesion of the gallbladder, particularly in patients with apparently sessile lesions by ultrasound. Although OCG does not replace CT scanning, the latter is less accurate than commonly appreciated for gallbladder carcinoma, only 57% sensitive in one study (12), and provides even less information on the smaller (potentially surgically curable) lesions that may be outlined by OCG. Gallstones are found in 70–90% of patients with gallbladder carcinoma; conversely, only approximately 1% of patients with gallstones develop carcinoma (13). Anatomic variations including duplication of the gallbladder may be appreciated by OCG. Even more rare, agenesis of the gallbladder is difficult to diagnose preoperatively (14). Recognition of the common and uncommon noncalculous conditions is critical to avoiding pitfalls in surgical management.

Oral Cholecystography in Conjunction with Nonsurgical Therapy

Perhaps the greatest resurgence of oral cholecystography is in conjunction with nonsurgical therapy. Although laparoscopic cholecystectomy is the treatment of

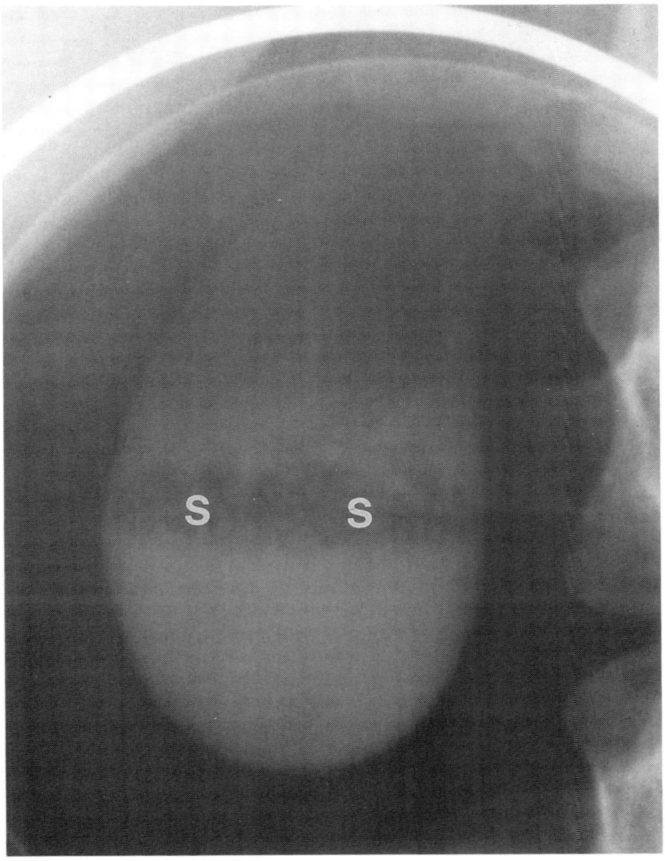

Figure 5. Buoyancy of cholesterol stones (S) on OCG in the upright position. (Copyright Robert Zeman, M.D.; used by permission.)

choice for symptomatic gallstones, a selected minority of patients either are not surgical candidates or opt against surgery. Oral cholecystography permits sizing and counting stones prior to attempts at nonoperative management of stones (1) following oral bile acid therapy, (2) following chemotherapy with methyl tert-butyl ether (MTBE) or ursodiol infusion, and (3) following extracorporeal shock wave lithotripsy (ESWL) procedures. Visualization of the gallbladder demonstrating a patent cystic duct is a standard prerequisite for therapy. Patient selection is important in nonsurgical management of gallbladder calculi. Both chemolytic and lithotripsy therapy are more effective in patients with a small stone burden defined by number and size of stones. The Munich criteria were devised as selection criteria for biliary lithotripsy protocols, but may be applied to chemolitholytic therapy. These criteria require either a single stone 30 mm or less, or up to three stones with the same aggregate volume as the single larger stone. In post-treatment follow-up, determination of fragment number and of size are equally important in assessing the need for retreatment or further therapy. To generalize from the many studies

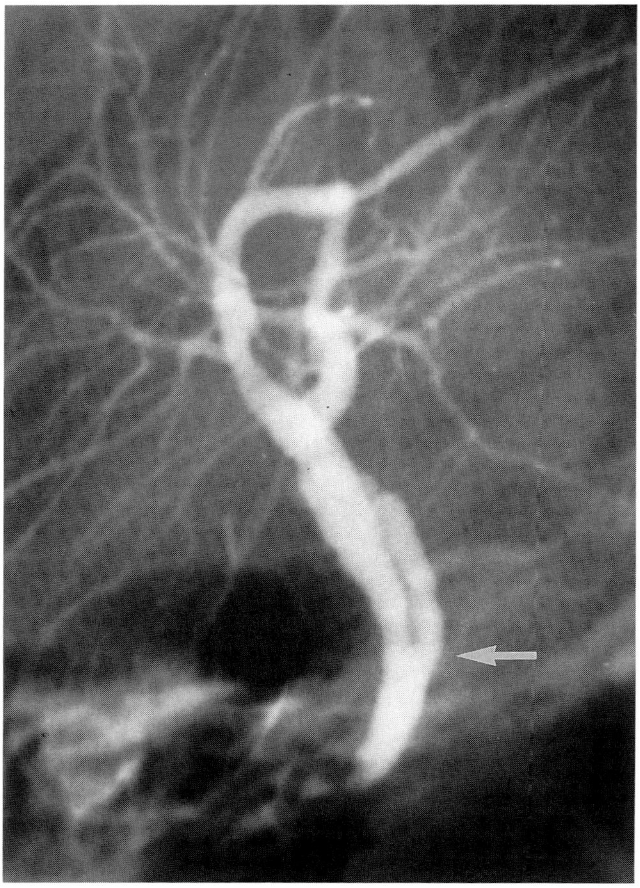

Figure 6. Cystic duct with low takeoff (arrow) from the common bile duct visualized by ERCP. (Copyright Robert Zeman, M.D., used by permission.)

comparing OCG and ultrasound for their contributions to nonoperative management of gallstones, ultrasound appears to be more sensitive (fewer false negatives) than OCG. Ultrasound, however, is limited in accurately counting and sizing stones, because stones are often contiguous or overlapping, which hampers quantification (15–20). Oral cholecystography may be better than ultrasound for both screening and determining size and number of fragments following ESWL for gallstones; a discrepancy among three radiologists concerning whether a patient was eligible for retreatment in 15% of OCG studies versus 45% of ultrasound studies has been reported (16). Others dispute the advantage of OCG in this regard (17, 18). Oral cholecystography, however, has the important advantage prior to initiating therapy of demonstrating patency of cystic duct, which is prerequisite to success with either chemolitholysis (to provide access) or lithotripsy (to provide egress). Future nonoperative trials may utilize both OCG and ultrasound. Of note, no chemolytic agents are effective on calcium. Thus the demonstration of floating stones (Fig. 5), which are

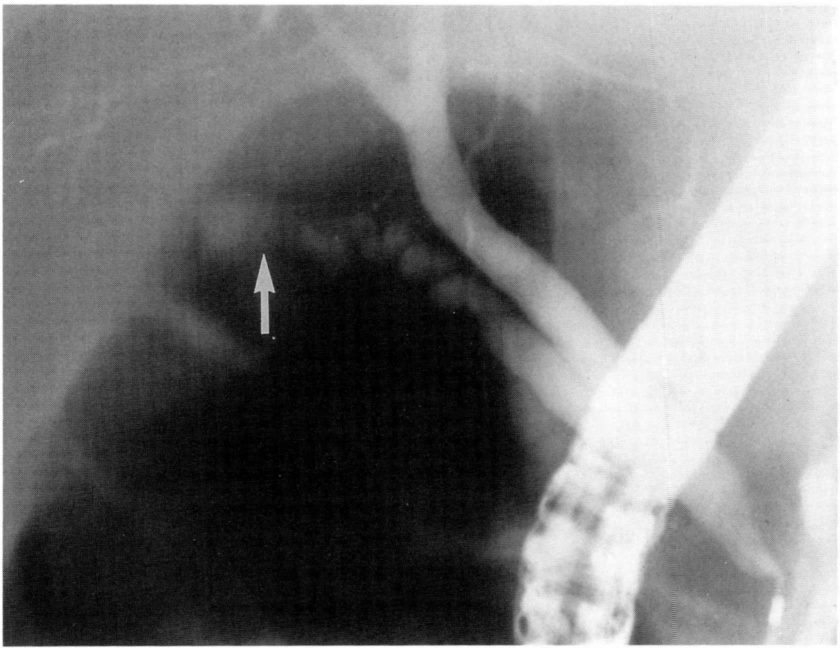

Figure 7. Gallbladder carcinoma with irregular termination of cystic duct (arrow) on ERCP.

cholesterol stones with a significantly lower calcium salt content (21), has therapeutic implications. The buoyant stones have higher cholesterol content and are more amenable to dissolution therapy with ursodiol (21–24). OCG is better able to demonstrate buoyancy, perhaps due to the increased specific gravity of bile produced by the cholecystographic agent.

Cholecystography will also be utilized more in the future for its ability to demonstrate gallbladder function following any of the nonsurgical gallbladder therapies. Meal-stimulated oral cholecystography has been used to assess gallbladder function following percutaneous endoscopic polypectomy (25). Abnormal gallbladder visualization following biliary lithotripsy often indicates need for cholecystectomy (26).

ENDOSCOPIC RETROGRADE CHOLANGIOPANCREATOGRAPHY

Endoscopic retrograde cholangiopancreatography is primarily utilized for demonstration of biliary ductal pathology, and remains the superior method in this regard.

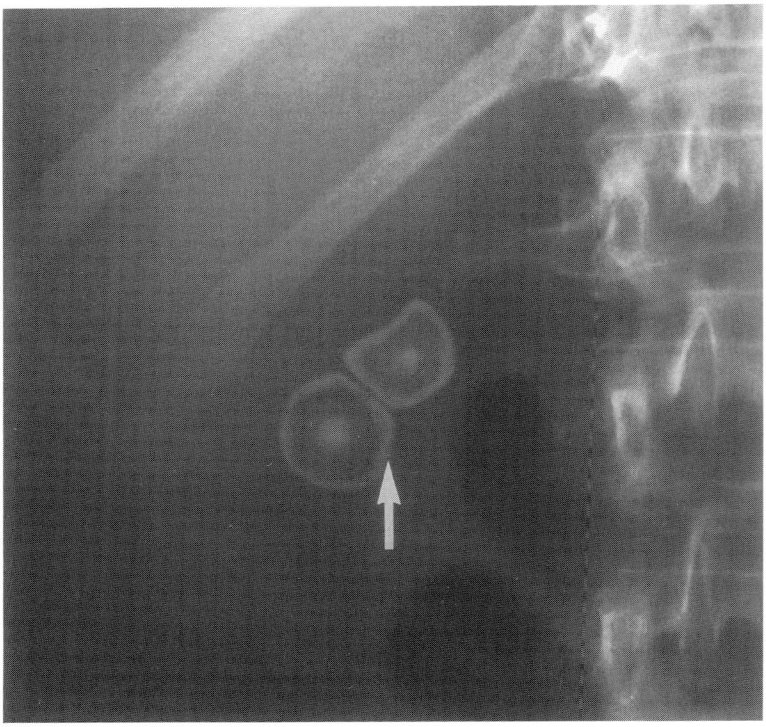

Figure 8. Calcification of gallstones (arrow) seen in the right upper quadrant on plain abdominal radiograph. (Copyright Robert Zeman, M.D.; used by permission.)

The technique for ERCP is described in Chapter 13. When the cystic duct is patent and allows contrast filling of the gallbladder, ERCP can provide useful information on gallbladder disease and potential therapy. Gallbladder calculous disease may be accessed retrograde via the patent cystic duct. If the cystic duct is dilated, a basket can be passed into the gallbladder for stone extraction. Similarly, ERCP may be utilized to retrieve stones for crystal analysis. Torsion of the gallbladder, agenesis, and congenital duplication can be demonstrated by ERCP as well as by OCG (27). Appreciation of a short cystic duct or low takeoff from the common bile duct can be critically important in surgical resection if demonstrated by ERCP (Fig. 6). Endoscopic retrograde cholangiopancreatography demonstrates gallbladder carcinoma in 76% of cases (12) (Fig. 7), and may help in planning operative therapy. In the same study, CT scan was reported as only 57% sensitive, and ultrasound 68% sensitive.

OTHER IMAGING TECHNIQUES

Diagnostic Cholecystography/Percutaneous Transhepatic Cholangiography

Diagnostic cholecystography with sonographic guidance and fluoroscopic control for transhepatic injection directly into the gallbladder may be utilized to provide

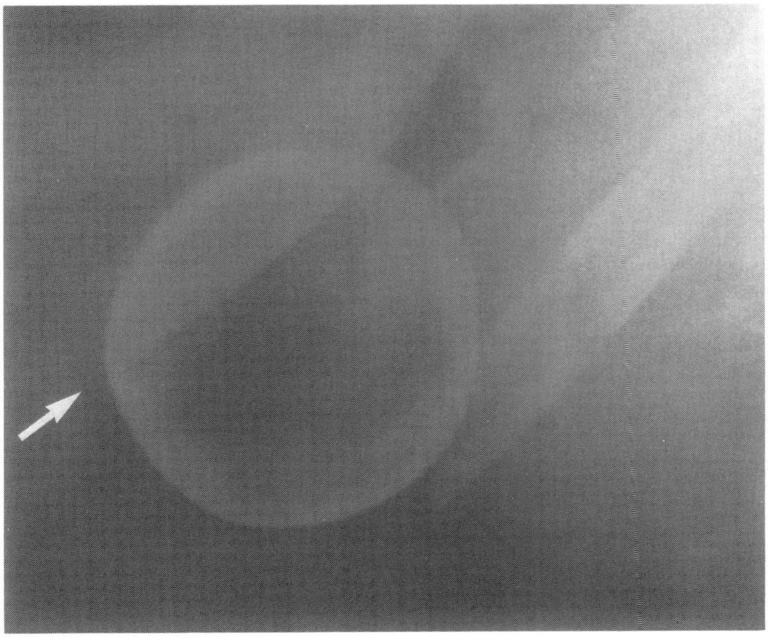

Figure 9. Porcelain gallbladder (arrow) on plain abdominal radiograph. (Copyright Robert Zeman, M.D.; used by permission.)

direct imaging when the gallbladder is inaccessible by conventional means. The technique is comparable to that of percutaneous transhepatic cholangiography elaborated in Chapter 12. The gallbladder is usually well opacified if not obstructed. Intravenous cholangiography may also be performed.

Abdominal Radiography

Diagnostic information on the gallbladder may also be fortuitously obtained from conventional radiographs of the abdomen or right upper quadrant. Abdominal radiographs (flat plate: kidney, ureter, bladder) allow direct visualization of radiolucent stones (approximately 10–15% of gallstones), owing to sufficient calcium carbonate and calcium phosphate (Fig. 8). Calcification of the gallbladder (porcelain gallbladder) can also be demonstrated (Fig. 9). The presence of a porcelain gallbladder almost universally indicates calculous disease, imparts a 10–25% risk of malignancy, and is an indication for cholecystectomy (13). Other rare but clinically useful findings include hydrops of the gallbladder; emphysematous cholecystitis, indicative of gangrene and impending perforation; the Mercedes-Benz sign (Fig. 10), caused by nitrogen gas-containing fissures resulting from cholesterol crystal shrinkage within gallstones; and demonstration of limy bile syndrome, also termed milk of calcium bile (20). This last condition is caused by calcium carbonate precipitation in bile yielding a radiopaque gallbladder or bile ducts visible on plain roentgenogram.

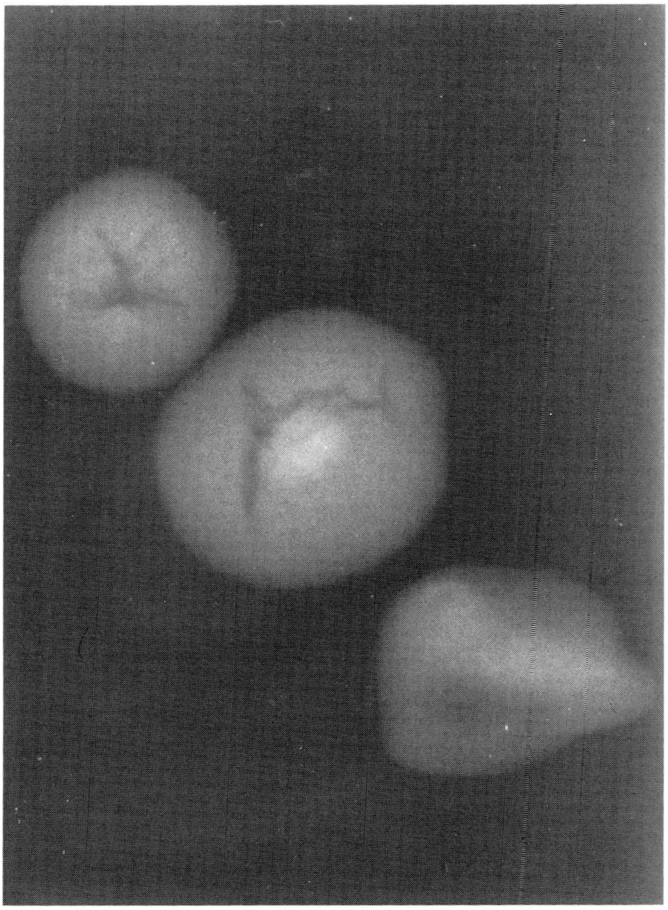

Figure 10. Mercedes–Benz sign with triradiate gas shadow of nitrogen within fissure of cholesterol crystal stone visualized on specimen radiograph. (Copyright Robert Zeman, M.D.; used by permission.)

Limy bile syndrome may be a complication of long-term total parenteral nutrition and implies a chronically obstructed gallbladder (13, 28).

In summary, the oral cholecystogram remains an important study in gallbladder imaging. In a recent review of 205 patients including both calculous and noncalculous disease, OCG diagnosed 87% of pathologically confirmed disease (7). Equivocal sonographic findings or right upper quadrant symptoms in sonogram-negative patients warrant consideration of OCG. Diagnosis of chronic cholecystitis may be based on OCG nonvisualization. Noncalculous disease is often best imaged by OCG. Nonsurgical therapies utilize OCG to quantify stone burden and to follow treatment. Endoscopic retrograde cholangiopancreatography and percutaneous cholecystography are similarly adjuncts for gallbladder imaging in specific cases. Abdominal radiographs as well may demonstrate gallbladder pathology. In imaging potential surgical patients, these techniques complement standard sonographic imaging and scintigraphy.

REFERENCES

1. Graham EA, Cole WH, Copher GH. Visualization of the gallbladder by the sodium salt of tetrabromophthalein. *JAMA*. 1924;82:1777.
2. Feld R, Kurtz AB, Zeman RK. Imaging the gallbladder: a historical perspective. *AJR*. 1991;156:737–740.
3. Shea JA, Berlin JA, Escarce JJ, Clarke JR, Kinosian BP, Cabana MD, Tsai WW, Horangic N, Malet PF, Schwartz JS, Williams SV. Revised estimates of diagnostic test sensitivity and specificity in suspected biliary tract disease. *Arch Intern Med*. 1994;154: 2573–2581.
4. Zeman RK, Burrell MI. Biliary imaging techniques. In: Zeman RK, Burrell MI, eds. *Gallbladder and Bile Duct Imaging: A Clinical Radiological Approach*. New York: Churchill Livingstone; 1987:47–104.
5. Amberg JR, Leopold GR. Is oral cholecystography still useful? *AJR*. 1988;151:73–74.
6. Renfrew DL, Witte DL, Berbaum KS, Barloon TJ. Comparison of oral cholecystography and ultrasonography for evaluating chronic cholecystitis using patient outcome as the reference standard. *Invest Radiol*. 1993;28:404–408.
7. Gelfand DW, Wolfman NT, Ott DJ, Watson NE, Chen YM, Dale WJ. Oral cholecystography versus gallbladder sonography: a prospective, blinded reappraisal. *AJR*. 1988;151:69–72.
8. Evens RG. The value of oral cholecystography. Letter. *AJR*. 1988;151:1251.
9. Brugge WR. Motor function of the gallbladder: measurement and clinical significance. *Semin Roentgenol*. 1991;26:226–231.
10. DaSilva AL, DaSilva RG. Delayed (modified) oral cholecystography in the study of biliary dyskinesia. *Arq Gastroenterol*. 1994;31:87–91.
11. Jones RS. Carcinoma of the gallbladder. *Surg Clin North Am*. 1990;70:1419–1428.
12. Oikarin H, Päivänsalo M, Lähde S, Tikkakoski T, Suramo I. Radiological findings in cases of gallbladder carcinoma. *Eur J Radiol*. 1993;17:179–183.
13. Lichtenstein JE. The gallbladder: what if it's not stone disease? *Semin Roentgenol*. 1991;26:209–215.
14. Donnelly PK. Non-functioning or non-existent gallbladder? *Br J Clin Pract* 1990; 44:416–417.
15. Torres WE, Baumgartner BR, Jones MT, Steinberg HV, Peterson JE. Comparison of ultrasonography and oral cholecystography in biliary lithotripsy. I. Screening patients. *Invest Radiol*. 1991;26:633–635.
16. Baumgartner BR, Jones MT, Torres WE, Nelson RC, Peterson JE. Comparison of ultrasonography and oral cholecystography in lithotripsy. II. Determining retreatment. *Invest Radiol*. 1991;26:636–639.
17. Brakel K, Lameris JS, Nijs HGT, Ginai AZ, Terpstra OT. The value of ultrasound in predicting non-visualization of the gall-bladder on OCG: implications for imaging strategies in patient selection for non-surgical therapy of gallstones. *Clin Radiol*. 1991;43:186–189.
18. Brakel K, Lameris JS, Nijs HGT, Ginai AZ, Terpstra OT. Accuracy of ultrasound and oral cholecystography in assessing the number and size of gallstones: implications for non-surgical therapy. *Br J Radiol*. 1992;65:779–783.
19. Maglinte DTT, Torres WE, Laufer I. Oral cholecystography in contemporary gallstone imaging: a review. *Radiology*. 1991;178:49–58.
20. Turner MA. Diagnostic methods and pitfalls in the gallbladder. *Semin Roentgenol*. 1991;26:197–208.

21. Malet PF, Baker J, Kahn MJ, Soloway RD. Gallstone composition in relation to buoyancy at oral cholecystography. *Radiology.* 1990;177:167–169.
22. Ros E, Valderrama R, Bru C, Bianchi L, Teres J. Symptomatic versus silent gallstones. Radiographic features and eligibility for nonsurgical treatment. *Dig Dis Sci.* 1994; 39:1697–1703.
23. Schoenfield LJ, Marks JW. Oral and contact dissolution of gallstones. *Am J Surg.* 1993;165:427–430.
24. Lanzini A, Northfield TC. Pharmacologic treatment of gallstones (practical guidelines). *Drugs.* 1994;47:458–470.
25. Ji ZL, Chen HR, Wang EH, Yang DT, Gao NR, Yang JZ, Liu BY. Percutaneous endoscopic polypectomy of gallbladder polyps. *Endoscopy.* 1994;26:609–612.
26. Torres WE, Baumgartner BR, Casarella WJ. Abnormalities of the gallbladder after extracorporeal shock-wave lithotripsy: imaging findings. *AJR.* 1992;159:325–327.
27. Desai HP, Gold BM, Burakoff R. Intermittent positional torsion of the gallbladder demonstrated on ERCP. *Gastrointest Endosc.* 1993;39:572–573.
28. Fowler CL, Soriano J, Ferry GD, Margraf LR, Harberg FJ. Limy bile syndrome. *J Pediatr Surg.* 1993;28:1568–1569.

6

SURGICAL SUMMARY: GALLBLADDER DISEASE

David C. Brooks, M.D.
Harvard Medical School
Boston, Massachusetts

Gallbladder disease is the most common elective intra-abdominal disease encountered by the general surgeon (Fig. 1). Cholecystectomy has been the mainstay of therapy for this disease since the 1880s when the first cholecystectomy was performed by Langenbach (1). Today, well over 500,000 cholecystectomies are performed yearly in the United States (2), making it the most common elective gastrointestinal operation performed in the country. The diagnosis of symptomatic cholelithiasis is generally straightforward. Certainly the diagnosis of cholelithiasis is straightforward. More difficult is determining which of those patients with demonstrated gallstones require surgical intervention. That decision has changed in the half century since World War II. In the past, surgery was recommended for all patients with stones. Currently, however, cholecystectomy is not recommended for patients with asymptomatic gallstones, except in unusual situations, because it has been well documented that less than 50% of all patients with gallstones will eventually develop symptoms.

DEMOGRAPHICS

Gallstones continue to be found predominantly in females, with a ratio of approximately 4:1. As the population ages, the incidence of gallstones rises in the male and may be equivalent to that of women in the elderly. Certain ethnic groups (some North American natives, Northern European populations, for example) have a significantly higher incidence than the norm. A family history may therefore have significant impact on the subsequent development of gallstones. Because the sex hormones are implicated in gallstone disease, both for the tendency to increase

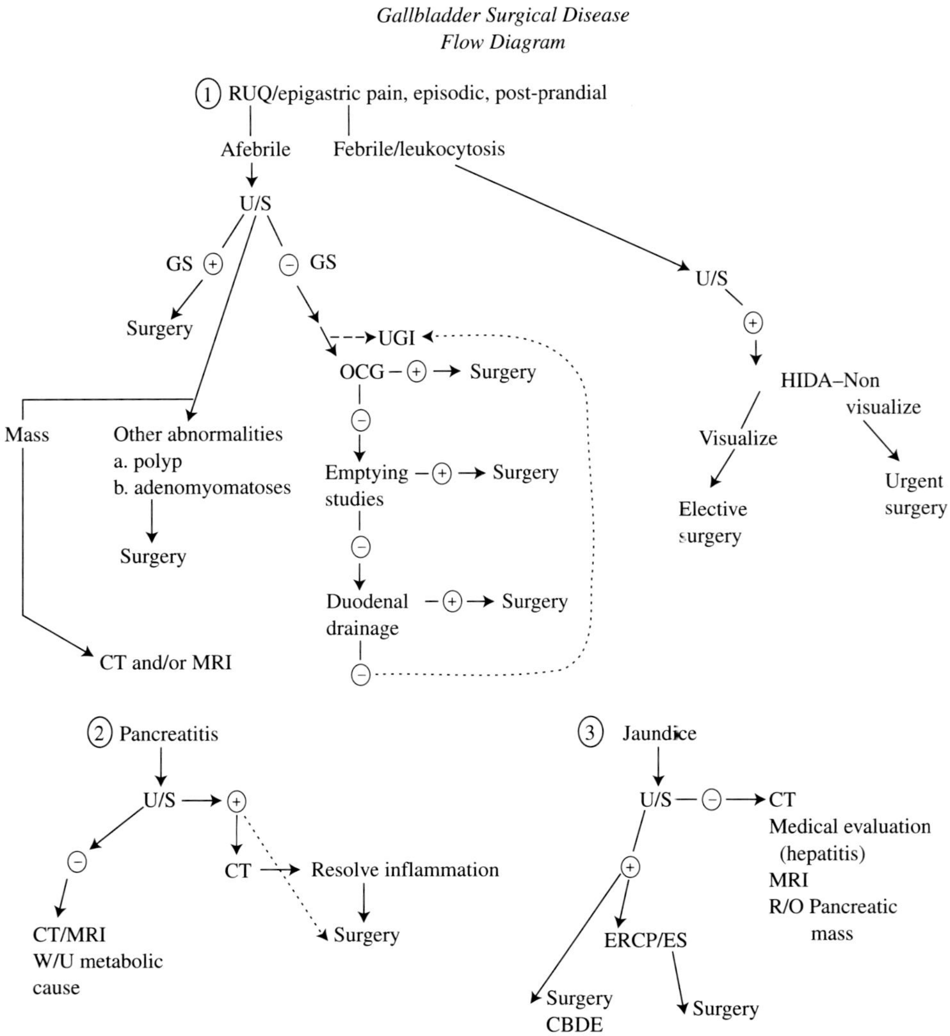

Figure 1. Overview of a surgical approach to gallbladder disease. GS: Gallstone, CBDE: common bileduct; ES: Endoscopic sphincterotomy.

cholesterol levels in bile and for their inhibitory effect on smooth muscle, the disease is naturally more common in women during their childbearing years.

The role of cholesterol saturation in the bile is well-documented. Additionally, motility changes within the gallbladder also have importance in the development of gallstones (3). Finally, nucleating events within the gallbladder may predispose to stones via the promotion of micellar formation (4).

GENERAL HISTORY

Surgical management of gallstone disease has changed remarkably in the decade since the introduction of laparoscopic cholecystectomy. This occurred nearly simultaneously in Europe and the United States in the late 1980s (5, 6). For the previous century, cholecystectomy through a generous right upper quadrant, midline, or right paramedian incision was the standard for the management of symptomatic cholelithiasis. Efforts to introduce nonsurgical forms of therapy have been unsuccessful. The dismal results from both the national cooperative study in gallstone dissolution (7) and the use of extracorporeal lithotripsy (8) in conjunction with oral dissolution treatment confirm the superiority of surgery in the management of this disease.

The remarkable success of laparoscopic cholecystectomy has maintained surgery as the primary form of therapy for patients with symptomatic gallstones who can tolerate general anesthesia. This accounts for the vast majority of patients, well in excess of 98%. Laparoscopic surgery is currently the treatment of choice in more than 85% of patients with gallstones and can be performed with acceptable morbidity and mortality rates. The only significant risk associated with the surgery is common bile duct injury, a complication which, though it occurred during classical or open cholecystectomy, probably occurred at a slightly lower incidence than during the laparoscopic technique (0.4 versus 0.2%) (9).

HISTORY OF IMAGING

The diagnosis of symptomatic cholecystitis has evolved in the century since the operation was first performed. Initially, the operation was reserved for patients with significant complications of gallstones, particularly infectious or obstructive sequelae. Reliable imaging of the gallbladder did not occur until the 1920s when the oral cholecystogram (OCG) was introduced (10). The OCG remained the standard form of imaging until the late 1960s when ultrasonography was introduced (11). Since that time there have been a variety of imaging modalities applied to the gallbladder and the biliary tree. Some have shown tremendous improvement in diagnosis; others remain to be tested against the traditional and reliable methods. This surgical summary focuses exclusively on the diagnosis of gallbladder disease, rather than imaging techniques for the remaining portions of the intra- and extrahepatic biliary tree.

ULTRASOUND

Choosing the proper diagnostic tool for specific disease processes requires an understanding of the pathophysiology and anatomic abnormalities that occur in each setting. The clinician forced to choose the appropriate test must intuitively understand the cost–benefit ratio of each test, its specificity and sensitivity, and whether the information it provides will hasten the final diagnosis. In gallbladder disease the single test that most frequently fulfills all these criteria is the abdominal ultrasound. Each radiographic test is presented with a discussion of its role in the management of specific disease entities.

Chronic Cholecystitis

Ultrasound is unquestionably the primary radiographic examination for the overwhelming majority of patients with cholelithiasis. In more than 85% of patients this test, combined with a complete history and physical, is sufficient to make the diagnosis and suggest the appropriate therapy. The presenting signs and symptoms of symptomatic cholelithiasis are well described and include episodic right upper quadrant or epigastric pain following meals, particularly fatty meals. The onset of the pain is typically within 30–45 min after ingestion. The pain is labeled colic but in fact is a fairly constant pain located below the right costal margin or beneath the xyphoid process. Typical pain lasts for as much as 3–4 hr, but is never as short as several minutes. The pain may radiate, most typically to the right scapular region, but also in a band-like distribution across the entire upper abdomen.

Patients without prior symptoms frequently experience their first episode of pain in the late evening or night after eating a large dinner. In many cases, this prompts a visit to an emergency facility. This is particularly so in patients presenting with epigastric pain, who may be concerned that the pain represents a primary cardiac event. Evaluation in emergency facilities follows a typical algorithm that generally rules out a major cardiac event, establishes the degree of infectious problems such as leukocytosis, and leads to further imaging studies (Fig. 1).

Invariably, the first imaging study performed is an abdominal ultrasound if the presenting signs and symptoms are sufficiently suggestive of cholelithiasis. Within a short period the presence or absence of gallstones can be confirmed. Additionally, in centers with significant experience in ultrasonography, other ultrasonographic findings may be able to rule out an infectious cause by the absence of significant wall thickening in the gallbladder or pericholecystic fluid. Using these criteria, physicians may be able to make a fairly specific diagnosis in a relatively short period.

Alternatively, patients may present to their primary care physician with a story of the new onset of mild epigastric or right upper quadrant pain following meals, but without sufficient pain to warrant emergency room visits. Evaluations that include a thorough history and physical examination and that direct the physician toward the biliary tree generally suggest symptomatic biliary tract disease and prompt an ultrasound.

Typically, patients continue to manifest the disease in the fashion of their first attack. Thus those who have initially presented with colic tend to have similar episodes until the gallbladder is removed. Likewise, those who present with acute cholecystitis tend to have repeated episodes of inflammation and infection involving the gallbladder until it is removed surgically. In the same manner, patients who present with biliary pancreatitis continue to pass stones and cause secondary inflammation of the pancreas.

Acute Cholecystitis

A small percentage of patients present not with chronic biliary pain suggesting long-standing cholecystitis but rather with an acute process in which not only the history but the physical findings are notably different from chronic cholecystitis.

The mechanism of pain in patients with chronic cholecystitis or biliary colic is increased intravesical pressure, whereas the mechanism of pain in patients with acute cholecystitis is direct peritoneal inflammation and focal peritonitis. These different pathophysiological events provide the rationale for choosing different tests for the detection of each disease. In addition to an infectious etiology leading to focal peritonitis in acute cholecystitis, the cystic duct is almost uniformly obstructed, either by stones or by soft tissue edema. This phenomenon, which does not change the morphology of the gallbladder, does alter the physiology of the gallbladder. Specifically, the obstructed cystic duct does not permit either inflow or outflow of bile.

This fact provides the physiological basis for the use of nuclear medicine scanning (hepatic iminodiacetic acid, HIDA, or 99^{M}Tc-diisopropyliminodiacetic acid, DISIDA) to differentiate between acute and chronic cholecystitis. Ultrasonography is an operator-dependent study. Therefore, the interpretation of subjective findings such as wall thickening or pericholecystic fluid rests on the skill and the experience of the ultrasonographer. Nuclear medicine scanning, however, derives its diagnostic precision by simply demonstrating filling or nonfilling of the gallbladder. The latter constitutes an abnormal study and correctly diagnoses acute cholecystitis in more than 98% of cases.

This exceedingly reliable test, however, cannot be used indiscriminately. For example, a patient with the clinical diagnosis of chronic cholecystitis or biliary colic does not necessarily have an abnormal or nonfilling HIDA scan. Thus the inexperienced clinician using this modality for the diagnosis of chronic cholecystitis may be erroneously presented with a negative diagnosis. It is important that the clinician select the appropriate test for the clinical presentation. Nevertheless, the overwhelming number of patients (in excess of 99%) will be diagnosed either by one of these tests or by a combination of the two.

ACALCULOUS CHOLECYSTITIS

In rare situations, patients may present with acalculous cholecystitis. Acalculous cholecystitis accounts for less than 10% of patients with primary biliary tract disease. Although it can present in ambulatory patients without significant co-morbidities, it more typically presents in patients residing in hospital with significant other co-morbidities. Again, as in the case of chronic and acute cholecystitis, the diagnosis is suggested by the clinical situation to which are added the determining factors gained by radiographic imaging. Ultrasonography can suggest the possibility of acalculous cholecystitis in this situation, again by highlighting wall thickness or perivesicle fluid. The utility of nuclear medicine scanning is less clear because prolonged fasting may have left the gallbladder less likely to fill with the radionuclide by diffusion.

ADENOMYOMATOSIS

Adenomyomatosis is an uncommon condition characterized by thickening of the gallbladder epithelium and muscular wall. It is a benign condition and one that rarely is identified except in situations in which symptomatic colic-type symptoms are present. The condition mimics chronic cholecystitis and is frequently manifested by episodic pain in the right upper quadrant. The ultrasound is often characteristic and can identify the diagnosis. Classical radiographic signs are often identified and used to confirm the diagnosis.

Gallbladder Cancer

Though it is the most common carcinoma found in the gallbladder, gallbladder cancer is an exceedingly uncommon disease, occurring in no more than 1–2% of all gallbladder specimens (12). Certain preoperative ultrasonographic findings suggest the diagnosis preoperatively, including a localized thickening in the gallbladder wall, with or without the presence of gallstones. The disease is thought to be particularly common in porcelain gallbladders, which are frequently identified by flat plate or kidney, ureter, bladder roentgenographic series of the abdomen. Additionally, adjacent polypoid lesions of the gallbladder may be identified. These generally stand out as different from gallstones, though on occasion an impacted stone may mimic a polypoid lesion.

The surgeon operating on a patient with an unusual finding such as gallbladder wall thickening is obligated to evaluate the gallbladder fully prior to performing a traditional cholecystectomy, regardless of whether it is done through an open or a laparoscopic approach. If there is a high level of suspicion for gallbladder cancer the surgeon must decide early in the case whether to proceed with a typical cholecystectomy or to extend the incision into the liver parenchyma of the gallbladder. Preoperative scanning in questionable cases frequently assists in determining if there is a significant possibility of a neoplastic process.

Emptying Studies

In a small percentage of patients with typical biliary colic occurring in the postprandial setting, imaging studies fail to detect any stones within the gallbladder. In this situation there are several possibilities for determining the etiology of the pain. The simplest initial test is an upper gastrointestinal series (UGI) to rule out the possibility of occult or atypical peptic disease. Alternatively, this can be accomplished by upper endoscopy.

If gastric and duodenal evaluation fails to demonstrate an ulcer and if the persistence of symptoms suggests a biliary source, the physician may obtain emptying studies to confirm the possibility of motility abnormalities leading to the symptomatology. An ultrasonographic emptying study consists of an ultrasound after an all-night fast followed by the administration of either a fatty meal or cholecystokinin (CCK). The resulting diminution in gallbladder size in response to the stimulation of the meal or the CCK can help in localizing the symptoms to the gallbladder. An ejection fraction less than 65% is considered abnormal and may be used to confirm the indications for surgery.

Alternatively, duodenal drainage, aspiration of bile, and examination under a polarizing light also confirm pathology in certain cases in which the ultrasound does not demonstrate obvious stones. Cholesterol crystals have a characteristic appearance under polarizing light. Their presence in bile of symptomatic patients with documented stones is considered sufficient to warrant surgery.

NUCLEAR MEDICINE

Cholecystitis

Nuclear medicine scanning of the biliary tree is useful in providing functional definition of the degree of inflammation present in the gallbladder. It does not determine the presence or absence of stones. In equivocal clinical situations where the presence or absence of acute inflammation of the gallbladder (as opposed to simple investigation of stones) is important, technetium scanning of the gallbladder provides important information. If, upon administration of the tracer, prompt uptake does not occur in the gallbladder, the study is interpreted as confirming acute cholecystitis. If the cystic duct is obstructed either by a stone or by tissue edema in response to infection, the study is diagnostic of acute cholecystitis in more than 98% of cases (13).

Certain situations may complicate the apparent simplicity of this study. For instance, if there is a stone impacted in the neck of the gallbladder in the setting of chronic or subacute symptoms, the HIDA scan may give a false positive test, suggesting acute cholecystitis. Clearly, it is important as in any radiographic test to evaluate the study in the appropriate clinical setting. If there is insufficient clinical evidence to suggest acute versus chronic cholecystitis, the clinician will be ill-served by placing undue importance on an abnormal HIDA or DISIDA scan.

Common Bile Duct Evaluation

Nuclear medicine scanning has no role in the diagnosis and management on neoplastic disease of the gallbladder. However, nuclear medicine scanning can have an important role in the evaluation of the common bile duct following gallbladder surgery. It may, for instance, confirm the clinical impression of common bile duct obstruction by failing to demonstrate free flow of the contrast medium into the duodenum and small bowel. Although not definitive and not quantifiable, the absence of contrast in the small bowel may infer bile duct obstruction.

Equally useful in the postoperative setting, nuclear medicine scanning of the biliary tree can be used to identify either a bile leak from the cystic duct or from intrahepatic radicals that pass directly into the gallbladder, the so-called ducts of Luschka. Additionally, the HIDA or DISIDA scan may demonstrate iatrogenic injury to the bile duct after laparoscopic or open cholecystectomy. In many institutions, a nuclear medicine study is the first radiological test performed on patients who return to the hospital or clinic following gallbladder surgery with complaints of pain or postoperative dysfunction.

Emptying Studies

Finally, nuclear medicine determination of gallbladder emptying can be performed in a manner analogous to that mentioned above in the section on ultrasound. As in the ultrasound technique, the patient is studied after an overnight fast, scanned, and then administered either a fatty meal or CCK. Calculation of emptying fraction is determined and used to supplement the clinical impression of biliary disease.

COMPUTED TOMOGRAPHY

Benign Disease

Computed tomography (CT) scanning has little place in the evaluation of uncomplicated, benign gallbladder disease. The ability to detect stones is less reliable than ultrasound and does not have the functional component that can be gained from nuclear medicine scanning. There are, however, indications for use of CT scanning in certain situations; the degree of calcification within gallbladder stones can be reliably determined. Although not important for routine surgical care of the patient with symptomatic gallstones, it does have a role when alternative treatments are used. For instance, if lithotripsy or oral dissolution therapy is being considered, a CT scan with appropriate measurements of stone density may assist the clinician in choosing this type of therapy. Gallstones with any degree of calcification, even those not evident on a plain film of the abdomen, do not respond to oral dissolution therapies. In fact, this may be the primary reason that success rates for dissolution therapy have been so low. Even small amounts of calcified debris left in the gallbladder after bile salt treatment increase the chance of recurrence of stones. Nevertheless, oral dissolution therapy and/or lithotripsy are used so infrequently in current management of gallstones that CT scanning for stone disease probably has a very small role.

Neoplasia

Computed tomography scanning can provide important information in staging and planning when gallbladder neoplasia is suspected. Stage I tumors are invariably identified as an incidental finding at the time of cholecystectomy and probably require no further surgical intervention. More advanced stages can be identified by CT scanning if adequate suspicion is raised during the initial ultrasound exam (14). The incidence of gallbladder cancer, however, is so low that preoperative identification is unusual except in very advanced cases.

MAGNETIC RESONANCE SCANNING

The role of magnetic resonance scanning of the right upper quadrant and in particular the gallbladder remains to be seen. Its role in uncomplicated cholelithiasis is negligible, and in malignant or neoplastic disease it can be used similarly to CT scanning to define the extent of the lesion and adjacent organ involvement in selected cases.

OTHER IMAGING MODALITIES

A number of other types of examination are available to assist in the recognition and management of gallbladder disease. Many are used infrequently or of primarily historical interest. Nevertheless, a complete evaluation of their utility is useful to provide an overview of available gallbladder imaging techniques.

Oral Cholecystography

Prior to the introduction of B-scale ultrasonography, the classic radiological examination for identification of an abnormal gallbladder was the oral cholecystogram (OCG). As ultrasonography became more sophisticated and more widely used, OCG faded into the background. Currently, the main indication for OCG is in the evaluation of a patient being proposed for lithotripsy or oral bile salt dissolution therapy. The OCG is the most definitive technique for identifying a patent cystic duct. Patency of the cystic duct is mandatory for successful treatment using nonsurgical techniques. Without a patent cystic duct the stone debris cannot be emptied from the gallbladder and its persistence can and will lead to stone reformation.

Occasionally, in patients with typical symptoms of biliary colic but without demonstrable gallstones on ultrasound, nonfilling of the gallbladder on double-dose OCG can be used to identify an abnormal gallbladder. This indication, however, is uncommon and used only rarely.

Endoscopic Retrograde Cholangiopancreatography

Though endoscopic retrograde cholangiopancreatography (ERCP) is the standard for identification of pathology within and around the common bile duct and the common hepatic duct, there is essentially no role for ERCP in the identification and management of uncomplicated gallbladder disease and cholelithiasis. Some innovative techniques are currently being evaluated to cannulate the cystic duct and gallbladder during ERCP but the practicality and utility of this technique need further investigation.

Even in complicated disease, there does not appear to be, as yet, a role for routine or even occasional ERCP. If there is preoperative concern suggesting a major anatomic abnormality or variant, it is conceivable that preoperative ERCP might have a role. This is so uncommon, however, that I have had no experience with this in more than 1,500 cholecystectomies in the past 6 years.

Percutaneous Transhepatic Cholangiography

Percutaneous transhepatic cholangiography (PTHC) has essentially no role in the diagnosis of uncomplicated gallbladder disease. This examination, like ERCP, has its greatest impact in extrahepatic biliary tract pathology rather than in the study of the gallbladder itself. In certain cases of established gallbladder cancer where the extent of impingement of the disease on the proximal bile duct is in question and the bile duct is not readily accessible to ERCP, PTHC may have a role.

SUMMARY

The single most useful imaging study for gallbladder disease is the abdominal ultrasound. In the vast majority of cases, the abdominal ultrasound yields an appropriate diagnosis, whether the disease is chronic cholecystitis, acute cholecystitis, or gallbladder neoplasia. It is certainly the first test that should be employed if gallbladder disease is suspected.

Following ultrasound in importance is nuclear medicine scanning. When the clinical picture is equivocal or confusing, HIDA or DISIDA scanning reliably differentiates chronic from acute cholecystitis. It has no use, however, in the uncomplicated patient presenting with episodic right upper pain who is not thought to have an acute inflammatory process in the gallbladder. Nuclear medicine scanning can also be of use in the postoperative period to evaluate leaks or obstruction to the bile duct without resorting to invasive procedures such as ERCP or PTHC.

Neoplastic disease is best initially diagnosed with ultrasound, primarily because patients most typically present with episodes of colic or persistent right upper quadrant pain. Once a neoplastic process is suspected, however, cross-sectional body imaging by CT or MR scanning is most important to define the disease.

Functional tests such as emptying studies should be reserved for the truly equivocal case in which functional abnormalities of motility are suspected as a cause of pain.

REFERENCES

1. Brooks DC. Newer concepts in the management of biliary tract disease. *Surg Rounds.* 1989;12:37–48.
2. Friedman GD, Kannel WB, Dawber TR. The epidemiology of gallbladder disease: observations in the Framingham study. *J Chronic Dis.* 1966;19:273–292.
3. Pauletzki J, Althaus R, Holl J, Sackman M, Paumgartner G. Gallbladder emptying and gallstone formation: a prospective study of gallstone recurrence. *Gastroenterology.* 1996;111:765–771.
4. Stolk MFJ, Van Erpecum KJ, Renooij W, et al. Gallbladder emptying in vivo, bile composition, and nucleation of cholesterol crystals in patients with cholesterol gallstones. *Gastroenterology.* 1995;108:1882–1888.
5. Perissat J, Collet DR, Belliard R. Gallstones: laparoscopic treatment, intracorporeal lithotripsy followed by cholecystostomy or cholecystectomy—a personal technique. *Endoscopy.* 1990;21:373–374.
6. Reddick EJ, Olsen DO. Laparoscopic laser cholecystectomy: a comparison with minilap cholecystectomy. *Surg Endosc.* 1989;3:131–133.
7. Schoenfield LJ, Lachin JM, et al. Chenodiol (chenodeoxycholic acid) for dissolution of gallstones: The National Cooperative Gallstone Study: a controlled trial of efficacy and safety. *Ann Intern Med.* 1981;95:257–282.
8. Sackmann M, Pauletzki J, Sauerbruch T, Holl J, Schelling G, Paumgartner G. The Munich gallbladder lithotripsy study. Results of the first 711 patients. *Ann Intern Med.* 1991;114:290–296.
9. The Southern Surgical Club. A prospective analysis of 1,518 laparoscopic cholecystectomies performed by Southern U.S. surgeons. *N Engl J Med.* 1991;324:1073–1078.
10. Graham EA, Cole WH, Copher GH. Visualization of the gallbladder by the sodium salt of tetrabromophthalein. *JAMA.* 1924;82:1777.
11. Crade M, Taylor KJW, Rosenfield AT, et al. Surgical and pathological correlation of cholecystosonography and cholecystography. *AJR.* 1978;131:227–229.
12. Piehler JM, Critchlow RW. Primary carcinoma of the gallbladder. *Surg Gynecol Obstet.* 1978;147:929–942.

13. Samuels BF, Freitas JE, Bree RL, et al. A comparison of radionuclide hepatobiliary imaging and real-time ultrasonography for the detection of acute cholecystitis. *Radiology.* 1983;147:207–210.

14. Tsukada K, Hatakeyama K, Kurosaki I, et al. Outcome of radical surgery for carcinoma of the gallbladder according to the TNM stage. *Surgery.* 1996;120:816–822.

II

THE BILIARY TREE

7

ULTRASOUND OF THE BILIARY TREE

Susan M. Ascher, M.D., and Brian Garra, M.D.
Georgetown University Medical Center
Washington, DC

Ultrasound is often the initial screening modality of choice for evaluating the biliary tree. It is both sensitive and accurate in the detection of bile duct dilatation. Ultrasound is a cost-effective, comprehensive exam capable of evaluating the entire abdomen without any known contraindications. This chapter addresses the use of ultrasound in the evaluation of the intra- and extrahepatic bile ducts. Normal anatomy is presented, followed by a discussion of pathological entities. Finally, future applications are raised.

NORMAL ANATOMY: INTRAHEPATIC BILE DUCTS

Ultrasound excels at imaging the fluid-filled tubular structures of the biliary tree. Although the ducts usually lie anterior to the portal venous radicals, other orientations are not uncommon. This is not problematic; routine color and duplex imaging reliably distinguishes the intrahepatic bile ducts from the vascular structures residing in the portal triads (Fig. 1) (1). The right and left hepatic ducts that course toward the porta hepatis are also routinely imaged.

DILATED INTRAHEPATIC BILE DUCTS

The finding of dilated intrahepatic ducts is very specific for active biliary obstruction. There are four criteria that allow dilated intrahepatic ducts to be distinguished from portal veins: (1) alteration in the normal appearance of the portal triads; (2) irregularity of bile duct walls; (3) stellate confluence of tubular structures; and (4) acoustic enhancement behind dilated bile ducts (2, 3). Of these, the first criterion

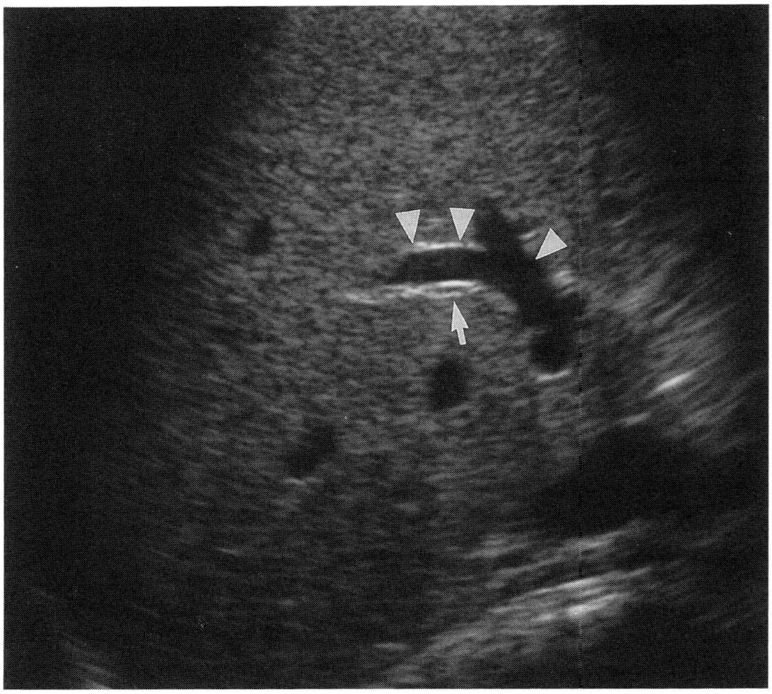

(A)

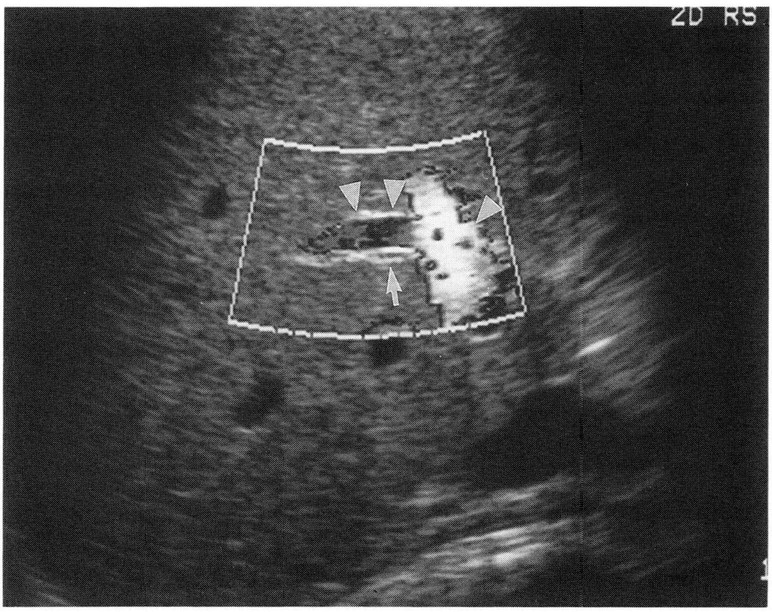

(B)

Figure 1. Normal intrahepatic duct. Two-dimensional (A) and color flow (B) transverse ultrasounds demonstrate the nearly imperceptible normal caliber intrahepatic bile duct (arrow, A and B) posterior to a portal venous radical (arrowheads, A and B). Variability in the orientation between the biliary tree and portal venous structures is not unusual and underscores the importance of color flow imaging (B).

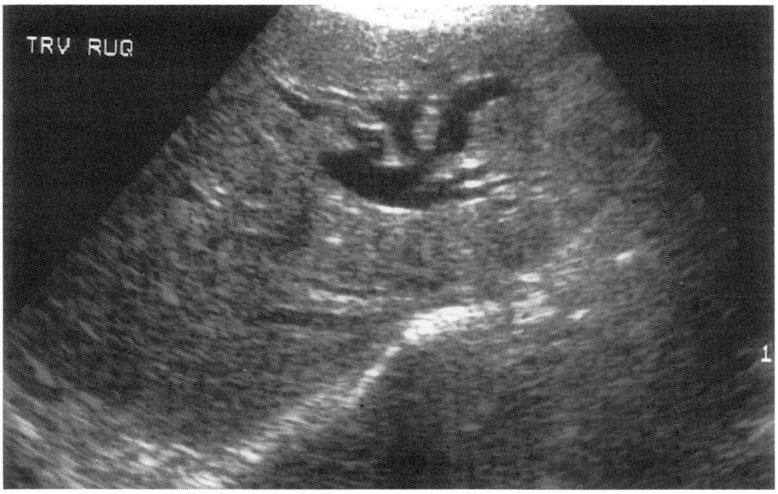

Figure 2. Intrahepatic biliary duct dilatation. Transverse ultrasound shows the parallel anechoic channels of dilated intrahepatic bile ducts and normal portal venous radicals.

is the most reliable. When intrahepatic ducts dilate, two or more tubular structures are seen in the expected location of the portal vein (Fig. 2). Typically the dilated ducts measure 2 mm or more in diameter and are more than 40% of the diameter of the accompanying vein lying within the same portal triad. The second criterion reflects the tortuosity and irregularity of the bile ducts when dilated; in contradistinction, the walls of the portal veins are always smooth. In the majority of patients, dilated intrahepatic bile ducts converge in a spoke-wheel or stellate pattern and show the characteristic acoustic enhancement associated with fluid-filled structures, the third and fourth criteria, respectively. Acoustic enhancement is not seen with vascular structures because the protein content of blood attenuates the sound beam (4). Moreover, the advent of color flow and Doppler imaging easily allows differentiation between vascular structures and bile ducts.

Although the ultrasound findings of intrahepatic bile duct dilatation are very specific, they are not equally sensitive. Up to 23% of patients with biliary obstruction have normal sized intrahepatic ducts. Additionally, the level of hyperbilirubinemia and duration of jaundice do not correlate with the presence or absence of intrahepatic biliary dilatation (5).

PATHOLOGY OF INTRAHEPATIC BILE DUCTS

Dilatation of the intrahepatic bile ducts is typically a manifestation of extrahepatic duct obstruction; however, several intrinsic intrahepatic biliary processes including neoplastic and inflammatory, and/or calculi, may cause duct dilatation.

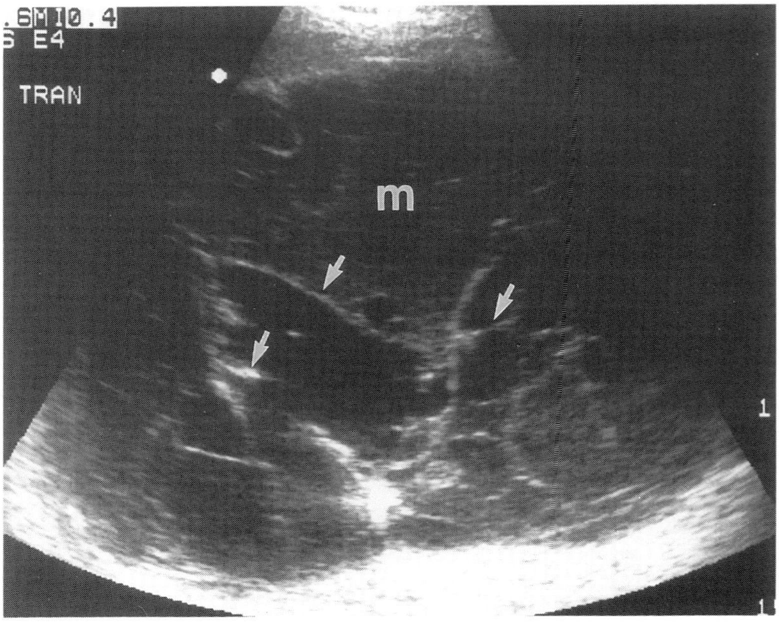

Figure 3. Biliary cystadenoma. Transverse ultrasound shows a complex cystic mass (m) within the liver. Septations (arrows) are typical of these rare tumors.

Neoplastic

Cholangiocarcinoma, the most common bile duct malignancy, is rarely confined to the intrahepatic ducts. Rather, cystadenoma and cystadenocarcinoma are tumors, although rare, that originate in the intrahepatic biliary tree and may produce dilatation. They occur in middle-aged women and patients who present with abdominal pain, mass, and/or jaundice. Their ultrasound appearance is nonspecific: multiple or single cystic masses with septa and/or papillary excrescences (Fig. 3) (6). They may also calcify. The differential diagnosis includes hemorrhagic or infected cysts, echinococcal cyst, abscess, hematoma, and cystic metastasis. Although percutaneous aspiration may allow differentiation of a primary biliary neoplasm from the other etiologies, surgical resection is necessary for distinguishing cystadenoma from its malignant counterpart.

Cholangitis

Sclerosing cholangitis and AIDS cholangitis may produce similar ultrasound findings. There is bile duct wall thickening (Fig. 4) (7–10). When this becomes pronounced, luminal compromise results. The patient's alkaline phosphatase and bilirubin may elevate, despite minimal duct dilatation. The imaging differential diagnosis includes primary and metastatic tumors, though these entities tend to be more focal. Moreover, history is very important; greater than 50% of patients with sclerosing cholangitis have ulcerative colitis and patients with AIDS cholangitis usually have

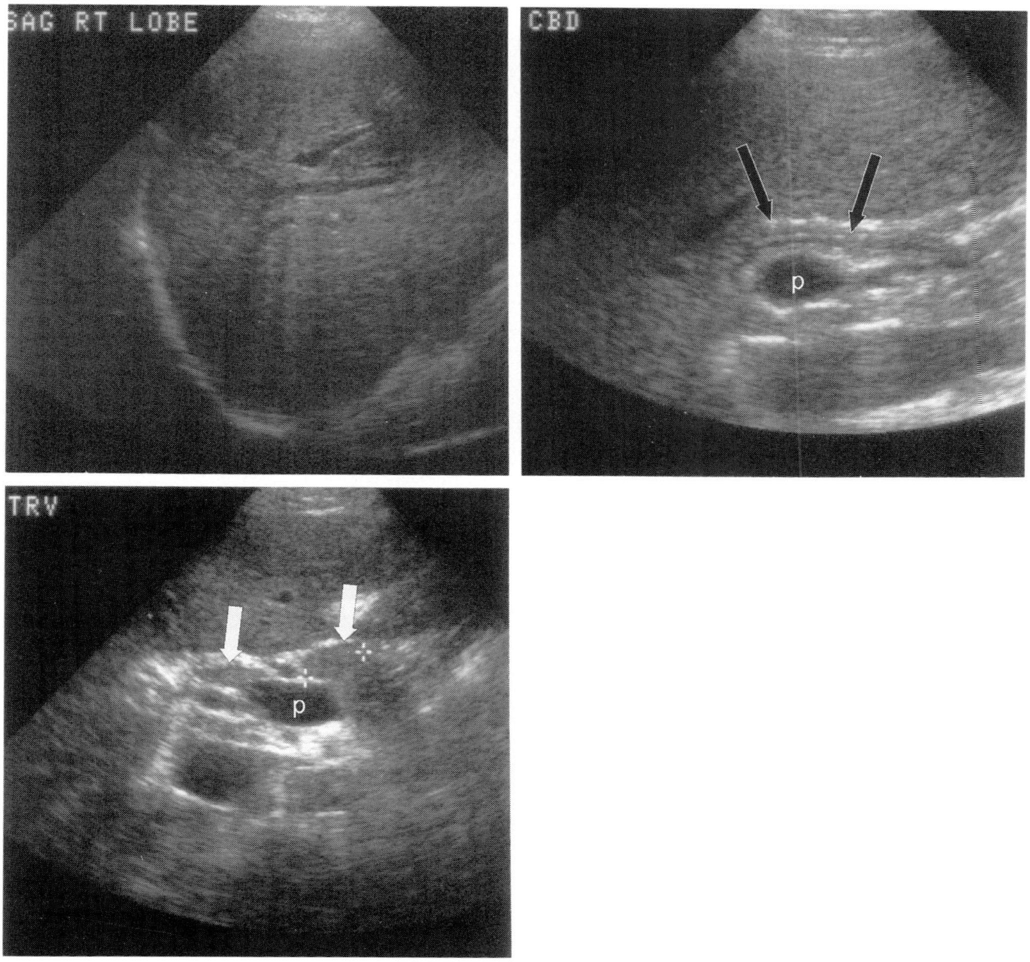

Figure 4. Sclerosing cholangitis. Sagittal (A), oblique (B), and transverse (C) ultrasound images show mild intrahepatic duct dilation (A), a thickened, but normal-caliber common bile duct (arrows, B) and periportal lymphadenopathy (arrows, C). (p = portal vein). (Images courtesy of Caroline Reinhold, M.D., Montreal General Hospital).

other HIV disease manifestations (3). Ultrasound has not fared well in defining intrahepatic duct manifestations of primary sclerosing cholangitis, though common bile duct involvement and advanced disease manifested by portal hypertension are detectable. In cases complicated by cholangiocarcinoma, marked nonsegmental intrahepatic duct dilatation and a mass lesion characterize the ultrasound findings.

Calculi

Oriental cholangiohepatitis is the most common cause of intrahepatic biliary calculi (11). As the name implies, this disease is typically seen in Asians, but may occur in any patient with prolonged biliary stasis. Subsequent infection leads to calcium bilirubinate crystal precipitates that coalesce to form soft stones, giving rise to another name for this entity, recurrent pyogenic cholangitis. The stones reside in both the intra- and extrahepatic bile ducts and may form a cast of the biliary tree (12). At ultrasonography, the calculi are of medium echotexture and produce variable amounts of acoustic shadowing (Fig. 5). The differential diagnosis is therefore extensive and includes blood, pus, sludge, and neoplasm. Nonetheless, the diagnosis of Oriental cholangitis should be entertained when echogenic material is distributed thoughout the biliary tree, especially because the surgical management is markedly different in this condition as compared with choledocholithiasis. Computed tomography may offer complementary information about the extent of disease. Computed tomography is also helpful for evaluating recurrent pyogenic cholangitis in patients with post-biliary–enteric anastomosis, because the intrahepatic gas obscures evaluation by sonography.

Caroli's Disease

Caroli's disease is a rare condition often associated with infantile polycystic kidney disease and hepatic fibrosis. It is characterized by segmental nonobstructive dilatation of the intrahepatic ducts. The ducts have a saccular or cystic morphology. Patients with Caroli's disease may develp pyogenic cholangitis, liver abscess, and/or stones. The most characteristic ultrasound finding is focal irregular intrahepatic duct dilatation (13, 14). Other features particular to Caroli's disease include complete or partial bridging of the duct walls and intraductal soft tissue protrusions (13, 14). In a patient with infantile polycystic kidney disease these ultrasound findings are pathognomonic.

NORMAL ANATOMY: EXTRAHEPATIC BILIARY TREE

The common hepatic duct (CHD) is reliably imaged in the porta hepatis. It is formed by the junction of the right and left intrahepatic ducts and lies anterior to the undivided right portal vein (Fig. 6). Interposed between, and perpendicular to, the right portal vein and the CHD is the hepatic artery. The common bile duct (CBD) is formed from the union of the CHD and cystic duct. The CBD then runs within the hepatoduodenal ligament with the main portal vein and the proper hepatic artery. In the proximal hepatoduodenal ligament the portal vein is posterior and the CBD and proper hepatic artery course anterolaterally and anteromedially, respectively. This relationship changes as these structures descend in the ligament; the CBD travels posteriorly within the pancreas to enter the duodenum (Fig. 7) and the portal vein travels anteriorly to its origin at the junction of the superior mesenteric and splenic veins.

The caliber of the normal CHD and CBD has generated much debate in the radiology literature; measurements range from 4 to 8 mm and controversy exists regarding the caliber of normal ducts following cholecystectomy (Fig. 8) (Tables 1 and 2) (15–23). It is accepted that the normal CBD may increase slightly with advancing age (22). Futhermore, the CHD and CBD may dilate after biliary surgery in the absence of duct obstruction (19, 21). Serial scanning may show a return to a more normal caliber duct in some cases. This transient dilatation may be related to localized biliary ileus or temporary duct compression from edema in the periductal fat of the hepatoduodenal ligament.

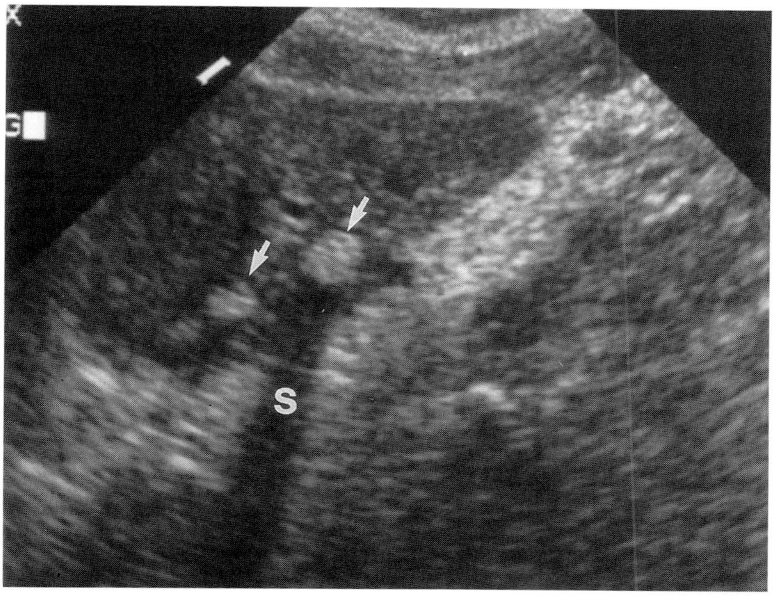

(A)

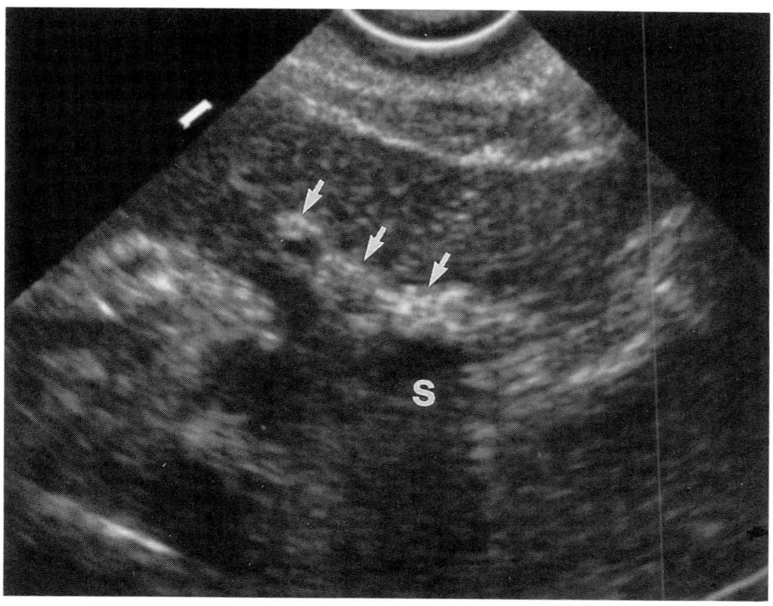

(B)

Figure 5. Recurrent pyogenic cholangitis in a patient with *Clonorchis senesis* infestation. Longitudinal (A) and transverse (B) ultrasounds show echogenic material (arrows, A and B) within the intrahepatic biliary tree in the left lobe of the liver. Note the acoustic shadowing (S, A and B) produced by the soft calcium bilirubinate precipitates.

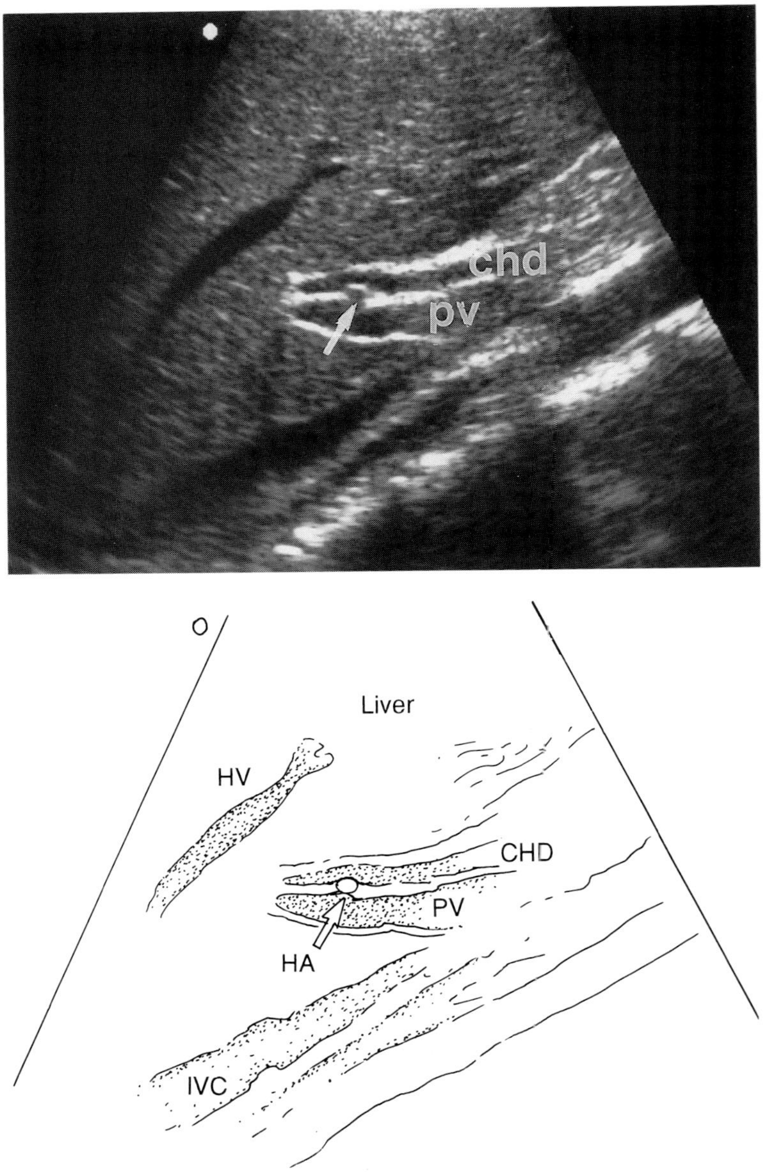

Figure 6. Normal common hepatic duct (CHD). Oblique ultrasound shows the usual relationships between the CHD anteriorly, the portal vein (PV) posteriorly and the hepatic artery (arrow) in cross-section interposed between the two.

DILATED EXTRAHEPATIC DUCTS

In the setting of biliary obstruction the extrahepatic ducts dilate preferentially. This is a function of Laplace's law and, in many cases, the inability of the intrahepatic ducts to dilate readily in the setting of fibrotic or infiltrated hepatic parenchyma.

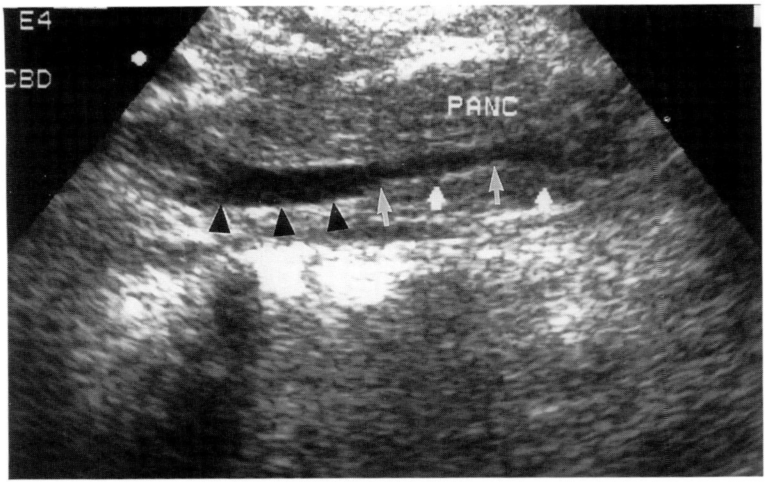

Figure 7. Normal CBD. Longitudinal ultrasound shows the normal caliber CBD (black arrowheads) as it tapers to traverse the pancreas (white arrows) (panc = pancreas).

Therefore, the diameter of the CHD is the most sensitive parameter for diagnosing biliary obstruction. Biliary obstruction is suggested if the diameter of the CHD is greater than or equal to 8 mm (Fig. 9) (3).

PATHOLOGY OF EXTRAHEPATIC BILE DUCTS

Although some ultrasound laboratories report being able to distinguish medical from surgical jaundice in more than 90% of cases, an understanding of potential imaging pitfalls and atypical cases is necessary for both the imager and referring clinician (24). Anatomic variability in the course of the hepatic duct and position of the hepatic artery occurs not infrequently (25, 26). These variations could potentially lead to mistakes in interpretation and have a negative impact on management; however, the routine use of duplex and color imaging renders this concern moot. Air in the biliary tree from surgery or a fistula is problematic for ultrasound interrogation. It produces "dirty shadowing" and obscures biliary anatomy; these patients are best evaluated with computed tomography (CT) or cholangiography (Fig. 10). More problematic are patients with dilatation of the biliary tree without jaundice. In these patients partial or intermittent obstruction may be present. In rare cases complete obstruction can occur with a significant time delay in the development of clinical symptoms. In patients with anicteric dilatation, the alkaline phosphatase and ultrasound findings may be more sensitive than bilirubin levels (27). Conversely, a patient with obstructive jaundice may not manifest duct dilatation. This has been noted in some patients with cholangitis, partial obstruction, or intermittent obstruction from choledocholithiasis (5, 28).

In these instances where the presence of biliary obstruction is questionable, a provocative test with a fatty meal may be performed. Patients are scanned before

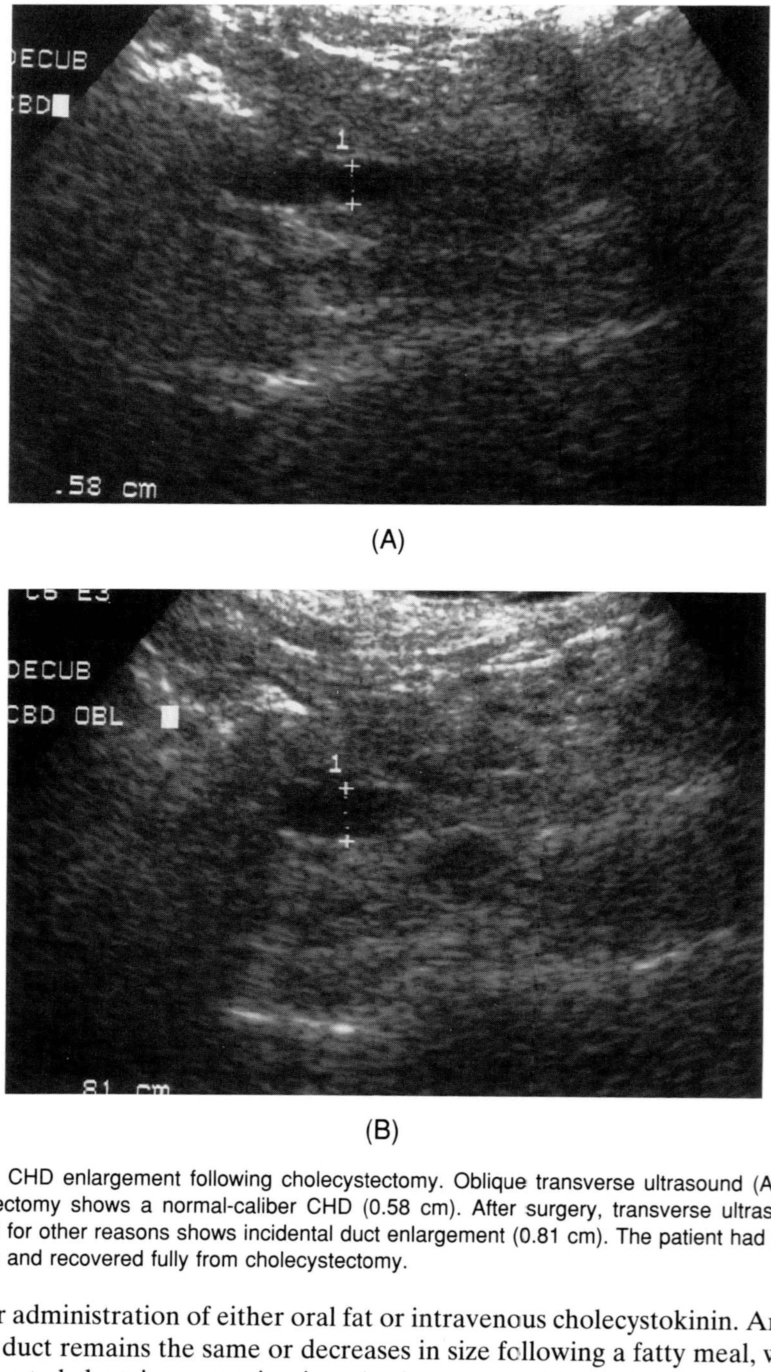

Figure 8. CHD enlargement following cholecystectomy. Oblique transverse ultrasound (A) prior to cholecystectomy shows a normal-caliber CHD (0.58 cm). After surgery, transverse ultrasound (B) performed for other reasons shows incidental duct enlargement (0.81 cm). The patient had no biliary symptoms and recovered fully from cholecystectomy.

and after administration of either oral fat or intravenous cholecystokinin. An unobstructed duct remains the same or decreases in size following a fatty meal, whereas an obstructed duct increases in size. A change of caliber of 2 mm or more is considered significant, though some investigators believe a 1-mm change is also significant (29, 30). In patients with partial CBD obstruction, fatty-meal testing has a sensitivity of 74% and a specificity of 100% (30). The significance of a duct that is initially dilated and fails to change in size following provocative testing is

Table 1. Normal common hepatic duct caliber

Reference	Diameter (mm)	Study Description
Weill et al. (15)[a]	4	100 jaundiced patients. 4-mm diameter allowed differentiation of nonobstructive jaundice from the obstructive variety
Cooperberg (16)[a]	4	100 healthy volunteers
	4–9	8 asymptomatic volunteers after cholecystectomy
Grahm et al. (17)[a]	4	56/67 asymptomatic volunteers after cholecystectomy
	5	4/67
	6–10	7/67

[a]Prospective study.

Table 2. Normal common bile duct caliber

Reference	Diameter (mm)	Study Description
Sample et al. (5)[a]	5	143 jaundiced patients. Medical jaundice was reliably differentiated from surgical jaundice when 5 mm was used as the upper normal limit for the CHD and CBD
Behan and Kazam (18)[a]	8	67 adults studied with ultrasound and cholangiography. Good correlation ($r = .86$, $p < .001$) between CBD diameters
Paruleker (19)[a]	4.1	73 normal adults
	(7.7)	20 asymptomatic patients postcholecystectomy (>1 year)
Mueller et al. (20)[a]	6	40 patients evaluated before and after (10.8 months) cholecystectomy. 37/40 asymptomatic patients had a normal CBD caliber before and after surgery
Niederau et al. (21)[a]	4	95% of healthy volunteers ($n = 73$)
	7	100% of healthy volunteers
	11	95% of asymptomatic postcholecystectomy volunteers ($n = 55$)
Wu et al. (22)[a]	1–10	256 healthy adult volunteers
	3.3	<21 years
	4.7	21–30 years
	4.8	31–40 years
	5.5	41–50 years
	5.8	51–60 years
	6.4	>60 years

[a]Prospective study.

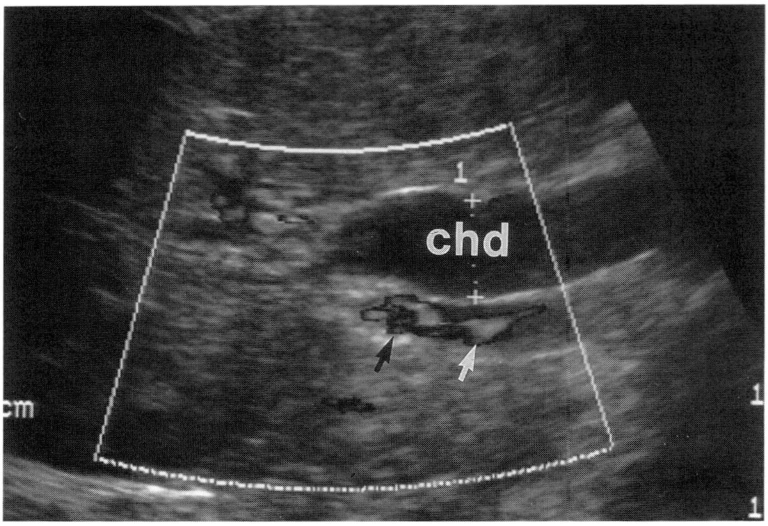

Figure 9. CHD dilatation. Oblique ultrasound shows a markedly dilated CHD. Color flow imaging easily differentiates the dilated duct from the posteriorly located portal vein (arrows).

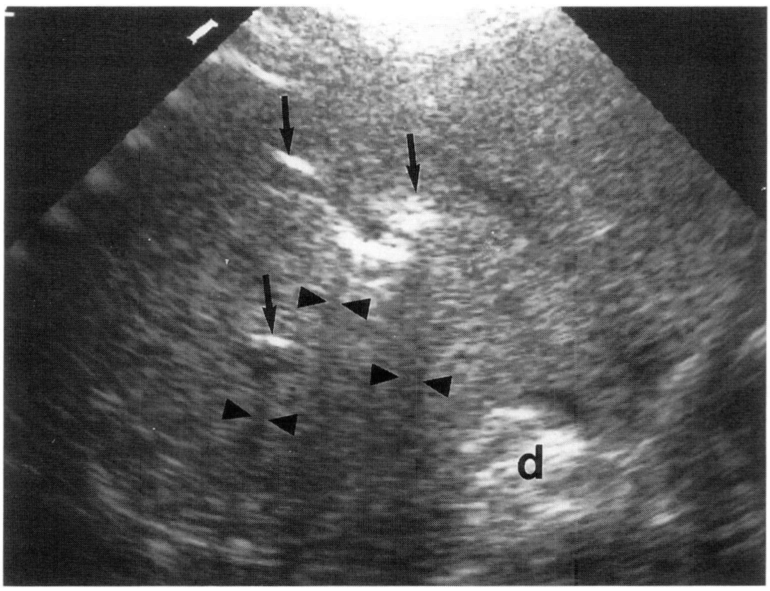

Figure 10. Pneumobilia. Transverse ultrasound demonstrates echogenic air within the biliary tree (arrows) in a post-sphincterotomy patient. Pneumobilia produces "dirty shadowing" (arrowheads) and may obscure ultrasound evaluation of the bile ducts (d = air-filled duodenum).

controversial (31). Moreover, critically ill patients may not be able to mount a response to a fatty meal, irrespective of the presence or absence of CBD obstruction (3).

Biliary tree ultrasound has two goals: (1) to determine the presence or absence of biliary obstruction and (2) if present, to determine the cause and level of obstruction. This information is important. It has an impact on what, if any, other diagnostic examinations should be performed and it is used to direct therapy. With current technology, the level and cause of biliary obstruction can be determined in 92 and 71% of cases, respectively (32). The level of obstruction can be conveniently divided into the porta hepatis, suprapancreatic CBD, or intrapancreatic CBD.

Porta Hepatis Obstruction

Porta hepatis obstruction is usually the result of primary or secondary neoplasms, including adenopathy. The sonographic features are characterized by intrahepatic duct dilatation with sparing of the CBD. Depending on the level of obstruction, the cystic duct and gallbladder may or may not be involved. Similarly, if the disease process involves either the right or left biliary tree, duct dilatation may be focal.

Cholangiocarcinoma

Cholangiocarcinoma is a rare tumor that occurs in the larger bile ducts. When located in the hilar area, as in 10–25% of cases, it is referred to as a Klatskin tumor (3). The diagnosis should be suggested when the caliber of the CBD is normal and dilated intrahepatic ducts that do not coalesce at the hilum are imaged (33, 34). The tumor is rarely visualized owing to its small size, though occasionally there is local invasion of the liver and porta hepatis (Fig. 11) (33, 34). Characterizing and staging of these hilar neoplasms with conventional and duplex sonography has met with mixed results. Chaotic portal flow, portal vein occlusion, and high-frequency-shift Doppler signals were found in 20, 10, and 7% of bile duct tumors, respectively (35). In another study, bile duct dilatation and the level of obstruction was documented by conventional ultrasound in 100% of cases and in 86% of cases the tumor itself was imaged. Depth of local tumor extension was correctly identified in up to 68% of patients. With the addition of duplex sonography, vascular patency was correctly determined in 86% of patients (36). Other diagnostic possiblilties include cholangitis, benign stricture, benign bile duct tumor, and metastasis.

Mirizzi Syndrome

Mirizzi syndrome is the name given to extrinsic compression of the CHD by a stone impacted in the cystic duct. It can occur in patients who have a low cystic duct inserting into the CHD. The classic ultrasound findings, although rare, include intrahepatic duct dilatation, a normal CBD, and a large stone in the gallbladder neck or cystic duct (37). If the ultrasound is negative or equivocal in a patient with suspected Mirizzi syndrome, a CT scan or cholangiogram should be performed.

Parasitic Infestation

Parasites can also lead to extrahepatic biliary dilatation. In cases of ascariasis, aggregates of worms in the gallbladder and biliary tree may be seen (38). In addition

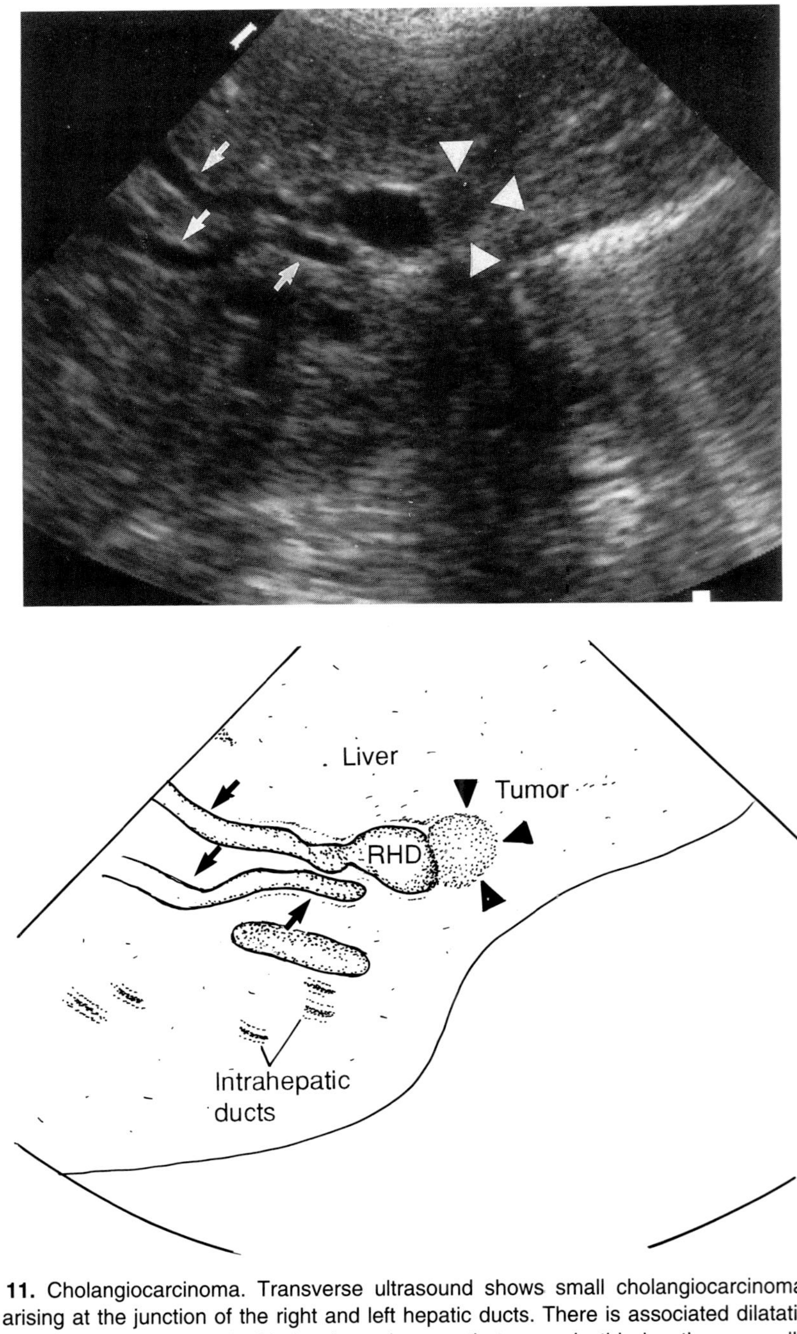

Figure 11. Cholangiocarcinoma. Transverse ultrasound shows small cholangiocarcinoma (arrowheads) arising at the junction of the right and left hepatic ducts. There is associated dilatation of the intrahepatic biliary tree (arrows). Cholangiocarcinomas that occur in this location are called "Klatskin tumors."

to aiding diagnosis, ultrasound is also useful for monitoring response to therapy. It can assess "worm burden." *Clonorchis sinensis* is a liver fluke endemic to peoples of the Far East. Though it usually resides in the intrahepatic biliary tree, it can, on occasion, infest the extrahepatic ducts as well. At ultrasound, intrahepatic duct dilatation may be seen in association with increased echogenicity and duct wall thickening. Occasionally, the echogenic worms may be seen in the extrahepatic biliary tree (39). Patients with biliary infestation are at increased risk for cholangiocarcinoma and recurrent pyogenic cholangitis (Fig. 5).

Suprapancreatic Common Bile Duct Obstruction

Suprapancreatic obstruction occurs above the pancreas, but below the porta hepatis. Depending on its severity and duration, the suprapancreatic CBD dilates with variable dilatation of the intrahepatic biliary tree. Malignancy is the most common cause of suprapancreatic CBD obstruction. Ultrasound may image the primary tumor or metastases including adenopathy. Rarely, an intraluminal mass is seen. Inflammatory strictures and calculi are uncommon causes of obstruction of the suprapancreatic CBD.

Intrapancreatic Common Bile Duct Obstruction

Obstruction of the biliary tree occurs most frequently at the level of the pancreatic head. This leads to dilatation of the CBD and the CHD as well as variable dilatation of the intrahepatic ducts. Neoplasms, calculi, and inflammatory strictures are the most common etiologies for intrapancreatic CBD obstruction.

Pancreatic Carcinoma

Pancreatic head masses frequently compromise the CBD. Tumors that measure 2.5 cm are reliably imaged (3). The tumors are overwhelmingly hypoechoic. Smaller masses may be inferred if a dilated CBD and pancreatic duct, the "double duct" sign, are present (Fig. 12) (40). As with cholangiocarcinoma, changes in portal venous flow and high-frequency-shift Doppler signals may be detected in some patients (35). Focal pancreatitis may mimic neoplasm. Doppler wave forms and ancillary findings of adenopathy and hepatic metastases can help distinguish the two entities, as can clinical history.

Choledocholithiasis

The ability of ultrasound to detect choledocholithiasis has been a source of debate in the radiological literature. The different sensitivities reported reflect differences in equipment, ultrasonographers, and patient populations (Table 3) (41–47). At present, ultrasonographic visualization of choledocholithiasis is possible in at least 70% of patients (3, 12). By meticulous scanning technique, altering patient position, and provocative fatty meal administration, the sensitivity of ultrasound in detecting distal choledocholithiasis approaches 86% (46). Classic findings include a shadowing echogenic focus in a dilated CBD (Fig. 13).

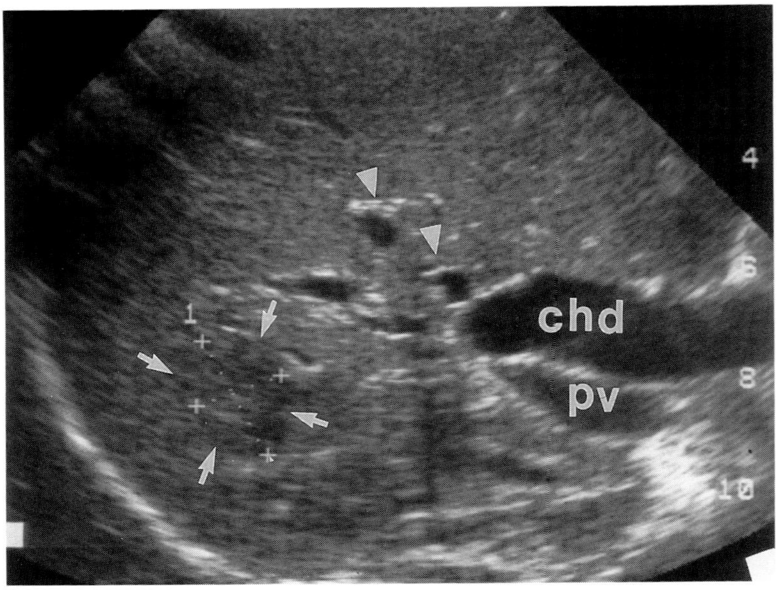

(A)

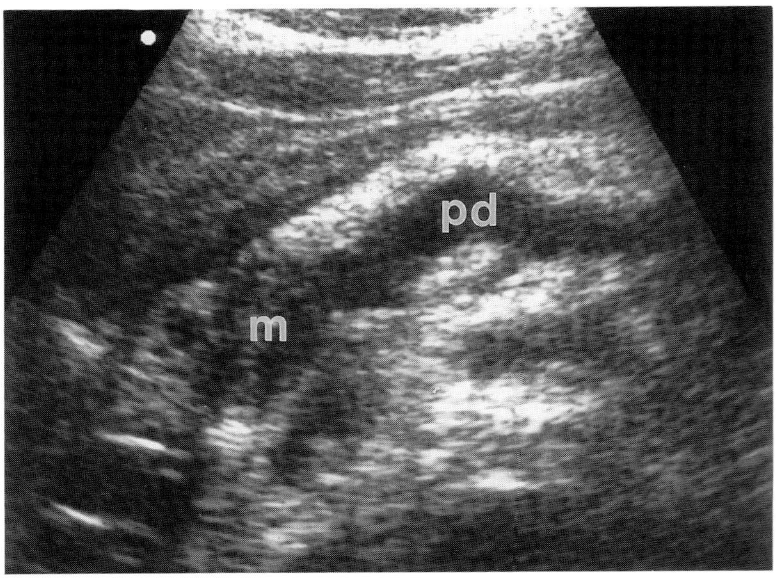

(B)

Figure 12. "Double duct" sign in a patient with pancreatic carcinoma. Oblique ultrasound (A) shows marked dilatation of the common hepatic duct (CHD) and intrahepatic ducts (arrowheads) in this patient with pancreatic carcinoma. A hypoechoic hepatic metastasis (arrows) is also noted (PV, portal vein). Transverse ultrasound (B) at a lower level shows the hypoechoic primary tumor (m) in the head of the pancreas with dilatation of the pancreatic duct (pd).

Table 3. Ultrasound for the detection of choledocholithiasis

Reference	Study Description
Quinn et al. (41)[a]	71 patients with CBD obstruction. 85% accuracy rate for detecting choledocholithiasis
Gross et al. (42)[b]	90 patients underwent ultrasound and ERCP. Ultrasound was 25% sensitive, 89% specific, with a 50% positive predictive value and 73% negative predictive value for choledocholithiasis
Cronan et al. (43)[b]	87 patients with biliary symptomatology were evaluated with ultrasound prior to surgery. Ultrasound had a sensitivity of 13% and a positive predictive value of 92% for detecting choledocholithiasis. All true positive ultrasound diagnoses were in patients with a dilated CBD
Mitchell and Clark (44)[a]	49 and 32 patients were evaluated with ultrasound and CT, respectively. For the detection of choledocholithiasis ultrasound had a sensitivity of 8% and an accuracy of 19%; CT had a sensitivity of 87% and an accuracy of 84%
Epstein et al. (45)[a]	138 patients with proven choledocholithiasis. Ultrasound accuracy was 22% and most cases (87%) were detected in patients with CBD dilatation
Pasanen et al. (47)[b]	220 patients evaluated with ultrasound, CT, and ERCP. The sensitivity was 22.2, 24, and 78.9%, respectively. The differences in sensitivity between ultrasound and ERCP and between CT and ERCP were statistically significant ($p < .0001$)

[a]Retrospective study.
[b]Prospective study.

Strictures

Strictures are difficult to define at ultrasound. In some cases an abrupt caliber change can be seen; rarely is the cause of stricture apparent. In patients with HIV disease, AIDS cholangitis may lead to stricture formation. In the appropriate clinical setting, distal CBD wall thickening with associated proximal dilatation should suggest the diagnosis (9). Moreover, an echogenic nodule in the distal CBD, the imaging manifestation of edema of the papilla of Vater, is found in two-thirds of patients with AIDS-related cholangitis (Fig. 14) (10). Mural thickening of the CBD is the ultrasound hallmark of primary sclerosing cholangitis (Fig. 4) (48). This is a more reliable indicator of primary sclerosing cholangitis with a sensitivity of 74% than duct dilatation (48). Other findings include focal regions of periportal echogenicity, ductal dilatation above a dominant stricture, and abnormalities of the gallbladder wall. Some investigators have advocated that once the diagnosis is made by endoscopic retrograde cholangiopancreatography, ultrasound is a valuable method in following the disease and imaging complications.

Choledochal Cyst

Choledochal cyst is a congenital anomaly of the extrahepatic biliary tree. It has been subdivided according to its morphology. The most common form, Type I, is

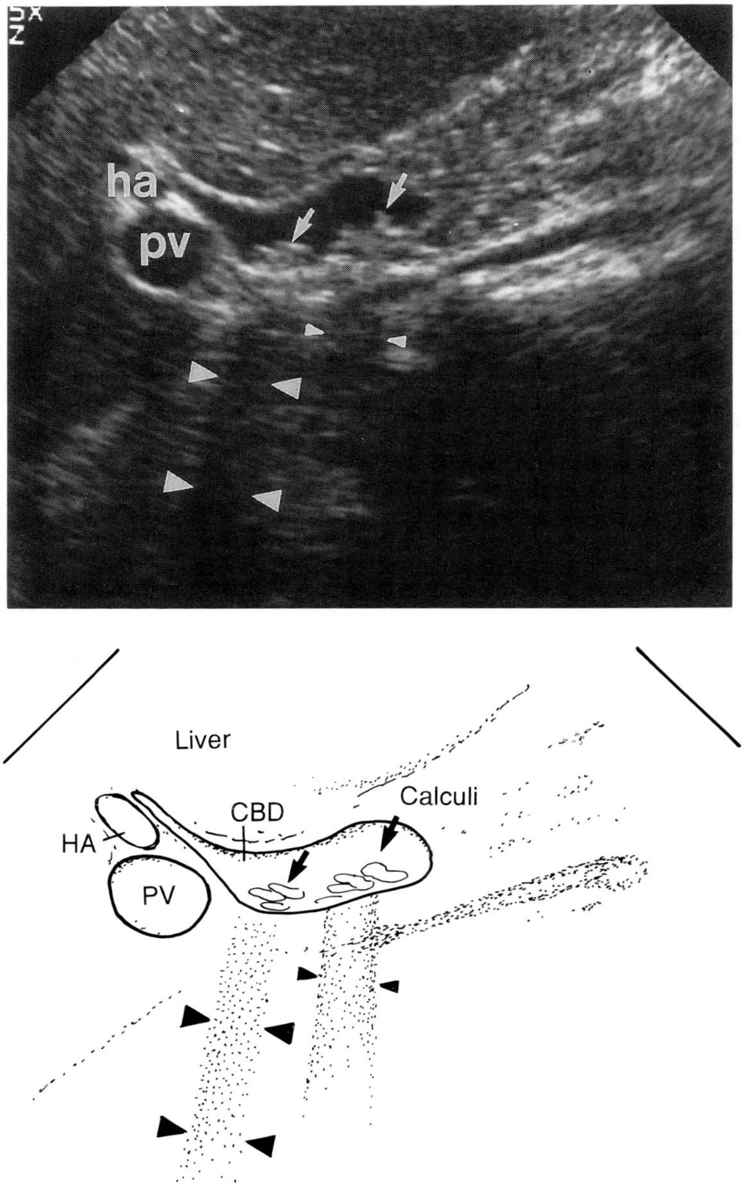

Figure 13. Choledocholithiasis. Oblique ultrasound shows shadowing (arrowheads) echogenic calculi (arrows) within a dilated extrahepatic biliary tree (PV = portal vein, HA = hepatic artery).

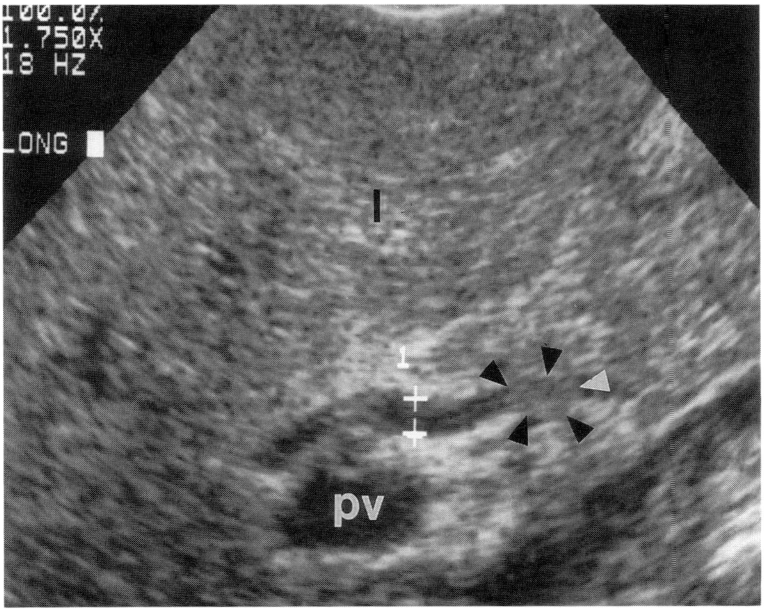

Figure 14. AIDS cholangitis. Longitudinal ultrasound shows dilatation of the common hepatic and common bile ducts. An echogenic nodule (arrowheads) in the distal CBD is typical of AIDS cholangitis. It is thought to reflect edema of the papilla of Vater (pv = portal vein; l = liver).

fusiform dilatation of the CBD. Types II and III, a diverticulum originating from the wall of the CBD and a choledochocele, respectively, are quite rare. The ultrasound findings reflect the type of cyst present (Fig. 15). The differential diagnosis includes pancreatic pseudocyst, hepatic cyst, and enteric duplication cyst. By demonstrating the relationship of the cyst to the biliary tree, ultrasound can suggest the correct diagnosis.

LAPAROSCOPIC ULTRASOUND

Laparoscopic cholecystectomy has been gaining momentum for managing cholelithiasis (49). However, even its most ardent supporters recognize that reduced intraoperative exposure of relevant anatomy including anatomic variations, discrepancy between three-dimensional structures displayed on a two-dimensional monitor, and inability to palpate critical structures are all important limitations. These factors may contribute to the greater incidence of bile duct injuries with resultant obstruction or leakage during laparoscopic cholecystectomy compared with those during open cholecystectomy, 0.5 and 2.7%, respectively (50). Because of this increased morbidity, routine intraoperative cholangiography has been advocated by some (51). Critics argue that it entails radiation exposure to the patient and personnel, adds substantially to anesthesia time, requires specialized equipment, may cause duct injury, and is unsuccessful in 10% of patients (52). In an effort to overcome some limitations

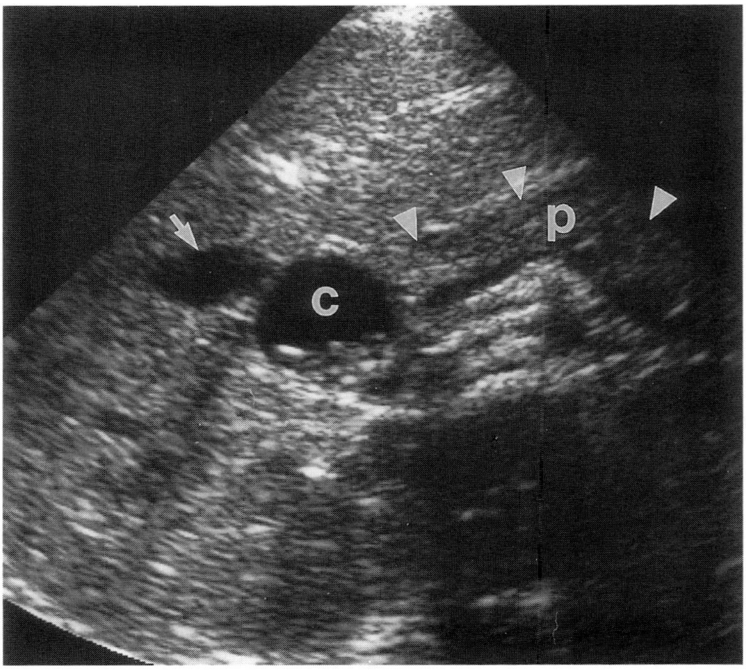

Figure 15. Choledochal cyst. Transverse ultrasound shows a cyst (c) with echogenic debris interposed between a dilated extrahepatic biliary tree (arrow) and the pancreas (arrowheads, p). At ERCP this proved to be a choledochal cyst.

of laparoscopic cholecystectomy without relying on routine intraoperative cholangiography, ultrasound transducers for laparoscopes have been developed (53). Alternatively, catheter-based ultrasound probes initially intended for intravascular applications have been recruited to assist laparoscopic cholecystectomy (54).

Irrespective of which system is employed, the techniques are somewhat comparable. The catheter-based or laparoscopic ultrasound probe is placed through a right subcostal or epigastric trocar and "dragged" along the biliary tree (54). For laparoscopic probes, longitudinal images of the extrahepatic bile ducts are obtained by applying the apparatus against the liver and using the hepatic parenchyma as a sonographic window (53, 55). Both methods have met with some success.

Using a rigid or deflectable probe fitted with a side-viewing 7.5-MHz linear array transducer, laparoscopic sonography was able to identify the inferior vena cava and the portal and superior mesenteric veins in 92 of 92 cases (100%); the cystic artery was identified in only one-third of patients (33%) (55). The CBD was visualized in all cases from the hilum to the suprapancreatic portion, whereas the intrapancreatic portion and the papilla were seen in 87 of 92 cases (95%) (55). Choledocholithiasis and cystic duct stones were identified in 3 of 92 patients (55). As with transabdominal ultrasound, air in the biliary tree from prior sphincterotomy precluded laparoscopic interrogation in one patient.

The catheter-based ultrasound systems use a higher-frequency transducer, 12.5-MHz, to survey the extrahepatic biliary tree, the tradeoff being better spatial resolution with a more limited ultrasonographic field of view. In 20 patients undergoing

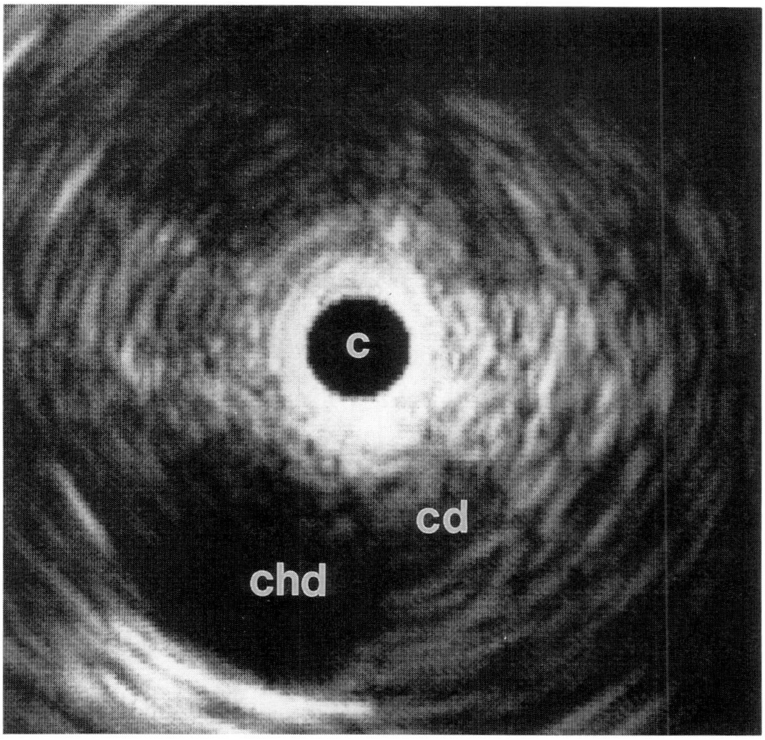

Figure 16. Cystic duct and common hepatic duct (CHD) junction. Transverse transmural ultrasound shows the cystic duct (cd) joining the common hepatic duct (chd).

laparoscopic cholecystectomy, the CHD in the vicinity of the cystic duct was seen in all patients; the junction of the cystic duct with the hepatic duct was seen in nine patients (Fig. 16) (54). The hepatic artery, cystic artery, and portal vein were identified in 10, 5, and 14 patients, respectively (54). There were no intraoperative ultrasound findings to suggest frank duct injury and no patient had clinical evidence to support bile leak at follow-up. Because no retained CBD calculi were imaged in these patients, a pig model implanted with human calculi in the suprapancreatic portion of the CBD was evaluated. The catheter-based ultrasound system performed well (Fig. 17); CBD stones appeared as expected, echogenic shadowing foci, and the size of the calculi were in agreement with their known dimensions determined prior to placement in the porcine CBD (54).

Laparoscopic and catheter-based sonography offer high-quality images of the extrahepatic biliary tree. Advancement in sonographic technology should lead to a wide selection of dedicated ultrasound probes with end and/or side-view transducers coupled with Doppler and color flow capabilities.

FUTURE DIRECTIONS

Transabdominal ultrasound remains the imaging modality of choice for screening the biliary tree. Continued advances in color and duplex (e.g., power Doppler)

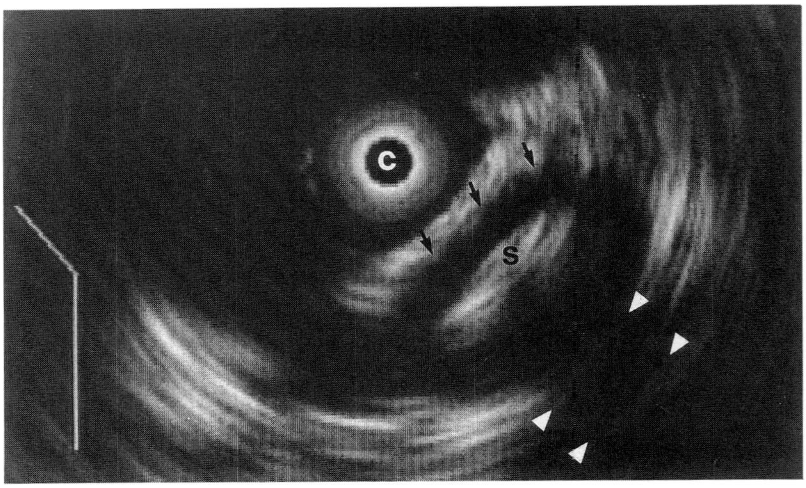

Figure 17. Porcine common bile duct implanted with human gallstones. Transverse transmural ultrasound of porcine CBD (arrows) containing a human gallstone (s) with associated acoustic shadowing (arrowheads) (c = catheter, CBD = common bile duct).

imaging will further strengthen its role. Recently the feasibility of ultrasound interrogation of the biliary tree via a percutaneous transhepatic biliary fistula was proved. By placing an ultrasound probe directly within the biliary tree, the investigators were able to evaluate the intra- and extrahepatic bile ducts, the portal vein, and the hepatic artery (56). Moreover, in patients with bile duct cancer they were able to diagnose the depth of invasion with a 93% accuracy rate (56). Although the patient population was small, this work suggests that intraductal ultrasound may be an important modality for staging biliary malignancy in the future.

REFERENCES

1. Bressler EL, Rubin JM, McCracken S, et al. Sonographic parallel channel sign: a reappraisal. *Radiology* 1987;164:343–346.
2. Laing FC, London LA, Filly RA. Ultrasonographic identification of dilated intrahepatic bile ducts and their differentiation from portal venous structures. *J Clin Ultrasound* 1978;6:90–94.
3. Laing FC. Rumack CM, Wilson SR, Charboneau JW, eds. "The Gallbladder and Bile Ducts" in *Diagnostic Ultrasound,* St. Louis: Mosby Year Book; 1991:106–144.
4. Filly RA, Sommer FG, Minton MJ. Characterization of biological fluids by ultrasound and computed tomography. *Radiology* 1980;134:167–171.
5. Sample WF, Sarti DA, Goldstein, LI, et al. Gray-scale ultrasonography of the jaundiced patient. *Radiology* 1978;128:719–725.
6. Byung IC, Lim JH, Han MC, et al. Biliary cystadenoma and cystadenocarcinoma: computed tomography and sonographic findings. *Radiology* 1989;171:57–61.
7. Carroll BA, Oppenheimer DA. Sclerosing cholangitis: sonographic demonstration of bile duct wall thickening. *AJR*. 1982;139:1016–1018.

8. Singcharoen T, Baddeley H, Benson M, et al. Primary sclerosing cholangitis: sonographic findings. *Aust Radiol.* 1986;30:99–102.
9. Dolmatch BL, Laing FC, Federle MP, et al. AIDS-related cholangitis: radiographic findings in nine patients. *Radiology.* 1987;163:313–316.
10. Da Silva, Bourdghene, Leconte I, Delage Y, Grange JD, Bigot JM. Sonography in AIDS-related cholangitis: prevalence and cause of an echogenic nodule in the distal end of the common bile duct. *AJR* 1993;160:1205–1207.
11. Federle MP, Cello JP, Laing FC, et al. Recurrent pyogenic cholangitis in Asian immigrants. *Radiology.* 1982;143:151–156.
12. Laing FC. Ultasound diagnosis of choledocholithiasis. *Semin Ultrasound CT MR.* 1987; 8:103–113.
13. Marchal GJ, Desmer VJ, Proesmans WC, et al. Caroli's disease: high-frequency ultrasound and pathologic findings. *Radiology.* 1986;158:507–511.
14. Mittelstaedt CA, Volberg FM, Fisher GJ, et al. Caroli's disease: sonographic findings. *AJR.* 1980;136:585–587.
15. Weill F, Eisencher A, Zeltner F. Ultrasonic study of the normal and dilated biliary tree. *Radiology.* 1978;127:221–224.
16. Cooperberg PL. High-resolution real-time ultraound in the evaluation of the normal and obstructed biliary tract. *Radiology.* 1978;129:477–480.
17. Grahm MF, Cooperberg PL, Cohen MM, et al. The size of the normal common hepatic duct following cholecystectomy: an ultrasonographic study. *Radiology.* 1980;135: 137–139.
18. Behan M, Kazam E. Sonography of the common bile duct: value of the right anterior oblique view. *AJR* 1978;130:701–709.
19. Paruleker SG. Ultrasound evaluation of common bile duct size. *Radiology.* 1979; 133:703–703.
20. Mueller PR, Ferrucci JT, Simeone JF, et al. Postcholecystectomy bile duct dilatation: myth or reality? *AJR.* 1981;136:355–358.
21. Niederau C, Muller J, Sonnenberg A, et al. Extrahepatic bile ducts in healthy subjects, in patients with cholelithiaisis, and in postcholecystectomy patients: a prospective ultrasonic study. *J Clin Ultrasound.* 1983;11:23–27.
22. Wu CC, Ho YH, Chen CY. Effect of aging on common bile duct diameter: a real-time ultrasonographic study. *J Clin Ultrasound.* 1984;12:473–478.
23. Ferrucci JT, Adson MA, Mueller PR, et al. Advances in the radiology of jaundice. *AJR.* 1983;141:1–20.
24. Koenigsberg M, Wiener SN, Walzer A. The accuracy of sonography in the differential diagnosis of obstructive jaundice: a comparison with cholangiography. *Radiology.* 1979;133:157–165.
25. Jacobson JB, Brody PA. The transverse common duct. *AJR.* 1981;136:91–95.
26. Berland LL, Lawson TL, Foley WD. Porta hepatis: sonographic discrimination of bile ducts from arteries with pulsed Doppler with new anatomic criteria. *AJR.* 1982;138: 833–840.
27. Zeman RK, Taylor KJW, Burrell MI, et al. Ultrasound demonstration of anicteric dilatation of the biliary tree. *Radiology.* 1980;134:689–692.
28. Muhletaler CA, Gerlock AJ Jr, Fleischer AC, et al. Diagnosis of obstructive jaundice with nondilated bile ducts. *AJR.* 1980;134:1149–1152.
29. Simeone JF, Butch RJ, Mueller PR, et al. The bile ducts after a fatty meal: further sonographic observations. *Radiology.* 1986;160:29–31.

30. Darwesh RM, Dodds WJ, Hogan WJ. Fatty meal sonography for evaluating patients with suspected partial commond duct obstruction. *AJR.* 1988;151:63–68.
31. Wilson SA, Bosink BB, van Sonnenberg E. Unchanged size of a dilated common bile duct after fatty meal: results and significance. *Radiology.* 1986;160:29–31.
32. Laing FC, Jeffrey RB Jr, Wing VW. Biliary dilatation: defining the level and cause by real-time ultrasound. *Radiology.* 1986;160:39–42.
33. Meyer DG, Weinstein BJ. Klatskin tumors of the bile ducts: sonographic appearance. *Radiology.* 1983;148:803–804.
34. Machan L, Muller NL, Cooperberg PL. Sonographic diagnosis of Klatskin tumors. *AJR.* 1986;147:509–512.
35. Garber SJ, Lees WR. The characterization of pancreatic and bile duct tumours by duplex Doppler. *Clin Radiol.* 1992;45:181–184.
36. Looser C, Stain SC, Baer HU, Triller J, Blumgart LH. Staging of hilar cholangiocarcinoma by ultrasound and duplex sonography: a comparison with angiography and operative findings. Br J Radiol. 1992; 65:871–877.
37. Jackson VP, Lappas JC. Sonography of the Mirizzi syndrome. *J Ultrasound Med.* 1984;143:591–596.
38. Cerri BB, Leite GJ, Simoes JB, et al. Ultrasonographic evaluation of ascaris in the biliary tract. *Radiology.* 1983;146:753–754.
39. Lim JH. Radiologic findings of clonorchiasis. *AJR.* 1990;155:1000–1008.
40. Zeman RK, Burrell MI. *Biliary Obstruction—Specific Disease Entities in Gallbladder and Bile Duct Imaging: A Clinical Radiologic Approach.* New York: Churchill Livingstone, 1987:471–592.
41. Quinn MF, Ralls PW, Boswell WD, et al. Predicting the cause of common bile duct obstruction with sonographic data analysis of binary variables. *Invest Radiol.* 1982; 17:316–323.
42. Gross BH, Harter LB, Gore RM, et al. Ultrasonic evaluation of common bile duct stones. Prospective comparison with endoscopic retrograde cholangiopancreatography. *Radiology.* 1983;146:471.
43. Cronan JJ, Mueller PR, Simeone JF. Prospective diagnosis of choledocholithiasis. *Radiology.* 1983;146:467–469.
44. Mitchell SE, Clark RA. A comparison of computed tomography and sonography in choledocholithiasis. *AJR.* 1984;142:729–733.
45. Einstein DM, Lapin SA, Ralls P, Halls JM. The insensitivity of sonography in the detection of choledocholithiasis. *AJR.* 1984;142:725–728.
46. Dong B, Chen M. Improved sonographic visualization of choledocholithiasis. *J Clin Ultrasound.* 1987;15:185–190.
47. Pasanen P, Partanen K, Pikkarainen P, Alhava E, Pirinen A, Janatuinen E. Ultrasonography, CT, and ERCP in the diagnosis of choledochal stones. *Acta Radiol.* 1992;3:53–56.
48. Marjorie CBL, Smits NJ, Phoa SSKS, Reeders JWAJ, Jansen PLM. Primary sclerosing cholangitis: sonographic findings. *Abdom Imaging.* 1993;20:109–112.
49. Ascher SM, Evans SRT, Zeman RK. Laparoscopic cholecystectomy: ultrasound of the extrahepatic biliary tree and the natural history of postoperative transabdominal ultrasound findings. *Semin Ultrasound CT MRI.* 1993;14:331–337.
50. Hunter JG. Avoidance of bile duct injury during laparoscopic cholecystectomy. *Am J Surg.* 1991;162:71–76.
51. Balachandran S, Goodman P, Saydjari R, et al. Operative cholangiography in patients undergoing laparoscopic cholecystectomy: unique radiographic findings. *AJR.* 1992; 159:65–67.

52. Berci G, Sakeir JM. The Los Angeles experience with laparoscopic cholecystectomy. *Am J Surg.* 1991;161:345–349.
53. Jakimowicz JJ. Technical aspects of intraoperative ultrasound applicable to laparoscopic ultrasound. *Endosc Surg Allied Technol.* 1994;2:119–126.
54. Ascher SM, Evans SRT, Goldberg JA, et al. Intraoperative bile duct sonography during laparoscopic cholecystectomy: experience with a 12.5-MHz catheter-based US probe. *Radiology.* 1992;185:493–496.
55. Bezzi M, Melino B, Orsi F, Di Nardo F, Silecchia G, Basso N, Passariello R, Rossi P. Laparoscopic sonography during abdominal laparascopic surgery: technique and imaging findings. *AJR.* 1995;165:1193–1198.
56. Kuroiwa M, Tsukamoto Y, Naitoh Y, et al. New techniques using intraductal ultrasonography for the diagnosis of bile duct cancer. *J Ultrasound Med.* 1994;13;189–195.

8

COMPUTED TOMOGRAPHY OF THE BILIARY TREE

Robert K. Zeman, M.D.
University of Vermont College of Medicine
Burlington, VT

Susan M. Ascher, M.D.
Georgetown University Medical Center
Washington, DC

Computed tomography (CT), especially helical (spiral) CT, has made great strides in its ability to detect abnormalities of the upper abdomen (1). It plays an important role in the evaluation of patients with biliary tract disease. Along with other noninvasive cross-sectional studies, CT is used as a screening technique to select those patients who need more invasive procedures such as cholangiography, percutaneous biopsy, laparoscopy, or open surgical exploration. This chapter reviews the diagnostic approach, technical aspects, normal anatomy, and CT findings in the evaluation of patients with suspected biliary obstruction (2).

DIAGNOSTIC APPROACH

Computed tomography is used in the initial evaluation of patients who have a history suggestive of progressive jaundice with other symptoms suggesting chronicity such as weight loss or back pain. In this group of patients malignancy is likely (2). Ultrasound is used for screening when the diagnosis of obstruction is less certain on clinical grounds, or when cholecystitis or choledocholithiasis is suspected as the source of the patients' symptoms. Ultrasound is less expensive than CT, but adds little to the diagnostic work-up in patients who are likely to have neoplasm, especially pancreatic carcinoma. Computed tomography offers sensitivity comparable to that of transabdominal ultrasound in allowing the recognition of intrahepatic duct dilatation, and is far superior to ultrasound for evaluation of abnormalities affecting the distal common bile duct. It is commonly performed to detect and help stage pancreatic carcinoma, cholangiocarcinoma, gallbladder carcinoma, and lymphoma. It allows determination of the presence of advanced disease and whether the obstruction is intra- or extrahepatic, and suggests the likely diagnosis. If advanced, widespread disease is present, there is often little more to do but perform percutaneous biopsy and establish biliary drainage (2).

In patients with biliary obstruction, CT should be performed before endoscopic retrograde cholangiopancreatography (ERCP) and stent placement. Assessment of surrounding tissue planes and major vessels is far easier when a stent is not present. Even nonmetallic stents produce streak artifacts and degrade the image. Because it is not necessary to administer oral barium in evaluating pancreatobiliary disease, ERCP can be performed almost immediately after CT should it be needed.

Patients with metastases from remote primary tumors, which have spread to involve the liver, biliary tract, and pancreas, are surviving longer due to progress in palliative alternatives. In this setting biliary obstruction is commonly diagnosed upon CT prior to the onset of symptoms or jaundice. Dilated bile ducts on routine, follow-up CT scans performed as part of the patient's ongoing care are not uncommon. Obstruction typically results from adenopathy involving the porta hepatis or peripancreatic lymph nodes or from segmental biliary obstruction due to hepatic metastases.

Computed tomography provides the most effective means for guiding biopsies of the pancreas, liver, and adjacent lymph nodes. Although in many instances the imaging appearance of abnormalities in this region is not specific, the judicious use of percutaneous biopsy has proved safe and efficacious in large numbers of patients. Histological biopsies using 18- to 20-gauge needles, or "biopsy guns," are becoming commonplace. If the stomach or intestine must be breached, a 22-gauge needle is used for cytology only. In our experience, even when evaluation is limited to cytology, the diagnosis may be made in approximately 90% of patients who subsequently prove to have malignancy.

TECHNICAL ISSUES

The quality of the CT examination greatly depends on the radiologist, as well as the quality and speed of the CT instrument available within the institution. It is often stated that ultrasonography is highly operator-dependent. In the age of helical (spiral) CT, we are finding that CT is even more operator-dependent. The scanning techniques and contrast administration methods must be optimized in the setting of pancreatobiliary disease. The use of old equipment or cutting corners on the examination technique lowers costs, but greatly compromises the clinical relevance and reliability of the interpretation results. It is vital that the radiologist understand the clinical issues in pancreatobiliary disease and work closely with the gastroenterologist, oncologist, and surgeon.

Although conventional CT scans performed in 10-mm increments allow crude assessment of the biliary tract and pancreas, helical (spiral) CT has dramatically improved our ability to see fine detail in these structures (3, 4). Conventional scanners use a "stop-and-go" approach to imaging. An individual section is acquired, the table is advanced, and then the table is stopped to acquire the next section.

This often leads to misregistration artifact resulting from the patient being asked to hold his or her breath for the acquisition of each individual section. It may take 3 min or more for a conventional scan of the abdomen. During a helical scan, the table moves *during* the X-ray exposure and acquisition of CT data. This results in a helically shaped volumetric data set. The entire upper abdomen may usually be scanned in 30 sec or less. Scanning speed has resulted in the ability to scan the entire liver, biliary tract, and pancreas with thin collimation, although the circulating level of intravenous contrast material is at its peak.

Because the helical acquisition is volumetric, the spacing or interval between reconstructed sections may be varied and selected by the user even after the scan acquisition has been completed. If the reconstruction spacing that is selected is less than the collimation, overlapping sections result. The ability to relocate scan sections offers great advantage for visualization of small pancreatic or biliary tumors. Small lesions that straddle two adjacent slices may not be well visualized owing to volume averaging; however, a section centered precisely on the lesion may show it in greater detail. Short segments of vascular encasement may also be evaluated using closely spaced, overlapping reconstruction of the helical CT data. Overlapping sections may be used as the source data for three-dimensional (3D) rendering of the bile ducts and mesenteric vessels. At least 50% overlap (that is, 5-mm "thin" sections reconstructed at 2-mm intervals) allow for artifact-free 3D models. Overlapping reconstruction does not result in any greater radiation exposure to the patient than nonoverlapping reconstruction.

For pancreatobiliary imaging, 5-mm or less collimation should be used. "Thicker" sections often make it difficult to diagnose small lesions or detect common duct stones.

ANATOMIC CONSIDERATIONS

On contrast-enhanced helical CT scans, the hepatic arteries and the portal veins must be well opacified. Normal-size intrahepatic ducts are not identifiable. Occasionally the right or left hepatic duct may be visualized (5). The hepatic duct is usually no more than 2–3 mm in diameter. It is important not to confuse small amounts of fat surrounding the hepatic vessels with dilated ducts. Similarly, patients who have ascites, a recent history of abdominal trauma, or recent liver transplant may have hepatic lymphedema (6); this is manifest as a low-attenuation halo, circumferentially surrounding the portal veins. This also may mimic, but should not be confused with dilated bile ducts which reside anterior to the vessels.

Within the porta hepatis, the common hepatic duct will be seen anterior to the hepatic artery and portal vein (7) (Fig. 1). In the axial plane the hepatic artery may actually be seen coursing laterally through the section. The common hepatic duct should not exceed 0.6 cm in diameter (8, 9). Despite earlier controversy, it is now clear that the duct caliber should not increase from prior uncomplicated cholecystectomy (10). The duct wall should be less than 1.5 mm in thickness (11). In patients who have sclerosing cholangitis, the duct wall may be thickened. As the common bile duct descends into the pancreas, its diameter is variable, but usually greater than that of the common hepatic duct. Once within the pancreatic substance, the duct migrates progressively posteriorly on its way to the ampulla of Vater. At the

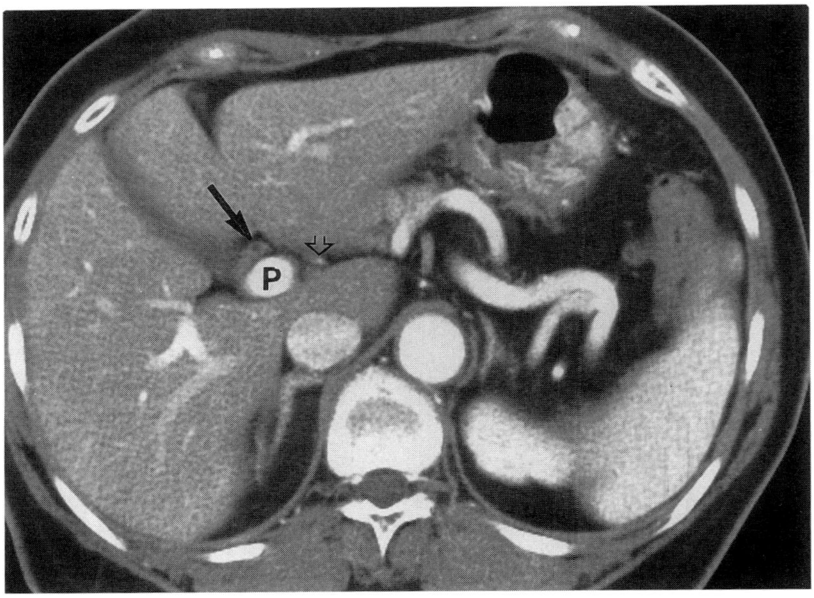

Figure 1. Normal common hepatic duct. Contrast-enhanced helical scan shows the normal caliber common hepatic duct (arrow) anterior to the portal vein (P). The normal duct is seen in this location in more than 90% of patients. The hepatic artery is also visualized (open arrow).

level of the ampulla, the duct may actually be seen crossing the pancreaticoduodenal space to enter the duodenal wall. This space separates the pancreatic head from the duodenum and is normally filled with fat, multiple retroduodenal veins, and small lymph nodes. The gastroduodenal artery may be seen anterior to the common bile duct on sections through the pancreatic head (Fig. 2).

When the bile duct is obstructed, its caliber increases. In general, duct caliber is greatest in patients with long-standing obstruction and markedly elevated bilirubin levels. Minimal dilatation is common in patients with low-grade obstruction, and may even occur prior to the development of significant hyperbilirubinemia (12). Because of Laplace's law, the extrahepatic duct usually dilates sooner and to a greater extent than the intrahepatic ducts (13). Unfortunately, in the setting of intermittent or ball-valve obstruction, as occurs with choledocholithiasis, dilatation of the ducts may not be a prominent feature (14). The radiologist must carefully follow the bile duct from section to section to look for subtle caliber or contour changes. It is important to scrutinize any transition zones present (15, 16). When the duct is abruptly narrowed or amputated, this often suggests the presence of neoplasm as the underlying cause. Stones within the duct typically produce a bull's-eye appearance owing to bile surrounding the stone just above its equator (17). Many of the characteristic appearances that have been observed on cholangiography over the years also apply to analysis of the duct contour on CT (Fig. 3).

At times the axial sections do not give a clear picture of the 3D relationships. Tubular structures such as the bile ducts and splanchnic vessels can be difficult to trace from section to section. We now have the ability to display 3D anatomy

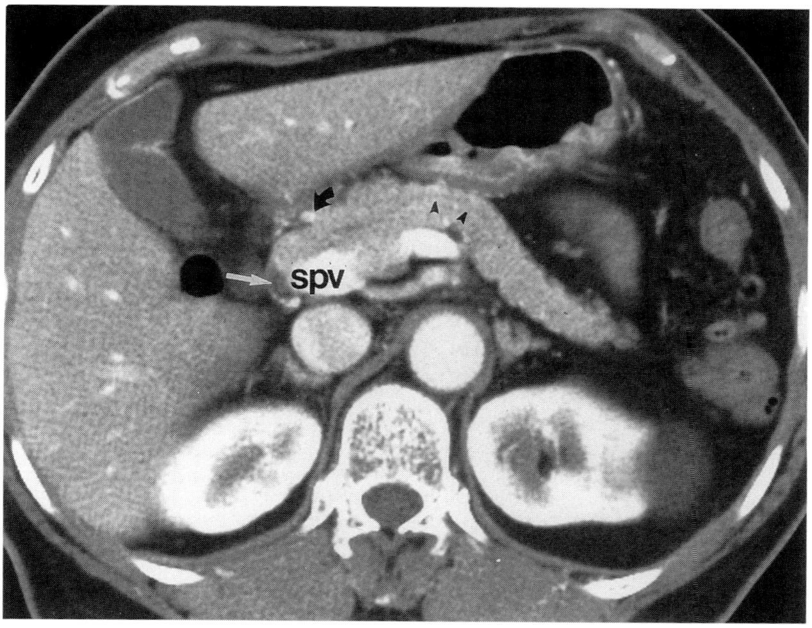

Figure 2. Normal common bile duct and gastroduodenal artery. Contrast-enhanced helical CT shows a borderline-sized distal common bile duct (arrow) coursing through the section The duct typically resides at the lateral edge of the pancreatic parenchyma, just lateral to the splenoportal confluence (spv). The faint enhancement just posterior to the duct is due to retroduodenal veins that are closely applied. The gastroduodenal artery (curved arrow) and normal-sized pancreatic duct (arrowheads) are also identified.

for surgical planning (18, 19). The overlapping section data are volumetrically reconstructed and post-processed to display only structures of a specific attenuation. Although 3D rendering is not necessary in every case, it can help the radiologist evaluate the vascular and biliary anatomy in patients with pancreatobiliary neoplasms (see Fig. 6 below and Chapter 22). It also may be useful for the surgeon considering biliary bypass or pancreatic resection. This technology should be available as an adjunct when needed.

CHARACTERIZATION OF SPECIFIC ETIOLOGIES OF OBSTRUCTION

Because many patients' initial imaging evaluations are with a cross-sectional study, it makes sense to classify the diseases that may obstruct the biliary tract based on cross-sectional findings. This can be done in many ways, but it is useful to categorize pancreatobiliary diseases on CT as follows: diseases that usually produce mass effect, diseases that occasionally produce mass effect, or diseases that seldom produce mass effect (2, 20) (Fig. 4).

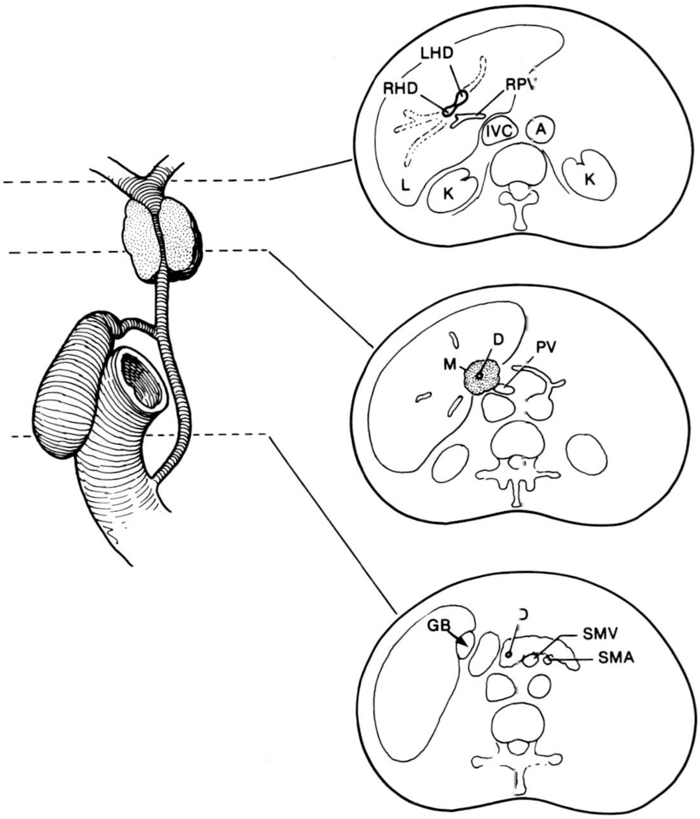

(A)

Figure 3. Schematic depiction correlating cholangiographic appearance with cross-sectional findings. (A) Cholangiocarcinoma. (B) Pancreatic or ampullary carcinoma. (LHD = left hepatic duct, RHD = right hepatic duct, RPV = right portal vein, L = liver, IVC = inferior vena cava, K = kidney, A = aorta, D = bile duct, M = mass due to tumor, PV = main portal vein, GB = gallbladder, SMV = superior mesenteric vein, SMA = superior mesenteric artery, PD = pancreatic duct). (Copyright Robert Zeman, M.D.; used by permission.)

Diseases that Usually Produce Mass Effect

There are three common diseases that produce bulky mass effect as they obstruct the biliary tract. These are pancreatic carcinoma, metastatic disease to the liver or peribiliary lymph nodes, and gallbladder disease such as gallbladder carcinoma or Mirizzi syndrome.

Focal enlargement of the pancreas is the hallmark of pancreatic carcinoma on cross-sectional studies (21–23). As the resolution of these studies has improved, it is increasingly common to identify small tumors that cause only focal attenuation changes (24). The vast majority of tumors, however, result in enlargement of the gland when tumor is present. Because most pancreatic adenocarcinomas arise in the pancreatic head, most obstruct the pancreatic duct and bile duct. Concomitant involvement and obstruction of both ducts has been called the "double duct sign"

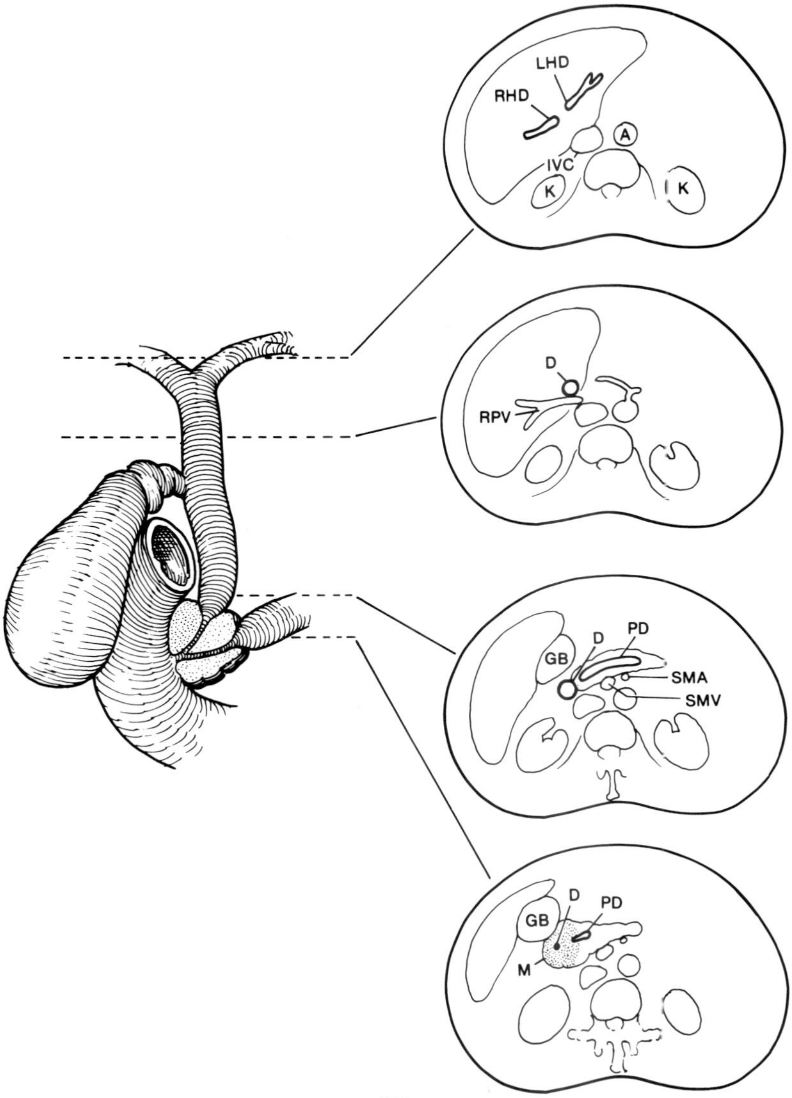

(B)

Figure 3. *(Continued)*

(Fig. 5). This sign is not specific for ampullopancreatic carcinoma: chronic pancreatitis may produce similar changes in 10–15% of cases (25). In addition to the presence of the "double duct sign," the diagnosis of carcinoma is suggested by the presence of focally reduced attenuation within the gland and enlargement of the gland contour. On CT carcinoma tends to be of low attenuation, and enhances with iodinated contrast material less than normal pancreas.

Evaluation of the pancreas is fully covered in Chapter 22. It is important to recognize the impact of new techniques for pancreatic cancer evaluation. Helical

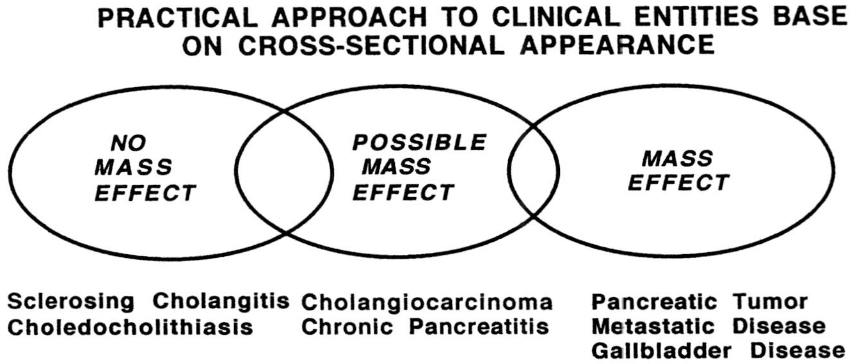

Figure 4. Presence or absence of mass effect on cross-sectional studies may be used to categorize diseases that may produce biliary obstruction.

(spiral) CT has had great impact on the ability to visualize small tumors and to detect more accurately vascular involvement as compared to conventional CT. This is especially true in detecting subtle arterial encasement. The splanchnic vessels may be displayed as a 3D model to help the surgeon formulate the surgical plan (18). In many instances the 3D model more dramatically depicts the degree and length of vascular encasement than the axial sections. When thrombus or vascular narrowing is present, the lesion is unlikely to be resectable. In more subtle cases, however, there is no substitute for direct surgical visualization. The bile ducts may also be displayed as a 3D model, affording the surgeon a view that simulates the operative field, and reveals the length of bile duct available for creation of a surgical anastomosis (19) (Fig. 6).

In many practices metastatic disease is the second most common cause of biliary obstruction associated with mass effect (26). Involvement anywhere from the intrahepatic ducts to the distal common bile duct may occur. The three most common sites of involvement are the intrahepatic ducts (encased by adjacent hepatic metastases), the common hepatic duct (compressed or invaded by porta hepatis adenopathy), and the distal bile duct (obstructed by pancreaticoduodenal lymph nodes) (27). Computed tomography readily demonstrates the level of obstruction. When hepatic metastases obstruct the intrahepatic ducts, foci of dilated ducts are seen to terminate in a focal mass. Hepatoma may give rise to a similar appearance in patients without a history of metastatic disease. Obstruction of the common hepatic duct by adenopathy in the porta hepatis appears as a soft-tissue mass-producing dilatation of the common hepatic and intrahepatic ducts (Fig. 7). Although the appearance may mimic that of a cholangiocarcinoma, the latter tends not to produce as great a mass effect as adenopathy in this region. Metastatic adenopathy is often associated with enlarged nodes in other regions. Common primary sites include tumors of gastrointestinal origin, lymphoma, lung carcinoma, and breast carcinoma. Ovarian and renal cell carcinoma may also obstruct the biliary tract. When metastases involve the bile ducts, they are almost always associated with soft-tissue mass effect. Frank invasion into the ducts may also occur and give rise to intraluminal polypoid masses.

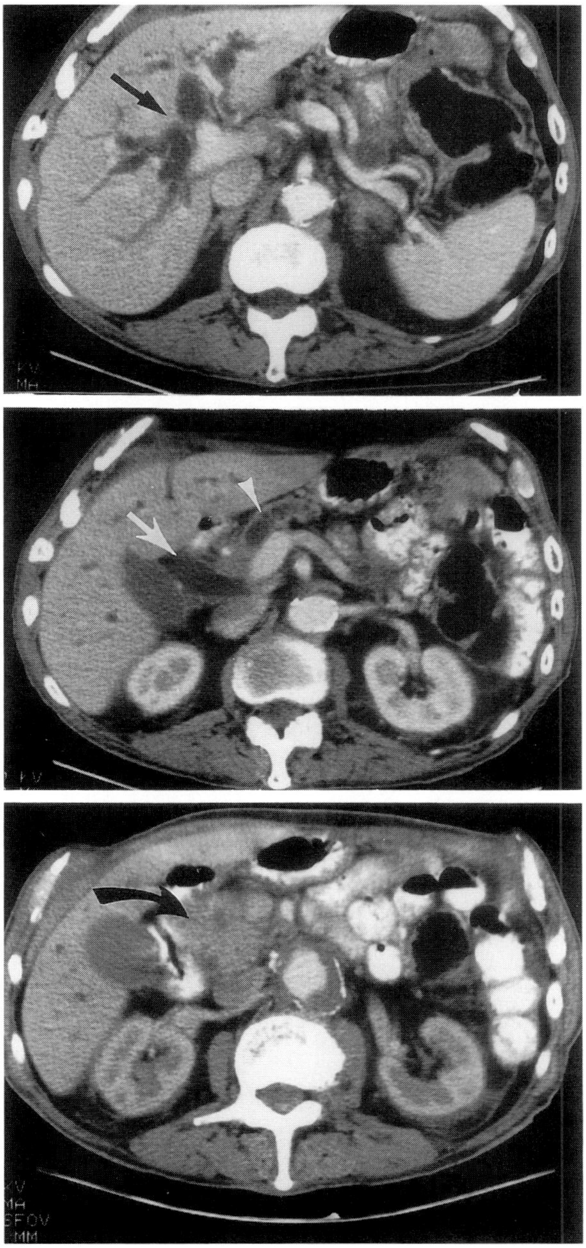

Figure 5. Pancreatic carcinoma resulting in the "double duct sign" on CT. Dilated intrahepatic ducts (arrow, top frame) are identified as water-density tubular structures within the liver. The ducts converge on a dilated common bile duct (arrow, middle frame). At the same level, a dilated pancreatic duct (arrowhead) is also identified. Scans just caudad to this level reveal the presence of a pancreatic mass (curved arrow, bottom frame). The mass caused abrupt amputation of the bile duct and pancreatic duct. This finding has been called the "double duct sign" and is suggestive of carcinoma.

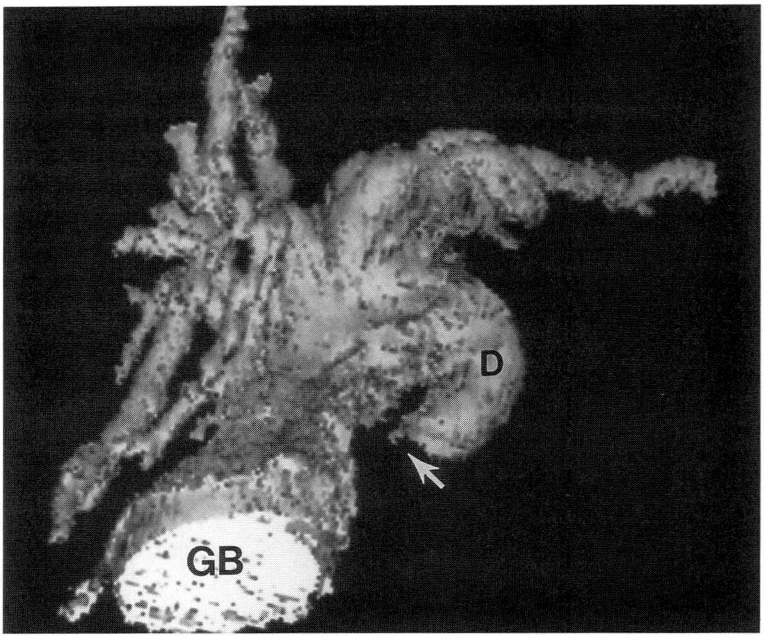

Figure 6. Three-dimensional rendering of bile duct in pancreatic carcinoma from helical CT data. Shaded surface display reveals intrahepatic and common bile ductal dilatation (D). In this patient a "high" pancreatic carcinoma has caused amputation of the duct (arrow). A Courvoisier gallbladder (GB) is also noted. Courtesy of Radiology (19).

The third most common cause of biliary obstruction associated with mass effect is gallbladder disease. Carcinoma of the gallbladder may obstruct the bile duct by direct extension through the gallbladder wall or extension into the cystic duct. Direct invasion into the liver frequently occurs at the time of presentation. Gallbladder carcinoma is presented in depth in Chapter 2. Gallbladder sarcomas are rare but may grow via the cystic duct into the common hepatic duct. This can result in a large polypoid mass protruding into the duct. Metastatic disease to the gallbladder, such as occurs with melanoma, can also rarely obstruct the bile duct, but tends to occur only in the latter stages of the disease.

Mirizzi syndrome (acute cholecystitis with erosion of a cystic duct stone directly into the common hepatic duct) results in simultaneous acute cholecystitis and biliary obstruction (28). Computed tomography demonstrates biliary dilatation, thickening and/or low-attenuation edema in the gallbladder wall, and pericholecystic inflammatory changes suggestive of acute cholecystitis (see Chapter 2). The inflammatory mass that results may actually protrude into the common hepatic duct and mimic a polypoid tumor on cholangiography. In severe cases, the entire right upper quadrant may become engulfed in inflammation, distorting the surgical biliary anatomy.

Diseases that Occasionally Produce Mass Effect

Cholangiocarcinoma in most patients produces subtle mass effect (29, 30). Many tumors are 1–2 cm in diameter and are detected on CT only after careful scrutiny

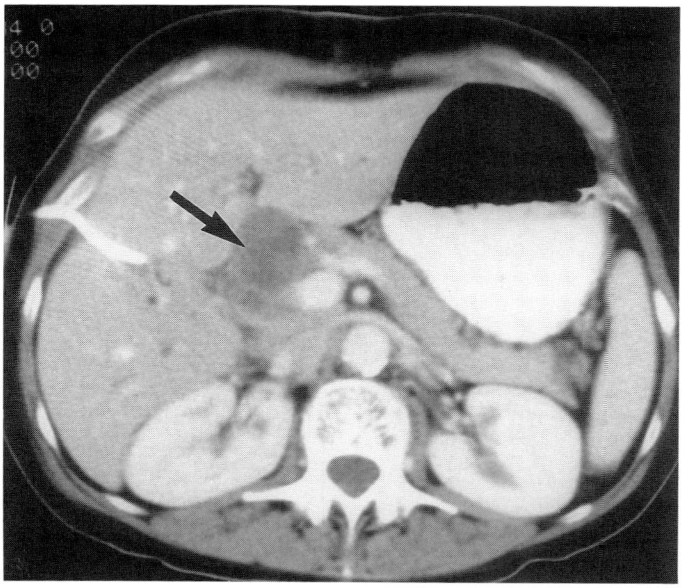

(A)

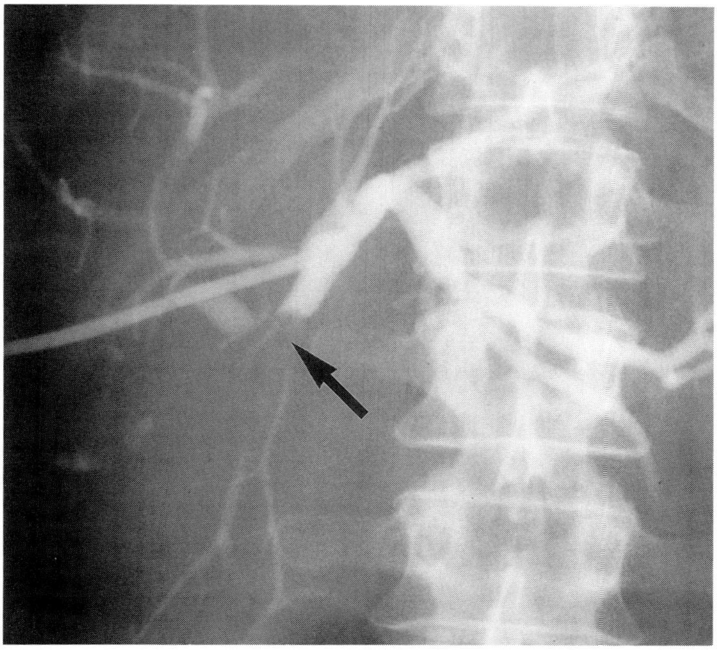

(B)

Figure 7. Lymphoma producing biliary obstruction due to bulky adenopathy in the porta hepatis. (A) CT scan reveals a bulky mass (arrow) in the porta hepatis. Mild duct dilatation was present despite the presence of a percutaneously placed biliary drainage catheters. (B) Cholangiogram shows high-grade obstruction of both the right and left hepatic ducts (arrow). Splaying of the ducts and their abrupt termination suggests malignancy. In this patient with known lymphoma, porta hepatis adenopathy caused this high-grade obstruction. The mass melted away with chemotherapy. (Copyright Robert Zeman, M.D.; used by permission.)

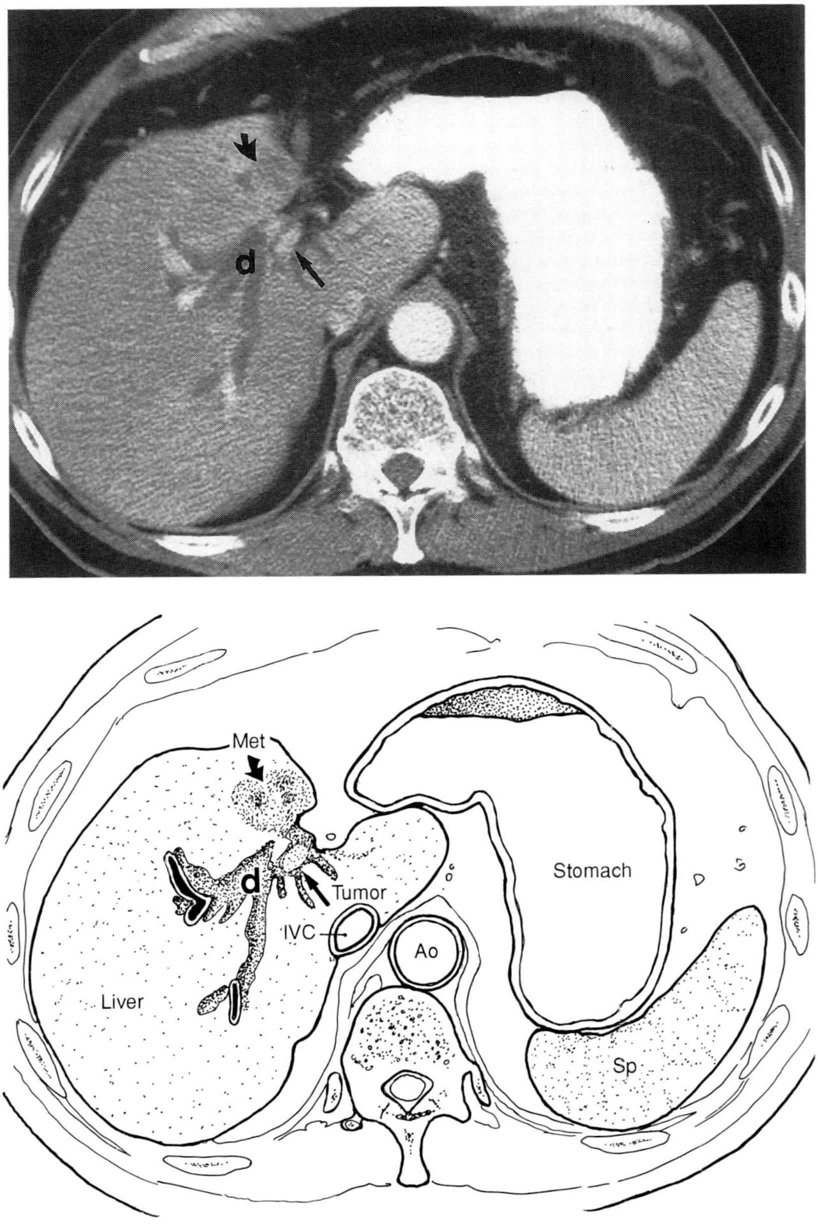

(A)

Figure 8. Cholangiocarcinoma. (A) Contrast-enhanced helical CT scan and drawing demonstrate dilated intrahepatic ducts and right hepatic duct (d), which terminate in a 1.5-cm enhancing mass (arrow). The appearance is suggestive of cholangiocarcinoma. A focal liver lesion (curved arrow) is also present. (B) Percutaneous transhepatic cholangiogram confirms obstruction of the right hepatic duct (arrow) with isolation of the right and left ductal systems. The diagnosis of cholangiocarcinoma was subsequently confirmed, and the lesion seen in the left lobe on CT proved to be a metastasis (next page).

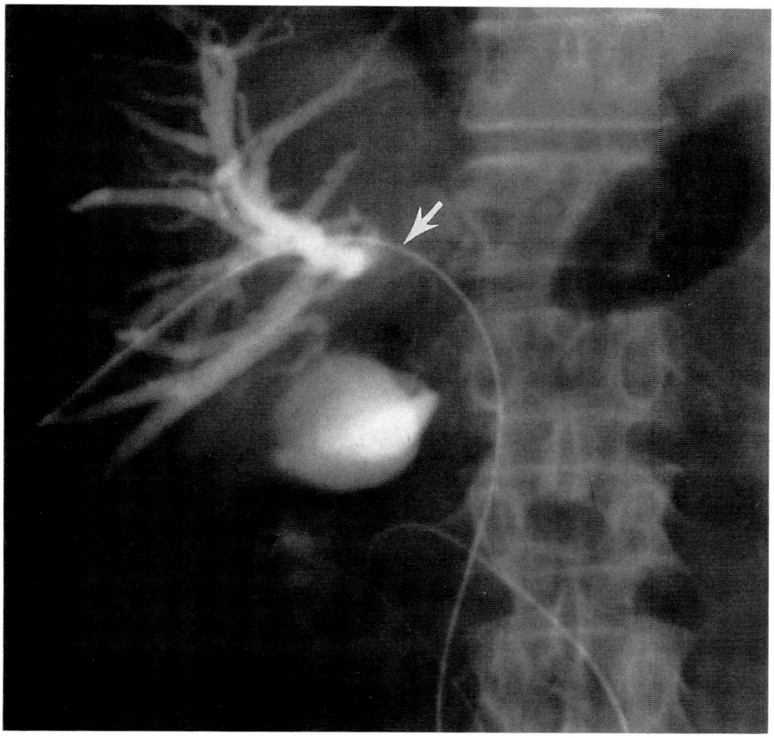

(B)

Figure 8. *(Continued)*

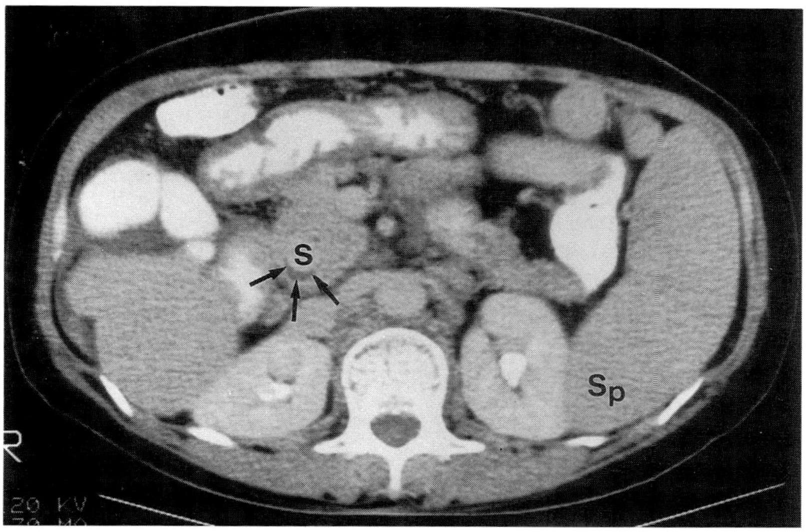

Figure 9. CT scan demonstrating choledocholithiasis. A high-attenuation stone is identified within the distal common bile duct (S). A low-attenuation halo of bile is identified surrounding the stone (arrows). This corresponds to the meniscus commonly seen on cholangiograms (Sp = enlarged spleen).

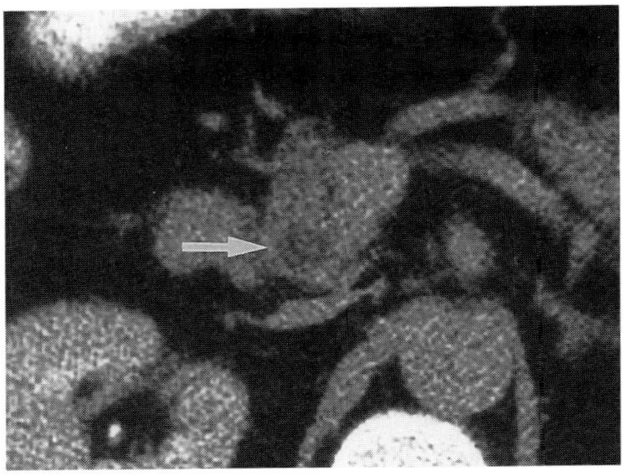

(A)

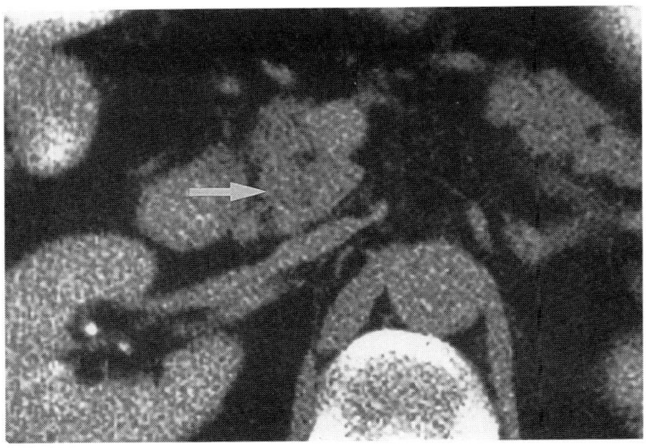

(B)

Figure 10. Reconstruction of overlapping sections to visualize better a common duct stone. (A) Section through the intrapancreatic portion of the bile duct (arrow) reveals a duct caliber of approximately 1 cm. No definite stone is identified within the duct. (B) 7 mm below the section shown in A, the duct appears of higher attenuation (arrow). Although the appearance suggests that of a stone, it could also be due to partial volume averaging with the pancreatic parenchyma and other soft tissues of the papilla. (C) Reconstruction of overlapping sections resulted in this image, between those shown in A and B. At this level, a densely calcified nidus (arrowhead) is identified within the stone. Use of overlapping reconstruction bolstered our confidence in diagnosing a common duct stone in this patient (next page). (D) ERCP confirms the presence of a common bile duct stone(s) (next page).

of the duct caliber and contour (Fig. 8). Most tumors produce a focal stenosis of the duct, but some may actually be multicentric. Polypoid and scirrhous forms also occur. The tumor may show increased or decreased attenuation compared to the liver on dynamic scans. Alternatively many cholangiocarcinomas are isoattenuated compared to liver. Because of this and the small size of many of these tumors, the diagnosis is often subtle. Delayed images 5–10 min after the contrast injection may demonstrate increased attenuation in these tumors owing to slow vascular flow (31).

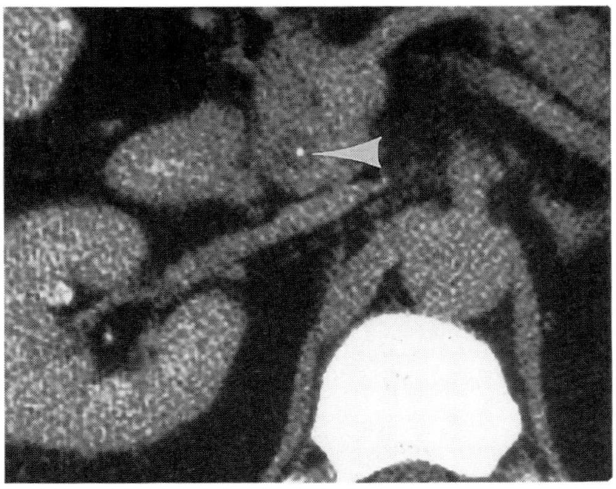

(C)

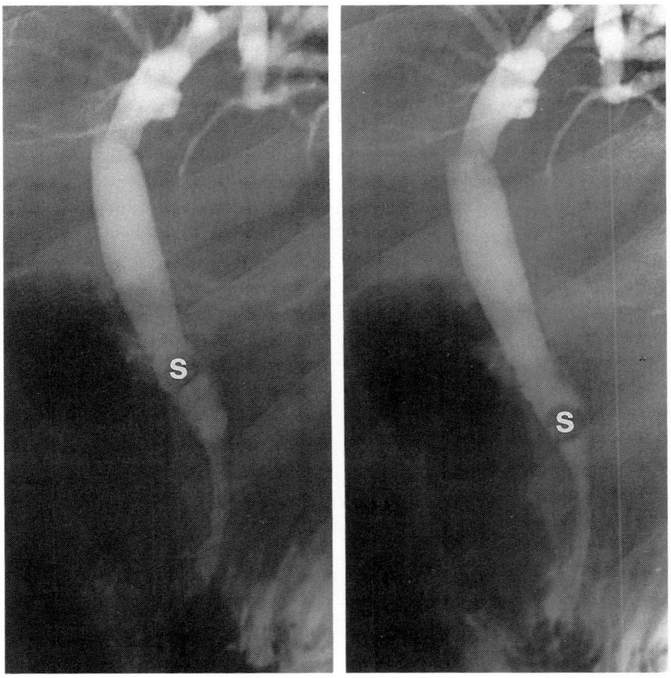

(D)

Figure 10. *(Continued)*

Roughly 50% of cholangiocarcinomas occur at the bifurcation and have earned the eponym Klatskin tumor. When the tumor occurs in this location, it produces dilatation of the right and left hepatic ducts. Computed tomography scans (and for that matter cholangiograms) must be carefully analyzed to determine the cephalad edge of the tumor. If the tumor has isolated the right and left hepatic ducts, it is usually not resectable (30). Three-dimensional display of CT data can nicely depict

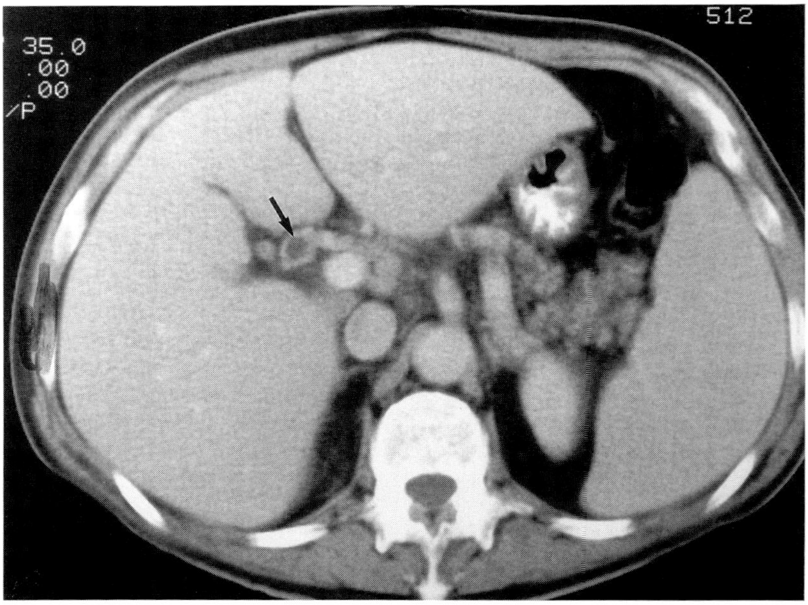

(A)

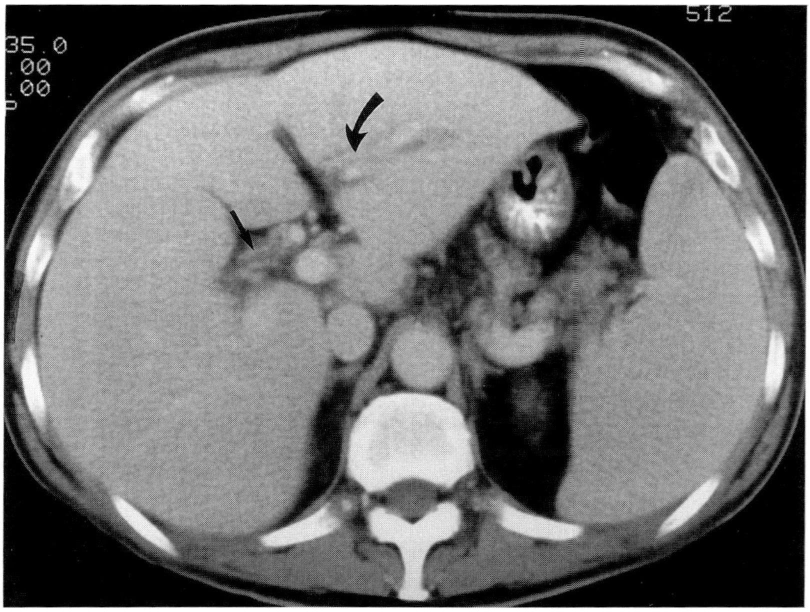

(B)

Figure 11. CT scan demonstrating changes of sclerosing cholangitis. (A) Contrast-enhanced CT scan demonstrates smooth symmetrical thickening of the right hepatic duct (arrow). (B) There also appear to be several isolated "pockets" of dilated ducts within the left lobe (curved arrow) and thickening of the right hepatic duct (arrow). The findings are suggestive of sclerosing cholangitis. In many patients with sclerosing cholangitis, abnormalities are seen on CT scan; however, scanning does not reliably determine the full extent of the disease in most patients.

the ducts for surgical planning in this context. If the portal vein is frankly encased by the tumor, resection is also unlikely. Because cholangiocarcinoma may spread to the liver, it is important to conduct a complete scan of the liver as part of the patient's CT study. The association of cholangiocarcinoma with sclerosing cholangitis, pyogenic (Asian) cholangiohepatitis, and other causes of biliary stasis such as choledochal cyst are well known.

Carcinoma of the ampulla and other small tumors of the choledochoduodenal junction are not well seen on cross-sectional studies. On CT inadequate distension of the duodenum is the main reason for failure to detect these tumors. Water and an effervescent agent help visualize the duodenum. Using this approach, wall invasion may be better seen by "negatively" opacifying the duodenum than with the standard use of barium. Barium will work, however, if good distension is achieved. Endoscopic ultrasound is generally superior to CT in assessing the extent of ampullary lesions (32).

Diseases that Seldom Produce Mass Effect

Choledocholithiasis is the most common cause of biliary obstruction without mass effect. The CT detection of choledocholithiasis requires careful analysis of the duct contents on thin 5-mm sections. The vast majority of common duct stones contain sufficient calcium bilirubinate to be radiodense on CT. Because of their density, most stones may be detected even when the duct is not dilated. In the most recent series on this topic using conventional CT, Baron found 76% sensitivity for CT of common duct stones (17). He found the best indicators of choledocholithiasis were dense intraluminal calcification and a "target sign" within the duct (Fig. 9). The latter refers to the appearance that results from a CT section being taken just above the equator of a stone within the dilated duct. A halo of bile surrounding the stone produces a target-like appearance. The experienced radiologist will follow the bile duct from section to section to detect subtle changes in attenuation of the lumen that may indicate the presence of a stone.

Reconstruction of overlapping sections using helical CT data holds much promise for improving the accuracy of stone detection with CT. Sections just above or below a stone may not detect the characteristic high attenuation of a stone because of volume averaging. A section through the center of the stone would be much more likely to depict the stone's attenuation accurately (Fig. 10). Data on the accuracy of helical CT in choledocholithiasis are still needed, however.

Sclerosing cholangitis is another disease that seldom produces mass effect on cross-sectional studies (33), with the possible exception of patients with multifocal fibrosclerosis (34). Most patients with sclerosing cholangitis have significant thickening of the extrahepatic duct wall (11) and focal "pockets" of dilated intrahepatic ducts on CT (Fig. 11). The duct wall thickening is usually symmetrical. Eccentric thickening is worrisome for cholangiocarcinoma, which can occur as a secondary complication of sclerosing cholangitis. Lobar atrophy and a nodular hepatic surface with caudate enlargement, indicative of secondary biliary cirrhosis, is present in long-standing disease. Adenopathy in the porta hepatis is often associated with primary sclerosing cholangitis. Ductal pseudodiverticula, although common, are below the resolution of CT or ultrasound. When it comes to mapping the extent of disease, looking for subtle evidence of progression, and identifying classic ductal pseudoulcerations, there is still no substitute for direct cholangiography.

There is an important interplay between the cross-sectional and radionuclide studies in patients with biliary disease. Although the radiologist needs to understand the technical aspects of performing these studies, he or she must also be committed to understanding the nature of the diseases that affect the biliary tree. A close working relationship between the gastroenterologist, radiologist, and surgeon will ensure optimal use of imaging procedures. The more efficient use of tests and their clinical relevance will increasingly become the recurrent theme of the future.

REFERENCES

1. Zeman RK, Brink J, Costello P, Davros WJ, Richmond B, Silverman PM, Vieco P. *Helical/Spiral CT: A Practical Approach.* New York: McGraw Hill Inc.; 1994.
2. Zeman RK, Burrell MI. Gallbladder and bile duct imaging. In *A Clinical Radiologic Approach.* New York: Churchill Livingstone; 1987.
3. Zeman RK, Fox SH, Silverman PM, Davros WJ, Carter LM, Griego D, Weltman DI, Ascher SM, Cooper CJ. Helical (spiral) CT of the abdomen. *AJR* 1993;160:719–725.
4. Zeman RK, Zeiberg AS, Davros WJ, et al. Routine helical CT of the abdomen: Image quality considerations. *Radiology.* 1993;189:395–400.
5. Liddell RM, Baron RL, Ekstrom JE, Varnell RM, Shuman WP. Normal intrahepatic ducts: CT depiction. *Radiology.* 1990;176:633–635.
6. Koslin DB, Stanley RJ, Berland LL, et al. Hepatic perivascular edema: CT appearance. *AJR.* 1988;150:111.
7. Sexton CC, Zeman RK. Correlation of computed tomography, sonography, and gross anatomy of the liver. *AJR.* 1983;141:711–718.
8. Cooperberg PL, Li D, Wong P, Cohen MM, Burhenne HJ: Accuracy of common hepatic duct size in the evaluation of extrahepatic biliary obstruction. *Radiology.* 1980; 135:141–144.
9. Graham MF, Cooperberg PL, Cohen MM, Burhenne HJ. The size of the normal common hepatic duct following cholecystectomy: An ultrasonographic study. *Radiology.* 1980; 135:137–139.
10. Mueller PR, Ferrucci JT, Jr., Simeone JF et al. Post cholecystectomy bile duct dilatation: Myth or reality? *AJR.* 1981;136:355–358.
11. Schulte SJ, Baron RL, Teefey SA, et al. CT of the extrahepatic bile ducts: wall thickness and contrast enhancement in normal and abnormal ducts. *AJR.* 1990;154:79–85.
12. Zeman RK, Taylor KJW, Burrell MI et al. Ultrasound demonstration of anicteric dilatation of the biliary tree. *Radiology.* 1980;134:689–692.
13. Zeman RK, Dorfman GS, Burrell MI et al. Disparate dilatation of the intrahepatic and extrahepatic bile ducts in surgical jaundice. *Radiology.* 1981;138:129–136.
14. Cronan JJ, Mueller PR, Simeone JF, O'Connell RS, vanSonnenberg E, Wittenberg J, Ferrucci JT Jr. Prospective diagnosis of choledocholithiasis. *Radiology.* 1983;146:467–469.
15. Pedrosa CS, Casanova R, Rodriquez R. Computed tomography in obstructive jaundice: I. The level of obstruction. *Radiology.* 1981;139:627–634.
16. Pedrosa CS, Casanova R, Lezana AH, Fernandez MC. Computed tomography in obstructive jaundice. II. The cause of obstruction. *Radiology.* 1981;139:635–645.

17. Baron RL: Common bile duct stones. Reassessment of criteria for CT diagnosis. *Radiology.* 1987;162:419–424.
18. Zeman RK, Davros WJ, Berman PM, et al. Three-dimensional models of the abdominal vasculature based on helical CT: usefulness in patients with pancreatic neoplasms. *AJR.* 1994;162:1425–1429.
19. Zeman RK, Berman PM, Silverman PM, Cooper C, Garra BS, Patt R, Ascher S. Helical CT of the biliary tract: Three-dimensional rendering without use of cholangiographic contrast. *Radiology.* 1995;196:865–867.
20. Zeman RK, Ascher SM, Patt RH. New approaches for pancreatobiliary disease: Helical (spiral) CT, MR imaging and endoluminal US. *Radiology.* 1993;189:73.
21. Taylor KJW, Buchin PJ, Viscomi GN, Rosenfield AT. Ultrasonographic scanning of the pancreas: Prospective study of clinical results. *Radiology.* 1981;138:211–213.
22. Freeny PC, Marks WM, Ryan JA, Traverso LW. Pancreatic ductal adenocarcinoma: diagnosis and staging with dynamic CT. *Radiology.* 1988;166:125–133
23. Ward EM, Stephens DH, Sheedy PR II. Computed tomographic characteristics of pancreatic carcinoma: an analysis of 100 cases. *Radiographics.* 1983;3:547–565.
24. Zeman RK. Helical CT of the pancreas. *Radiol. Clin North Am.* 1995;33:887–902.
25. Ralls PW, Halls JM, Renner I, Juttner H. Endoscopic retrograde cholangiopancreatography (ERCP) in pancreatic disease. A reassessment of the specificity of ductal abnormalities in differentiating benign from malignant disease. *Radiology.* 1980;134:347–352.
26. Zeman RK, Burrell MR, Dorfman GS, Stein S, Garra BS, Jaffe MH. Silverman PM. The protean manifestations of metastatic disease involving the biliary tract. *Radiology.* 1988;169:300.
27. Zeman RK, Schiebler M, Clark LR et al. The clinical and imaging spectrum of pancreaticoduodenal lymph node enlargement. *AJR.* 1985;144:1223–1227.
28. Clemmet AR, Lowman RM. The roentgen features of the Mirizzi syndrome. *AJR.* 1965;4:480–483.
29. Thorsen MK, Quiroz F, Lawson TL, Smith DF, Foley WD, Stewart ET. Primary biliary carcinoma. CT evaluation. *Radiology.* 1984;152:479–483.
30. Nesbit GM, Johnson CD, James EM, et al. Cholangiocarcinoma. Diagnosis and evaluation of resectability by CT and sonography as procedures complimentary to cholangiography. *AJR.* 1988;151:933–938.
31. Itai Y, Araki T, Furui S, Yashiro N, Ohtomo K, Iio M, computed tomography of primary intrahepatic biliary malignancy. *Radiology.* 1983;147:485–490.
32. Tio TL, Guido NJ, Tytgat GNJ, Rolf JLM, Cikot TL, Paul RA, Sars TL. Ampullopancreatic carcinoma: Preoperative TNM classification with endosonography. *Radiology.* 1990;175:455–461.
33. Teefey SA, Baron RL, Rohrmann CA, Shuman WP, Freeny PC. Sclerosing cholangitis: CT findings. *Radiology.* 1988;169:635–639.
34. Clark A, Zeman RK, White EM et al: Pancreatic pseudotumors associated with multifocal idiopathic fibrosclerosis. *Gastrointest Radiol.* 1987;13:30–32.

9

NUCLEAR MEDICINE IN BILIARY TREE EVALUATION

Harvey A. Ziessman, M.D.
*Georgetown University Medical Center
Washington, DC*

Robert K. Zeman, M.D.
*University of Vermont College of Medicine
Burlington, VT*

The unique ability of cholescintigraphy to image physiology, particularly bile drainage, in contrast to anatomy, for example, bile duct dilatation, makes it a very useful diagnostic imaging modality in the evaluation of patients with suspected biliary tract disease.

BILIARY OBSTRUCTION

The terms surgical jaundice, biliary obstruction, and bile duct dilatation are not synonymous. Biliary obstruction can be seen in the absence of hyperbilirubinemia or jaundice. The latter is usually a late manifestation of biliary obstruction (1–3). Obstruction does not always result in dilatation of the bile ducts (4–6) and dilatation can be present in the absence of obstruction.

The pathophysiological sequence of events in high-grade biliary obstruction progresses in a predictable manner: obstruction, increased intraductal pressure, reduced bile flow, biliary duct dilatation, increased cellular permeability, and fibrogenesis leading to hepatocellular damage (biliary cirrhosis) (7, 8). Because these events require finite time, ductile dilatation may not become evident until 24–72 hr after the initiating event, even in high-grade obstruction (9). Extrahepatic ductal dilatation occurs more rapidly in the previously cholecystectomized patient because the gallbladder is not available for decompression.

The pathogenesis and natural history of low-grade and intermittent obstruction such as that caused by choledocholithiasis has not been as well documented or studied as high-grade obstruction; however, clinical experience suggests that the symptomatology, clinical presentation, time course, and perhaps even the outcome are different.

The noninvasive imaging work-up of patients with biliary obstruction usually starts with ultrasonography. A clinical suspicion of obstruction often can be confirmed by the anatomic observation that the biliary tree is dilated. When obstruction is the result of choledocholithiasis, the obstructing calculi can be seen only rarely. The amount of dilatation varies widely and is directly related to the duration, degree, and etiology of the obstruction. Dilatation is most prevalent in long-standing obstruction, especially when secondary to malignant etiologies (10). Although the degree of dilatation is not directly proportional to the serum bilirubin, the largest, most dilated ducts tend to occur in deeply jaundiced patients. In early obstruction, the ducts may not be dilated. Benign causes of low-grade obstruction often do not cause significant dilatation of the biliary tract (11–13). Ductal dilatation may also be restricted by edema and scarring due to infection or cirrhosis.

The overall sensitivity of ultrasonography for making the diagnosis of biliary obstruction has been variously reported to be between 80 and 99% (14–17). This wide range is due primarily to the varied patient populations studied, for example, whether or not, and to what extent, patients with late-stage painless jaundice were included in the study compared to those with more subtle manifestations of biliary obstruction. Consequently, there are many clinical situations in which the diagnosis of obstruction cannot be made by the anatomic observation of dilatation. Here physiological imaging with cholescintigraphy can be quite helpful.

A very different clinical situation exists in patients who have had previous obstruction or biliary duct instrumentation, because the caliber of the biliary ducts often remains enlarged in the postoperative period. When these patients have suspected persistent or recurrent obstruction, functional imaging with cholescintigraphy is required to determine if the biliary tree is patent or obstructed. Because cholescintigraphy images the physiological process, obstruction to biliary flow can be seen from its onset, regardless of whether the ducts are dilated or not. In the setting of dilated ducts but no obstruction, biliary flow is normal.

A discordance between functional imaging with cholescintigraphy and anatomic imaging with ultrasonography has been well documented by numerous clinical investigations (18, 19). In one report of 125 patients being evaluated for biliary obstruction, biased toward patients with early- or low-grade obstruction and mild hyperbilirubinemia, 23% had discordant sonography and scintigraphy; that is, one study suggested biliary obstruction and the other did not (19). Thirteen patients had early obstruction due to neoplasm or low-grade obstruction secondary to choledocholithiasis or biliary stricture. These patients did not show sonographic evidence of ductal dilation whereas cholescintigraphy demonstrated abnormal bile flow in all 13 cases, emphasizing that functional abnormalities may precede morphologically evident disease. An additional seven patients showed ductal dilatation on sonography but had normal bile flow on cholescintigraphy. These patients all had dilated ducts from prior common duct exploration or chronic passage of stones.

METHODOLOGY

Although the first radiopharmaceutical approved for clinical use (Tc 99m dimethyl-IDA or lidofenin) did not produce diagnostic images in patients with a serum bilirubin greater than 5 mg/dl, both of the Tc 99m IDA radiopharmaceuticals now used in the United States, *mebrofenin* and *disofenin* (see Chapter 3), permit visualization of the biliary tree at serum bilirubin levels as high as 20–30 mg/dl.

After intravenous injection of Tc 99m IDA, the patient is imaged supine for 1 hr with the gamma camera placed anteriorly. The study is acquired on computer as continuous 1-min frames. Images are commonly formatted on radiographic film every 2–10 min. Delayed images or intervention with cholecystokinin may be required, as discussed below. The computer-acquired study (1-min images for 60 min) can be displayed in a cinematic mode on computer. This movie display can sometimes be quite helpful diagnostically.

IMAGE INTERPRETATION

Cancerous and noncancerous causes of biliary tract obstruction produce significantly different findings in hepatobiliary imaging (20). Tumors typically cause high-grade obstruction and often secondary hepatocyte dysfunction, whereas choledocholithiasis most often produces a picture of partial obstruction with little or no secondary liver dysfunction. On occasion, malignant tumors cause only partial obstruction and choledocholithiasis can result in complete obstruction. Pancreatitis tends to cause only mild partial obstruction and no or minimal liver dysfunction.

Cholescintigraphy in patients with high-grade common duct obstruction of recent onset usually shows good hepatic extraction or uptake, but no excretion of the radiolabeled bile into the biliary tree; that is, a persistent hepatogram (liver scan), is seen (Fig. 1). The high intraductal back pressure prevents excretion of the radiolabeled bile into the biliary ducts. This pattern is quite characteristic and the diagnosis can usually be made by the end of 1 hr of imaging. Delayed images even up to 24 hr often remain unchanged. If the obstruction is high grade but incomplete, delayed images (4–24 hr) may show some degree of excretion into biliary structures.

In a patient with partial common duct obstruction, cholescintigraphy demonstrates the radiolabeled bile entering the biliary tree, but flow is impeded and biliary-to-bowel transit often delayed beyond the normal 1-hr diagnostic cutoff time (Fig. 2). In the past, delayed biliary-to-bowel transit has been used as the primary criterion to make the diagnosis of partial obstruction. However, as many as 50% of patients with partial common duct obstruction have normal biliary-to-bowel transit at 60 min. On the other hand, greater than 20% of normal patients (21), 50% of patients who have been pretreated with cholecystokinin (CCK) prior to cholescintigraphy (22), and about 5% of patients with chronic cholecystitis have delayed biliary-to-bowel transit beyond the 60-min time period (23). Several other criteria are more specific for the diagnosis of partial common duct obstruction and should be sought. These imaging findings include the presence of intraluminal filling defects (not commonly seen, but best detected on cinematic display), segmental bile duct narrowing, prominent bile collection above the narrowing, persistent

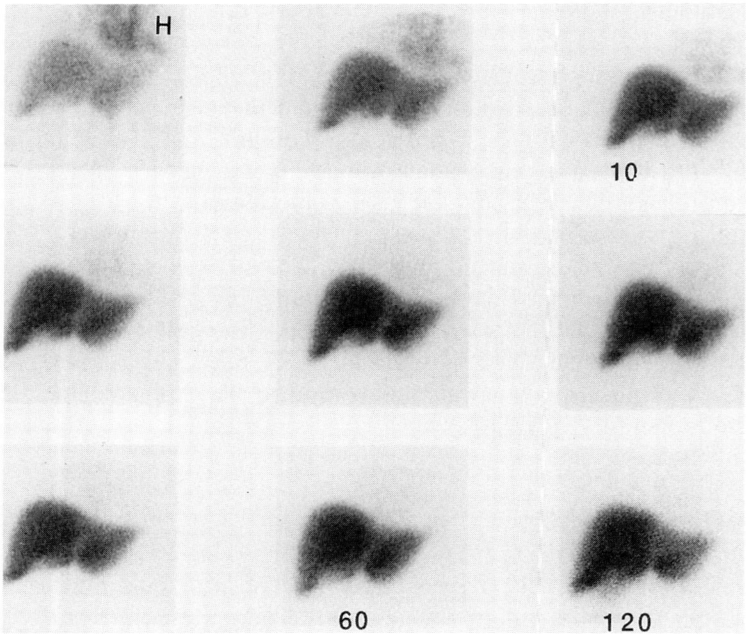

Figure 1. High-grade common duct obstruction. Good hepatic extraction is manifested by prompt disappearance of blood pool radiotracer from the heart (H) and near maximal uptake by the liver within 10 min. However, no excretion into any biliary structures is seen.

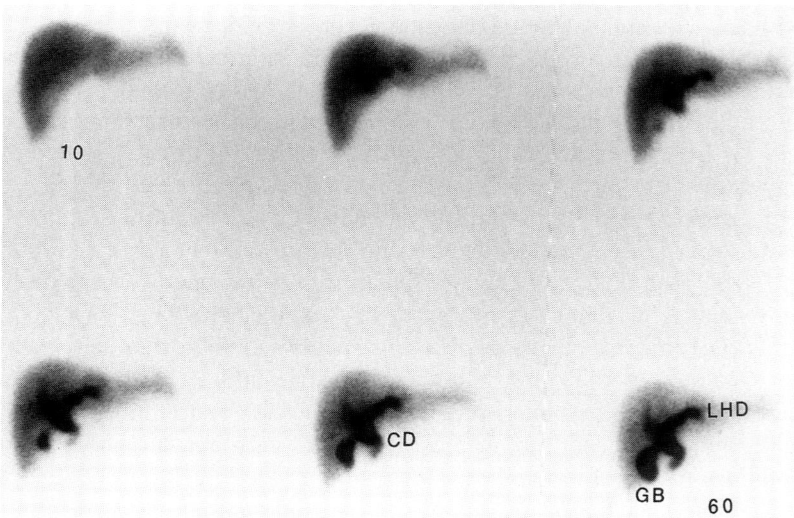

Figure 2. Partial common bile duct obstruction. Over the course of 60 min, the gallbladder (GB) fills. The common bile duct (CD) appears to be dilated and has an apparent cutoff distally with prominent biliary retention. No biliary activity is seen to enter the bowel at 60 min. The left hepatic duct (LHD) and to a lesser extent other intrahepatic ducts also appear prominent with biliary retention.

pooling after delayed imaging at 2 hr or after CCK infusion, and poor gallbladder contraction (19, 24). Segmental obstructions can also be easily identified on cholescintigraphy.

Functional causes of delayed biliary-to-bowel transit can be differentiated from true obstruction by having the patient change position or walk around, and/or by obtaining delayed images at 2–4 hr. A more rapid and reproducible method is to give CCK intravenously. In a nonobstructed patient, the sphincter of Oddi relaxes, followed by prompt biliary-to-bowel transit. If the gallbladder is not diseased, it contracts. If the common duct is truly obstructed, little or no change in bile duct retention occurs after CCK. An obstructed patient often has poor gallbladder contraction due to the high intraductal back pressure. A patient with chronic cholecystitis but no ductal obstruction has poor gallbladder contraction, but prompt biliary-to-bowel transit due to relaxation of the sphincter.

In the setting of severe hepatocyte dysfunction, it can occasionally be difficult to differentiate between primary hepatocellular disease with delayed transit and biliary obstruction with secondary hepatocyte dysfunction. However, image analysis can usually differentiate between the two. Primary parenchymal disease is manifested by poor liver uptake and delayed background (blood pool) clearance, whereas primary obstruction with secondary hepatocyte dysfunction has a lesser degree of dysfunction and evidence of a prominent ductal pattern.

Quantitative methods using computer-generated time–activity curves have been advocated to assist differentiating obstruction from parenchymal dysfunction (25–28). Various semiquantitative and quantitative techniques are most useful when used in conjunction with image analysis. Semiquantitative grading scales (1 to 4+) have used heart/liver ratios at specific time periods, ductal patterns (such as normal, prominent, cutoff), time of first biliary-to-bowel clearance, and so on, whereas others have used more quantitative indices derived from liver and bile duct time–activity curves, for example, half-emptying times and percent radiotracer clearance from common bile duct at specific time intervals. More recently, mathematical deconvolutional techniques have been successfully used in this differential diagnosis (29, 30).

POSTOPERATIVE BILIARY TRACT

Cholescintigraphy has also proved useful in the evaluation of the postoperative patient with suspected complications of biliary tract surgery, biliary enteric anastomoses, laparoscopic cholecystectomy, and gallstone lithotripsy (31–35) and in the differential diagnosis of the postcholecystectomy syndrome (36, 37).

Biliary Leaks and Obstruction

The rate of bile duct injury has increased two- to threefold as laparoscopic cholecystectomy has become the procedure of choice for elective cholecystectomy for chronic cholecystitis, compared to the very low rate seen reported with open cholecystectomy (38).

Although ultrasonography can demonstrate a fluid collection, it cannot determine its etiology and source. Cholescintigraphy can diagnose the site of leakage and

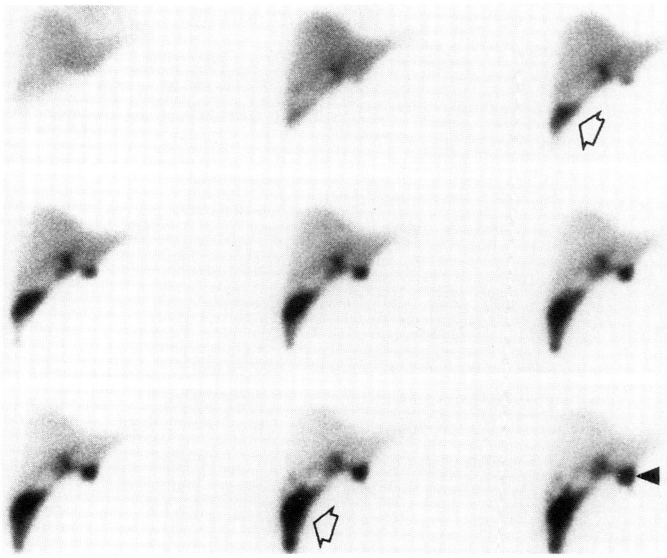

Figure 3. Postoperative biliary leak in a 50-year-old woman with abdominal discomfort after an elective laparoscopic cholecystectomy. Bile is seen to accumulate rapidly in the region of the gallbladder fossa and extends inferiorly below the right lobe of the liver (open arrowheads). Focal accumulation is also noted inferior to the left lobe (closed arrowhead). No common duct or biliary-to-bowel transit is seen.

estimate how rapid the leak is (Fig. 3) (39). This information can aid the surgeon in deciding whether surgical intervention or more conservative careful observation would be the appropriate therapy (40). Follow-up studies can be used to confirm resolution or persistence of the leakage. Cholescintigraphy can determine whether a fluid collection seen on computed tomography (CT) is of biliary origin. Prior to percutaneous drainage of a biloma, cholescintigraphy can ensure that central biliary obstruction is not present. With obstruction, it is unlikely that bile leakage can be effectively treated by percutaneous drainage without addressing the underlying cause of obstruction. Obstruction, whether due to retained or recurrent stones or stricture, can be diagnosed by cholescintigraphy in the postoperative patient by criteria similar to the nonoperated patient. This is discussed in detail below.

Bile leakage seen on cholescintigraphy appears as a progressively increasing pericholecystic collection of radiotracer and/or as free bile in the abdomen (41). Bile can accumulate perihepatically, over the dome of the liver, in the subdiaphragmatic space, and in the colonic gutters. Delayed imaging up to 24 hr may be required to detect a small or slow leak (42, 31). Patient repositioning may be necessary to confirm the presence of a small leak. Peritoneal tubing, drains, and drainage bags may exhibit tracer accumulation and should be imaged as well (43).

BILIARY DIVERSION SURGERY

Cholescintigraphy can aid in the evaluation of postoperative biliary–enteric anastomoses, both for detection of early complications and for long-term follow-up (32,

44, 45). Biliary leaks can be detected, the functional patency of the anastomosis determined, and recurrent obstruction diagnosed. Because there are many different biliary diversion procedures that can be performed, it is helpful for the surgeon to familiarize the imager with the patient's postoperative anatomy to aid in image interpretation in the setting of distorted anatomy.

Postoperative recurrent obstruction can be difficult to diagnose because clinical and laboratory findings may be ambiguous. Alkaline phosphatase is frequently persistently elevated even in patients with a normal postoperative biliary tract. The presence of cholangitis may not necessarily represent recurrent or treatable obstruction; for example, segmental biliary obstruction not bypassed at the time of surgery may result in recurrent low-grade obstruction.

Contrast cholangiography has limitations in evaluation of these patients. It may not be possible to reach the biliary tract via ERCP if a long Roux-en-Y loop has been created as part of the anastomosis. Percutaneous transhepatic cholangiography is an invasive procedure with associated morbidity. There is a definite role for the noninvasive study to establish which patients will benefit from cholangiography.

Ultrasonography has a high incidence of nondiagnostic exams, up to 67% in one series (46), frequently due to gas in the anastomotic bowel segment or refluxed biliary air, a finding that does not guarantee patency of the biliary tract. Biliary dilatation may be present even when obstruction has been adequately relieved by surgery. In one series, 22% of patients had a persistently dilated biliary tree yet did not have recurrent obstruction (44).

Cholescintigraphy is the only noninvasive method that can distinguish obstructed dilated ducts from those that are chronically dilated, but not obstructed. Base-line cholescintigraphy and ultrasonography several weeks after surgery allow detection of subtle deterioration in biliary drainage. If the ducts remain dilated or obscured by refluxed biliary air, cholescintigraphy should be used for long-term follow-up.

POSTCHOLECYSTECTOMY SYNDROME

Recurrent abdominal pain following cholecystectomy can be due to a number of different biliary etiologies that include common duct stricture, recurrent or retained common duct stones, stone formation in a prominent cystic duct, or sphincter of Oddi dysfunction. Of course, symptoms may also be of a nonbiliary origin. It can be difficult to distinguish between the various causes of pain in the postcholecystectomy patient.

A postoperative *cystic duct remnant* can act like a small gallbladder and become diseased, producing symptoms identical to those of acute and/or chronic cholecystitis. Cystic duct remnants are not uncommon, occurring in one series in 14% of 125 symptomatic postcholecystectomy patients (32). However, there is controversy as to whether this entity is a common or rare cause of clinical symptoms (47). The presence of a remnant does not prove that the pain originates there. However, cholescintigraphy can be helpful in identifying stasis in a cystic duct remnant (48).

Retained or *recurrent common duct stones* and *inflammatory fibrosis* are common causes of the postcholecystectomy pain syndrome. Cholescintigraphy confirms the diagnosis of obstruction by noting bile flow rather than duct size. In addition to the scintigraphic diagnostic findings described for partial obstruction, duct dynamics are important to note. Because the gallbladder is not present to act as an alternative reservoir for bile, duct dynamics directly predicts the adequacy of biliary drainage. With obstruction, one sees unchanging or increasing, rather than the normally decreasing, radioactivity within the common duct between 1 and 2 hr after injection (37). Quantitative cholescintigraphy can further increase the diagnostic confidence in confirming or excluding the diagnosis of obstruction (25, 27).

Sphincter of Oddi dysfunction is an important but poorly understood clinical syndrome presenting as intermittent abdominal pain and transient liver function abnormalities following cholecystectomy. Other terms used to describe this syndrome include papillary stenosis, biliary spasm, and biliary dyskinesia. It occurs in about 14% of patients with postcholecystectomy pain (49). Symptoms are presumably caused by a partial or intermittent common duct obstruction, but without an obvious mechanical cause, such as stricture or stone. This obstruction may be the result of a fixed obstruction (papillary stenosis) or a functional obstruction (biliary dyskinesia). The dysfunction is not felt to be related to the cholecystectomy per se, but to a preexisting condition, perhaps damage from prior passage of stones or traumatic duct exploration. The treatment is usually either surgery or endoscopic sphincterotomy (50–52). Pharmacological therapies are under investigation (53).

Until 1970, no imaging method could determine if postcholecystectomy pain was due to recurrent biliary disease. Exploratory laparotomy and the inability to pass a Bakes dilator greater than 3 mm in diameter were the sole criteria used to establish the presence of sphincter stenosis. The development of fiber optic endoscopy and endoscopic retrograde cholangiopancreatography (ERCP) has made it possible to determine if a specific anatomic cause of biliary obstruction is present. If after dilation of the biliary duct upon ERCP, there is delayed drainage of contrast material beyond 45 min, the diagnosis of sphincter stenosis is suggested. However, this finding is nonspecific.

Endoscopic biliary manometry is increasingly used to make this diagnosis. Sphincter of Oddi pressure of greater than 40 mm Hg is generally considered abnormal (54). Although manometry is considered specific for the diagnosis of sphincter dysfunction, it is invasive, technically difficult, not possible to perform in many patients, prone to a wide range of subjective interpretative errors, and in some cases affected by medications given during ERCP. Additionally, it is not widely available. Questions have been raised about the technique's reproducibility (55). Pancreatitis is a serious complication. A noninvasive alternative would be desirable.

Real-time ultrasonography is used to evaluate the postcholecystectomy biliary tract (56). However, diagnosis relies on duct size, and as discussed, significant pathology may be present in the absence of ductal dilatation. Fatty meal or CCK-stimulated sonography has been used to evaluate borderline or marginally dilated bile ducts (25, 57). However, it is still not a particularly sensitive technique (67%) (25).

Conventional cholescintigraphy has a useful role to play in evaluation of the postcholecystecomy patient (36, 37). The radionuclide study allows physiological assessment of duct drainage, which correlates well with the washout of contrast material from the biliary tract observed on ERCP. In a prospective study of patients with the postcholecystectomy syndrome, cholescintigraphy accurately (>90%) detected patients with anatomic causes of obstruction and sphincter of Oddi dysfunction (37). The most common scintigraphic pattern was that of prominent ductal

Table 1. Accuracy of quantitative cholescintigraphy for diagnosis of sphincter of Oddi dysfunction

Investigators	Year	Reference	Sensitivity (%)	Specificity (%)
Darwesh et al.	1988	25	67	85
Kloiber et al.	1988	27	93	64
Peng et al.	1994	79	88	80
Sostre et al.	1991	60	100	100

activity without evidence of washout on images at 2 hr compared to 1-hr images. Resolution of this abnormal pattern was seen in patients on follow-up studies even though the ducts remained dilated. More recent cholescintigraphic studies have used quantitative parameters of Tc 99m IDA uptake and clearance to confirm this diagnosis and to determine the effectiveness of therapy (25, 27, 58, 59) (Table 1).

A particularly intriguing recent investigation utilized an infusion of CCK in all patients at the start of cholescintigraphy (60). The rationale was to "stress" the capacity of the biliary ducts. Importantly, the investigators used both image analysis and quantitative parameters to calculate a semiquantitative diagnostic score. Manometry was used as the standard. Out of 26 patients, all obstructed patients were separated from nonobstructed patients with a 100% accuracy.

Although manometry and ERCP have been used in investigative studies as the standard, the true standard should be the patient's clinical response to treatment in combination with a repeat noninvasive study giving objective evidence of whether there was improvement compared to the preoperative study. For example, a good response to surgery would be consistent with resolution of the patient's symptoms *and* an improvement in the biliary duct's half-emptying time (Fig. 4). This type of data, however, is quite limited (25, 58). Further studies are needed to define better the relative accuracy and role of ultrasonography, scintigraphy, manometry, and ERCP using outcome results with patients classified clinically.

A clinical classification of these patients has been proposed and is gaining acceptance (61). Type I patients have abnormal liver function studies, a dilated common bile duct, and slow drainage of contrast at ERCP. Type II patients have only one or two of these features, whereas type III patients are those with suggestive pain, but normal duct size, drainage time, and liver function tests. Biliary obstruction is highly probable in Type I. Sphincter ablation is appropriate treatment, and these patients may not need manometry, scintigraphy, or ultrasonographic CCK-stimulated testing. In Type II and III patients, confirmatory evidence from manometry or scintigraphy is necessary to justify risks of sphincter ablation.

LIVER TRANSPLANT EVALUATION

The vascular, hepatobiliary, and intestinal phases of cholescintigraphy provide valuable diagnostic information about the post-liver transplant patient. The radionuclide

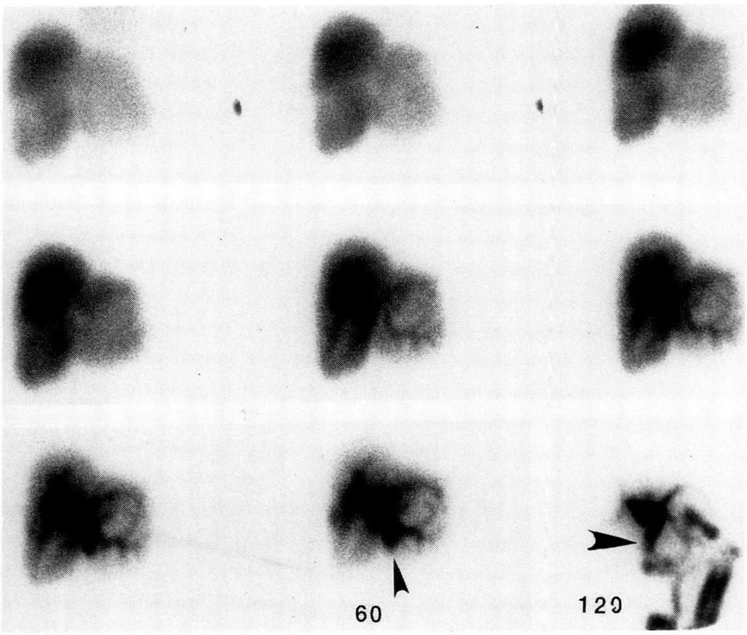

(A)

Figure 4. Sphincter of Oddi dysfunction in a 46-year-old female postcholecystectomy patient with recurrent abdominal pain. ERCP excluded mechanical obstruction. Manometry showed elevated sphincter of Oddi pressure (48 mm). Cholescintigraphy pre- and postsphincterotomy was performed. (A) Preoperative study. Sequential images over 60 min show prominent intrahepatic biliary retention and apparently dilated common hepatic duct (arrowhead). At 120 min, radiotracer has entered the common duct and has an apparent cutoff (arrowhead) at the sphincter of Oddi with proximal dilatation and retention. (B) Postsphincterotomy study. There is still prominent radiotracer retention within the common duct (arrowhead). However, hepatic parenchymal clearance at 60 min and biliary-to-bowel transit have improved significantly from the base-line study (Fig. 4A). (C) Time–activity curves for the liver and common bile duct prior to (top) and after (bottom) surgery. Preoperatively the liver curve (A) was continually upsloping during the entire 60-min study. After surgery, uptake peaked at about 20 min and then decreased thereafter (B). Similarly the common bile duct showed continuous rise of activity preoperatively (C), but postoperatively peaked at about 25 min and declined thereafter in a more normal pattern (D, next page). Both sets of curves show significant improvement (next page).

angiogram can evaluate blood flow to the liver, and dynamic images over 1–2 hr can detect a postoperative bile leak or extrahepatic biliary obstruction (62, 63).

Differentiation of rejection from other complications can sometimes be suggested by clinical symptoms and liver function tests. However, in the absence of liver biopsy, the diagnosis of rejection is often made by exclusion. Rejection causes a reduction in hepatocyte function that can be noted on Tc99 IDA imaging; however, the changes are nonspecific (64–66) and can be seen with intraheptic cholestasis. Quantitative deconvolution techniques have been successfully used to differentiate between pure hepatocellular dysfunction and liver allograft rejection (67, 68).

Regional infarction of the liver can be manifested as segmental hypoperfusion.

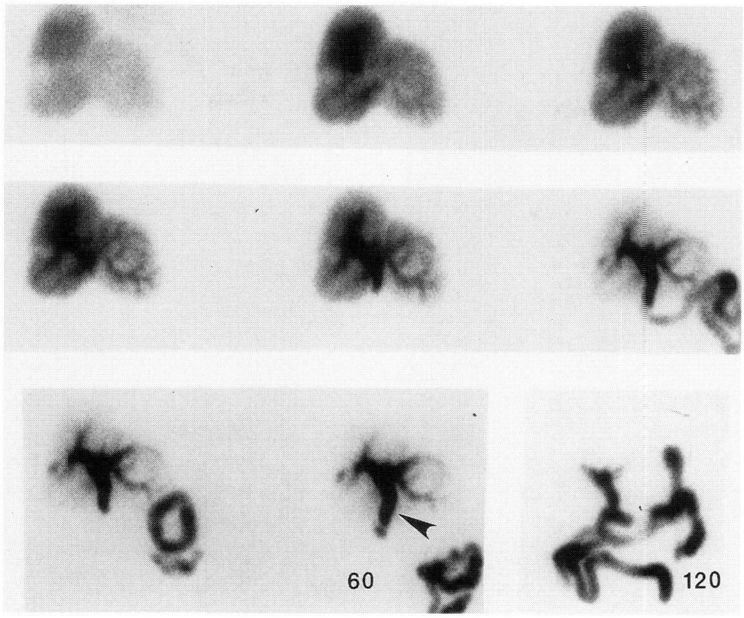

(B)

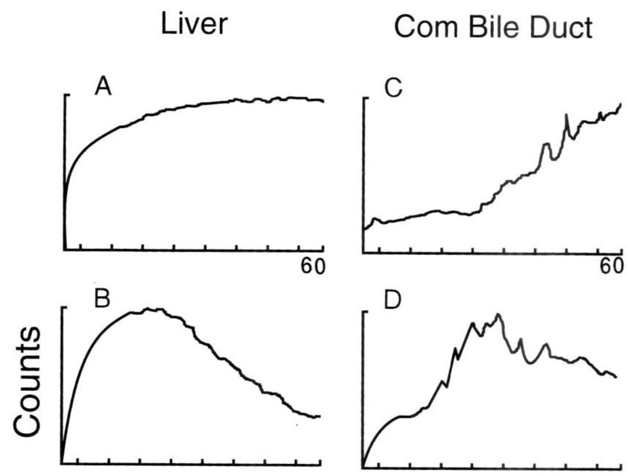

(C)

Figure 4. *(Continued)*

More global ischemia appears as decreased hepatic uptake and decreased blood pool clearance, similar to that seen with hepatocyte dysfunction. Focal infectious processes can be localized as a space-occupying lesion, in contrast to diffuse infection that would have a nonspecific hepatocyte dysfunction pattern.

Cholescintigraphy may be most useful in monitoring a patient's response to therapy (65, 69). It has also been found useful in predicting recovery of poorly functioning grafted livers (70).

TRAUMA

The evaluation of trauma requires interplay between cholescintigraphy and anatomic imaging modalities. Post-traumatic lesions that must be differentiated include hepatic laceration, hematoma, bile duct transection, extrahepatic biliary leakage, intrahepatic biloma formation, and performation of the gallbladder. Computed tomography and ultrasonography are used to detect liver parenchymal injuries. However, only biliary scintigraphy can demonstrate communication between the biliary tree and space-occupying lesions that represent biloma formation (40, 71–76).

Bile leakage is a common occurrence following penetrating and blunt trauma (70). It may initially be occult and detected only after clinical deterioration or discharge of bilious material from surgical bed drains. Cholescintigraphy can be used to follow the quantity of bile leakage and assess resolution in those patients treated conservatively (39).

Cholescintigraphy can also be used to follow resolution of a space-occupying process. In a patient with biloma formation who is not clinically improving despite diminished biliary leakage on cholescintigraphy, secondary abscess formation must be considered. In addition, seeing a persistent parenchymal defect that is not diminishing in size on scintigraphic exam also suggests the need for cross-sectional imaging.

CHOLEDOCHAL CYST

The term choledochal cyst is a misnomer; it is not a cyst but rather a congenital dilatation of the biliary-duct. This occurs most commonly in the extrahepatic biliary system, especially the common bile duct, but dilatation may occur intrahepatically (Caroli's disease). A common clinical presentation is that of obstruction, but choledochal cysts also may present as an abdominal mass, jaundice, pain, cholangitis, or bile peritonitis. The classic clinical triad of jaundice, abdominal mass, and pain is seen in only 20–30% of cases. The typical scintigraphic findings consist of early photopenia in the region in question with late filling (often greater than 1 hr) and retention of radiotracer for a prolonged period (Fig. 5). Filling occurs within 1 hr in more than 50% of patients, by 12 hr in 75%, and by 24 hr in 85%; the remaining 15% never fill (76). In these latter cases the diagnosis cannot be confirmed with cholescintigraphy.

BILIARY ATRESIA

The clinical and laboratory diagnosis of biliary atresia is very difficult. A definitive diagnosis of biliary atresia is usually made by percutaneous transhepatic cholangiography, laparotomy, or laparoscopy. Cholescintigraphy has proved to be quite useful in differentiating biliary atresia from other causes of neonatal jaundice. A patent biliary tree can rule it out by demonstrating passage of radiotracer into the bowel. Studies have demonstrated good sensitivity (97%) and specificity (88%) for making the diagnosis of biliary atresia (77). The diagnosis is typically made when no intestinal activity is seen by 24 hr after injection. Hepatocyte clearance is relatively

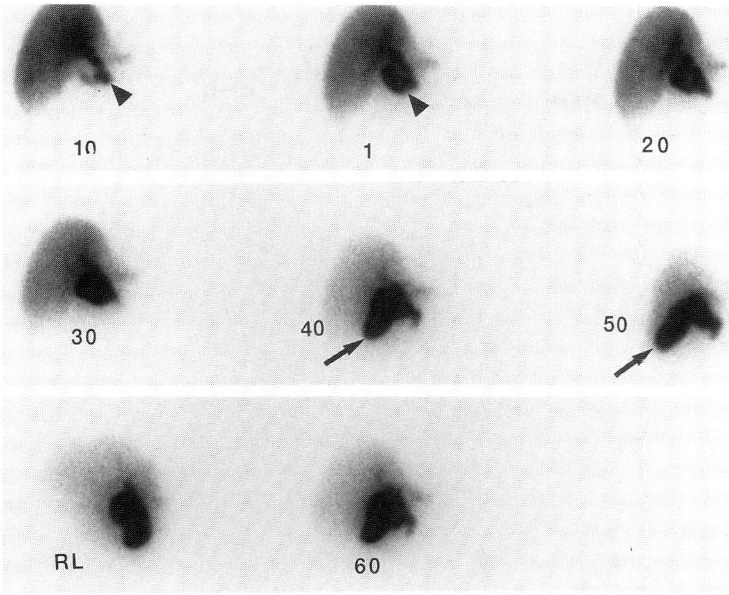

(A)

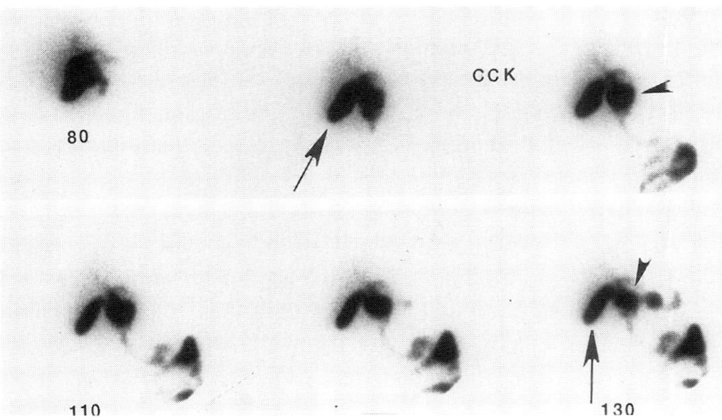

(B)

Figure 5. Choledochal cyst. Middle-aged male alcoholic with history of pancreatitis admitted with abdominal pain and mass thought to be a pseudocyst on CT but a choledochal cyst could not be ruled out. (A) A choledochal cyst (arrowheads) begins to fill as early as 10 to 15 min. By 40–50 min the gallbladder (arrow) visualizes and the choledochal cyst continues to fill. RL, right lateral. (B) By 90 min two distinct structures can be seen more clearly, the gallbladder (arrow) and the choledochal cyst (arrowheads). With the administration of CCK, the gallbladder contracts and some biliary-to-bowel transit is noted with decreasing size of the choledochal cyst (arrowhead at 130 min). This was an asymptomatic choledochal cyst. The patient did have a pancreatic pseudocyst that caused his pain.

preserved. In contrast, studies are interpreted as compatible with neonatal hepatitis when there is impairment in hepatocyte uptake and clearance, but radiotracer reaches the bowel by 24 hr. Patients should be pretreated with phenobarbital for 5–7 days prior to cholescintigraphy to maximize the accuracy of the study (78).

REFERENCES

1. Zeman R, Taylor KJW, Burrell MI, Gold J. Ultrasound demonstration of anicteric dilatation of the biliary tree. *Radiology.* 1980;134:689–692.
2. Weinstein DP, Weinstein BJ, Brodmerkel GJ. Ultrasonography of biliary tract dilation without jaundice. *AJR.* 1979;132:729–734.
3. Weinstein BJ, Weinstein DP. Biliary tract dilation in the nonjaundiced patient. *AJR.* 1980;134:899–906.
4. Muhletaler CA, Gerlock AJ Jr, Fleischer AC, James AE Jr. Diagnosis of obstructive jaundice with nondilated bile ducts. *AJR.* 1980;134:1149–1152.
5. Beinart C, Efremidis S, Cohen B, Mitty HA. Obstruction without dilation. Importance in evaluating jaundice. *JAMA.* 1981;245:353–356.
6. Thomas JL, Zornoza J. Obstructive jaundice in the absence of sonographic biliary dilation. *Gastrointest Radiol.* 1980;5:357–360.
7. Klingensmith WC III, Whiteney WP, Spitzer VM, et al. Effect of complete biliary-tract obstruction on serial hepatobiliary imaging in an experimental model: concise communication. *J Nucl Med.* 1981;22:866–868.
8. Zeman RL, Taylor KJW, Rosenfield AT, et al. Acute experimental biliary obstruction in the dog: sonographic findings and clinical implications *AJR.* 1981;136:965–967.
9. Zeman RK, Burrell MI, Gold JA, Russo Jr R. The intrahepatic and extrahepatic bile ducts in surgical jaundice: Radiological evaluation and therapeutic implications. *Crit Rev Diag Imaging.* 1984;21:1–36.
10. Lapis JL, Orlando RC, Mittelstaedt CA, Staab EV. Ultrasonography in the diagnosis of obstructive jaundice. *Ann Intern Med.* 1978;89:61–63.
11. Shuman WP, Rogers JV, Rudd TG, et al. Low sensitivity of sonography and cholescintigraphy in acalculous cholecystitis. *AJR.* 1984;142:531–534.
12. Cronan JJ, Mueller PR, Simeone JF, et al. Prospective diagnosis of choledocholithiasis. *Radiology.* 1983;146:467–469.
13. Gross BH, Harter LP, Gore RM, et al. Ultrasonic evaluation of common bile duct stones: prospective comparison with endoscopic retrograde cholangiopancreatography. *Radiology.* 1983;146:471–474.
14. Sample WF, Sarti DA, Goldstein LL, et al. Grayscale ultrasonography of the jaundiced patient. *Radiology.* 1978;128:719–725.
15. Cooperberg PL. High resolution real time ultrasound in the evaluation of the normal and obstructed biliary tract. *Radiology.* 1978;129:477–480.
16. Neiman HL, Mintzer RA. Accuracy of biliary duct ultrasound: comparison with cholangiography. *AJR.* 1977:129:979–982.
17. Taylor KJW, Rosefield AT, Spiro HM. Diagnostic accuracy of gray scale ultrasonography for the jaundiced patient. *Arch Intern Med.* 1979;139:60–63.
18. Kaplun L, Weissmann HS, Rosenblatt RR, et al. The early diagnosis of common bile duct obstruction using cholescintigraphy. *JAMA,* 1985;254:2431–2434.
19. Zeman RK, Lee C, Jaffe MH, Burrell MI. Hepatobiliary scintigraphy and sonography in early biliary obstruction. *Radiology,* 1984;153:793–798.

20. Klingensmith WC, Kuni CC, Fritzberg AR. Cholescintigraphy in extrahepatic biliary obstruction. *AJR.* 1982;139:65–70.
21. Williams W, Krishnamurthy GT, Brar HS, Bobba VR. Scintigraphic variations of normal biliary physiology. *J Nucl Med.* 1984;25:160–165.
22. Kim CK, Palestro CJ, Solomon RW, et al. Delayed biliary-to-bowel transit in cholescintigraphy after cholecystokinin treatment. *Radiology.* 1990;176:553–556.
23. Weissmann HS, Sugarman LA, Badia JD, et al. Improving the specificity and accuracy of Tc-99m IDA cholescintigraphy with delayed views. *J Nucl Med.* 1980;21:17.
24. Krishnamurthy GT, Bobba VR, McConnell D, et al. Quantitative biliary dynamics: introduction of a new noninvasive scintigraphic technique. *J Nucl Med.* 1983;24:217–223.
25. Darweesh RMA, Dodds WJ, Hogan WJ. Efficacy of quantitative hepatobiliary scintigraphy and fatty-meal sonography for evaluating patients with suspected partial common duct obstruction. *Gastroenterology.* 1988;94:779–786.
26. Joshi SN, George EA, Perillo. Quantitative temporal analysis of 99mtechnetium p-isopropyl-iminodiacetic acid (PIPIDA) as a measure of hepatic function in health and disease. *Gastroenterology.* 1981;81:1045–1051.
27. Kloiber R, AuCoin R, Hersfield NB, et al. Biliary obstruction after cholecystecomy: diagnosis with quantitative cholescintigraphy. *Radiology.* 1988;169:643–647.
28. Krishnamurthy GT, Lieberman DA, Brar HS. Detection, localization and quantitation of degree of common bile duct obstruction by scintigraphy. *J Nucl Med.* 1985;26: 726–735.
29. Brown Paul H, Juni JE, Lieberman DA, Krishnamurthy GT. Hepatocyte versus biliary disease: a distinction by deconvolutional analysis of technetium-99m IDA time-activity curves. *J Nucl Med.* 1988;29:623–630.
30. Juni JE, Reichle R. Measurement of hepatocellular function with deconvolutional analysis: Application in the differential diagnosis of acute jaundice. *Radiology.* 1990;177:171–175.
31. Estrada WN, Zanzi I, Ward R, et al. Scintigraphic evaluation of postoperative complications of laparoscopic cholecyectomy. *J Nucl Med.* 1991;323:1910–1911.
32. Weissman HS, Gliedman ML, Wilk PJ, et al. Evaluation of the post-operative patient with 99m Tc-IDA cholescintigraphy. *Semin Nucl Med.* 1982;12:27–52.
33. Pasmans HLM, Go PMHYH, Gouma DJ, et al. Scintigraphic diagnosis of bile leakage after laparoscopic cholecystectomy: a prospective study. *Clin Nucl Med.* 1992;17:697–700.
34. George JK, Velchik MG. Biliary complications of gallstone lithotripsy detected by Tc-99m DISIDA scintigraphy. *Clin Nucl Med.* 1991;16:157–159.
35. Walker AT, Shapiro A, Brooks DC, et al. Bile duct disruption and biloma after laparoscopic cholecystectomy: imaging evaluation. *AJR.* 1992;258:785–789.
36. Lee RGL, Gregg JA, Korxhetz AM, et al. Sphincter of Oddi stenosis: diagnosis using hepatobiliary scintigraphy and endoscopic manometry. *Radiology.* 1985;156:793–796.
37. Zeman RK, Dobbins J, Gorelick F, et al. Postcholecystectomy syndrome: Evaluation using biliary scintigraphy and endoscopic retrograde cholangiopancreatography (ERCP). *Radiology.* 1985;156:787–792.
38. NIH Consensus Development Panel on Gallstones and Laparoscopic Cholecystectomy. *JAMA.* 1993;269:1018–1024.
39. Weissman HS, Chun KJ, Frank M, et al. Demonstration of traumatic bile leakage with cholescintigraphy and ultrasonography. *AJR.* 1979;133:843–847.
40. Horattas MC, Lewis RD, Fenton AH, Awender HM. Modern concepts in Nonsurgical Management of Traumatic Biliary fistulas. *J Trauma.* 1994;36:180–189.

41. Rayter Z, Tonge C, Bennett C, et al. Ultrasound and HIDA: Scanning in evaluating bile leaks after cholecystectomy. *Nucl Med Commun.* 1991;12:197–202.

42. Rozran RS, Preston DF, McMillan JH. Hepatobiliary imaging for demonstration of bile leaks. *Clin Nucl Med.* 1984;9:189–192.

43. Ziessman HA, Atlas of cholescintigraphy. In: Ziessman HA, VanNostrand D, eds. *Selected Atlases of Gastrointestinal Scintigraphy,* New York: Springer-Verlag; 1992:1–34.

44. Zeman RK, Lee C, Stahl RS, et al. Ultrasonography and hepatobiliary scintigraphy in the assessment of biliary-enteric anastomoses. *Radiology.* 1982;145:109–115.

45. Rosenthal L, Fonseca C, Arzoumanian A, et al. 99m Tc-IDA hepatobiliary imaging following upper abdominal surgery. *Radiology.* 1979;130:375–378.

46. Sample WF, Sarti DA, Goldstein LI, et al. Gray-scale ultrasonography of the jaundiced patient. *Radiology.* 1978;128:719–727.

47. Way LW, Sleisenger MH. Postoperative syndromes. In *Gastrointestinal Disease,* 4th ed. Sleisenger MH, Fordtran, JS, eds. Philadelphia: W.B. Saunders Company; 1989:1729–1733.

48. D'Alonzo W, Velchik MG. Post-cholecystectomy syndrome due to a cystic duct remnant diagnosed by hepatobiliary scintigraphy. *Clin Nucl Med.* 1984;9:719–720.

49. Steinberg WM. Sphincter of Oddi dysfunction: a clinical controversy. *Gastroenterology.* 1988;95:1409–1415.

50. Schein CJ, Beneventano TC. Choledochoduodenal junction stenosis in the postcholecystecomy syndrome. *Surgery.* 1968;64:1039–1046.

51. Moody FG, Becker JM, Potts JR. Transduodenal sphincteroplasty and transampullary septectomy for postcholecystectomy pain; *Ann Surg.* 1983;197:627–636.

52. Geenen JE, Hogan WJ, Dodds WJ, et al. The efficacy of endoscopic sphincterotomy after cholecystectomy in patients with sphincter of Oddi dysfunction. *N Engl J Med.* 1989;320:82–87.

53. Sand J, Nordback I, Koskinen M, et al. Nifedipine for suspected type II sphincter of Oddi dyskinesia. *Am J Gastroenterol.* 1993;88:530–535.

54. Geenen JE, Hogan WJ. Endoscopic access to the papilla of Vater. *Endosc Suppl* 1980 (supplement):47–56.

55. Thune A, Scicchitano J, Roberts-Thomson I, Toouli J. Reproducibility of endoscopic sphincter of Oddi Mannometry. *Dig Dis Sci.* 1991;36:1401–1407.

56. Parulekar SG. Ultrasound evaluation of common bile duct size. *Radiology.* 1979;133: 703–707.

57. Simeone JF, Mueller PR, Ferrucci, JT et al. Sonography of the bile ducts after a fatty meal: an aid in detection of obstruction. *Radiology.* 1982;143:211–216.

58. Shaffer EA, Hersfield NB, Logan HK, Kloiber R. Cholescintigraphic detection of functional obstruction of the sphincter of Oddi. Effect of papillotomy. *Gastroenterology.* 1986;90:728–733.

59. Pace RF, Chamberlain MJ, Passi RB. Diagnosing papillary stenosis by technetium-99m HIDA scanning. *Can J Surg.* 1983;26:191–193.

60. Sostre S, Kaloo AN, Spiegler EJ, et al. A noninvasive test of sphincter of Oddi dysfunction in postcholecystectomy patients: the scintigraphic score. *J Nucl Med.* 1992;33:1216–1222.

61. Ruffolo TA, Lehman GA. HIDA imaging in postchoecystectomy symdrome-clinical value or romancing the stone? *Am J Gastroenterol.* 1991;86:1092–1093.

62. Mochizuki T, Tauxe WN, Dobkin J, et al. Detection of complications after liver transplantation by technetium-99m mebrofenin hepatobiliary scintigraphy. *Ann Nucl Med.* 1991;5:103–107.

63. Gelfand MJ, Smith HS, Ryckman FC, et al. Hepatobiliary scintigraphy in pediatric liver transplant recipients. *Clin Nucl Med.* 1992;17:542–549.

64. Loken MK, Ascher NL, Boudrea RJ, et al. Scintigraphic evaluation of liver transplant function. *J Nucl Med.* 1986;27:451–459.

65. Hawkins RA, Hall T, Gambhir SS, Busuttil RW, et al. Radionuclide evaluation of liver transplants. *Semin Nucl Med.* 1988;18:199–212.

66. Busuttil RW, Goldstein LI, Danovitch GM, et al. Liver transplantation today. *Ann Intern Med.* 1986;104-377-81.

67. Merion RM, Campbell DA Jr, Dafoe DC, et al. Observations on quantitative scintigraphy with deconvolutional analysis in liver transplantation. *Transplant Proc.* 1988;20:695–697.

68. Juni JE, Thrall JH, Froelich JW, et al. A appended curve technique for deconvolutional analysis—method and validation. *Eur J Nucl Med.* 1988;14:403–407.

69. deJonge MWC, Pauwels EKJ, Hennis PJ, et al. Cholescintigraphy and Tc-99m diethyl IDA for the detection of rejection of auxiliary liver transplants in pigs. *Eur J Nucl Med.* 1983;8:485–488.

70. Karademir S, Csete ME, Jurim O, et al. Role of 99m Tc labeled DISIDA scan in the assessment of marginal liver grafts after orthopic transplantation. *Clin Transplant.* 1994;8:54–58.

71. Zeman RK, Lee C, Stahl RS, et al. Strategy for the use of biliary scintigraphy in noniatrogenic biliary trauma. *Radiology.* 1984;151:771–777.

72. Sty JR, Starshak RJ, Hubbard AM. Radionuclide hepatobiliary imaging in the detection of traumatic biliary tract disease in children. *Pediatr Radiol.* 1982;12:115–118.

73. Caride VJ, Gibson DW. Noninvasive evaluation of bile leakage. *Surg Gynecol Obstet.* 1982;154:517–520.

74. Christensen PB, Oestek-Joergensen E, Schoubye J, Pedersen SA. Scintigraphy with 99m Tc-(2,6 diethylacentanilides) acid as a diagnostic test in traumatic lesions of the liver and biliary tract. *Gastrointest Radiol.* 1981;6:43–46.

75. Kuni CC, Klingensmith WC, Kowep LJ, Fritzberg AR. Communication of intrahepatic cavities with bile ducts: demonstration with Tc-99m diethyl IDA imaging. *Clin Nucl Med.* 1980;5:349–351.

76. Sty JR, Babbitt DP, Squires W. Tc-99m IDA hepatobiliary imaging: a fractured liver. *Clin Nucl Med.* 1979;4:493–494.

77. Campanovo E, Buck JL, Drane WE. Scintigraphic features of choledochal cyst. *J Nucl Med.* 1989;30:622–627.

78. Gerhold JP, Klingensmith WC, Kuni CC, et al. Diagnosis of biliary atresia with radionuclide hepatobiliary imaging. *Radiology.* 1983;146:499–504.

79. Majd M, Reba RC, Altman RP. Effect of phenobarbital on Tc-99m scintigraphy in the evaluation of neonatal jaundice. *Semin Nucl Med.* 1981;11:194–204.

80. Peng NJ, Lai KH, Tsay DG, et al. Efficacy of quantitative cholescintigraphy in the diagnosis of sphincter of Oddi dysfunction. *Nucl Med Commun.* 1994;15:899–904.

10

MAGNETIC RESONANCE CHOLANGIOPANCREATOGRAPHY

Eric K. Outwater, M.D.
Thomas Jefferson University Hospital
Philadelphia, Pennsylvania

Magnetic resonance cholangiopancreatography (MRCP) is a method of imaging the biliary tree and pancreatic ducts. The principle that underlies this technique is that the bile and pancreatic secretions within the ductal systems have markedly prolonged T2 values compared to solid tissues within the upper abdomen. Therefore, heavily T2-weighted sequences demonstrate maximal contrast between the fluid and the surrounding soft tissue. With the correct imaging parameters, solid tissue displays virtually no signal, whereas fluid-containing structures still retain considerable signal intensity, thus providing maximal contrast between fluid-containing structures and surrounding soft tissue. Because these sequences can be acquired as a volume acquisition, the resulting data set can be used for a three-dimensional reconstruction of the biliary tree and pancreatic duct. Other applications of this technique have been used to image the urinary tract and cerebrospinal fluid-filled thecal sac (1,2). The sequences used in MRCP depend upon marked differences in T2 values between the fluid and surrounding soft tissue, actual flow within the ducts is not relevant (3).

TECHNICAL CONSIDERATIONS

The two types of sequences that have been used for MRCP images include fast spin echo (FSE) or steady-state free procession (SSFP) gradient echo sequences. The latter display the obstructed biliary tree with images that are relatively free of any motion artifact, and have been shown to portray the level of obstruction accurately (4), yet they yield a fairly low signal-to-noise ratio and thus requires a fairly thick section and large field of view. Imaging of smaller ducts is compromised; specifically, the ability to image the normal, undilated biliary and pancreatic ducts has been limited.

Other investigators have demonstrated that FSE sequences can show the biliary tree in both obstructed systems and normal individuals using a non-breath-hold technique, relying on signal averaging to compensate for motion degradation (5). Obstruction of the biliary tree and the pancreatic duct is demonstrated, although motion can be a limiting factor in visualizing the branches of the intrahepatic biliary tree. Reinhold et al. (6), however, have shown that this type of FSE sequence reliably depicts more branching of the biliary and pancreatic ducts than the gradient echo sequence. The use of a surface coil can allow the use of a much smaller field of view for higher-resolution images. Several investigators have established that this is an accurate technique for evaluation of the biliary and pancreatic tree (5–7).

Three-dimensional FSE imaging may offer certain advantages over 2D acquisitions. First, 3D acquisitions improve signal-to-noise ratios over 2D acquisitions, other relevant factors being equal. Second, 3D acquisitions often offer the opportunity for thin partitions to be obtained, thus increasing the image resolution when reconstruction projections are made in other than the plane of acquisition. Recent studies have demonstrated that the FSE acquisitions are useful for imaging the biliary tree (8, 9). Another approach involves acquisition of the entire relevant volume encompassing the biliary tree and pancreatic ducts in a single slab, that is, a single image. This offers the advantage of excellent signal-to-noise ratio but does not allow projection of the volume in multiple planes without separate acquisitions (10). Another disadvantage with this technique is that intraductal filling defects can be obscured by overlying fluid.

A number of technical innovations may increase the capability of MRCP sequences. These include multicoil arrays for imaging the upper abdomen to improve spatial resolution and refinements of the FSE technique to reduce examination times (e.g., breathing independent T2 weighted single shot echo-train spin-echo sequences).

CLINICAL ADVANTAGES AND APPLICATIONS

Actual opacification of the biliary and pancreatic ducts requires percutaneous cholangiography and the more widely used ERCP. Endoscopic retrograde cholangiopancreatography, of course, yields pancreaticograms of unparalleled resolution. The greatest advantage of ERCP is that therapeutic interventions such as stent placement, stone removal, or papillotomy can be performed at the time of the diagnosis. Though generally safe, ERCP is not without significant risks. Pancreatitis occurs in 1–5% of cases, biliary sepsis is a risk in obstructed ductal systems, and risks of intubation include bleeding, perforation, and aspiration. Relative disadvantages of ERCP include sedation or anesthesia, failure to cannulate or opacify the CBD or pancreatic duct in 5–15% of the cases, failure to opacify the pancreatic duct or common bile duct distal to a complete obstruction, and expense of greater than $3000 at some institutions. Consistently technically adequate studies require considerable training and experience (11, 12).

In contrast, MR imaging of the biliary and pancreatic ducts risks no complications in properly screened patients. Sedation and analgesia are avoided, although mild sedation may be needed to combat claustrophobia. The volume acquisition visualizes all obstructed segments (Fig. 1) and simultaneously images biliary and pancreatic ducts. Volume data sets permit 3D reconstruction and viewing in multiple

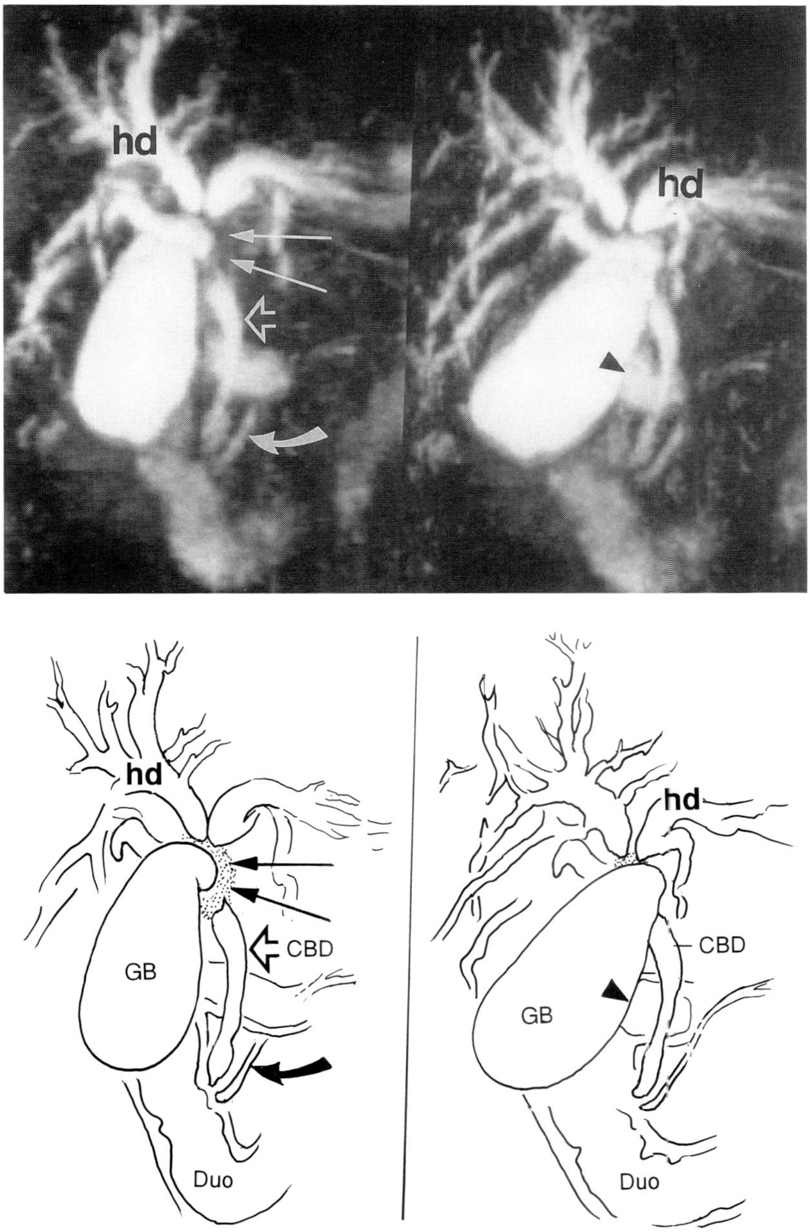

Figure 1. MR cholangiographic demonstration of multiple biliary ductal obstructions. Two MIP reconstructions from the 3D data set show dilatation of the intrahepatic bile ducts with separate occlusions of the common hepatic duct (arrows) and left and right hepatic ducts (hd) by a Klatskin tumor. Note that the mid common bile duct (open arrow) and pancreatic duct (curved arrow) are normal. The location of the duodenal bulb that overlies the common bile duct and pancreatic duct is marked by an arrowhead.

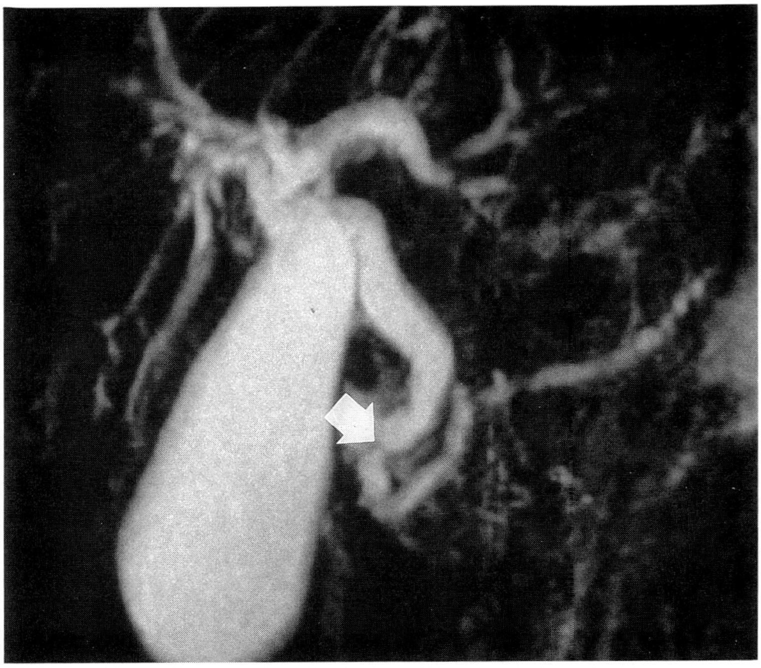

(A)

Figure 2. Benign stricture demonstrated by MR cholangiography. (A) MIP reconstruction demonstrates the dilatation of the common bile duct and intrahepatic ducts. The distal common bile duct shows a focal narrow stricture (arrow). The pancreatic duct is not dilated. These findings are compatible with benign stricture. (B) ERCP demonstrates a focal web in the distal common bile duct (arrow, next page).

perspectives, including projections similar to conventional radiographic studies performed with contrast material. As opposed to ERCP, structures are displayed in their in vivo state without distension of the lumen under pressure.

It is important to realize that the ductal system itself is not selectively displayed by MRCP technique. Rather, it is any and all fluid with sufficiently long T2 to obtain signal intensity at the imaging parameters employed. Bowel contents, cysts, ascites, and other fluid in the upper abdomen will be imaged as well. Anything that shortens the T2 of the bile or pancreatic secretions, such as blood, proteinaceous debris, or calculi may appear as focal nonvisualization of the duct. Gallbladder bile itself has a T2 much shorter than that of water (13–15). A potential concern is that, given the limited resolution of the images, any of these substances within the lumen of the biliary tree or pancreatic duct may give the false impression of obstruction, narrowing, or calculi.

With the reconstructed MRCP images, the maximum intensity projection (MIP) reconstructions represent degraded data. Some of the information on the individual source images is lost when displaying the whole volume in the MIP format. Potential for error occurs if the reconstructed images alone are used for interpretation, rather than as an overall layout of the pancreatic and biliary tree. A specific example of this is the identification of small intraluminal filling defects such as calculi. If fluid surrounds the calculus, the higher-signal-intensity fluid is registered by the MIP

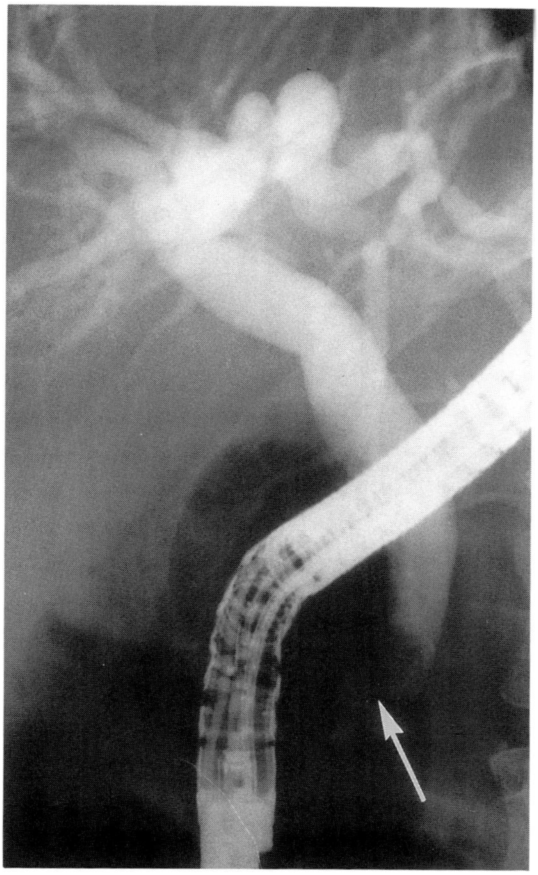

(B)

Figure 2. *(Continued)*

technique and the intraluminal filling defect may be completely inapparent on the reconstructed images. Therefore it is critical to rely on the individual source images for interpretation.

Clinical applications for MRCP include the identification of the site and cause of biliary obstruction, diagnosis of chronic pancreatitis by characteristic changes in

Table 1. Diagnostic performance of MR cholangiography for diagnosis of biliary obstruction

N	Sensitivity (%)	Specificity (%)	Accuracy	Abnormality Evaluated	Reference
21	87	100	90	Various	9
39	86	100	87	Level of obstruction	4
24	93	100	96	Level of obstruction	7
126	91	100	94	Obstruction	18
126	94	81	98	Choledocholithiasis	18
126	86	98	97	Malignant obstruction	18

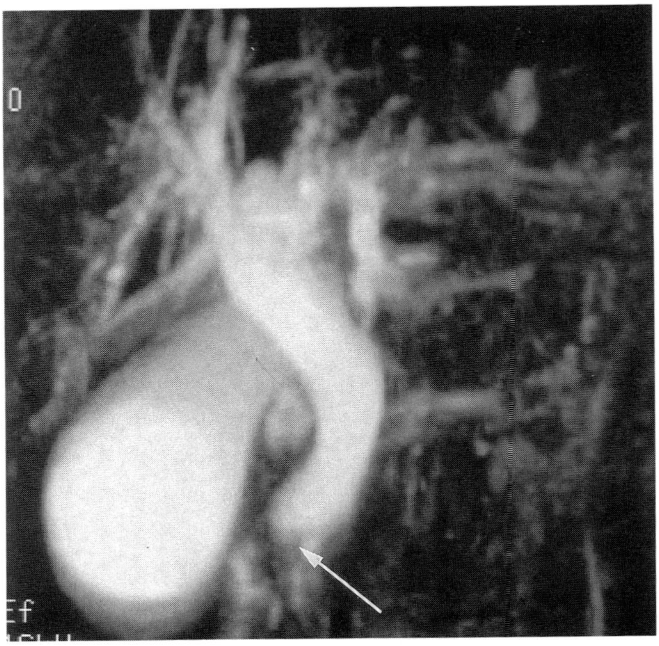

(A)

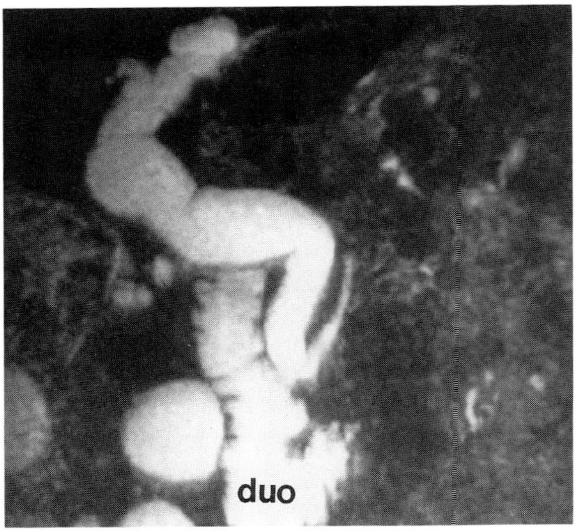

(B)

Figure 3. Difficulty in distinguishing benign from malignant ampullary strictures with MR cholangiography. MR cholangiography with MIP reconstructions of 3D data sets show ampullary strictures due to ampullary carcinoma (*A*) and benign ampullary stricture (B). Note that subtle irregularity of the distal CBD in (A) (arrow) is the only clue that this stricture is malignant. (C) ERCP image corresponding to MRCP in (B) shows CBD dilatation without tumor (duo, duodenum, next page).

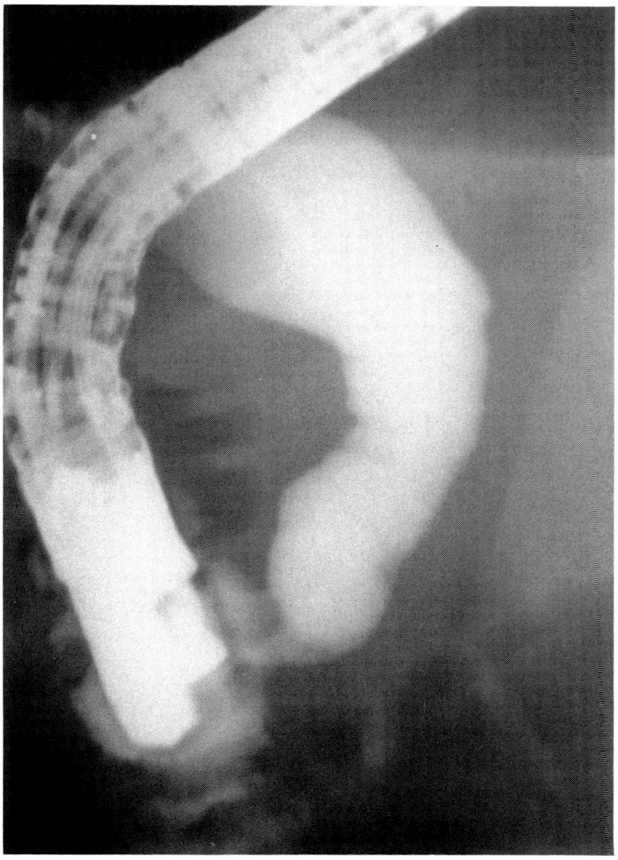

(C)

Figure 3. *(Continued)*

the pancreatic ductal system, and diagnosis of choledocholithiasis. The diagnosis of biliary obstruction with MRCP is fairly straightforward (Figs. 1, 2), because the dilated ductal system proximal to an obstruction is easier to visualize with MRCP technique than the thinner normal caliber ducts. Many studies have demonstrated that MRCP can identify the level of obstruction and the probable cause in the vast majority of patients (3–6, 8, 16, 17). Accuracy of identification of the level of obstruction and the cause of obstruction is in excess of 90% in most studies (3, 5, 6, 8, 9, 16) (Table 1). Criteria for distinguishing benign from malignant causes of biliary obstruction are similar to those used for conventional cholangiography. Because the sphincter lumen is not visualized directly by MRCP, difficulty may be encountered in distinguishing benign from malignant strictures at this site (Fig. 3).

COMMON BILE DUCT CALCULI

Magnetic resonance cholangiopancreatography has also been used to detect common bile duct calculi. In a small study of 10 patients with choledocholithiasis, stones could be detected in a nonblinded fashion in all cases (18). Stones were seen in all cases in the study of Barish et al. (8) and 5/7 cases reported by Macaulay et al. (6). Ultrasound (19, 20) and computed tomography (CT) (21) are insensitive for the diagnosis of choledocholithiasis. All biliary calculi reported to date were hypointense compared to the surrounding bile on MRCP studies. This is important in light of the variable appearance of calculi on CT (21, 22).

PANCREATIC ABNORMALITIES

Magnetic resonance cholangiopancreatography can also be used to detect pancreatic abnormalities such as pancreatic ductal obstruction from carcinoma, and dilatations and strictures that indicate the presence of chronic pancreatitis. Endoscopic retrograde cholangiopancreatography is performed in suspected chronic pancreatitis for several reasons: (1) to detect ductal abnormalities that may support the diagnosis of chronic pancreatitis in those patients in whom a clinical diagnosis is uncertain, (2) for presurgical evaluation of the ampulla, possible pancreas divisum, and any areas of ductal narrowing, calculi, and dilatation that would alter the approach in partial pancreatectomy, (3) to further characterize masses detected by ultrasound or CT, and (4) for interventional techniques such as removal of common bile duct stones, obtaining cytological material, stricture dilatation, or removal of pancreatic duct calculi (11, 23–25). Ultrasound and CT are insensitive for the diagnosis of chronic pancreatitis, because calcifications are present in a minority of cases (26–28). Furthermore, the differentiation of carcinoma from fibrotic masses of chronic pancreatitis is difficult with CT or ultrasound (27, 29); this differentiation is easier based on pancreatographic information (30, 31).

Takahara et al. and Soto et al. have found agreement between MRCP and ERCP in between 70 and 92% of cases, with 83–100% agreement for ductal dilatation indicating the presence of chronic pancreatitis; 92–100% of filling defects within the pancreatic ducts were demonstrated with MRCP. These findings would imply that moderate to severe cases of pancreatitis can be detected with MRCP. The MRCP method may have difficulty in detecting minor narrowing of the ducts, particularly in the side branches. The significance of relatively minor changes, especially in the side branches, is questionable because these are frequent findings in patients without clinical chronic pancreatitis (11). Delineation of the pancreatic duct can be combined with other imaging methods such as fat-saturated T1-weighted images or gadolinium-enhanced images to identify pancreatic parenchymal abnormalities that might indicate the presence of chronic pancreatitis (32–35).

PANCREATIC CYSTS AND BILIARY ANOMALIES

Other important findings important to note on MRCP are the presence of pancreatic cysts and other fluid collections, and congenital abnormalities of biliary development. Pancreas divisum is an important anomaly to note in patients who have acute pancreatitis of obscure cause or repeated episodes of acute pancreatitis. The key finding in making this diagnosis is the continuation of the main pancreatic duct into the duct of Santorini and hence into the minor papilla (Fig. 4) (10). Given the

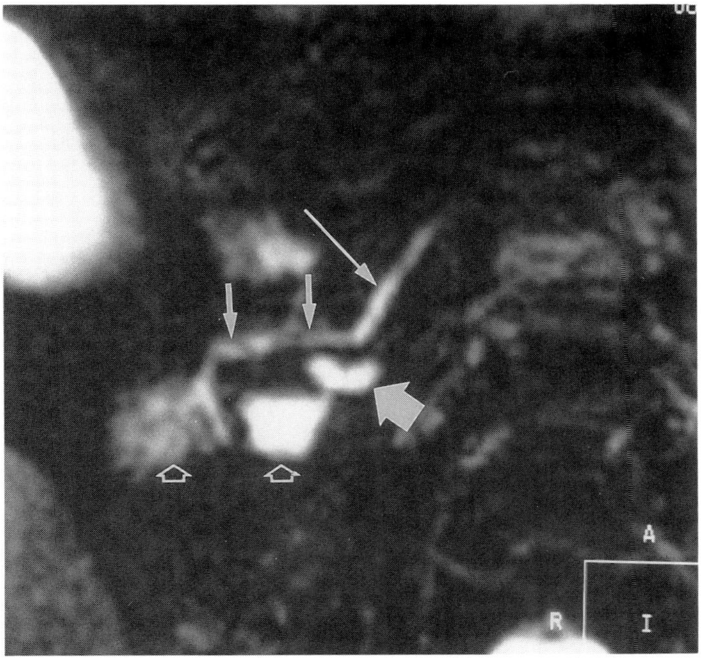

(A)

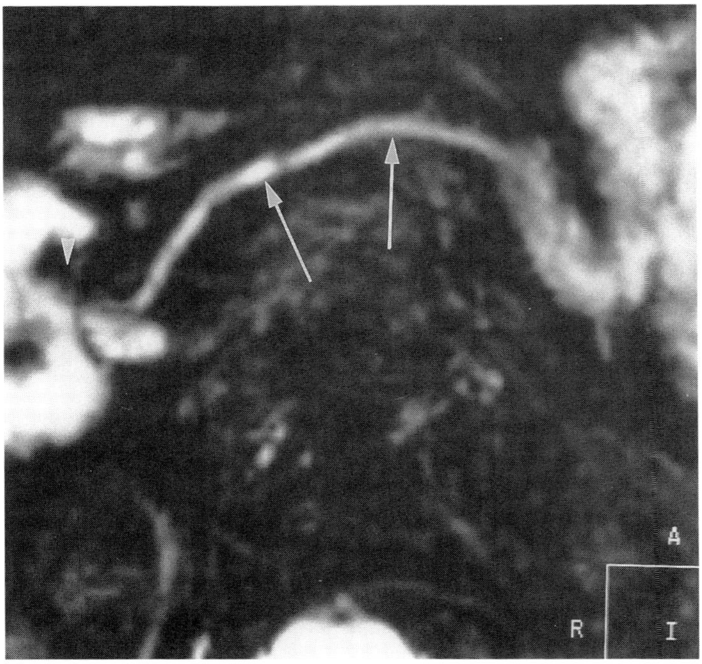

(B)

Figure 4. Pancreas divisum. Two reconstructions of selected axially acquired MRCP images show the main pancreatic duct (long arrows) draining into the duct of Santorini (short arrows). Note that the main duct runs anteriorly to the CBD (broad arrow), rather than the normal medial route. Open arrows denote the duodenum.

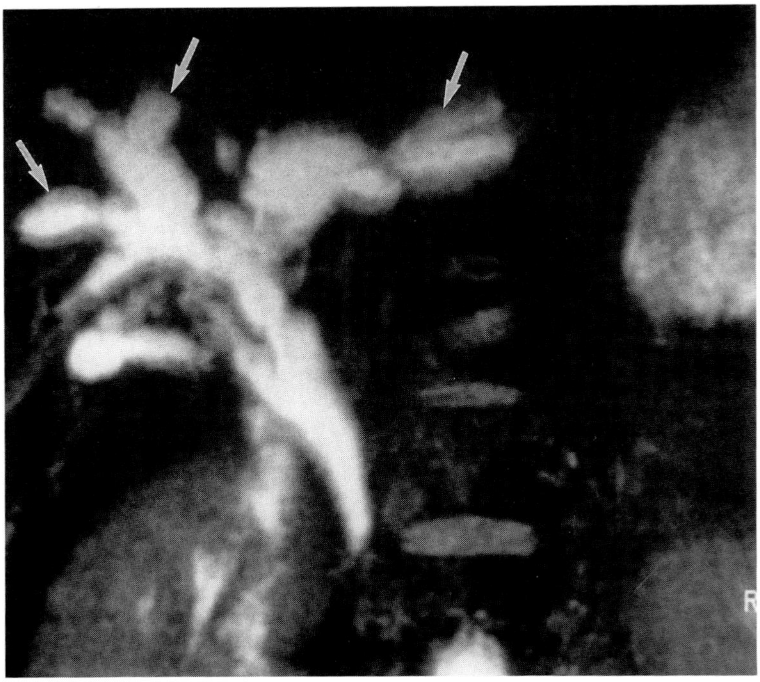

Figure 5. Caroli's disease demonstrated on MR cholangiography. MIP reconstruction from 3D data set shows saccular dilatations (arrows) of the intrahepatic biliary tree and dilatation of the common bile duct with narrowed tapering, findings consistent with type IV choldedochal cyst (38) or Caroli's disease.

variations in anatomy, it may be difficult to make this diagnosis unless both the minor duct and the major duct are well displayed. Congenital abnormalities such as choledochal cysts and choledochocele are easily detected with MRCP (Fig. 5). Similarly, peripancreatic fluid collections and pancreatic pseudocysts are easily displayed with this technique. Identification of ductal connections to the pseudocyst may be difficult in a nondilated ductal system but can be identified in some cases.

SUMMARY

MRCP may best be considered an adjunct to a complete MR imaging evaluation of the pancreatic and biliary systems. This includes FSE techniques with more conventional TEs to image the pancreas, fat-suppressed T1-weighted images for greater sensitivity in detecting focal or diffuse pancreatic signal abnormalities, and dynamic gadolinium contrast enhancement (Fig. 6) (32, 36, 37). Magnetic resonance cholangiopancreatography may be valuable not because it can generate images of equal quality to ERCP, but because it can serve as an adjunct to an examination that can achieve what ERCP cannot: the diagnosis of mass lesions in the pancreas,

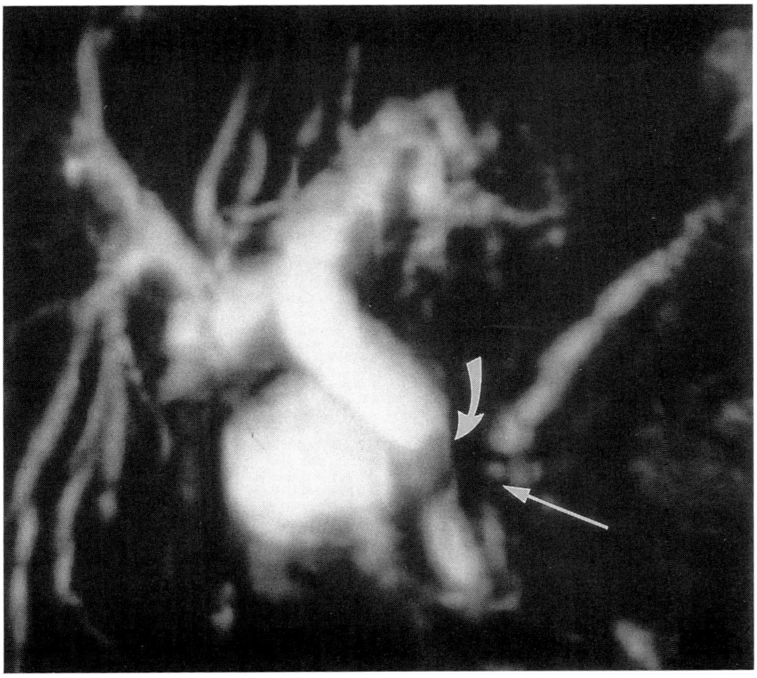

Figure 6. Diagnosis of small pancreatic tumor. MR cholangiography shows intrahepatic biliary dilatation with a focal stricture of the common bile duct (curved arrow) and pancreatic duct (straight arrow), the so-called double duct sign.

parenchymal inflammation, peripancreatic adenopathy, metastases in the liver, detection and characterization of pancreatic pseudocysts, and the detection of vascular stenoses, thromboses, and occlusions, as well as the detection of pancreatic duct stenoses and dilatations. After this type of a comprehensive examination, ERCP can be applied in a more selective manner with fewer overall complications, with the purpose of diagnosis in those patients where MRI has failed to answer the specific clinical questions, or in those patients that require therapeutic endoscopic intervention.

REFERENCES

1. Roy C, Saussine C, Jahn C, et al. Evaluation of RARE-MR urography in the assessment of ureterohydronephrosis. *J Comput Assist Tomogr.* 1994;18:601–608.
2. VanDyke CW, Modic MT, Beale SM, Amartur S, Ross JS. 3D MR myelography. *J Comput Assist Tomogr.* 1992;16:497–500.
3. Outwater EK, Gordon SG. Imaging the pancreatic and biliary ducts with MR (editorial). *Radiology.* 1994;192:19–21.
4. Hall-Craggs MA, Allen CM, Owens CM, et al. MR cholangiography: clinical evaluation in 40 cases. *Radiology.* 1993;189:423–427.

5. Outwater EK. MR cholangiography with a fast spin-echo sequence. *JMRI.* 1993;3:131.
6. Reinhold C, Guibaud L, Genin G, Bret PM. MR cholangiopancreatography: comparison between two-dimensional fast spin-echo and three-dimensional gradient-echo pulse sequences. *JMRI.* 1995;4:379–384.
7. Macaulay SE, Schulte SJ, Sekijima JH, et al. Evaluation of a non breath-hold MR cholangiography technique. *Radiology.* 1995;196:227–232.
8. Soto JA, Barish MA, Yucel EK, et al. Pancreatic duct: MR cholangiopancreatography with a three-dimensional fast spin-echo technique. *Radiology.* 1995;196:459–464.
9. Barish MA, Yucel EK, Soto JA, Chuttani R, Ferrucci JT. MR cholangiopancreatography: efficacy of three-dimensional turbo spin-echo technique. *AJR.* 1995;165:295–300.
10. Laubenberger J, Buchert M, Schneider B, Blum U, J. H, Langer M. Breath-hold projection magnetic resonance-cholangio-pancreaticography (MRCP): a new method for the examination of the bile and pancreatic ducts. *MRM.* 1995;33:18–23.
11. Axon ATR. Endoscopic retrograde cholangiopancreatography in chronic pancreatitis: Cambridge classification. *Radiol Clin North Am.* 1989;27:39–50.
12. Shimizu S, Tada M, Kawai K. Diagnostic ERCP. *Endoscopy.* 1992;24:95–99.
13. Bakan DA, Barnhart JL. Determination of parameters effecting proton relaxation of hepatic and gallbladder biles in dogs. *Hepatology.* 1988;8:341–346.
14. Hricak H, Filly RA, Margulis AR, Moon KL, Crooks LE, Kaufman L. Work in progress: nuclear magnetic resonance imaging of the gallbladder. *Radiology.* 1983;147:481–484.
15. Loflin TG, Simeone JF, Mueller PR, et al. Gallbladder bile in cholecystitis: in vitro MR evaluation. *Radiology.* 1985;157:457–459.
16. Schuster DM, Pedrosa MC, Robbins AH. Magnetic resonance cholangiography. *Abdom Imaging.* 1995;20:353–356.
17. Meakem TJ, Holland GA, McDermott VGM et al. Fast spin echo multicoil magnetic resonance cholangiography: initial experience. Proceedings of the Twelfth Annual Scientific Meeting of the Society of Magnetic Resonance in Medicine; August 14–20, 1993; New York, NY.
18. Guibaud L, Bret PM, Reinhold C, Atri M, Barkun ANG. Diagnosis of choledocholithiasis: value of MR cholangiography. *AJR.* 1994;163.
19. Gross BH, Harter LP, Gore RM, et al. Ultrasonic evaluation of common bile duct stones: Prospective comparison with endoscopic retrograde cholangiopancreatography. *Radiology.* 1983;146:471–474.
20. Cronan JJ, Mueller PR, Simeone JF, et al. Prospective diagnosis of choledocholithiasis. *Radiology.* 1983;146:467–469.
21. Barakos JA, Ralls PW, Lapin SA, et al. Cholelithiasis: evaluation with CT. *Radiology.* 1987;162:415–418.
22. Jeffrey RB, Federle MP, Laing FC, Wall S, Rego J, Moss AA. Computed tomography of choledocholithiasis. *AJR.* 1983;
23. Frey CF, Suzuki M, Isaji S, Zhu Y. Pancreatic resection for chronic pancreatitis. *Surg Clin North Am.* 1989;69:499–528.
24. Parikh NJ, Geenen JE. Current role of ERCP in the management of benign pancreatic disease. *Endoscopy.* 1992;24:120–124.
25. Malfertheiner P, Buchler M. Correlation of imaging and function in chronic pancreatitis. *Radiol Clin North Am.* 1989;27:51–64.
26. Ferrucci JT, Wittenberg J, Black EB, Kirkpatrick RH, Hall DA. Computed body tomography in chronic pancreatitis. *Radiology.* 1979;130:175–182.
27. Neff CC, Simeone JF, Wittenberg J, Mueller PR, Ferrucci JT Jr. Inflammatory pancreatic masses. *Radiology.* 1984;150:35–38.

28. Alpern MB, Sandler MA, Kellman GM, Madrazo BL. Chronic pancreatitis: ultrasonic features. *Radiology.* 1985;155:215–219.

29. Shimizu H, Ida M, Takayama S, et al. The diagnostic accuracy of computed tomography in obstructive biliary disease: a comparative evaluation with direct cholangiography. *Body CT.* 1981;138:411–416.

30. Plumley TF, Rohrmann CA, Freeny PC, Silverstein FE, Ball TJ. Double duct sign: reassessed significance in ERCP. *AJR.* 1982;138:31–35.

31. Schlauch D. Double-duct-sign—is it always cancer? *Endoscopy.* 1993;25:489–490.

32. Mitchell DG, Shapiro M, Schuricht A, Barbot D, Rosato F. Pancreatic disease: findings on state-of-the-art MR images. *AJR.* 1992;159:533–538.

33. Semelka RC, Ascher SM. MR imaging of the pancreas. *Radiology.* 1993;188:593–602.

34. Semelka RC, Simm FC, Recht MP, Deimling M, Lenz G, Laub GA. MR imaging of the pancreas at high field strength: comparison of six sequences. *J Comput Assist Tomogr.* 1991;15:966–971.

35. Semelka RC, Shoenut JP, Kreoeker MA, Micflikier AB. Chronic pancreatitis: MR imaging features before and after administration of gadopentetate dimeglumine. *JMRI.* 1993;3:79–82.

36. Semelka RC, Shoenut JP, Kroeker MA, et al. Bile duct disease: prospective comparison of ERCP, CT, and fat suppression MRI. *Gastrointest Radiol.* 1992;17:347–352.

37. Gabata T, Matsui O, Kadoya M, et al. Small pancreatic adenocarcinomas: efficacy of MR imaging with fat suppression and gadolinium enhancement. *Radiology.* 1994;193:683–688.

38. Rizzo RJ, Szucs RA, Turner MA. Congenital abnormalities of the pancreas and biliary tree in adults. *Radiographics.* 1995;15:49–68.

11

INTRAOPERATIVE CHOLANGIOGRAPHY

Stephen R. T. Evans, M.D., and Mohsen Shabahang, M.D.
Georgetown University Medical Center
Washington, DC

Among all patients undergoing cholecystectomy, 5–10% are reported to harbor asymptomatic common bile duct stones (1, 2). Before the 1930s when Mirizzi first described intraoperative cholangiography (IOC), 30–65% of patients undergoing cholecystectomy were subjected to a common bile duct exploration based on clinical criteria such as jaundice, elevated liver function tests, and pancreatitis (3, 4). With the advent of IOC, the rate of common bile duct explorations decreased to 25% and the rate of positive studies, those in which choledocholithiasis was diagnosed, increased from 25 to 65% (4, 5). Soon after the introduction of this procedure into North America in the 1950s, controversy over its routine versus selective use developed. The advocates of routine IOC argued that the procedure led to the identification of unsuspected stones in 3–5% of patients (6). Proponents of selective use pointed to the 4% false positive studies that led to unnecessary common bile duct explorations and claimed that most of the unsuspected stones discovered by IOC would have remained asymptomatic. This controversy has escalated with the more widespread use of laparoscopic cholecystectomy. In view of the increased rate of common bile duct injuries associated with laparoscopic cholecystectomy, IOC was thought to be important in clarifying the anatomy of the region that would be helpful to surgeons, especially those less experienced with the technique. The widespread use of endoscopic retrograde cholangiopancreatography (ERCP) made the debate more complicated because it offered an alternative diagnostic and therapeutic alternative. Presently, fewer than half the centers in the United States perform IOC on a routine basis. In this chapter, technical aspects of the procedure are reviewed, the arguments for routine versus selective IOC are discussed in the context of laparoscopic cholecystectomy, cost effectiveness is analyzed, and finally IOC is contrasted to other modalities such as ERCP and intraoperative ultrasound.

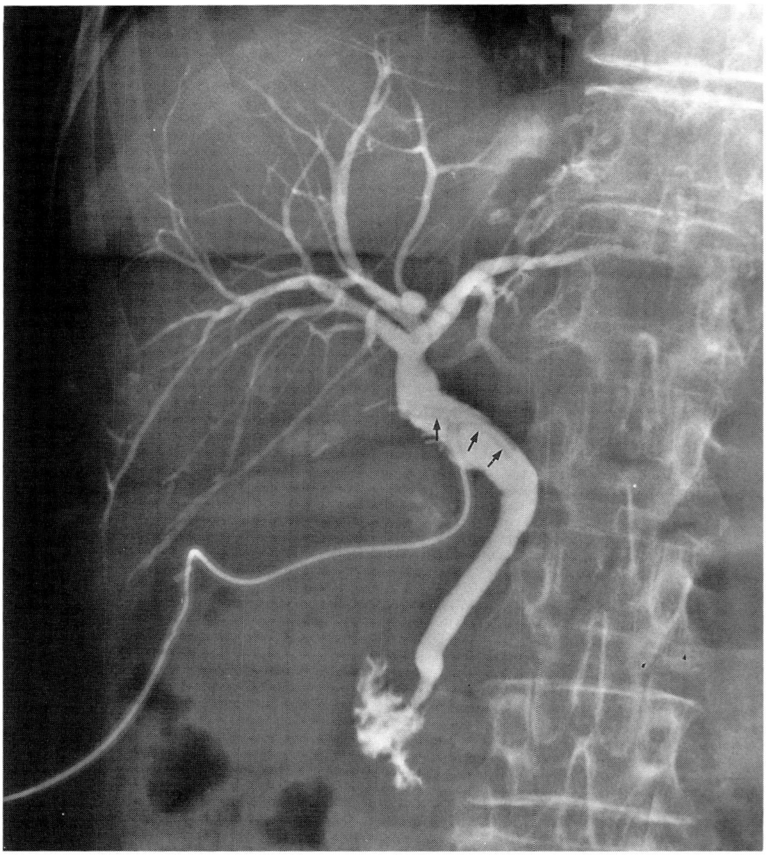

Figure 1. Intraoperative cholangiogram obtained in an open cholecystectomy using a T-tube (arrows) inserted into the common bile duct. The biliary tree including the common bile duct and intrahepatic ducts are clearly depicted.

TECHNICAL CONSIDERATIONS

The main objective of IOC is the visualization of the biliary tree, including the common bile duct, right and left hepatic ducts, intrahepatic ducts, and unimpeded flow into the duodenum (7, 8) (Fig. 1). Laparoscopic IOC can be performed via a variety of techniques. The procedure may be done using the same ports as for cholecystectomy or through a separate needle site. Several types of catheters are available, including balloon tipped or flat tipped (Fig. 2). The former do not require any instruments or clips to hold them in place whereas the latter do. The scope is introduced through the subumbilical cannula while the retractors are inserted into the ports located in the anterior axillary and midclavicular lines. The gallbladder fundus is retracted cephalad while a second grasper introduced through the midclavicular line retracts the infundibulum laterally. This exposes the cystic duct and creates a right angle to the common bile duct. An occluding clip is placed at the junction of the gallbladder and the cystic duct. A transverse incision is made just

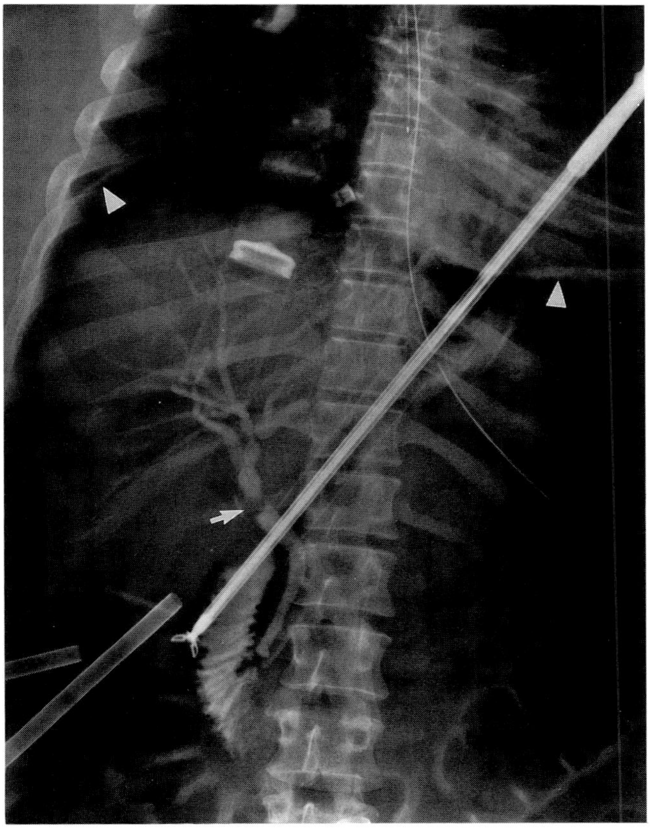

Figure 2. Laparoscopic intraoperative cholangiogram done using a balloon tipped catheter. The balloon tip (arrows) is seen as a lucency in the common bile duct which may be confused with a stone. Note the pneumoperitoneum (arrowheads).

beneath the clip using a laparoscopic scissor. The catheter is passed into the abdomen via another port lateral to the gallbladder. Precise positioning of the catheter is accomplished by the use of a grasper through the epigastric port. Once the catheter is securely in the cystic duct saline is injected to ensure the absence of any leakage. Then 15 ml of contrast medium is introduced and the image obtained (Fig. 3). This can be done either as a static radiograph or fluoroscopically. The latter is an overall superior technique offering the advantage of speed with better resolution, allowing for dynamic evaluation of the biliary tree, and lower frequency of false positive and false negative studies (6) (Fig. 4). After completion, the cystic duct is clipped distal to the incision. The reasons for failure in performing intraoperative cholangiograms range from the small diameter of the cystic duct to its tortuosity to the existence of prominent valves (9). An important point in the interpretation of the intraoperative cholangiogram is to ensure visualization of the entire biliary tree (10). An incomplete study is one of the main reasons for misinterpretation. Intraoperative cholangiogram adds 10–20 min to the procedure (6, 11). The added cost is estimated at approximately $700.

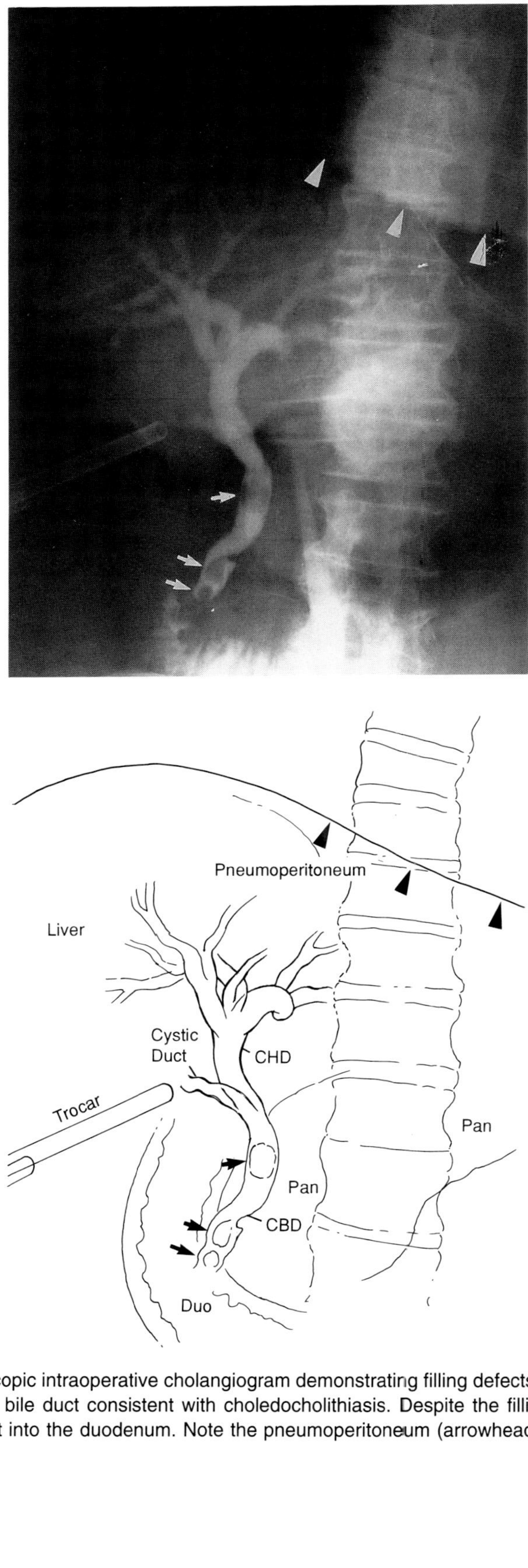

Figure 3. Laparoscopic intraoperative cholangiogram demonstrating filling defects (arrows) in the mid and distal common bile duct consistent with choledocholithiasis. Despite the filling defects, there is free flow of contrast into the duodenum. Note the pneumoperitoneum (arrowheads).

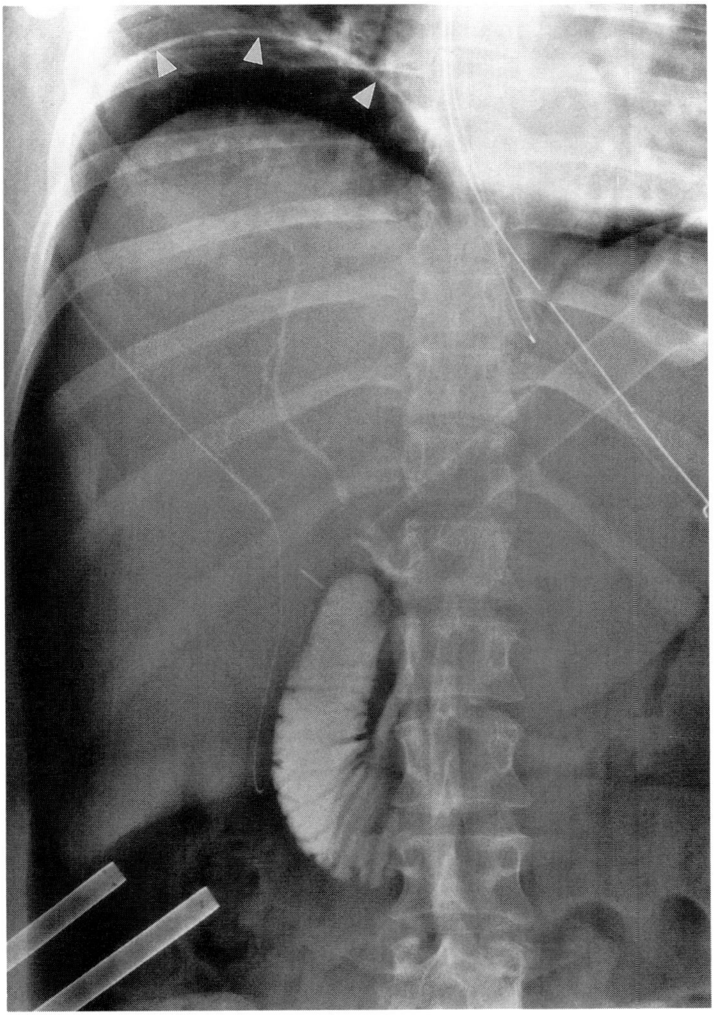

Figure 4. There is insufficient retrograde flow of contrast in this IOC with limited ability to detect any abnormalities in the proximal biliary tree. The quality of this film also points out some of the limitations of a static film versus fluoroscopic visualization. Note the pneumoperitoneum (arrowheads).

Intraoperative cholangiograms can also be obtained by cannulating the gallbladder instead of the cystic duct (12). In this case, the cholangiogram is done immediately after the insertion of the laparoscope. The catheter is inserted into the fundus of the gallbladder instead of the cystic duct. Some bile is aspirated and contrast is injected. The technique has not gained popularity because of the high risk of bile leakage.

INDICATIONS

The indications for IOC have been a source of controversy. The use of this procedure in patients undergoing laparoscopic cholecystectomy who present with the clinical

Table 1. Clinical criteria indicative of increased risk of choledocholithiasis

Dilated common bile duct (>12 mm)
Dilated cystic duct (>5 mm)
Pancreatitis
Cholangitis
Elevated bilirubin
Elevated alkaline phosphatase
Sonographic evidence of duct stones
Palpable common bile duct stones
Gallstones < 10 mm
Cholecystitis
Advanced age

criteria associated with choledocholithiasis (Table 1) is well accepted (11). However, the proponents of selective IOC believe that these studies should be obtained only in patients with these criteria, whereas advocates of routine IOC contend that by performing the study in every patient, the surgeon obtains a clear view of the biliary anatomy. This decreases the probability of iatrogenic injury and retained unsuspected common bile duct stones. The main question in this debate is whether the benefits of routine IOC are significant enough to justify the complications and cost. As Clair and Brooks point out, the false positive rate of routine IOC is 1–5%, which translates into 12,000 patients among about 600,000 undergoing cholecystectomy annually (11). These patients are subjected to laparoscopic common duct exploration or postoperative ERCP, both of which are associated with complications ranging from pancreatitis to cystic duct avulsion. The monetary cost is also significant. With an estimated $500–700 per procedure, the cost for 500,000 IOCs will be approximately $250 million. The following discussion illustrates these arguments in more depth.

ROUTINE INTRAOPERATIVE CHOLANGIOGRAPHY

Because laparoscopic cholecystectomy has replaced the conventional technique, the controversy over performing intraoperative cholangiograms on a routine versus selective basis has been rekindled. Because laparoscopy gives a two-dimensional image and precludes palpation of the common bile duct, IOC has been used not only to detect the presence of choledocholithiasis, but also to clarify anatomy and any injuries caused by the procedure. The proponents of routine IOC base their practice on three arguments: better anatomic delineation of the biliary tree and hence lower incidence of injury, identification of unsuspected calculi and injury, and increased familiarity of surgeons with the technique (especially for purposes of teaching) and interpretation of results (7, 13).

Many surgeons use IOC as a "road map" for a safe and successful laparoscopic cholecystectomy (14). This is thought to be especially important in cases where anatomic anomalies such as a short cystic duct or drainage of the cystic duct into the right hepatic duct exist. At Cedars-Sinai Medical Center in Los Angeles, Phillips et al. successfully performed IOCs on 53 of 58 patients (15). Among the 53 patients, five (8%) showed anatomic anomalies. In a series at the University of Maryland Medical Center, Flowers et al. reported a 2.6% incidence of anatomic variance in 364 patients undergoing laparoscopic cholecystectomy (16), and Campenhout et al. reported a 10% rate among 107 patients (17). Other arguments supporting the use of IOC as a "road map" focus on the fact that the laparoscope projects a two-dimensional image that is obtained in a plane parallel to that of the biliary tree. This renders the identification of the common bile duct more difficult, especially in patients with anatomic anomalies, obesity, or nonpliable livers that are difficult to rotate cephalad (6).

The second argument stressed by the proponents of routine IOC focuses on the importance of identifying a bile duct injury that occurs during the operation. This is based on the premise that recognition of the injuries at the time of the original operation would prevent septicemia, jaundice, or peritonitis (18). In a study of patients with biliary tract injuries following laparoscopic cholecystectomy from seven different institutions, Woods et al. noted immediate recognition and treatment occurring twice as often when IOCs were done (3). Proponents of routine IOC claim that the technique helps detect proximal injuries to the common bile duct and hence decreases the incidence of more severe duct injury, which may require hepaticojejunostomy (5).

Unsuspected choledocholithiasis detected by IOC differs from a rate of 2.6% in the Flowers series (16) to 7.5% in the Cedars-Sinai series (9) to 9.3% in the Campenhout series (17). Although most of these stones are extractable by ERCP postoperatively (or may be clinically insignificant), these authors believe that it is important to detect their existence before the development of symptoms.

Increased experience with the technique and interpretation of IOC may be important, as suggested by a reported 64% rate of misinterpretation (6). Increased experience during training may lead to a higher degree of proficiency and prevent misinterpretations, resulting in lower morbidity.

SELECTIVE INTRAOPERATIVE CHOLANGIOGRAPHY

In the era of open cholecystectomies and before the endoscopic extraction of retained common bile duct stones was possible, routine IOC had a false positive rate of 1% and led to a number of unnecessary common bile duct explorations (19). In a study by Pace et al. of 1351 cholecystectomies, it was determined that the rate of common bile duct explorations might have been 55% less if IOC had been done exclusively on patients suspect for choledocholithiasis, namely those with pancreatitis, dilated common bile duct, elevated bilirubin or alkaline phosphatase, or palpable common bile duct stones (19). In another study of open cholecystectomies done at the Universtiy of Arkansas Medical Center, the group of patients undergoing routine IOC had a higher rate of postoperative complications possibly due to a higher rate of common bile duct exploration (20). Hence a strong argument was made against performing the procedure routinely.

In the era of laparoscopic cholecystectomy, the proponents of selective IOC have not changed their criteria for the procedure and in fact rely more heavily on

ERCP in the case of the unsuspected retained stone. Arguments against routine IOC still persist. The reasons include the relatively high false positive rate when used routinely, absence of a significant difference in morbidity of laparoscopic cholecystectomy in groups undergoing routine versus selective IOC when careful dissection is done, and the hypothesis that many of the undetected stones will remain asymptomatic and if they do become symptomatic, ERCP and sphincterotomy can be utilized to extract the stone.

The false positive rate of IOC is about 1–5% (11). Proponents of selective IOC argue that if the procedure were limited to patients who meet the selective criteria (Table 1), the false positive rate would be much lower and hence would avoid unnecessary common bile duct explorations that may be associated with complications such as stricture formation (21).

The most significant argument made by the proponents of selective IOC pertains to the use of the procedure to create a "road map." Careful dissection of Calot's triangle with early mobilization of the anterior and posterior gallbladder peritoneal attachments, definitive visualization of the junction of the infundibulum and cystic duct, and caudad retraction of Hartmann's pouch with lateral retraction of the neck will minimize duct injury (1). In a study of 525 patients undergoing laparoscopic cholecystectomy, IOC was used on a selective basis only for patients with jaundice, pancreatitis, elevated liver function tests, and sonographic evidence of choledocholithiasis (4). In this group, Lorimer et al., reported no bile duct injuries or leaks. Additionally, a study from the Royal College of Surgeons in Dublin, in 300 laparoscopic cholecystectomies with selective IOC, only two injuries were reported, both of which were noted during the operation (2). Clair et al. reported one injury in a prospective study of 514 patients undergoing laparoscopic cholecystectomy with selective IOC (22). Opponents of routine IOC also point out that the argument made for use of routine IOC as a tool to gain a higher level of experience in interpreting the results of intraoperative cholangiograms is not valid. The success rate in groups doing routine and selective IOC is similar, ranging from 90–95% (11).

As has been alluded to above, surgeons who use IOC selectively utilize criteria such as those outlined in Table 1 to determine the need for the study. They argue that such selective use does not increase the risk of retained stones. Clair and Brooks studied a group of 1250 patients who had undergone laparoscopic cholecystectomy and selective IOC (11). The risk of retained stones in this group was less than 1%, which is similar to results published by those who perform IOC routinely. In a retrospective study of 495 patients undergoing laparoscopic cholecystectomy and selective IOC at Mayo Clinic, only 1.4% of these patients presented within 2 months after the operation with symptoms of choledocholithiasis (23). Robinson et al. argue that if IOC has been done routinely that number would have decreased to 0.6%. The authors note that in all of these patients with retained choledocholithiasis, ERCP and sphincterotomy were adequate for extracting the stones. These results are confirmed by a study of 1344 patients at Kaiser Permanente at Los Angeles where seven presented with retained stones (24). All seven underwent ERCP and stones were extracted successfully.

At the University of Paris, Huguier et al. proposed a scheme to determine the need for IOC in patients undergoing laparoscopic cholecystectomy (25). The authors believe patients with a low probability of having choledocholithiais (<2%) can be discriminated from those with a high probability (>32%) by using

Table 2. Studies supporting routing versus selective intraoperative cholangiography

Author	Year	Attempted IOC	Successful IOC	False Positive	Anomaly	Stones	Recommendation
Phillips et al. (15)	1990	58	53 (92%)	—	5 (9%)	6 (10%)	Routine
Berci et al. (14)	1991	415	373 (90%)	—	—	—	Routine
Flowers et al. (16)	1992	165	150 (91%)	3 (2%)	—	16 (10%)	Routine
Campenhout et al. (17)	1993	105	75 (71%)	—	8(8%)	10 (9%)	Routine
Clair et al. (22)	1993	36	30 (83%)	—	—	1 (2.8%)	Selective
Dorazio (24)	1995	98	—	6 (6%)	—	1 (1%)	Selective
Robinson et al. (23)	1995	161	—	2 (1.2%)	—	5 (3%)	Selective
Traverso et al. (10)	1994	624	535 (86%)	7 (1.3%)	105 (20%)	68 (13%)	Selective

five criteria: advanced age, dilated common bile duct above 12 mm, small gallstones (<10 mm), history of biliary colic, and chronic or acute cholecystitis. The scoring is based on the above-mentioned factors. The formula is as follows: $R = 0.04 \times \text{age} + 31.1$ (if the common bile duct diameter is >12 mm) + 1.2 (if gallstones measure <10 mm) +1 (if the patient has a history of colic) + 0.7 (if patient presented with cholecystitis), where R is the determinant of the patient's risk level. An R value of less than 3.5 puts the patient at a 2% risk level, a score of 3.5–5.9 is equivalent to about a 17% risk, and a score of greater than 5.9 increases the risk of choledocholithiasis to greater than 32%. More studies such as this will help to clarify further the clouded argument of selective versus routine use of IOC. Table 2 summarizes the findings of eight of the most recent studies supporting routine or selective IOC.

INTRAOPERATIVE CHOLANGIOGRAPHY VERSUS ENDOSCOPIC RETROGRADE CHOLANGIOPANCREATOGRAPHY

The more prevalent use of ERCP has altered the indications for IOC; ERCP can be used preoperatively in patients suspected of having choledocholithiasis or postoperatively in those thought to have retained common bile duct stones. Endoscopic retrograde cholangiopancreatography may not be as reliable as IOC in visualizing the common bile duct, especially the proximal portion (7). Despite this, some advocate the use of preoperative ERCP as a substitute for IOC.

In an attempt to compare the morbidity, mortality, length of hospital stay, or hospital cost among patients undergoing IOC or preoperative ERCP, Stiegmann et al. randomized 34 patients suspected of having choledocholithiasis (based on elevated serum bilirubin and alkaline phosphatase, increased common bile duct diameter, and sonographic evidence of stones) into these two treatment groups. No significant difference was noted in any of these variables between the two groups of patients. In view of the similarity in outcome between the two alternatives, the debate centers on the appropriateness of preoperative ERCP as a replacement for IOC.

Several studies have analyzed the outcome of preoperative ERCP in patients suspected of having choledocholithiasis. In a series of 400 patients at the Western General Hospital at Edinburgh, Scotland, 20% underwent preoperative ERCP based on clinical presentation indicative of choledocholithiasis (27). Fifty-six percent of the ERCPs were normal whereas 38% showed common bile duct stones. Postoperatively, 17 patients underwent ERCP with 12 having retained duct stones. All stones were extracted and in no case was there an indication for operative intervention. ERCP is not free of complications, but the rate is relatively low. In a prospective study of 1300 patients undergoing laparoscopic cholecystectomy at McGill University, Barkun reported a 1–3% risk of pancreatitis associated with ERCP (1). In the same study, of 106 patients who underwent preoperative ERCP based on clinical criteria, 50 (47%) were diagnosed with choledocholithiasis. Of the 50 patients, stones were extracted successfully in 45. The remaining five required common bile duct exploration. Intraoperative cholangiograms were done in 54 patients of which six were shown to have choledocholithiasis. Five of the six had undergone ERCP and unsuccessful attempts at extracting the stones. Only in one of these patients did IOC show a stone that had not been detected with selective use of preoperative ERCP. In a study of 1507 patients from three centers in England, the complication rate of ERCP was shown to be 2.7% (28). Of all the patients, 306 underwent ERCP for suspected choledocholithiasis; 161 (52%) of these patients were proved to have common bile duct stones. ERCP was successfully used in 128 of them to extract the stones. One percent of the patients were found to have retained stones in whom ERCP was used successfully to extract the stones. Finally, in their series of 300 patients undergoing laparoscopic cholecystectomy, Grace et al. performed preoperative ERCP on 27, of whom only seven (26%) had a positive study (2).

In view of the studies shown here, even in patient populations selected based on clinical criteria for choledocholithiasis, preoperative ERCP is associated with a high rate of normal results ranging from 48 to 74%.

INTRAOPERATIVE CHOLANGIOGRAPHY VERSUS LAPAROSCOPIC ULTRASONOGRAPHY

Recently, laparoscopic ultrasonography has been proposed as an alternative to IOC. This procedure is less invasive and does not require the injection of any contrast material. The ultrasound transducer is introduced through the epigastric or umbilical port and brought into contact with the region of the biliary tree under study (29). The time required for laparoscopic ultrasonography ranges from 3 to 18 min. The results of four different studies comparing laparoscopic ultrasonography with IOC were similar (29–32). These originated from Washington University, St. Vincent's Hospital in Indianapolis, University of Denver, and a combined study from Pisa, Italy and Dundee, Scotland. They all showed excellent detection of unsuspected stones in the extrahepatic biliary tree. In fact, in all four studies, laparoscopic ultrasonography was more sensitive than IOC in showing the unsuspected common bile duct stone. Also, this technique has a lower false positive rate. The specificity of laparoscopic ultrasonography is 100% compared to 76% for IOC

(31). However, the technique is not adequate for studying the proximal and distal regions of the biliary tree or in detecting anatomic anomalies. In view of the limitations of laparoscopic ultrasonography, it can be considered as an adjunct to but not a replacement for IOC.

Intraoperative cholangiography is a valuable technique for the visualization of the biliary tree, especially when used with fluoroscopy. The debate over routine versus selective use may be partially resolved when more prospective studies comparing the two approaches have been completed. In this era of cost containment and optimizing resource utilization, there must be rational justification for all costly procedures based on outcomes analysis. The use of clinical criteria indicative of choledocholithiasis may lead to a more cost-efficient and judicious utilization of the procedure. This is particularly true as surgeons' experience in performing laparoscopic cholecystectomy increases and the utility of IOC as a "road map" decreases. Other modalities such as ERCP or laparoscopic ultrasound may be useful as adjuncts to IOC, but at present are not replacements for it.

REFERENCES

1. Barkun JS, Fried GM, Barkun AN, et al. Cholecystectomy without operative cholangiography: implications for common bile duct injury and retained common bile duct stones. *Ann Surg.* 1993;218:371–379.
2. Grace PA, Qureshi A, Burke P, et al. Selective cholangiography in laparoscopic cholecystectomy. *Br J Surg.* 1993;80:244–246.
3. Woods MS, Traverso LW, Kozarek RA, et al. Biliary tract complications of laparoscopic cholecystectomy are detected more frequently with routine intraoperative cholangiography. *Surg Endosc.* 1995;9:1076–1080.
4. Lorimer JW, Fairfull-Smith RJ. Intraoperative cholangiography is not essential to avoid duct injuries during laparoscopic cholecystectomy. *Am J Surg.* 1995;169:344–347.
5. Phillips EH. Routine versus selective intraoperative cholangiography. *Am J Surg.* 1993;165:505–507.
6. Soper NJ, Brunt LM. The case for routine operative cholangiography during laparoscopic cholecystectomy. *Surg Clin North Am.* 1994;74:953–959.
7. Willekes CL, Edoga JK, Castronuovo JJ, Widmann WD, McLean ER, Chevinsky AH. Technical elements of successful laparoscopic cholangiography as defined by radiographic criteria. *Arch Surg.* 1995;130:398–400.
8. Gompertz RHK, Rhodes M, Lennard TWJ. Laparoscopic cholangiography: an effective and inexpensive technique. *Br J Surg.* 1992;79:233–234.
9. Sackier JM, Berci G, Phillips E, Carroll B, Shapiro S, Paz-Partlow M. The role of cholangiography in laparoscopic cholecystectomy. *Arch Surg.* 1991;126:1021–1026.
10. Traverso LW, Hauptmann EM, Lynge DC. Routine intraoperative cholangiography and its contribution to the selective cholangiographer. *Am J Surg.* 1994;167:464–468.
11. Clair DG, Brooks DC. Laparoscopic cholangiography: the case for a selective approach. *Surg Clin North Am.* 1994;74:961–966.
12. Kuster GGR, Gilroy S, Graefen M. Intraoperative cholangiography for laparoscopic cholecystectomy. *Surg Gynecol Obstet.* 1993;176:411–417.
13. Cantwell DV. Routine cholangiography during laparoscopic cholecystectomy. *Arch Surg.* 1992;127:483–484.

14. Berci G, Sackier JM, Paz-Partlow M. Routine or selected intraoperative cholangiography during laparoscopic cholecystectomy? *Am J Surg.* 1991;161:355–360.
15. Phillips EH, Berci G, Carroll B, Daykhovsky L, Sackier J, Paz-Partlow M. The importance of intraoperative cholangiography during laparoscopic cholecystectomy. *Am Surg.* 1990;56:792–795.
16. Flowers JL, Zucker KA, Graham SM, Scovill WA, Imbembo AL, Bailey RW. Laparoscopic cholangiography: results and indications. *Ann Surg.* 1991;215:209–216.
17. Campenhout IV, Prosmanne O, Gagner M, Pomp A, Deslandres E, Levesque HP. Routine operative cholangiography during laparoscopic cholecystectomy: feasibility and value in 107 patients. *AJR.* 1993;160:1209–1211.
18. Berci G. Biliary ductal anatomy and anomalies: the role of intraoperative cholangiography during laparoscopic cholecystectomy. *Surg Clin North Am.* 1992;72:1069–1075.
19. Pace BW, Cosgrove J, Breuer B, Margolis IB. Intraoperative cholangiography revisited. *Arch Surg.* 1992;127:448–450.
20. Hauer-Jensen M, Karesen R, Nygaard K, et al. Prospective randomized study of routine intraoperative cholangiography during open cholecystectomy: long-term follow-up and multivariate analysis of preditors of choledocholithiasis. *Surgery* 1993;113:318–323.
21. Keane FBV, Tanner WA, Gillen P. Operative cholangiography and laparoscopic bile duct exploration. *Br J Surg.* 1993;80:957–958.
22. Clair DG, Carr-Locke DL, Becker JM, Brooks DC. Routine cholangiography is not warranted during laparoscopic cholecystectomy. *Arch Surg.* 1993;128:551–555.
23. Robinson BL, Donohue JH, Gunes S, et al. Selective operative cholangiography: appropriate management for laparoscopic cholecystectomy. *Arch Surg.* 1995;130:625–631.
24. Dorazio RA. Selective operative cholangiography in laparoscopic cholecystectomy. *Am Surg.* 1995;61:911–913.
25. Huguier M, Bornet P, Charpak Y, Houry S, Chastang C. Selective contraindications based on multivariate analysis for operative cholangiography in biliary lithiasis. *Surg Gynecol Obstet. 1991;172:470–474.*
26. Stiegmann GV, Goff JS, Mansour A, Pearlman N, Reveille RM, Norton L. Precholecystectomy endoscopic cholangiography and stone removal is not superior to cholecystectomy, cholangiography, and common duct exploration. *Am J Surg.* 1992;163:227–230.
27. Madhavan KK, MacIntyre IMC, Wilson RG, Saunders JH, Nixon SJ, Hamer-Hodges DW. Role of intraoperative cholangiography in laparoscopic cholecystectomy. *Br J Surg.* 1995;82:249–252.
28. Welbourn CRB, Mehta D, Armstrong CP, Gear MWL, Eyre-Brook IA. Selective preoperative endoscopic retrograde cholangiography with sphincterotomy avoids bile duct exploration during laparoscopic cholecystectomy. *Gut* 1995;37:576–579.
29. Teefey SA, Soper NJ, Middleton WD, et al. Imaging of the common bile duct during laparoscopic cholecystectomy: sonography versus videofluoroscopic cholangiography. *AJR* 1995;165:847–851.
30. Pietrabissa A, di Candio G, Giulianotti C, Shimi SM, Cuschieri A, Mosca F. Comparative evaluation of contact ultrasonography and transcystic cholangiography during laparoscopic cholecystectomy: a prospective study. *Arch Surg.* 1995;130:1110–1114.
31. Barteau JA, Castro D, Arregui ME, Tetik C. A comparison of intraoperative ultrasound versus cholangiography in the evaluation of the common bile duct during laparoscopic cholecystectomy. *Surg Endosc.* 1995;9:490–496.
32. Stiegmann GV, Soper NJ, Filipi CJ, McIntyre RC, Callery MP, Cordova JF. Laparoscopic ultrasonography as compared with static or dynamic cholangiography at laparoscopic cholecystectomy. *Surg Endosc.* 1995;9:1269–1273.

12

PERCUTANEOUS TRANSHEPATIC CHOLANGIOGRAPHY AND BILIARY INTERVENTIONS

Steven V. Lossef, M.D.
Georgetown University Medical Center
Washington, DC

Interventional radiologists have made important contributions to the diagnosis and treatment of disorders of the bile ducts. The role of percutaneous biliary interventions has been redefined with the advent of modern endoscopic therapy and laparoscopic surgery. The purpose of this chapter is to outline the current indications and techniques for transhepatic management of biliary disease.

DIAGNOSTIC PERCUTANEOUS CHOLANGIOGRAPHY

Percutaneous transhepatic cholangiography (PTHC) has been used for delineation of biliary obstruction, stenosis, leakage, and stone disease for more than 30 years (1). However, advances in endoscopic retrograde cholangiopancreatography (ERCP) have reduced the need for purely diagnostic transhepatic cholangiograms; ERCP has the advantage of being less invasive than percutaneous procedures by eliminating the need to puncture the hepatic capsule. It provides information about both biliary and pancreatic ducts, and affords the capability for endoscopic stenting and stone extraction, if necessary. Percutaneous transhepatic cholangiography is currently indicated only when ERCP has failed or is unfeasible. Successful ERCP may be precluded by benign or malignant strictures of the esophagus or duodenum that prevent introduction of an endoscope. Postoperative changes following Roux-en-Y biliary–enteric bypass also may restrict endoscopic manipulation. Bulky tumor invading the ampulla may make endoscopic cannulation of the bile duct impossible.

Finally, high-grade strictures, bulky stones, or complete occlusions may limit the ability to opacify and evaluate the peripheral bile ducts endoscopically. Percutaneous diagnostic cholangiography may provide important information in such selected cases, and may also be a preamble to performing percutaneous interventions such as stent insertion, stone extraction, and stricture dilatation.

Percutaneous transhepatic cholangiography involves insertion of a 22-gauge Chiba needle (skinny needle) into an intrahepatic bile duct (1). Puncture of an intrahepatic duct is usually performed by making blind needle passes, which is relatively safe when a 22-gauge needle is employed. Ultrasound guidance is sometimes helpful, especially for left ductal punctures (2). Percutaneous transhepatic cholangiography is usually performed using local anesthetic and conscious sedation. Broad-spectrum intravenous antibiotics should always be administered prior to the procedure. Any abnormality of prothrombin time, partial thromboplastin time, and platelets should be corrected. Usually a right intrahepatic duct is punctured via a right midaxillary line approach through the right lateral tenth or eleventh intercostal space, below the pleural reflection. The needle is inserted and then slowly retracted while contrast is injected until the tip is positioned within a bile duct. The intrahepatic and extrahepatic ducts are then opacified. Radiographs are obtained in frontal and oblique projections. It may be necessary to roll the patient into the left lateral decubitus position temporarily to fill the left intrahepatic ducts. If strictures or stones are suspected to involve the left intrahepatic ducts predominantly, a subxiphoid approach to the left intrahepatic ducts may be utilized (2). Contrast should not be injected under pressure in the setting of bacterial cholangitis. Complications of percutaneous thin-needle cholangiography include sepsis, bleeding, pneumothorax, and bile peritonitis (1).

Percutaneous cholangiograms should be examined for the presence and location of ductal stenoses, occlusions, intraluminal filling defects, and/or bile leaks. If contrast flows freely through patent and intact bile ducts and no percutaneous interventions are necessary, the needle may be safely removed. If there is complete obstruction to bile flow, it is important to insert a percutaneous drainage catheter to prevent painful intraperitoneal leakage of bile through the needle tract. Percutaneous access should also be maintained if further interventional radiology procedures are required.

PERCUTANEOUS BILIARY DRAINAGE FOR MALIGNANT TUMORS

Percutaneous biliary drainage is indicated for palliation of pruritus and treatment of cholangitis in patients with unresectable tumors when ERCP has failed or is not feasible (3, 4). Such patients may be palliated and spared a major surgical bypass procedure. Patients with pancreatic carcinoma, cholangiocarcinoma involving the common bile duct or distal common hepatic duct, gallbladder carcinoma, ampullary carcinoma, and metastases or lymphoma involving the peripancreatic and porta hepatis regions may benefit from percutaneous drainage. Percutaneous drainage often proves superior to endoscopic drainage for high cholangiocarcinomas located in the proximal common hepatic duct and at the confluence of the right and left bile ducts (Klatskin tumors). Preoperative percutaneous biliary drainage is also indicated in selected patients with resectable cholangiocarcinomas because a palpa-

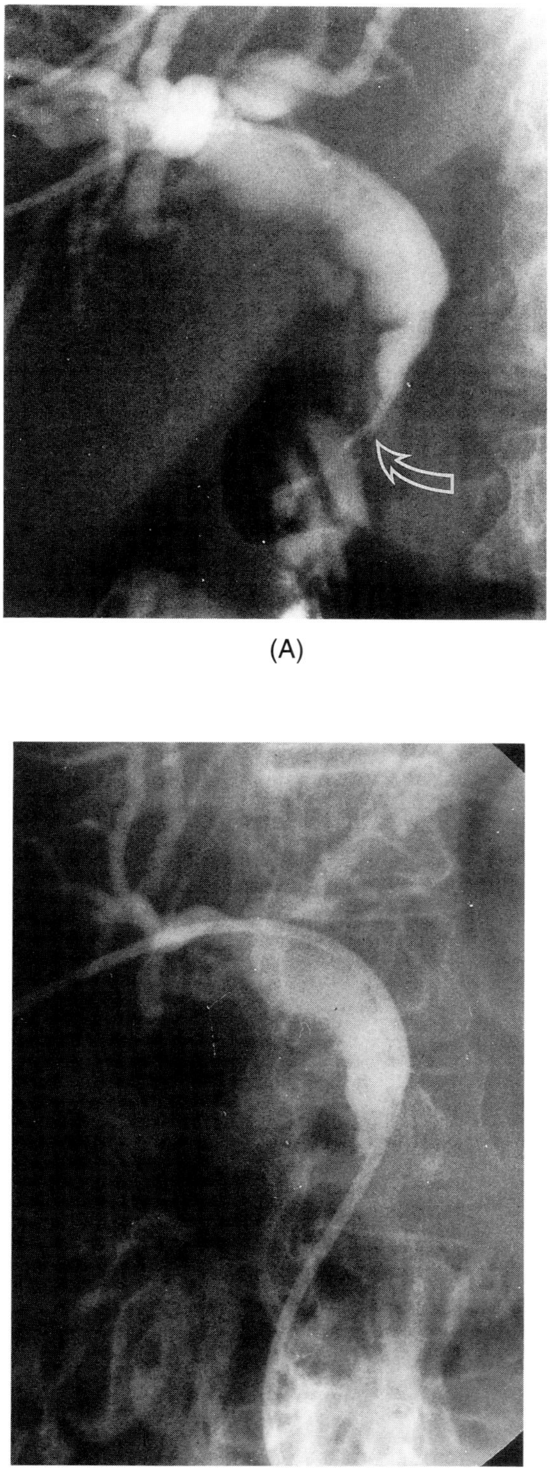

(A)

(B)

Figure 1. (A) Biliary obstruction and severe narrowing of the distal common bile duct (arrow) due to carcinoma of the pancreas. (B) An internal–external biliary drainage catheter inserted via a right ductal approach relieves the obstruction.

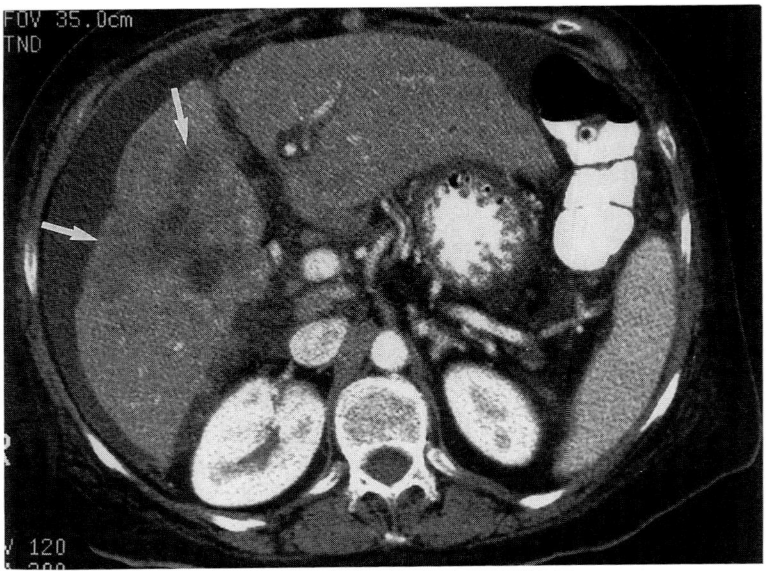

(A)

Figure 2. (A) A CT scan in a patient with biliary obstruction due to carcinoma of the gallbladder shows a bulky metastasis (arrows) in the right lobe of the liver and abundant ascites. These factors led to the choice of a left ductal approach for biliary decompression. (B) Cholangiogram shows narrowing of the central left intrahepatic ducts and obstruction of the common hepatic duct (next page). (C) An internal–external drainage catheter decompresses the right and left ducts and has its distal tip in the duodenum (page 180).

ble internal–external stent may aid in surgical dissections near the bifurcation of the hepatic ducts (5).

An abdominal CT scan and/or sonogram should be performed prior to percutaneous biliary drainage. This is helpful for planning the approach if bile duct dilatation is limited to only one hepatic lobe. Cross-sectional imaging also permits planning of a suitable percutaneous tract to avoid traversing any potentially necrotic or hemorrhagic intrahepatic masses. It may identify patients with multiductal obstruction caused by extensive bilobar metastases or infiltrating hepatic tumors, in whom insertion of multiple drainage catheters yields low practical utility. Finally, it allows detection of ascites or large right pleural effusions, factors that favor the choice of a left ductal approach.

Percutaneous Biliary Drainage Procedure

Any coagulation abnormalities are corrected and intravenous antibiotics are administered prior to performing biliary drainage. The initial puncture may be either right or left sided. Right hepatic approaches (Fig. 1) are technically easier because there are a larger number of bile ducts available per needle pass. However, a left ductal approach is preferable if there is abundant ascites, because intraperitoneal fluid is less likely to pool and leak around the more anteriorly placed tube when the patient rests in the supine position (Fig. 2). Left ductal punctures are also useful if there is a large right pleural effusion, because it eliminates the risk of traversing

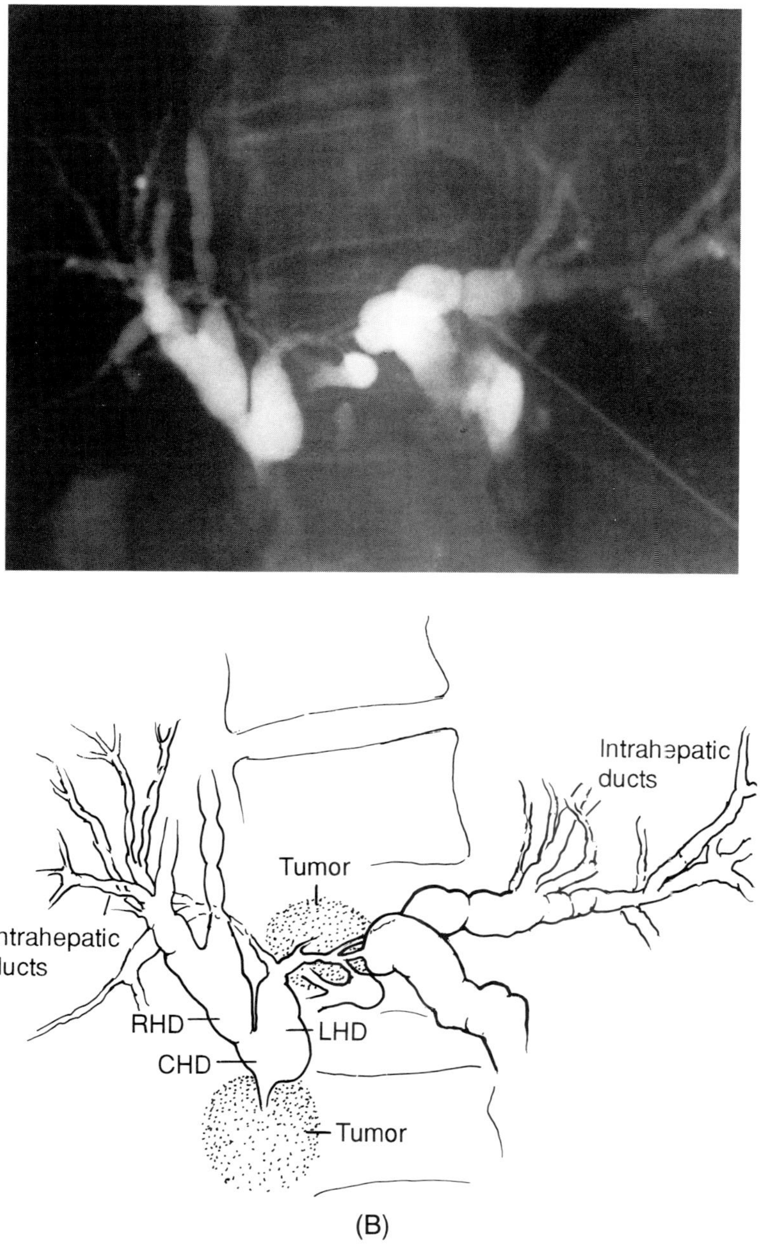

(B)

Figure 2. *(Continued)*

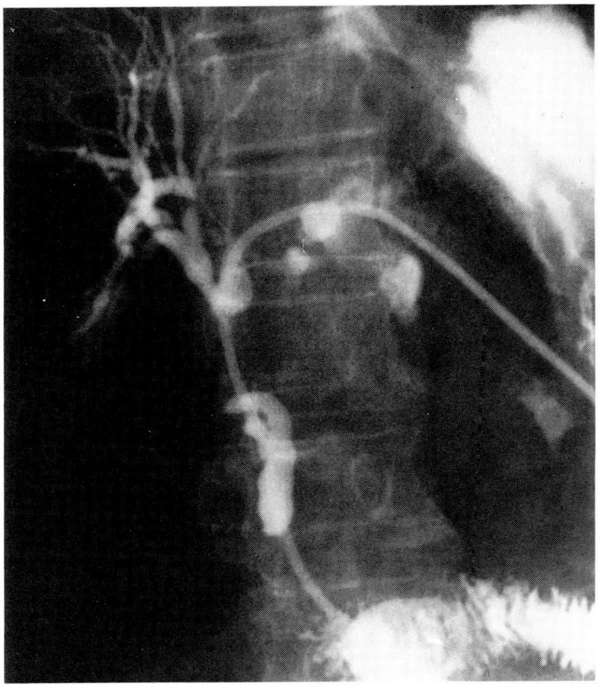

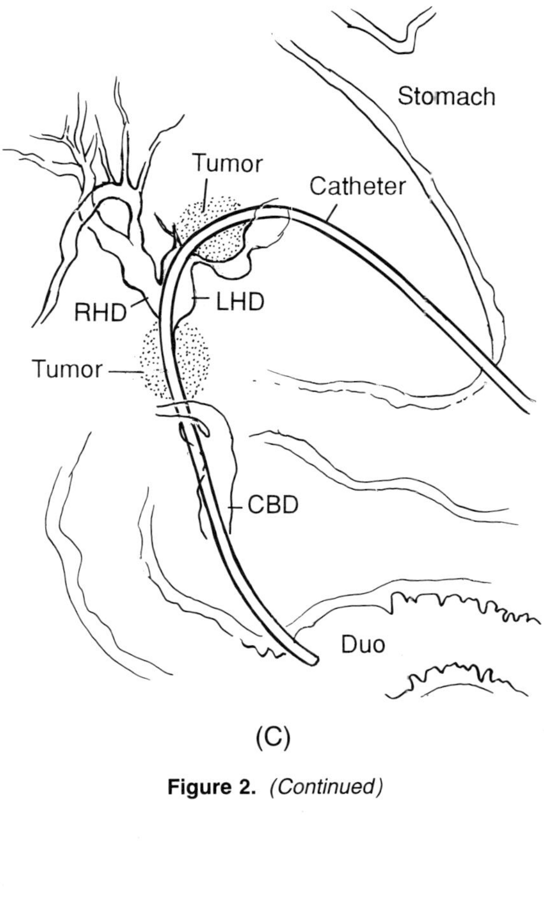

(C)

Figure 2. *(Continued)*

an expanded right pleural space. Left-sided approaches may be necessary if bulky tumor involves the right lobe of the liver or if there is isolated dilatation of the left intrahepatic ducts. It is usually necessary to drain only one lobe of the liver, even if there is isolation of the right and left ducts as in the case of a central cholangiocarcinoma (Klatskin tumor). However, insertion of separate right and left drainage catheters may be necessary for isolated right and left ducts in the setting of infectious cholangitis or persistent symptomatic jaundice (6).

A 22-gauge needle is used for the initial duct puncture to minimize the risk of hemorrhage if multiple needle passes are required. Central duct punctures should be avoided to minimize the risk of hemorrhage, bile leak, or eventual tumor encroachment on catheter side holes. After an 0.018-inch guide wire is advanced into the biliary ducts, a variety of devices (Cope and Neff devices, Cook, Bloomington, IN; Accu-Stick device, Medi-Tech, Watertown, MA) may be used to convert to a more substantial 0.035-inch guide wire. This permits serial tract dilation and insertion of an 8.5-French drainage catheter, internal–external stent, or internal metallic endoprosthesis.

External Drainage Catheter Insertion

External drainage requires minimal catheter manipulation and is indicated if the patient is septic or experiencing severe procedural related pain that cannot be controlled with usual doses of intravenous analgesics, or if initial attempts at crossing the obstruction with a guide wire and catheter are unsuccessful. External drainage is established by coiling a Cope-type nephrostomy tube at the confluence of the right and left bile ducts or in the common hepatic duct. If there is insufficient space to coil the catheter, the tip of the catheter may be advanced into a peripheral duct for more stable purchase pending subsequent internalization (7). Initially an 8.5-French drainage tube should be inserted to minimize patient discomfort during tract dilation. The patient can be externally decompressed for several days or weeks. This may permit resolution of infection, decrease in edema, and maturation of the percutaneous tract, allowing subsequent passage of a guide wire into the duodenum for internalization. Even if the occlusion remains impassable, the initial tube may be exchanged for a larger-caliber (10–12 French) external-drainage catheter, which will be less likely to become occluded by debris. Complications encountered following percutaneous biliary drainage include sepsis, bleeding, bile leak, catheter occlusion, and catheter dislodgement. Transcatheter embolization is indicated if hemobilia develops owing to erosion of a hepatic artery branch adjacent to the percutaneous drainage catheter with formation of a pseudoaneurysm.

Internal–External Catheter Insertion

Internal–external biliary drainage is established by advancing a guide wire across the occlusion and into the duodenum. Hydrophilic coated guide wires facilitate traversal of even the tightest stenoses. A multi-side-hole drainage catheter (Ring or Cope, Cook, Bloomington, IN) is then inserted with the proximal side holes in an intrahepatic duct or the common hepatic duct and distal side holes in the duodenum (Figs. 1, 2). An 8- or 10-French tube is initially inserted, and eventually exchanged for a 12-French catheter. The major advantage of placement of an internal–external tube is the ability to cap the tube, allowing bile to flow into the intestine to aid in digestion of lipids and fat-soluble vitamins, while maintaining external access for subsequent catheter exchanges. This is especially important for patients in whom endoscopic stent exchanges are impractical. An internal–external catheter also provides more secure anchoring, especially in minimally dilated ductal systems, and is less likely to become dislodged. An internal–external stent may be inserted alongside obstructed plastic internal biliary stents or through occluded metallic endoprostheses. An internal–external drainage catheter should not be capped in the presence of cholangitis or small bowel obstruction.

Internal Biliary Stent Insertion

Completely internal biliary stents eliminate the need for any external catheters and may be inserted percutaneously when endoscopic stenting is not possible. They are convenient and psychologically beneficial, but have the drawback of sacrificing percutaneous access for future catheter exchanges. In an effort to decrease the size of the percutaneous hepatic tract, combined "rendezvous" procedures have been developed, in which a transhepatic guide wire is grasped by a duodenoscope to facilitate otherwise impossible endoscopic stent insertions (8). Regardless of the method of insertion, plastic internal stents require periodic endoscopic exchange every 3 months, because of encrustation by sludge and biofilm.

The advent of the self-expanding Wallstent endoprosthesis (9) revolutionized internal stenting by allowing insertion of a 10-mm diameter metallic stent via an 8-French percutaneous sheath. A prospective randomized trial (10) showed that the median patency for the Wallstent (273 days) was superior to that of 10-French plastic internal stents (126 days). Metallic endoprostheses have virtually supplanted plastic internal endoprostheses in the current practice of interventional radiology. [The Wallstent (Schneider, Minneapolis, MN) is constructed of a stainless steel wire mesh and is self-expanding. It is flexible, negotiates curves, and permits parallel stenting of right and left bile ducts (11). Biliary side branches have been reported to remain patent despite insertion of a Wallstent as long as there is no direct tumor encasement (12).] Overlapping stents may be inserted for long occlusions. Wallstents should extend up to 1 cm into the duodenum for palliation of pancreatic carcinoma and low bile duct tumors (Fig. 3). Positioning of the stent above the ampulla is possible for high hepatic duct lesions, with the theoretical advantage of preserving the integrity of the sphincter of Oddi.

Patency rates for the Wallstent ranges from 76 to 89%, depending on the length of follow-up (series range from 2 to 22 months) and the stent location (9, 11, 13–15). Patency of the Wallstent was found to be higher for distal ductal tumors (89–95%) than for hilar malignancies (46–72%) in two studies (14, 16).

Narrowing or occlusion of the Wallstent may occur owing to extension of tumor above or below the stent ends, ingrowth through the interstices of the wire mesh, hyperplasia of mucosa or connective tissue, or impaction of sludge. Metallic stents become permanently incorporated into the wall of the bile duct within weeks and cannot be removed. They should be inserted only in patients with unresectable malignant disease who have relatively short expected survivals (6–9 months). Patients with long expected survivals may experience occlusion of the Wallstent and will require new percutaneous biliary access. Treatment of occlusions of an indwell-

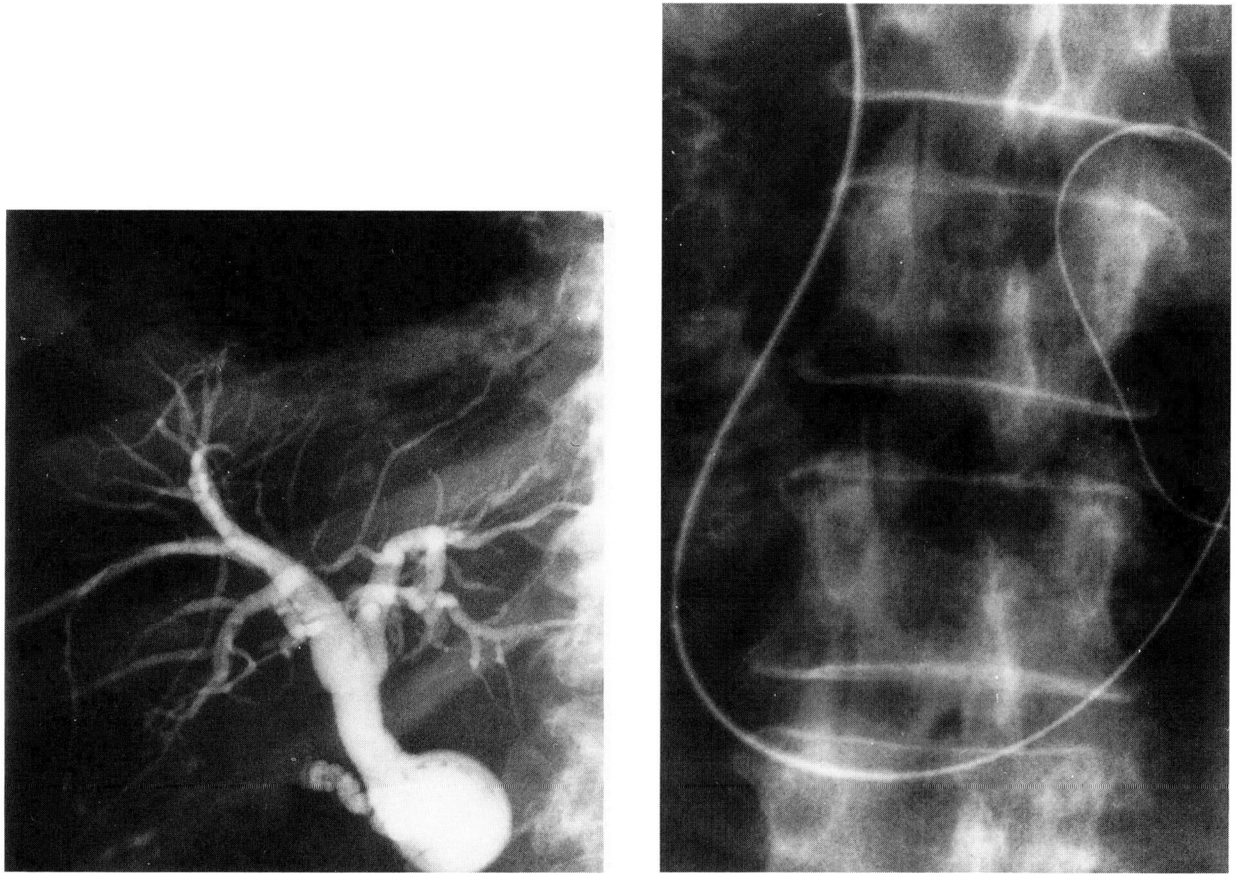

(A) (B)

Figure 3. (A) Injection via a right external biliary drainage catheter shows obstruction of the common bile duct due to carcinoma of the head of the pancreas. (B) A guide wire has been steered beyond the common bile duct obstruction and into the duodenum. (C) A balloon has been used to predilate the common bile duct prior to stent insertion (next page). (D) A Wallstent endoprosthesis has been inserted (open arrows), with its distal tip extending into the duodenum (next page).

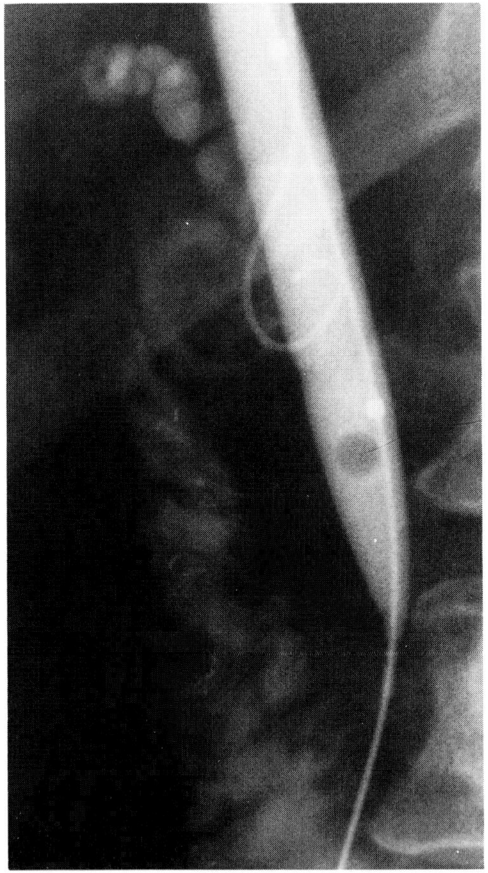

(C)

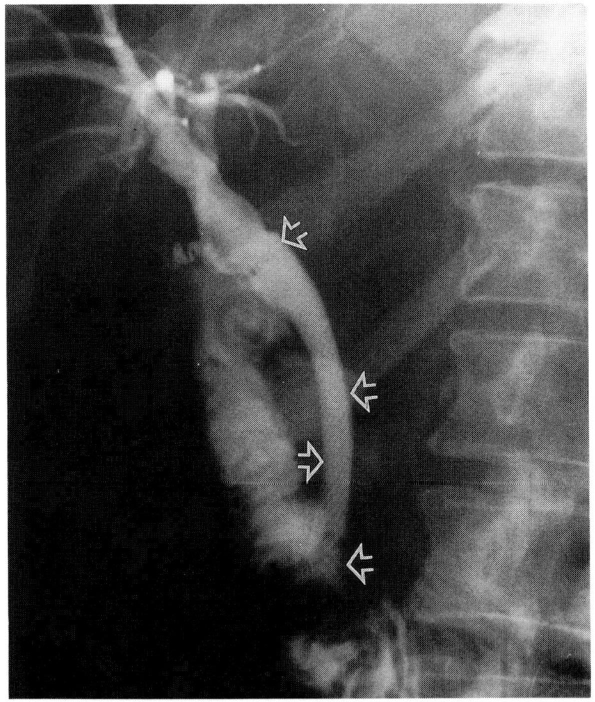

(D)

Figure 3. *(Continued)*

ing Wallstent consists of establishment of new percutaneous biliary access and introduction of a guide wire and internal–external drainage catheter through the occluded Wallstent into the duodenum. Internal–external stenting will then be necessary for the life of the patient, with periodic elective outpatient exchanges at 2- to 3-month intervals.

Potential complications encountered following insertion of the Wallstent include cholangitis, bleeding acalculus cholecystitis, and duodenal ulceration due to mucosal trauma from stent wires (15).

PERCUTANEOUS BILIARY DRAINAGE FOR BENIGN STRICTURES

The vast majority of benign biliary strictures are iatrogenic (17–22). Delayed biliary strictures may develop weeks or months following cholecystectomy (laparoscopic or open), and the initial trauma may have been unrecognized at the time of surgery. Benign anastomotic strictures may also develop months or years following biliary bypass surgery (hepatojejunostomy or hepaticojejunostomy (Figure 4)). Computed tomography and/or sonography should initially be performed to identify dilatation of the bile ducts and exclude the presence of stones, abscess, or recurrent tumor. Endoscopic retrograde cholangiopancreatography may initially be attempted in patients with biliary strictures who have not undergone Roux-en-Y biliary–jejunal anastomoses. Percutaneous biliary drainage is indicated if ERCP is unsuccessful or if Roux-en-Y bypass makes ERCP unfeasible. Percutaneous cholangiography provides important information on the location and extent of benign strictures. Percutaneous biliary drainage may be required for relief of cholangitis or pruritus and stabilization of the patient pending definitive surgical treatment of the stricture. A readily palpable internal–external catheter simplifies operative dissection for those patients who will undergo hepaticojejunostomy (5). Establishment of percutaneous drainage also provides access for those patients who will be treated primarily by balloon dilation.

Most benign biliary strictures may be percutaneously approached using a right ductal puncture. It may be necessary to insert tubes via both right and left ductal approaches if there are bilateral intrahepatic duct strictures, complex strictures of the hepatic bifurcation, or episodes of cholangitis with isolated right and left ducts. An attempt should be made to traverse the stricture with a hydrophilic guide wire and insert an internal–external drainage catheter. If it is not possible to traverse the obstruction, an external biliary drainage catheter should be inserted above the level of occlusion.

Patients with benign biliary strictures who are in good medical condition achieve the most durable result following surgical repair. In a retrospective study by Pitt and co-workers, successful outcomes at a mean follow-up of nearly 6 years (17) were statistically higher following surgical treatment with Roux-en-Y choledochojejunostomy or hepaticojejunostomy (88%), compared with percutaneous balloon dilation (55%), although costs were similar. The authors recommended surgical repair for benign postoperative strictures in most patients and reserve balloon dilation for patients who are at high risk for such lengthy surgical procedures. Strictures complicating laparoscopic cholecystectomy are often refractory to percutaneous balloon dilation, and surgical repair (Roux-en-Y hepaticojejunostomy) often provides the most durable result, especially in young and otherwise healthy

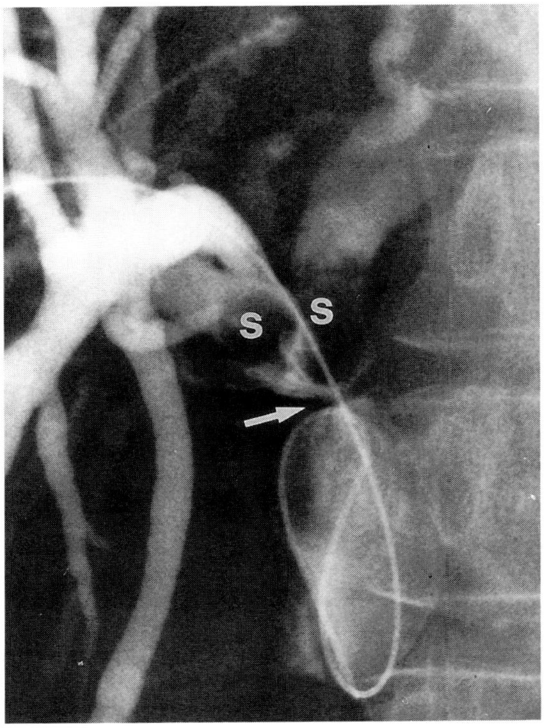

(A)

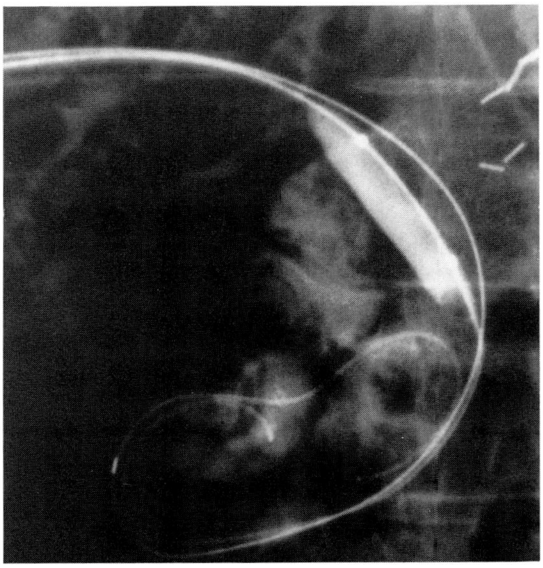

(B)

Figure 4. (A) A guide wire crosses a benign stricture of a hepaticojejunostomy anastamosis (arrow) which developed 12 years following a Whipple procedure. Stones (s) are present in the right and left ducts proximal to the tight stenosis. (B) A balloon is used to dilate the stricture percutaneously. (C) A basket (arrow) is used to extract and crush stones and debris (next page). (D) Final cholangiogram after balloon dilation and stone extraction shows widely patent anastamosis (next page).

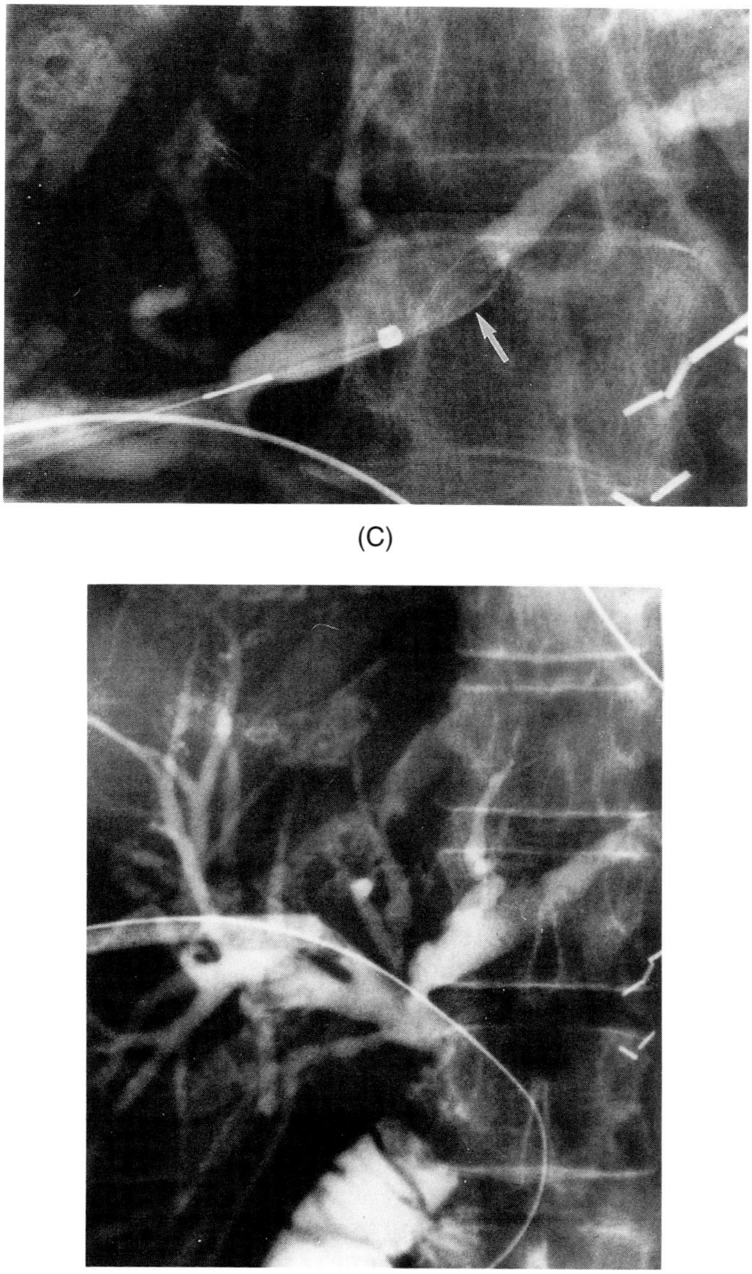

(C)

(D)

Figure 4. *(Continued)*

patients (23, 24). Millis and co-workers (18) hold that surgical reconstruction should be the standard therapy for primary bile duct strictures but they reported a 90% success rate for balloon treatment of surgical anastomotic strictures. They recommend that percutaneous balloon dilation be attempted for anastomotic strictures developing after biliary reconstruction prior to reoperation and revision. Even if primary surgical repair is intended rather than balloon dilation, insertion of unilateral or bilateral Ring or Cope internal–external stents serves as an aid in the surgical dissection of scarred hepatic ducts (5). Stents may be maintained postoperatively to facilitate optimal healing of the newly created anastomosis.

Percutaneous balloon dilation of benign strictures should be reserved for patients with primary strictures who are considered poor surgical candidates owing to coexisting medical or surgical conditions, or in patients with recurrent strictures at a biliary–enteric anastomosis. Favorable prognostic signs include onset of obstruction >2 years following surgery or trauma and short segmental involvement (19).

Percutaneous balloon dilation of benign strictures may be painful and should be performed with the assistance of anesthesia. A guide wire is advanced across the stenosis and a balloon is positioned using fluoroscopic guidance. The balloon diameter should match the caliber of uninvolved bile ducts adjacent to the stricture. Multiple 60-sec inflations are performed. Any coexisting intraductal stones or debris may be extracted using baskets or flushed into the intestine.

Management following balloon dilation and stenting varies widely (20–25). Many centers maintain a 10- to 12-French internal–external biliary drainage catheter across the dilation site for 6 months, with routine stent exchanges every 2–3 months. At the end of 6 months the stent is removed and exchanged for a vascular sheath over a guide wire. This allows contrast injection as the sheath is retracted, while guide-wire access is maintained. If there is wide patency, the guide wire and catheter are removed. If there is a mild residual stenosis, an external biliary drainage catheter is inserted with its tip positioned above the dilation site. This external drain may be capped for a trial period of 2–3 months, at which time a follow-up cholangiogram is performed. If the dilation site is still patent with only minimal residual narrowing and the patient has been asymptomatic, the tube may be removed. If there is any significant restenosis or recurrence of symptoms after the trial of capping of the external tube, redilation and long-term internal–external stenting may be required. If the patient is young and a good surgical candidate, definitive surgical treatment or anastomotic revision may be preferable. Metallic stents in patients with benign disease are to be avoided because they cannot be removed if they become occluded and may preclude subsequent surgical bypass. In the future, coated stents may provide a solution to the problem of long-term proliferation of mucosa and connective tissue within metallic endoprostheses.

A multicenter review reported the primary patency following balloon dilation to be 67% for benign anatomostic strictures and 76% for iatrogenic nonanastomotic strictures (20).

SCLEROSING CHOLANGITIS

Percutaneous Cholangiography for Evaluation of Sclerosing Cholangitis

Sclerosing cholangitis results in inflammation and fibrosis of intrahepatic and extrahepatic bile ducts and require percutaneous intervention. Patients with early or mild cases may be asymptomatic with only a mild elevation of liver function tests. The condition is generally progressive, and may cause jaundice, fever, chills, pruritus, and abdominal pain. Many patients eventually develop secondary biliary cirrhosis, with portal hypertension, variceal bleeding, and/or hepatic insufficiency. There is a strong association with ulcerative colitis and, to a lesser degree, Crohn's disease.

Abdominal CT or sonography is usually performed in symptomatic patients to exclude gallstones, mass lesions, or abscesses. Endoscopic retrograde cholangiopancreatography should then be performed to establish the diagnosis of sclerosing cholangitis and evaluate the extent of ductal involvement. Percutaneous thin-needle cholangiography (PTHC) should be performed only if ERCP is unsuccessful or nondiagnostic. It may be necessary to puncture ducts in both right and left hepatic lobes for a complete examination. Correlation with CT or sonography may be useful for planning a puncture route into an isolated ductal system. If flow-limiting, high-grade stenoses are identified on the diagnostic PTHC, the radiologist should be prepared to insert a percutaneous drainage catheter.

The cholangiographic findings of sclerosing cholangitis have been described by MacCarty and co-workers (25). The most characteristic findings are short strictures of the intrahepatic and extrahepatic bile ducts, usually measuring 1–2 cm in length. There may be a beaded appearance due to areas of dilatation alternating with annular stenoses. Other findings include band-like narrowings, outpouchings and diverticula, shaggy mural irregularity, pruning of the biliary tree, and eventually diffuse, confluent strictures. The entire biliary tree may be involved, but in 20% of patients the involvement is limited to the intrahepatic and proximal extrahepatic ducts. Intraductal debris or stones may be identified. The gallbladder and cystic ducts are usually not involved.

Cholangiocarcinoma may complicate sclerosing cholangitis, with a reported incidence of 12% (26). Cholangiographic findings that should raise the suspicion of malignant transformation include the presence of a polypoid mass or progression of strictures or dilatation on serial cholangiograms. Endobilary brush and/or percutaneous needle biopsy may be necessary for diagnosis.

Percutaneous Therapy for Sclerosing Cholangitis

Treatment of symptomatic strictures limited to the common bile duct, common hepatic duct, and hilar ducts should be initially be attempted endoscopically (27). Endoscopic techniques include dilation of strictures using 6–8 mm balloons and extraction of stones and debris trapped by strictures using baskets. If there are residual stenoses following endoscopic balloon dilation, endoscopically inserted internal plastic stents are required.

Percutaneous transhepatic interventions should be reserved for patients with symptomatic sclerosing cholangitis (pruritus or bacterial cholangitis) who have failed endoscopic therapy, have gastrojejunostomies that impede ERCP, or who have inaccessible strictures in peripheral right or left intrahepatic ducts. Attention should be directed to percutaneous balloon dilation of any high-grade, focal, "dominant" strictures (28). The initial tract should be planned to give optimal access to the stricture (Fig. 5). Right, left, or bilateral ductal punctures may be required. In some centers, a choledochojejunal Roux-en-Y loop (Hutson–Russel loop) is surgically created and approximated to the anterior abdominal wall for direct percu-

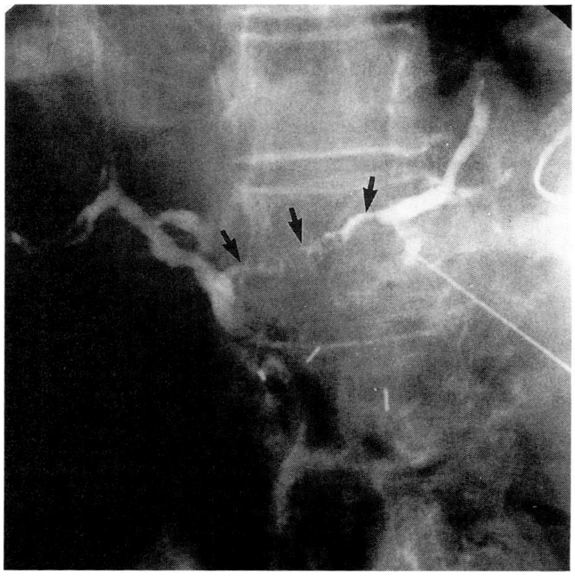

(A)

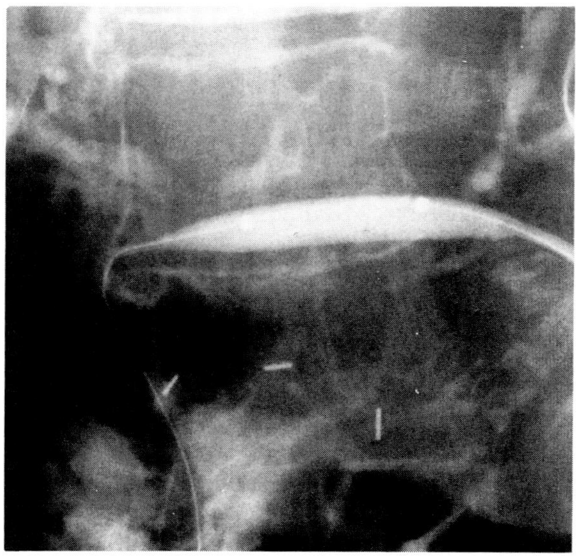

(B)

Figure 5. (A) Left percutaneous transhepatic cholangiogram in a patient with sclerosing cholangitis. There is severe stricturing of the left intrahepatic duct (arrows), which also contains multiple small stones (filling defects). (B) After extraction of the stones, a balloon is used to dilate the left ductal stricture. (C) Final result after dilation of the dominant stricture (next page).

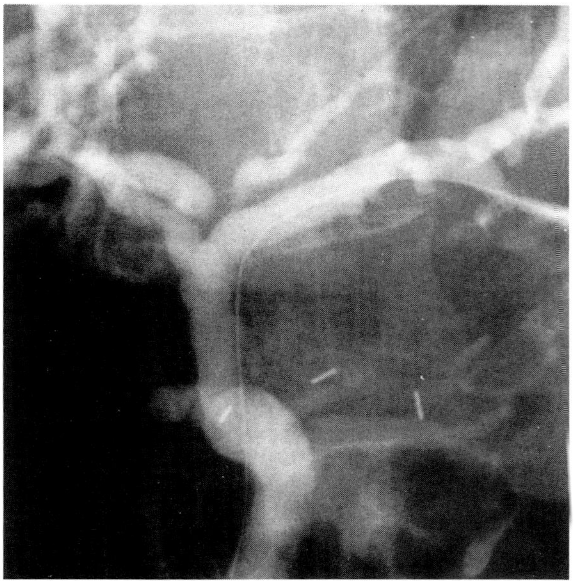

(C)

Figure 5. *(Continued)*

taneous access to the biliary tree (29). An attempt should be made to cross the dominant stricture(s) with a hydrophilic guide wire, and initially insert an 8-French internal–external stent. If there is active infection, an external drainage catheter should be initially inserted. If there is suspicion of malignant degeneration, brush or forceps biopsy may be performed. Biliary ductal shave biopsy using a Simpson atherectomy catheter may be considered if these are nonproductive, although the device is expensive, may not negotiate acutely angulated percutaneous tracts, and has a 10% risk of serious hemorrhage (30). After several days, the patient should be brought back for balloon dilation of strictures. This may be painful, so we routinely request the support of an anesthesiologist. Intrahepatic stones and concretions or debris should be extracted using baskets or flushed out of the system. A 12-French plastic internal–external drainage catheter is then inserted across the dilation site and may eventually be capped. We avoid using metallic endoprostheses in patients with sclerosing cholangitis because of a high rate of long-term stent occlusion. We usually maintain a capped internal–external tube for approximately 1 year and routinely exchange the catheter every 3 months. Removal of the access catheter should be considered only if there is continued patency at the dominant stricture site(s) at least 1 year. Strictures are often recurrent and may require repeat dilation and long-term internal–external stenting. The primary patency rate for percutaneous dilatation was only 50% in a series of 14 patients reported by Skolkin et al. (31) and 42% in a multicenter trail reported by Mueller et al. (20). However, these efforts may palliate symptoms and preserve adequate hepatic function pending liver transplantation.

BENIGN BILIARY STRICTURES SECONDARY TO CHRONIC PANCREATITIS

Chronic pancreatitis may result in benign stricturing of the common bile duct that may simulate malignant narrowing. Pancreatic carcinoma should be excluded. Percutaneous drainage may be necessary in patients with symptomatic jaundice when ERCP fails. Biliary strictures due to chronic pancreatitis respond poorly to balloon dilation owing to the severity of surrounding fibrosis (20, 32). Patients who fail to respond to balloon dilation may require surgery or long-term internal–external stenting.

INTERVENTIONAL RADIOLOGICAL MANAGEMENT OF BILE DUCT INJURIES

Most trauma to the bile ducts is iatrogenic, and there has been an increase in the incidence with the advent of laparoscopic surgery. Injuries may become apparent in the immediate postoperative period in the case of bile leaks or complete occlusions, or may develop over months when due to strictures. Patients may present with jaundice, fever, bile peritonitis, biliary fistula, or abdominal pain (33). Injuries related to cholecystectomy include clipping, ligation, or laceration of the common duct or an anomalous branch. Leakage from the cystic duct stump may result from a slipped ligature or clip. Delayed strictures may result from devascularization of the bile duct due to excessive dissection or thermal injury. Complications following biliary–enteric anastomoses include leakage at a hepaticojejunostomy anastomosis and stricture formation.

Noniatrogenic trauma to the bile ducts may occur following ballistic or penetrating trauma, but such patients usually undergo emergent exploratory surgery.

When traumatic injury is clinically suspected, ERCP should be the first procedure performed. If there is a transection or large bile leak, contrast injected during ERCP may preferentially flow into the subhepatic space without filling of the entire biliary tree. Because the exact location of the upper extent of an occlusion and the status of the confluence of the ducts is crucial for surgical decision making, it may be

Table 1. Bismuth classification of trauma to the bile ducts

Type I	Trauma to the main bile duct at least 2 cm below the hepatic bifurcation
Type II	Trauma to the main bile duct within 2 cm of the hepatic bifurcation
Type III	Destruction of the proximal hepatic duct distal to an intact hepatic bifurcation
Type IV	Partial or complete obliteration of the bifurcation of the right and left hepatic ducts
Type V	Trauma to a variant right hepatic duct branch or the proximal hepatic duct near its junction with a variant right hepatic duct branch

Reference: Chartrand-Lafebvre C, Dufresne MP, Lafortune M, Lapointe R, Dagenais M, Roy A. Iatrogenic injury to the bile duct: a working classification for radiologists. *Radiology.* 1994;193: 523–526.

necessary to perform PTHC. This is usually performed via a right ductal approach with a 22-gauge needle. If there is a biliary leak, the bile ducts may be nondilated and perseverance may be required to cannulate a suitable duct. It is important to search for any anatomic variations in hepatic duct branching, including aberrant right hepatic ducts and excluded ductal systems that do not communicate with the opacified ducts owing to obstruction or transection (24).

The Bismuth classification (Table 1) is surgically oriented and based upon the level of bile duct disruption, the integrity of the bifurcation of the right and left ducts, and the presence of trauma to any anatomic variants of the right hepatic duct (34). Radiologists should include this classification in their reports to facilitate communication with surgical colleagues. Although not incorporated into the Bismuth classification, several other factors should be described when interpreting the cholangiogram, including the degree of ductal narrowing, the length of the stricture, and the presence of biliary leakage or intrahepatic ductal stones.

Clipping or Ligation of an Extrahepatic Bile Duct

Percutaneous biliary drainage should be performed to relieve biliary obstruction and delineate the upper limit of the occlusion (23, 24, 33). An attempt should be made to traverse the obstruction with a hydrophilic guide wire and insert an internal–external drainage catheter. It may not be possible to traverse an obstruction caused by a tight surgical clip or suture ligature (Fig. 6). In this case, an external biliary drainage catheter should be inserted with its tip positioned above the level of occlusion. Eventual surgical reconstruction is usually required for most patients who prove to have complete occlusions of the bile duct. An attempt at balloon dilation and long-term stenting may be considered in selected patients who demonstrate a focal stenosis or who have multiple risk factors for reoperation.

Laceration or Transection of the Common Hepatic or Bile Duct

Unilateral or bilateral percutaneous biliary drainage catheters should be inserted (23, 24, 33, 36). An attempt should be made to advance a guide wire across the point of leakage and then into the distal common bile duct and duodenum. An internal–external catheter should be inserted, spanning the lacerated or transected segment of duct. The catheter(s) should be connected to external bag drainage to divert bile, in an attempt to "dry up" the operative site, resolve jaundice and cholangitis, and decrease local inflammation prior to definitive reconstructive surgery (33). Computed tomography or ultrasound-guided drainage of any associated bilomas may be necessary (35). Preoperative insertion of a palpable percutaneous drainage catheter often aids the surgeon during high dissections of scarred, traumatized, and inflamed common hepatic ducts (5, 33). Although major lacerations may seal with percutaneous drainage alone, surgical repair is often necessary because of late scarring and stricture formation. If surgical reconstruction is necessary, internal–external access may be continued for postoperative stenting of hepaticojejunal anastomoses.

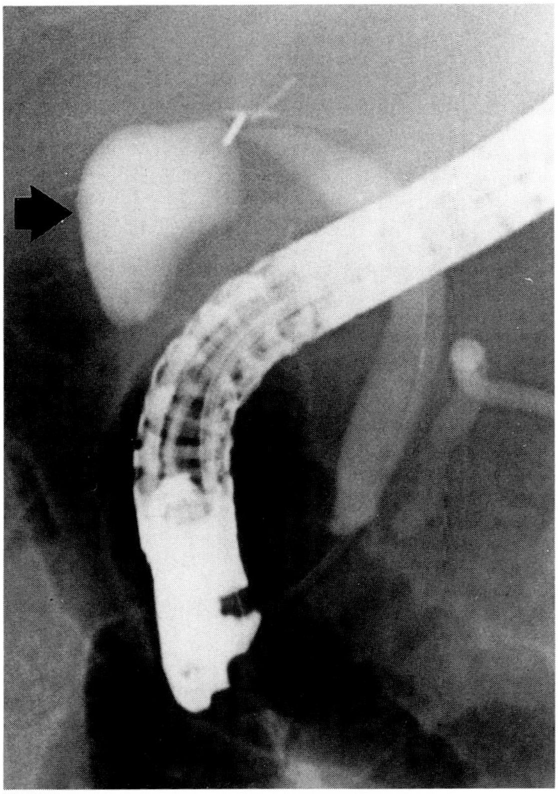

(A)

Figure 6. (A) ERCP in a patient who developed jaundice and fever several weeks following cholecystectomy. Obstruction of the bile duct by a surgical clip prevented successful endoscopic drainage. Contrast pools at the site of a bile duct leak (arrow). (B) A left external drainage catheter decompresses the biliary tree proximal to the site of the bile leak. A guide wire could not be advanced beyond surgical clips (open arrow) which ligated the common hepatic duct (next page).

Leakage from the Cystic Duct Stump

An internal–external biliary drainage catheter spanning the cystic duct stump may be percutaneously inserted if ERCP stenting is not possible (23). The stent should be opened to external drainage to maximize diversion of bile. At least 1 month should be allowed for complete closure of the cystic duct stump before catheter removal.

Leakage of a Hepaticojejunostomy Anastomosis

Most patients who have undergone recent biliary–enteric anastomoses have some form of internal–external stent spanning the anastomosis already in place. Catheter cholangiography will demonstrate any extravasation at the anastomotic site. If no indwelling percutaneous access is present in a patient with a suspected anastomotic

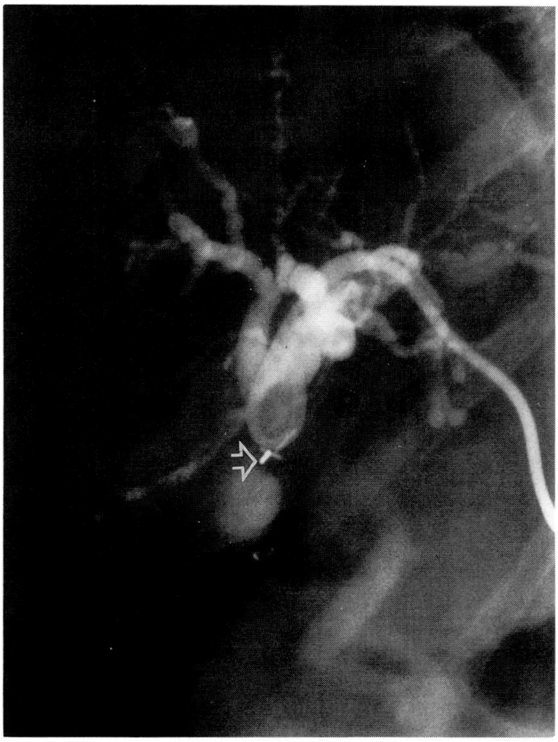

(B)

Figure 6. *(Continued)*

leak, PTHC should be performed. Patients may require long-term external drainage for diversion of bile. If an accessible biloma is present, CT-guided percutaneous drainage should be performed. If the location of the biloma is inaccessible to percutaneous drainage or the anastomosis appears completely disrupted, surgical exploration may be required.

Displaced T-tubes

Intraperitoneal leakage of bile may occur if surgically inserted T-tubes become displaced in the immediate perioperative period. If ERCP stenting is unsuccessful, percutaneous biliary drainage and internal–external stenting may be necessary if there is bile leak, residual stricture, or retained stones (36).

Management of Leaks following Hepatic Resections

Percutaneous biliary drainage and diversion of bile may be required for selected patients with intraperitoneal bile leaks or cutaneous fistulas following partial hepa-

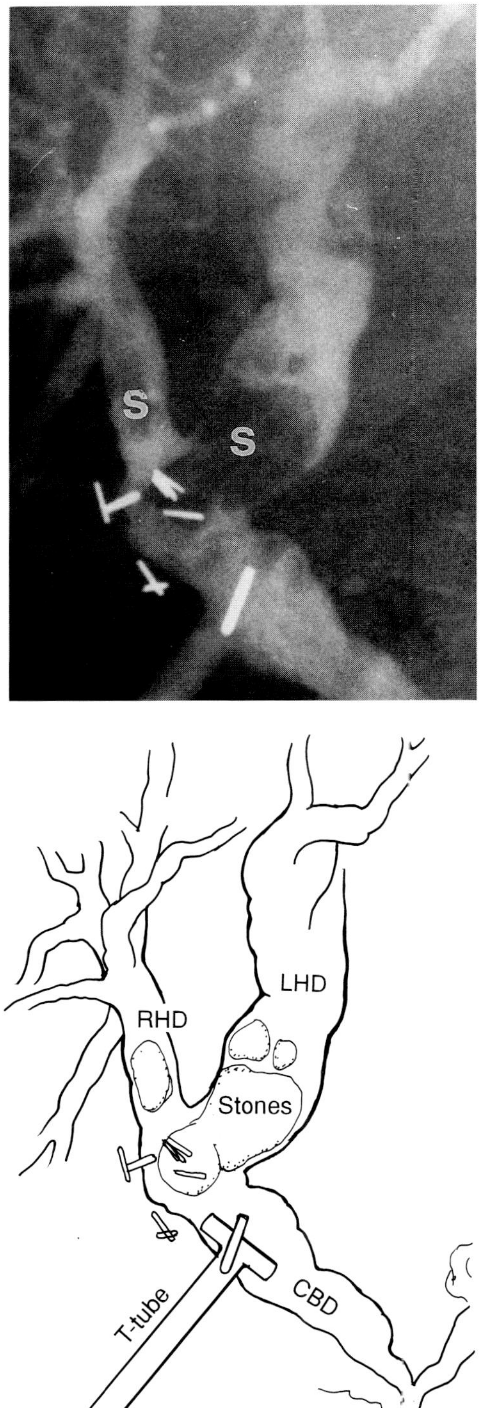

(A)

Figure 7. (A) T-tube cholangiogram shows bulky retained stones following cholecystectomy. (B) A stone extraction basket has been inserted after waiting 6 weeks for the T-tube tract to mature. (C, next page). Final cholangiogram after stone extraction (page 198).

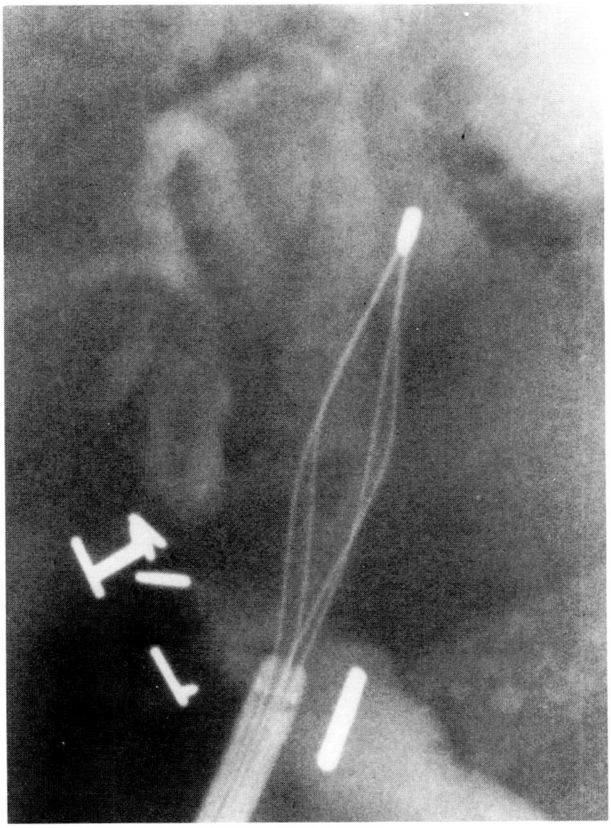

(B)

Figure 7. *(Continued)*

tectomy (36). Computed tomography- or ultrasound-guided drainage of intraabdominal bile collections may also be required. This may obviate reoperation.

PERCUTANEOUS EXTRACTION OF EXTRAHEPATIC BILIARY DUCT STONES

Percutaneous extraction of retained common bile ducts stones following open cholecystectomy and common duct exploration has been performed for more than two decades using T-tube tracts. Stone baskets are introduced after allowing a 6-week period for T-tube tract maturation, with successful extraction and fragmentation of retained stones in up to 95% of patients (37). Modern surgical practice has shifted from open to laparoscopic cholecystectomy, and T-tubes are now encountered only infrequently. Currently, a percutaneous transhepatic tract must be created and allowed to mature in order to remove retained stones following laparoscopic chole-

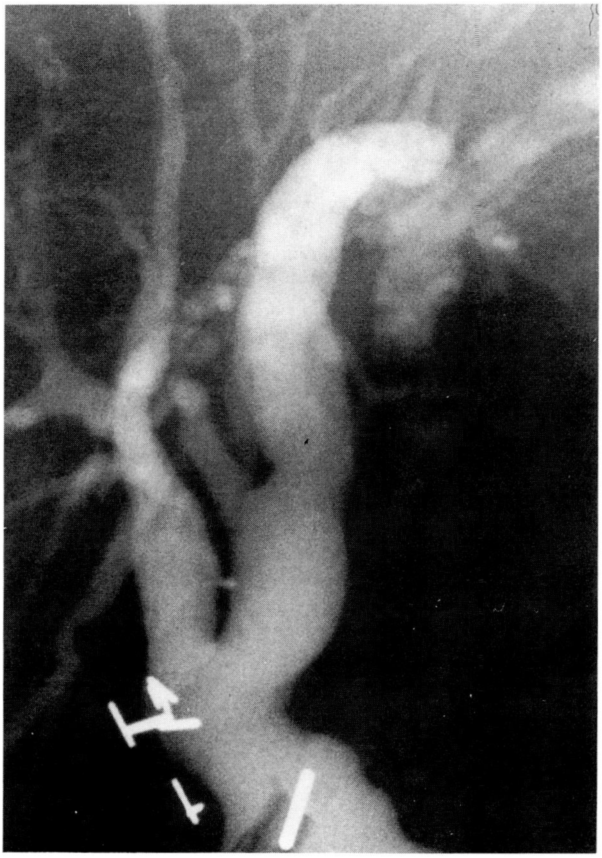

(C)

Figure 7. *(Continued)*

cystectomies. Endoscopic retrograde cholangiopancreatography and endoscopic retrograde basket extraction of retained common bile duct stones has proved to have effectiveness (76–90%) similar to percutaneous techniques (38, 39). Endoscopic retrograde extraction has the benefit of not requiring a percutaneous T-tube or transhepatic tract and is generally recommended as the initial technique for patient without T-tubes who have small- to moderate-sized extrahepatic stones. Percutaneous extraction should be reserved for cases when endoscopic extraction fails, such as when giant stones (>2.5 cm) cannot be crushed by mechanical lithotripsy or endoscopic electrohydraulic lithotripsy (40), or when stones are in inaccessible locations. Percutaneous extraction is preferable to endoscopy when a mature T-tube tract is already in place (41).

Most stones may be retrieved using standard baskets using a 14- to 16-French sheath introduced through a matured T-tube or transhepatic tract (Fig. 7). If the retained stone or fragments are too large or numerous for basket extraction, they may be fragmented and flushed into the duodenum (Fig. 8). Angiographic occlusion balloons may also be used to sweep stones from peripheral bile ducts into more accessible locations in the extrahepatic ducts or to push stones and fragments into the duodenum (42). If an endoscopic papillotomy has not already been performed, percutaneous dilation of the papilla may be accomplished with an 8-mm diameter balloon catheter (43). A 15-French flexible choledochoscope and electrohydraulic lithotripsy probe may be introduced via a percutaneous transhepatic or T-tube tract to fragment large or impacted stones that cannot be removed with conventional stone baskets (47). Tunable dye lasers have also been used to fragment retained stones in the common hepatic and bile ducts when percutaneous or endoscopic basket extraction fails (45). Both electrohydraulic and laser lithotripsy must be performed using direct choledochoscopic visualization of the stone (Fig. 9) to prevent perforation of the bile duct.

Stone extractions may be painful and assistance from the anesthesia service is recommended. A drainage catheter should be maintained in place for follow-up cholangiograms and to maintain access until all stone debris is eliminated from the biliary ducts.

PERCUTANEOUS INTERVENTIONS FOR INTRAHEPATIC STONES

Intrahepatic stones are uncommon in the Western Hemisphere and usually form because of stasis from benign strictures, sclerosing cholangitis, choledochal cysts, or biliary tumors (49). Intraductal stones due to Oriental cholangiohepatitis are discussed below.

Intrahepatic stones should ideally be removed at the same time the underlying stenosis is treated. Although ERCP may identify intrahepatic stones, endoscopic extraction techniques are often not effective in small peripheral ducts. Pitt and coworkers (46) describe a combined interventional radiology and surgery approach for treatment of intrahepatic stones. Underlying strictures of extrahepatic ducts are treated with a surgical biliary–enteric anastomosis with intraoperative choledochoscopy and stone extraction. Preoperative internal–external stent insertion by the interventional radiologist facilitates surgical dissection and provides high-quality cholangiograms for accurate stone localization. A percutaneous tract should be maintained postoperatively for extraction of any residual stones using fluoroscopic and choledochoscopic guidance. Primary percutaneous balloon dilation of strictures and basket extraction of intrahepatic stones may be elected for patients who are high surgical risks or who have already undergone hepaticojejunostomy. If stones are localized to a single duct, a direct peripheral puncture may be performed. If stones fill several ducts, puncture of a duct in the opposite lobe of the liver affords access (47), or multiple ducts may need to be punctured. If a T-tube tract with a direct course to the stone-bearing ducts is already in place, this may be used after allowing 6 weeks for maturation. Percutaneous flexible choledochoscopy (15–20 French) with electrohydraulic or laser lithotripsy may be used for complete stone extraction via percutaneous transhepatic, T-tube, or a subcutaneously implanted jejunal limb of a Roux-en-Y hepaticojejunostomy (47, 48). Patients usually require multiple procedures to attain a stone-free status, which may be achieved in up to 94% of patients using a combined surgical–radiological approach (46). Occasionally,

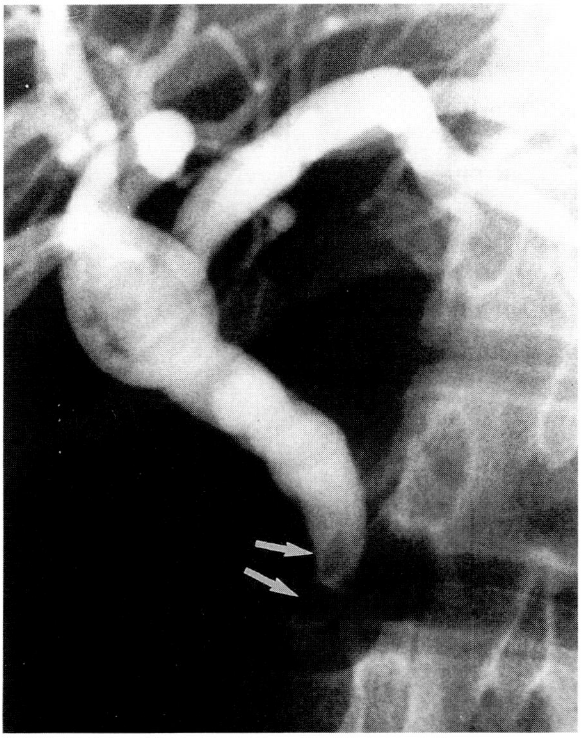

(A)

Figure 8. (A) A right transhepatic route was used to provide percutaneous access for two distal common bile duct stones (arrows) diagnosed 2 years following cholecystectomy. ERCP extraction had been unsuccessful. (B) A stone basket with a malleable tip (arrow) was used to push the stones across a sphincterotomy and into the duodenum (next page).

stones may be limited to one or two severely atrophic hepatic segments, in which case a partial hepatectomy may be preferable.

ORIENTAL CHOLANGIOHEPATITIS

Oriental cholangiohepatitis (recurrent pyogenic cholangitis) provides special challenges to the interventional radiologist and surgeon. This is a chronic condition characterized by recurrent episodes of cholangitis, pain, and jaundice (49). Multiple bilirubinate calculi fill dilated intrahepatic and extrahepatic bile ducts. There may be coexisting fibrosis and biliary strictures. There is a strong association with parasitic infections (*Ascaris lumbricoides* and *Clonorchis sinensis*), accounting for the high incidence in Asians. There is usually superinfection with gram-negative bacteria, and patients may present with suppurative cholangitis or liver abscess. If untreated, cirrhosis and portal hypertension may develop. There is also an increased incidence of cholangiocarcinoma which may reach 5–10%, attributable to bile stasis and

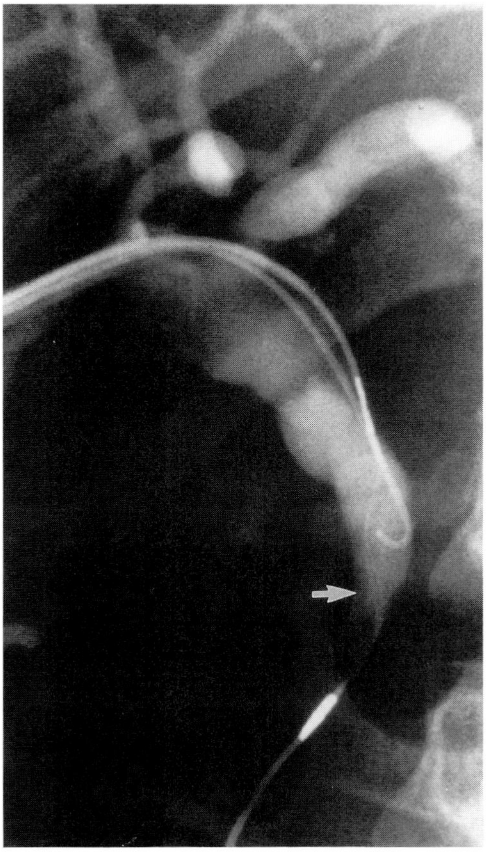

(B)

Figure 8. *(Continued)*

recurrent infection (50). Coexisting cholangiocarcinomas are often infiltrating and difficult to diagnose on cholangiography because of superimposed scarring and stricturing. Cholangiocarcinoma has also been reported to develop 2–14 years after successful removal of intrahepatic calculi (51) and should be considered in patients with recurrent symptoms or ductal dilatation.

Ultrasonography and CT are initially recommended for assessment of bile duct dilatation, localization of intrahepatic and extrahepatic stones, and determination of segmental or lobar hepatic atrophy (52). Any abscesses should be percutaneously drained. Initial treatment of suppurative cholangitis should be limited to simple external biliary drainage. Because primary percutaneous treatment often requires multiple sessions and access routes, combined surgical debulking and percutaneous interventions are preferable. Surgical treatment includes choledochostomy, hepaticocholedochostomy, and removal of stones with forceps, baskets, or a flexible choledochoscope with electrohydraulic or laser lithotripsy. Residual stones may be removed postoperatively using preshaped catheters and baskets via T-tube tracts

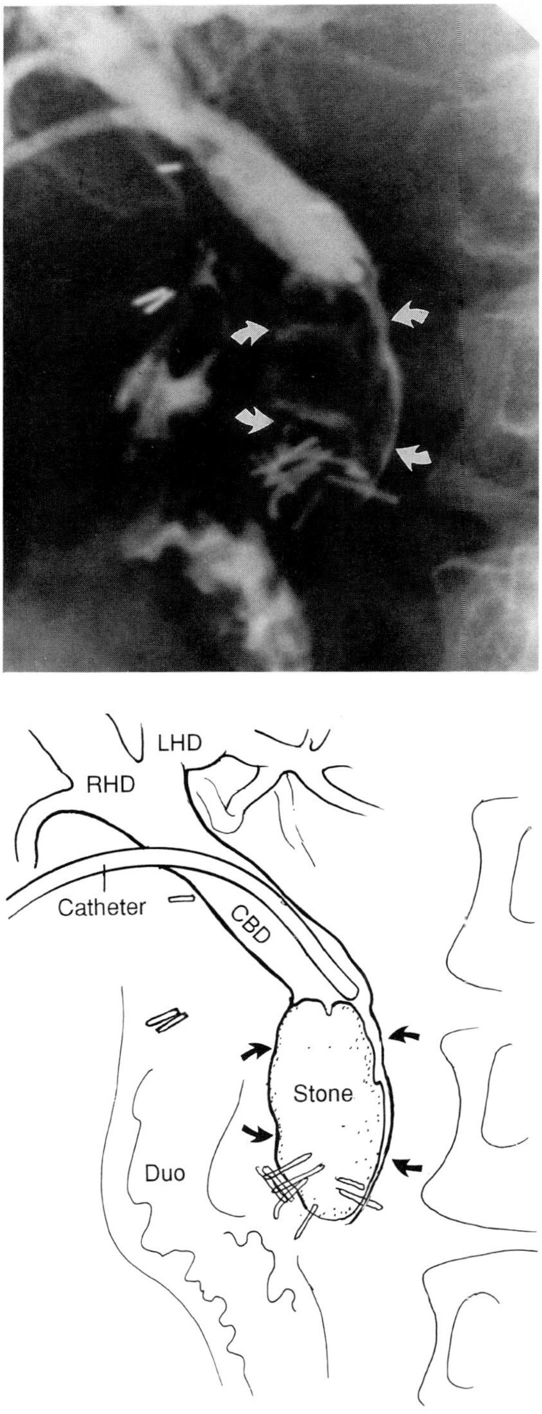

(A)

Figure 9. (A) A right ductal approach was used to access a 2 × 3 cm stone (outlined by arrows) impacted in the common bile duct. (B) A percutaneous balloon sphincterotomy is performed to allow stone fragments to pass into the duodenum (next page). (C) A 16-French flexible endoscope is used to apply an electrohydraulic lithotripsy probe directly to the stone surface (next page).

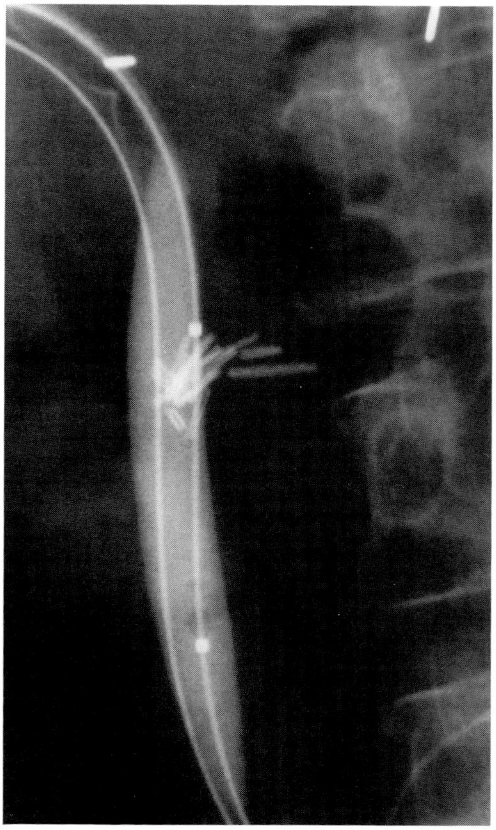

(B)

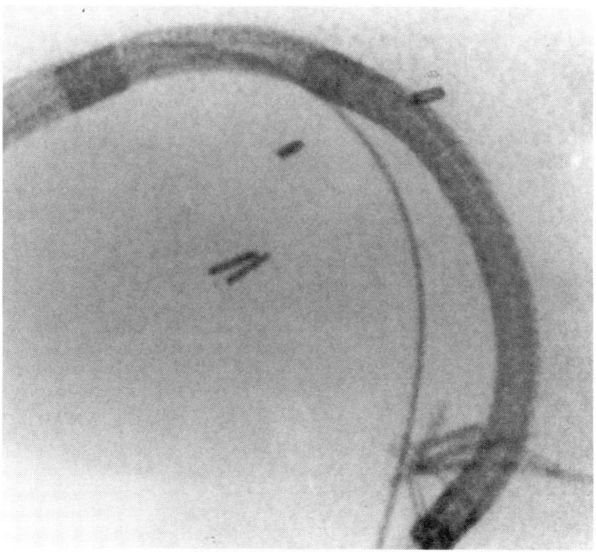

(C)

Figure 9. *(Continued)*

(53). Postoperative flexible choledochoscopy via T-tube tracts, percutaneous transhepatic routes, or hepaticocutaneous jejunostomies are also useful (52). Percutaneous balloon dilation of associated strictures is necessary for removal of all fragments. Adjunctive extracorporeal shock wave lithotripsy may be employed (53). Complete percutaneous clearance of stones was reported in 50–90% of patients (52, 53).

REFERENCES

1. Mueller PR, Harbin WP, Ferrucci JT, Wittenberg J, vanSonnenberg E. Fine-needle transhepatic cholangiography: reflections after 450 cases. *AJR.* 1980;136:85–90.
2. Mueller PR, Ferrucci JT, vanSonnenberg E, et al. Obstruction of the left hepatic duct: diagnosis and treatment by selective fine-needle cholangiography and percutaneous biliary drainage. *Radiology.* 1982;145:297–302.
3. Ferrucci JT, Mueller PR, Harbin WP. Percutaneous transhepatic biliary drainage: technique, results, and applications. *Radiology.* 1980;135:1–13.
4. Berquist TJ, May GR, Johnson CM, Adson MA, Thistle JL. Percutaneous biliary decompression: internal and external drainage in 50 patients. *AJR.* 1981;136:901–906.
5. Crist DW, Kadir S, Cameron JL. The value of preoperatively placed percutaneous biliary catheters in reconstruction of the proximal part of the biliary tree. *Surg Gynecol Obstet.* 1987;165:421–424.
6. Kaufman SL, Kadir S, Mitchell SE, Kinnison ML, Chang R. Left lobe of the liver: percutaneous biliary drainage. *Radiology.* 1989;170:191–194.
7. Mueller PR, vanSonnenberg E, Ferrucci JT. Percutaneous biliary drainage: technical and catheter related problems in 200 procedures. *AJR.* 1982;138:17–23.
8. Robertson DAF, Hacking CN, Birch S, Ayres R, Shephard H, Wright R. Experience with a combined percutaneous and endoscopic approach to stent insertion in malignant obstructive jaundice. *Lancet.* 1987;2:1449–1452.
9. Boguth L, Tatalovic S, Antonnucci F, Heer M, Sulser H, Zollikofer CL. Malignant biliary obstruction: clinical and histopathologic correlation after treatment with self-expanding metallic prostheses. *Radiology.* 1994;192:669–674.
10. Davids PHP, Groen AK, Rauws EAT, Tytgat GNJ, Huibregtse K. Randomized trial of self-expanding metal stents versus polyethylene stents for distal malignant biliary obstruction. *Lancet.* 1992;340:1488–1492.
11. LaBerge JM, Doherty M, Gordon RL, Ring EJ. Hilar malignancy: treatment with an expandable metallic transhepatic biliary stent. *Radiology.* 1990;177:793–797.
12. Nicholson DA, Chetty N, Jackson JE, Roddie ME, Adam A. Patency of side branches after peripheral placement of metallic biliary endoprostheses. *JVIR.* 1992;3:127–130.
13. Gordon RL, Ring EJ, LaBerge JM, Doherty MM. Malignant biliary obstruction: treatment with expandable metallic stents—follow-up of 50 consecutive patients. *Radiology.* 1992;182:697–701.
14. Laméris JS, Stoker J, Nijs HGT, et al. Malignant biliary obstruction: percutaneous use of self-expandable stent. *Radiology.* 1991;179:703–707.
15. Stoker J, Laméris JS. Complications of percutaneously inserted biliary wallstents. *JVIR.* 1993;4:767–772.
16. Becker CD, Glättli A, Maibach R, Baer HU. Percutaneous palliation of malignant obstructive jaundice with the Wallstent endoprosthesis: follow-up and reintervention in patients with hilar and non-hilar obstruction. *JVIR.* 1993;4:597–604.

17. Pitt HA, Kaufman SL, Coleman J, White RI, Cameron JL. Benign postoperative biliary strictures: operate or dilate. *Ann Surg.* 1989;210:417–427.
18. Millis JM, Tomkins RK, Zinner MJ, Longmire WP, Roslyn JJ. Management of bile duct strictures: an evolving strategy. *Arch Surg.* 1992;127:1077–1082.
19. Williams HJ, Bender CE, May GR. Benign postoperative biliary strictures: dilatation with fluoroscopic guidance. *Radiology.* 1987;163:629–634.
20. Mueller PR, vanSonnenberg E, Ferrucci JT, et al. Biliary stricture dilatation: multicenter review of clinical management in 73 patients. *Radiology.* 1986;160:17–22.
21. Galacher DJ, Kadir S, Kaufman SL, et al. Nonoperative management of benign postoperative biliary strictures. *Radiology.* 1985;156:625–629.
22. Moore AV, Ilescas FF, Mills SR, et al. Percutaneous dilatation of benign biliary strictures. *Radiology.* 1987;163:625–628.
23. Teratola SO, Savader SJ, Lund GB, et al. Biliary tract complications following laparoscopic cholecystectomy: imaging and intervention. *Radiology.* 1992;184:195–200.
24. Branum G, Schmitt C, Baillie J, et al. Management of major biliary complications after laparoscopic cholecystectomy. *Ann Surg.* 1993;217:532–541.
25. MacCarty RL, LaRusso NF, Wiesner RH, Ludwig J. Primary sclerosing cholangitis findings on cholangiography and pancreatography. *Radiology.* 1983;149:39–44.
26. MacCarty RL, LaRusso NF, May GR, et al. Cholangiocarcinoma complicating primary sclerosing cholangitis: cholangiographic appearances. *Radiology.* 1985;156:43–46.
27. Cotton PB, Nickl N. Endoscopic and radiologic approaches to therapy in primary sclerosing cholangitis. *Semin Liver Dis.* 1991;11:40–48.
28. May GR, Bender CE, LaRusso NF, Wiesner RH. Nonoperative dilatation of dominant strictures in primary sclerosing cholangitis. *AJR.* 1985;145:1061–1064.
29. Russel E, Yrizarry JM, Huber JS, et al. Percutaneous transjejunal biliary dilatation: alternate management for benign strictures. *Radiology.* 1986;159:209–214.
30. Schechter MS, Doemeny JM, Johnson JO. Biliary duct shave biopsy with use of the Simpson atherectomy catheter. *JVIR.* 1993;4:819–824.
31. Skolkin MD, Alspaugh JP, Casarella WJ, Chuang VP, Galambos JT. Sclerosing cholangitis: palliation with percutaneous cholangioplasty. *Radiology.* 1989;170:199–206.
32. Citron SJ, Martin LG. Benign biliary strictures: treatment with percutaneous cholangioplasty. *Radiology.* 1991;178:339–341.
33. vanSonnenberg E, D'Agostino HB, Easter DW, et al. Complications of laparoscopic cholecystectomy: coordinated radiologic and surgical management in 21 patients. *Radiology.* 1993;188:399–404.
34. Chartrand-Lafebvre C, Dufresne MP, Lafortune M, Lapointe R, Dagenais M, Roy A. Iatrogenic injury to the bile duct: a working classification for radiologists. *Radiology.* 1994;193:523–526.
35. Vaccaro JP, Dorfman GS, Lambiase RE. Treatment of biliary leaks and fistulae by simultaneous percutaneous drainage and diversion. *Cardiovasc Intervent Radiol.* 1991;14:109–112.
36. Kaufman SL, Kadir S, Mitchell SE, et al. Percutaneous transhepatic biliary drainage for bile leaks and fistulae. *AJR.* 1985;144:1055–1058.
37. Burhenne HJ. Percutaneous extraction of retained biliary tract stones: 661 patients. *AJR.* 1980;134:888–898.
38. Nussinson E, Cairns SR, Vaira D, Dowsett JF, Mason RR. A 10 year single center experience of percutaneous and endoscopic extraction of bile duct stones with T tube in situ. *Gut.* 1991;32:1040–1043.

39. Becker CD, Eigenmann F, Scheurer U, Halter F. Comparison of percutaneous and endoscopic retrograde removal of postoperative retained bile duct stones. *Cardiovasc Intervent Radiol.* 1993;16:144–149.
40. Classen M, Hagenmüller F, Frimberger E. Giant bile duct stones: non-surgical treatment. *Endoscopy.* 1988;20:21–26.
41. Cotton PB. Retained bile duct stones: T-tube in place: percutaneous or endoscopic management. *Am J Gastroenterol.* 1990;85:1075–1078.
42. Meranze SG, Burke DR, Hartz WH, McLean GK. Removal of retained common duct stones with angiographic occlusion balloons. *AJR.* 1986;146:383–385.
43. Centola CAP, Jander HP, Stauffer A, Russinovich NAE. Balloon dilatation of the papilla of Valer to allow biliary stone passage. *AJR.* 1981;136:613–614.
44. Burton KE, Picus D, Hicks ME, et al. Fragmentation of biliary calculi in 71 patients by use of intracorporeal electrohydraulic lithotripsy. *JVIR.* 1993;4:251–256.
45. Dawson SL, Mueller PR, Lee MJ, Saini S, Kelsey P, Nishioka NA. Treatment of bile duct stones by laser lithotripsy: results in 12 patients. *AJR.* 1991;158:1007–1009.
46. Pitt HA, Venbrux AC, Coleman J, et al. Intrahepatic stones: The transhepatic team approach. *Ann Surg.* 1994;219:527–537.
47. Bonnel DH, Liguory CE, Cornud FE, Lefebvre JP. Common bile duct and intrahepatic stones: results of transhepatic electrohydraulic lithotripsy in 50 patients. *Radiology.* 1991;180:345–348.
48. Yoshimoto H, Ikeda S, Tanaka M, Matsumoto S, Kuroda Y. Choledochoscopic electrohydrolic lithotrispy and lithotomy for stones in the common bile duct, intrahepatic ducts, and gallbladder. *Ann Surg.* 1989;210:576–582.
49. vanSonnenberg E, Casola G, Cubberley DA, et al. Oriental cholangiohepatitis: diagnostic imaging and interventional management. *AJR.* 146:327–331.
50. Sheen-Chen S, Chou F, Eng H. Intrahepatic cholangiocarcinoma in hepatolithiasis: a frequently overlooked disease. *J Surg Oncol.* 1991;47:131–135.
51. Chijiiwa K, Ichimaya H, Kuroki S, Koga A, Nakayama F. Late development of cholangiocarcinoma after the treatment of hepatolithiasis. *Surg Gynecol Obstet.* 1993;177:279–282.
52. Fan S, Choi T, Lo C, Mok F, Lai EC, Wong J. Treatment of hepatolithiasis: improvement of result by a systematic approach. *Surgery.* 1991;109:474–480.
53. Han JK, Choi BI, Park JH, Han MC. Percutaneous removal of retained intrahepatic stones with a pre-shaped angulated catheter: review of 96 patients. *Br J Radiol.* 1992;65:9–13.

13

ENDOSCOPIC RETROGRADE CHOLANGIOPANCREATOGRAPHY

Stephen W. Fry, M.D., and Firas H. Al-Kawas, M.D.
Georgetown University Medical Center
Washington, DC

Since endoscopic retrograde cholangiopancreatography (ERCP) was first introduced in 1970 (1), its role in the diagnosis and management of biliary disorders has grown significantly. Currently ERCP is an essential step in the evaluation and treatment of many biliary disorders.

CHOLEDOCHOLITHIASIS

Bile duct stones (CDS) are classified as primary if they actually form in the bile duct or secondary if associated with cholelithiasis. Primary stones are common in areas such as Southeast Asia, especially in association with recurrent pyogenic cholangitis (2). In Western countries primary CDS are less common and occur in patients with biliary stasis due to bile duct strictures or cystic dilatation of the biliary system. Some data suggest an association with juxtapapillary diverticula (3) or that foreign material such as surgical sutures (4) or clips (5) may act as nidi for stone formation. In the Western hemisphere secondary choledocholithiasis is much more common. On ERCP, CDS appear as filling defects and can vary in size and shape (Fig. 1).

Choledocholithiasis occurs in up to 15% of patients undergoing cholecystectomy for symptomatic cholelithiasis (6–8). The diagnosis and management of choledocholithiasis has changed dramatically in the age of laparoscopic cholecystectomy (LC). Previously, open common bile duct exploration (OCBDE) was the standard for the management of choledocholithiasis detected at the time of cholecystectomy. Laparoscopic removal of common duct stones is possible; however, it is time consum-

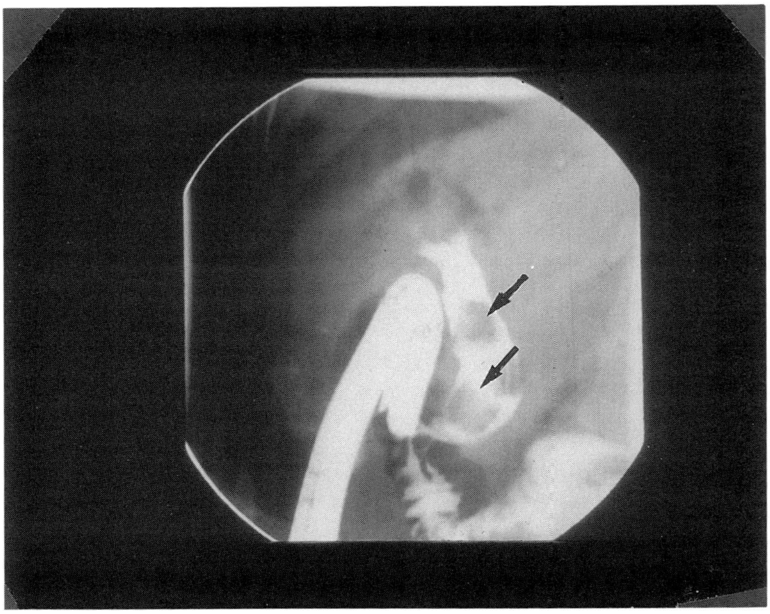

Figure 1. Choledocholithiasis. Cholangiogram demonstrating three filling defects (arrows) within the distal common bile duct consistent with stones.

ing and technically difficult and thus not performed by most surgeons. Stones can be successfully managed by ERCP in at least 90% of cases (9–11). Failures may result from anatomic reasons such as inaccessible papillae due to prior surgery, papillary stenosis, and inexperience. Post-Bilroth II gastrectomy presents a difficult problem. However, in expert hands the desired duct will be cannulated successfully in 60–90% of cases (12–13). The use of additional devices such as a needle knife has greatly enhanced success rates in all patients (14–16).

Although ERCP has assumed a pivotal role in the diagnosis and treatment of CDS the question remains as to when it should be utilized in relationship to LC. Erickson and Carlson (9) used decision analysis based on literature-derived data to compare four clinical strategies for using ERCP with LC: (1) preoperative ERCP, with sphincterotomy for choledocholithiasis; (2) selective preoperative ERCP for patients at high risk for choledocholithiasis, choledocholithiasis found at surgery treated by postoperative ERCP; (3) no preoperative ERCP, choledocholithiasis detected intraoperatively treated by postoperative ERCP; and (4) no preoperative ERCP, choledocholithiasis detected intraoperatively treated with OCBDE. Postoperative ERCP resulted in the lowest cost, procedure numbers, and hospital and back-to-work days. With high preoperative likelihood of choledocholithiasis, selective preoperative ERCP was a clinically equivalent strategy. A survey of the Society of American Gastrointestinal Endoscoping Surgeons indicated that 80% of surgeons preferred this approach (17).

Because of questions regarding the risk, efficacy, and cost of present techniques for diagnosing CDS before or during LC, it is important to identify those patients at the highest risk. The presence of jaundice, cholangitis, ultrasound- or CT-documented choledocholithiasis, or nonresolving acute gallstone pancreatitis clearly indicates a need for ERCP (18). A recent meta-analysis of 21 selected studies found that several individual parameters (clinical, laboratory, ultrasound) had specificities greater than 92%, but none had an acceptable sensitivity (19). The isolated presence of cholangitis or ultrasound evidence of CDS makes the diagnosis of CDS very likely, but because these findings are rarely seen in this population, clinicians must also consider the second tier of indicators, such as the isolated presence of a dilated duct on ultrasound, elevated bilirubin, clinical jaundice, or elevated alkaline phosphatase. Therefore, management of patients with a moderate risk of CDS based solely on the presence of these second-tier indicators is quite controversial because these abnormalities tend to have a low positive predictive value. On the other hand, a high negative predictive value was recently reported for age <60 combined with a normal serum bilirubin and the inability to visualize CDS on ultrasound (20).

Two randomized studies have demonstrated the need for urgent ERCP and subsequent endoscopic spincterotomy (ES) with stone removal for severe gallstone pancreatitis (21, 22). The Leicester group prospectively randomized 121 patients with gallstone pancreatitis to receive either conventional medical therapy or ERCP within 72 hr (21). All stones identified on ERCP were successfully removed and there were no complications associated with ERCP/ES. Three important findings came from this study: (1) urgent ERCP/ES can be safely performed by an experienced endoscopist in the setting of acute pancreatitis; (2) urgent ERCP/ES is associated with a significant reduction in morbidity (12 versus 61%), although this reduction in morbidity was seen only in patients with severe pancreatitis; (3) hospital stay was significantly shortened (median 9.5 versus 17 days) by urgent ERCP/ES. More recently, Fan et al. (22) randomized 127 patients with cholelithiasis and acute pancreatitis to urgent ERCP/ES (within 24 hr) or initial conservative management followed by selective ERCP/ES. There was no difference in outcome for those with mild prognostic scores but for those with "severe" scores, the morbidity and mortality rates for both groups were 54 and 13% and 18 and 3%, respectively. Several other studies have shown that recent or resolving gallstone pancreatitis is a poor predictor of CDS (23–26). These patients need not undergo preoperative ERCP because the CDS infrequently demonstrated by intraoperative cholangiography can be removed by ERCP postoperatively.

In summary, when there is a high index of suspicion for CDS, ERCP should be performed prior to cholecystectomy when possible. However, when there is less compelling evidence, then postoperative ERCP should be performed in those patients with stones demonstrated by an intraoperative cholangiogram. This approach will reduce cost and unnecessary patient risk.

Stone Extraction

Most CDS are 8–10 mm in size and thus well suited for endoscopic removal (27). Following ES (Fig. 2) stones <15 mm may be removed using a balloon-tipped catheter (Fig. 3). The stone is trapped below the balloon and extracted with traction. When dealing with multiple CDS it is best to attempt removal one at a time to avoid impaction in the distal duct. Alternatively, stones may be captured with a

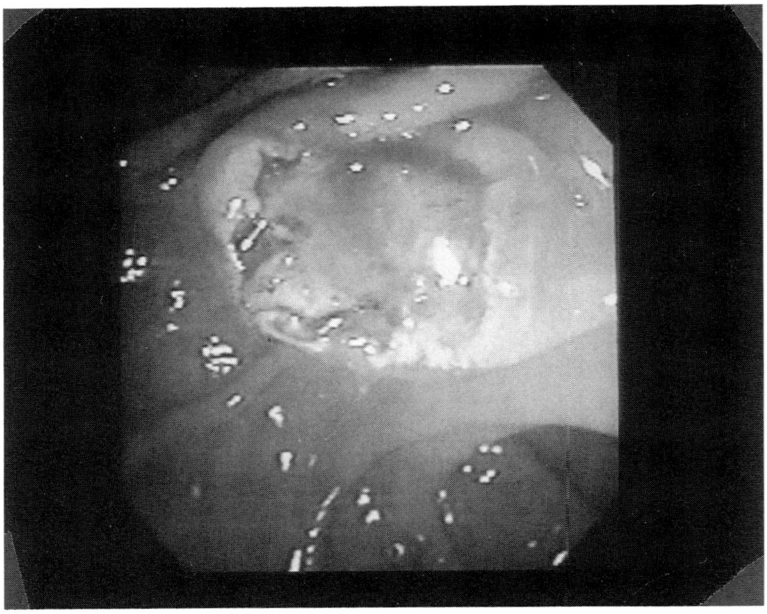

(A)

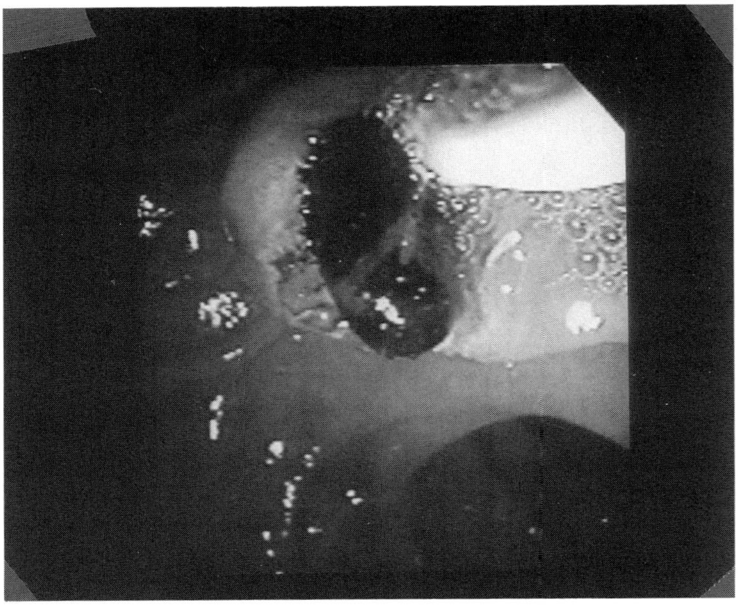

(B)

Figure 2. Endoscopic sphincterotomy. (A) Endoscopic view of a major papilla following sphincterotomy. (B) Endoscopic view of stone retrieval following sphincterotomy.

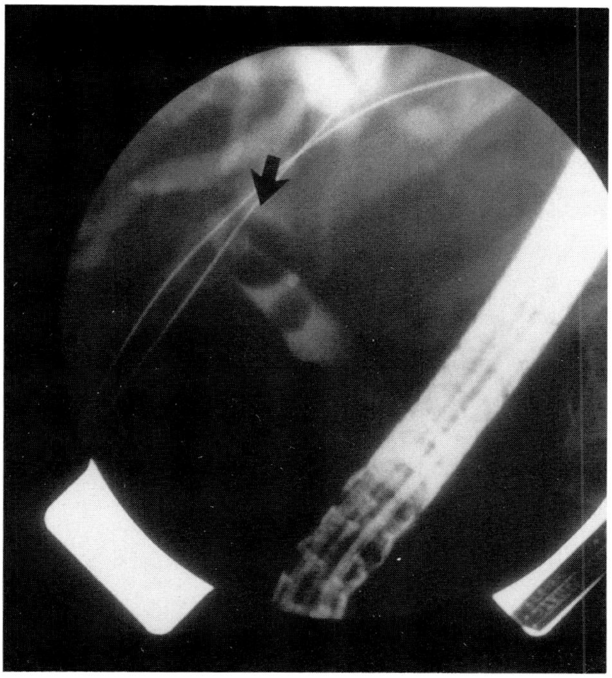

Figure 3. Balloon-tipped catheter extraction. Cholangiogram demonstrating balloon-tipped (arrow) catheter positioned proximal to a stone within the common hepatic duct.

Dormia basket and extracted. This is especially useful when dealing with stones >10 mm or small stones in a dilated bile duct.

Recently there has been a growing concern over the potential long-term effects of ES, prompting some authorities to suggest that small stones (<10 mm) be removed following endoscopic papillary balloon dilation (ED) rather than ES. This is achieved with a 8–10 mm hydrostatic balloon (Fig. 4). Several studies have demonstrated comparable clearance rates of small stones as well as similar complication rates (28–30). It would seem that this removal technique would be most appropriate in younger patients with small, secondary CDS.

The morbidity and mortality associated with ES performed for CDS is approximately 7 and 1.5%, respectively, and results primarily from bleeding, perforation, and pancreatitis (31). When subsequent drainage is inadequate cholangitis can ensue. Most bleeding is self-limited and rarely requires endoscopic intervention or transfusion. Most perforations are also successfully managed conservatively with antibiotics and careful observation. The risk of pancreatitis associated with ES is increased in the setting of nondilated bile ducts (32).

Mirizzi Syndrome

Mirizzi syndrome is defined as common hepatic duct obstruction caused by extrinsic compression from an impacted stone in the cystic duct (Fig. 5). This may be caused

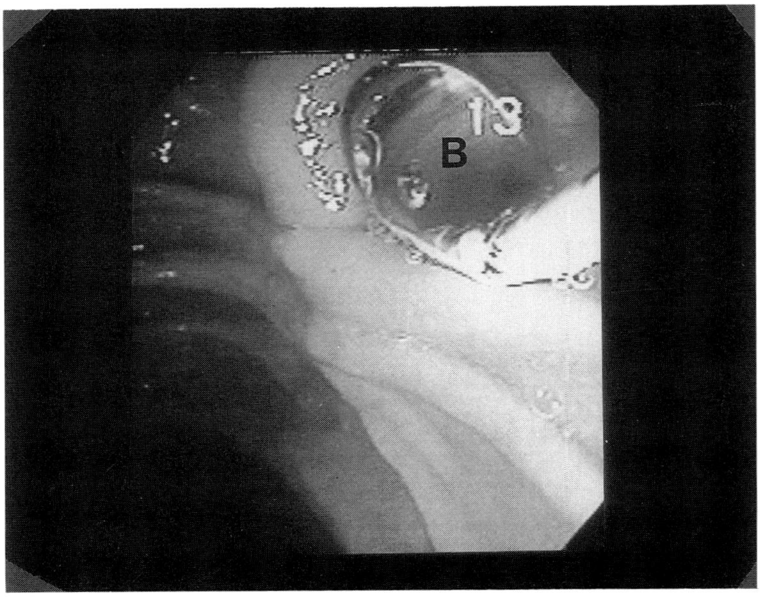

Figure 4. Papillary dilation. Endoscopic view of papillary dilation with an 8-mm hydrostatic balloon (B).

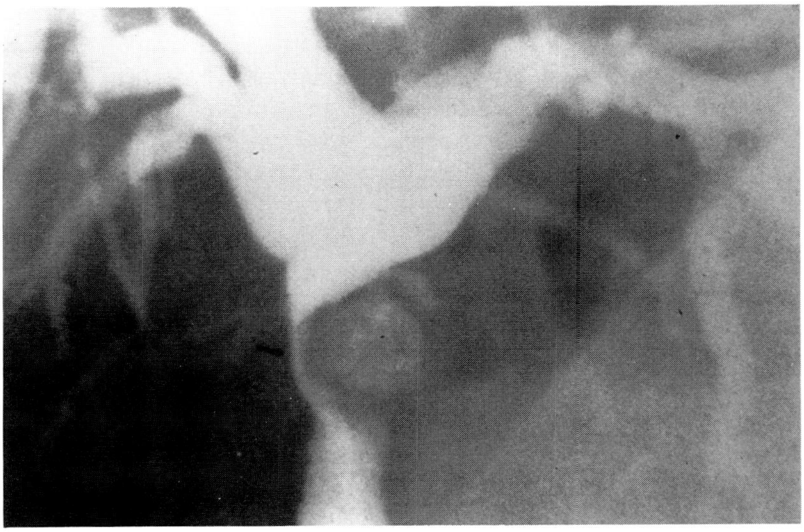

Figure 5. Mirizzi syndrome. Cholangiogram demonstrating extrinsic compression of the common duct (arrow) by a stone impacted in the distal cystic duct. (case courtesy of John Baillie, M.D.).

simply by compression from the stone or associated inflammation. Cholangiographic diagnosis depends on documentation of hepatic duct narrowing or obstruction with an adjacent cystic duct stone. The latter is often difficult but if there is no cystic duct opacification there should be a high index of suspicion. Common bile duct obstruction can be treated with biliary stenting (33) and subsequent laparoscopic cholecystectomy. Alternatively, Binmoeller et al. (34) used electrohydraulic lithotripsy under strict cholangioscopic guidance to treat successfully 14 of 14 patients with Mirizzi syndrome. Complete stone clearance was achieved with one session in 12 patients and in two sessions in two patients (both had multiple stones). One patient suffered a transient cystic duct leak thought to be due to pressure necrosis that responded to conservative management. This technique was suggested to be an effective and relatively safe alternative to surgery. Obviously this approach would be more acceptable in patients who can not or do not want to undergo cholecystectomy.

Acute Cholangitis

Acute cholangitis occurs when there is biliary obstruction and bacterial contamination of the duct. It may be associated with Charcot's triad (pain or tenderness over the liver, fever, and jaundice) or Reynold's pentad (pain, fever, jaundice, altered mental status, and shock) and is potentially life threatening. It is typically associated with CDS but may present with malignant or benign strictures, congenital anomalies, prior duct instrumentation, or surgery. Two retrospective series demonstrated endoscopic biliary drainage to be superior to surgery for acute calculus cholangitis (35, 36). These series presented several important points with regard to clinical management. Following antibiotics and stabilization, ERCP/ES should be performed within 24 hr. Nasobiliary drains or biliary stents should be used if there is any question concerning the adequacy of stone removal or subsequent drainage. Failed attempts at endoscopic biliary decompression should be immediately followed by percutaneous or surgical decompression. Patients with gallbladder in situ must be watched carefully for cholecystitis or empyema of the gallbladder. In the only prospective randomized study comparing endoscopic biliary drainage to surgical decompression for patients with acute calculus cholangitis there was a reported morbidity of 34% and mortality of 10% for endoscopic treatment compared with 66% and 32%, respectively, for surgical treatment (37). ERCP/ES is the treatment of choice for acute calculus cholangitis.

Choledocholithiasis and Pregnancy

Symptomatic CDS in a pregnant woman is a challenging problem. Although surgery can be performed with little risk to the mother it may be associated with an increased risk of fetal loss. Recent reports have shown ERCP/ES to be a safe and effective alternative (38–40). Radiation exposure to the fetus may be safely limited by the use of proper shielding and by capturing fluoroscopic images with a videoendoscopy system, rather than spot radiography (40).

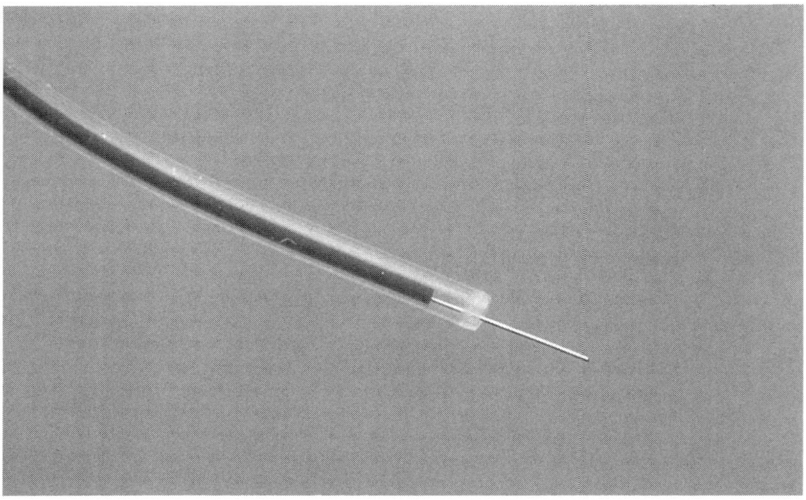

Figure 6. Needle knife sphincterotome.

Management of Difficult Bile Duct Stones

One of the first hurdles in the management of CDS is cannulation of the CBD. When free cannulation can not be achieved a precut sphincterotomy is warranted for further therapeutic intervention. Two types of precut sphincterotomes are currently employed by endoscopists. The first type is a pull type sphincterotome in which the wire extends to the tip of the catheter, and the second is a needle knife (Fig. 6). The needle knife is the most popular, with 80–90% success in selective cannulation of the bile duct. In expert hands the complication rate is similar to that with ES (41, 42). When this method is unsuccessful a "rendezvous" procedure may be attempted, in which a percutaneous transhepatic wire is inserted and grasped with a snare in the duodenum and pulled through the instrument channel. A sphincterotome may then be inserted into the bile duct over the guide wire and the procedure completed.

Following sphincterotomy 90% of CDS can be successfully removed using Dormia baskets and balloon-tipped catheters. The length of the sphincterotomy should be tailored to the size of the stone. Difficulty or failure to clear the common duct of stones usually occurs owing to large (>15 mm) stone size (43). Stones found proximal to biliary strictures also present a significant challenge. A mechanical lithotriptor or "crushing basket" has become the most useful endoscopic adjunct for large stone removal (Fig. 7). Using this technique the stone is captured in a wire basket that has been advanced through a metal sheath. Longitudinal traction is then applied by turning a crank handle so that the basket is withdrawn into the metal sheath, resulting in stone fragmentation (Fig. 8). A review of seven selected series involving 592 patients with CDS not amenable to standard removal techniques shows an overall duct clearance rate of 87% with mechanical lithotripsy (31). In the event of failure with mechanical lithotripsy other options may be considered, including intraductal lithotripsy with electrohydraulic or laser modalities (44, 45). The use of chemical dissolution with mono-octanoin or methyl *tert*-butyl ether has been associated with low success rates and is rarely used (46, 47).

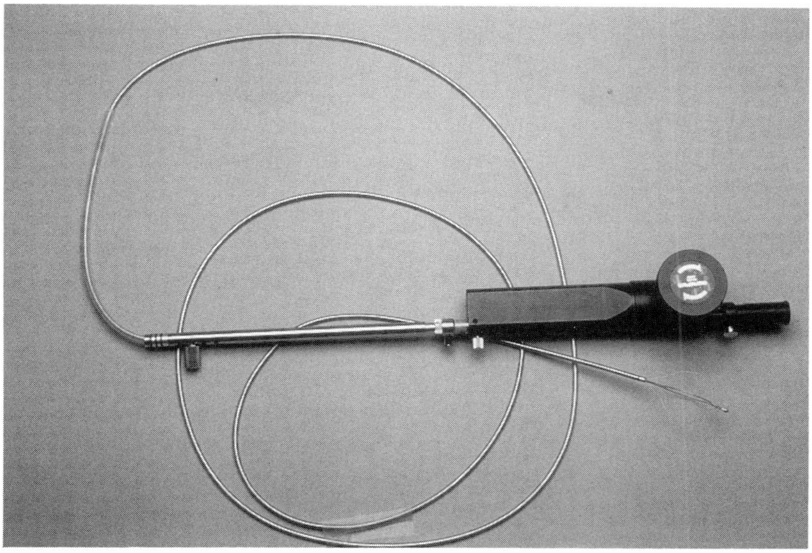

Figure 7. Mechanical lithotriptor.

Should endoscopic stone extraction fail, insertion of a biliary stent is indicated to prevent stone impaction and ensure adequate drainage. This is an excellent temporizing measure (48, 49) but is associated with significant long-term complications (48). Therefore permanent stenting should be restricted to patients that are unfit for surgery and/or with a limited life expectancy.

SPHINCTER OF ODDI DYSFUNCTION

Postcholecystectomy syndrome (PCS) is a misnomer because the clinical manifestations of this syndrome, intermittent epigastric or right upper quadrant abdominal pain, nausea, and vomiting have nothing to do with the event of the cholecystectomy. Sphincter of Oddi (SO) dysfunction (SOD) is found in only 1 to 10% of patients with PCS and may be caused by either SO stenosis or spasm (50). The standard for making the diagnosis is ERCP with SO manometry (SOM). Sphincter of Oddi dysfunction is defined by an elevated basal pressure (>40 mm Hg above the intraduodenal pressure) (Fig. 9). However, spasm may also be associated with tachyoddia (phasic contractions >7/min) and a paradoxical response to cholecystokinin.

Patients with suspected SOD may be separated into three groups based on liver function tests (LFTs) and the presence or absence of CBD dilatation (51) (Table 1). Sphincter ablation via ES has been shown to be effective in the treatment of confirmed SOD (52). Patients with Type 1 SOD do not require SOM prior to ES (53), but the efficacy of SOM in predicting a positive long-term response to ES in Type 2 patients was recently confirmed (54). Endoscopic sphincterotomy in patients with SOD appears to be associated with increased risk of complications compared to patients with stone disease.

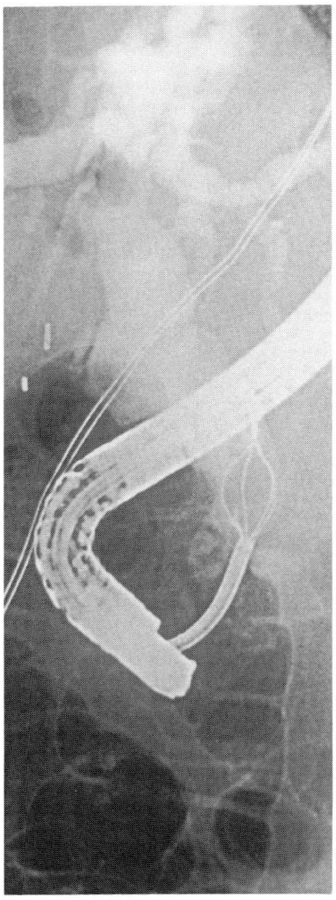

Figure 8. Mechanical lithotriptor. A stone is captured within the wire basket and crushed against the metal sheath.

MALIGNANT BILIARY STRICTURES

Biliary obstruction due to both primary and secondary malignancies is a major cause of jaundice. The initial imaging modality utilized in the work-up of these patients is often ultrasonography or CT scan. If a mass is detectable, an image-guided needle biopsy often yields a specific histological diagnosis. At other times, ductal dilatation rather than a distinct mass is seen with noninvasive imaging. This is when ERCP can be of great assistance both diagnostically and therapeutically. Malignant lesions of the bile duct may present in three ways: they narrow or obstruct the duct, produce a filling defect within the duct, or ulcerate (55).

Endoscopic Differentiation of Strictures: Benign versus Malignant

Symptoms associated with malignant biliary obstruction are often nonspecific and include anorexia, nausea, vomiting, and weight loss. Painless jaundice is typically thought to be due to malignancy until proved otherwise. Although painful jaundice is often related to choledocholithiasis, underlying malignancy, especially when at

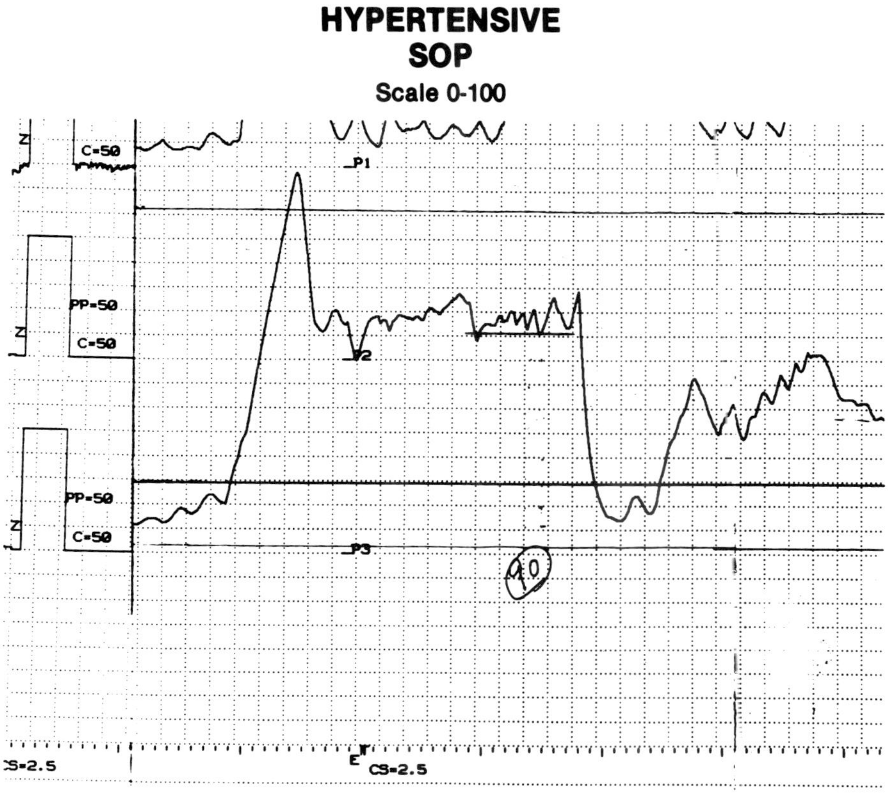

Figure 9. Sphincter of Oddi manometry. This tracing demonstrates a hypertensive sphincter of Oddi, with a base-line pressure greater than 40 mm Hg.

an advanced stage, may be responsible. Morphological characteristics of a stricture such as abruptness and irregularity on cholangiography may be suggestive of malignancy but certainly not diagnostic (Fig. 10). Even the classic "double duct sign" associated with pancreatic head malignancy where there is distal stricturing of both the CBD and the pancreatic duct may rarely be due to benign inflammatory pancreatic disease (56). Definitive diagnosis ultimately relies on obtaining represen-

Table 1. Groups of patients with suspected SOD and the prevalence of abnormal findings on manometry

Type	Clinical Findings	SOD on Manometry (%)
1	Abnormal LAE and dilated CBD	70
2	Abnormal LAE or dilated CBD	50
3	Normal LAE and CBD	<5

Patients in all three groups had biliary type symptoms. LAE, liver-associated enzymes. Adapted from Dodds.[5]

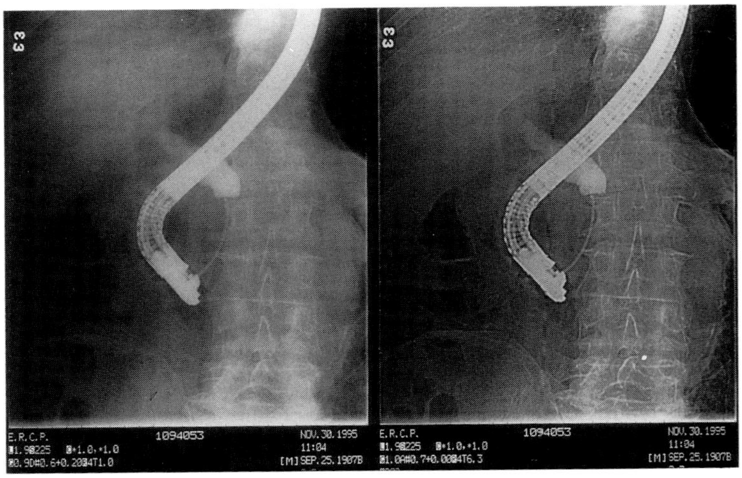

Figure 10. Malignant bile duct stricture. Cholangiogram demonstrating a mid-duct stricture, caused by a cholangiocarcinoma, with marked proximal dilatation of the intrahepatic ducts. A wire has traversed the stricture and is situated within the intrahepatic system.

tative tissue samples. ERCP provides the least invasive and safest technique for achieving this. Additionally, biliary obstruction may be caused by ampullary tumors with ERCP providing direct visualization, tissue sampling, and the ability to decompress the biliary system with the placement of biliary endoprosthesis (Fig. 11).

The nature of bile duct stenosis is critical in determining appropriate further therapy, be it surgical resection, chemotherapy, radiotherapy, or simple palliative decompression. Obviously, the least invasive technique for achieving this determination is desirable. Endoscopic bile collection for cytology alone has yielded very poor results leading to its abandonment (57). If bile collection is performed, prior dilation of the stricture may significantly increase the yield for obtaining diagnostic cytology (58). At the time of stent exchange, adherent stent material may provide cytological diagnosis (59, 60). Endobiliary brush cytology has a sensitivity ranging from 40 to 70% and a specificity near 100% (61–64). The addition of endobiliary biopsies to cytology was superior to brush cytology alone in some studies (62, 63). Endoscopic sphincterotomy is usually required to facilitate insertion of biopsy forceps. Some authors have suggested that the modest additional diagnostic yield does not warrant the increased risk associated with ES (62). Patients with biliary obstruction requiring decompression often undergo ES for therapeutic purposes, thus negating the argument against performing biopsy. However, a recently available malleable biopsy forceps was successfully introduced without a sphincterotomy in 87% of patients (65). Certainly patients with suspected intra-ampullary cancers should undergo ES allowing for aggressive intraductal biopsy, because these cancers have a favorable prognosis when detected early. Although sensitivities of individual sampling techniques tend to vary amongst investigators, several recent studies (Table 2) have reported an overall improvement in sensitivity when multiple sampling devices were used in the same patient (62, 63, 66, 67).

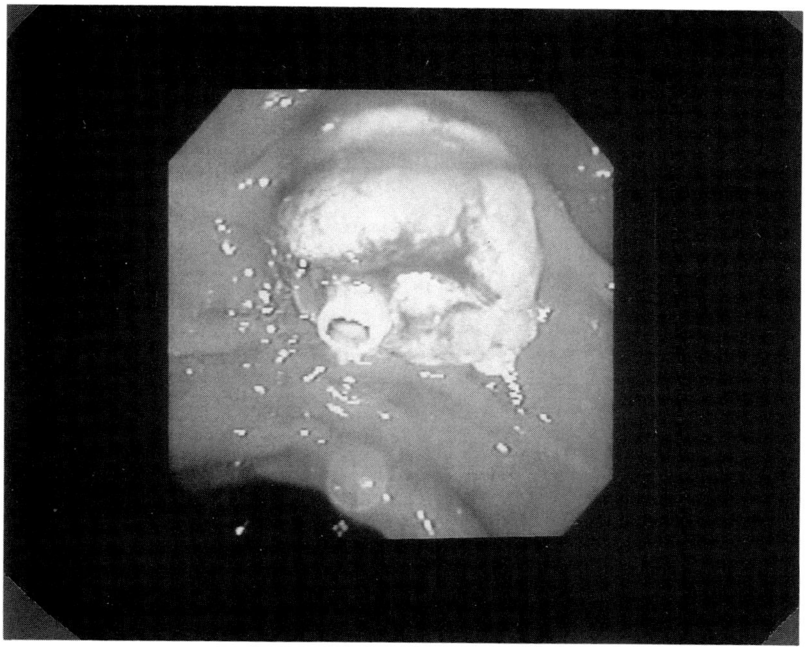

Figure 11. Ampullary carcinoma. This patient presented with biliary obstruction due to ampullary carcinoma. ERCP provided direct visualization of the etiology and biopsy for diagnosis. A plastic biliary stent was then placed for biliary decompression.

The extrabiliary origin of many cancers responsible for biliary obstruction makes them less accessible for tissue sampling (61, 68). Ponchon et al. (63), found that when they compared cancers that directly invaded the bile duct to those that extrinsically compressed the duct, the combination of cytology and biopsy had a sensitivity of 86 and 36%, respectively. Howell et al. (69) tried to overcome this barrier by performing endoscopic needle aspiration (ENA). They compared the sensitivity of ENA and brush cytology to evaluate 31 patients with biliary strictures

Table 2. Positive sampling frequency in malignant strictures undergoing simultaneous sampling methods

	Sensitivity of Tissue Sampling Techniques (%)				
Study	No. of Patients	Brush Cytology	Biopsies	ENA	Combined
Pugliese et al. (62)	64	53	53	—	61
Ponchon et al. (63)	134	35	43	—	63
Cunningham et al. (66)	20	50	45	—	70
Sherman et al. (67)	77	43	47	37	71[a]

[a]Combined brush cytology and biopsy yielded a sensitivity of 64%.

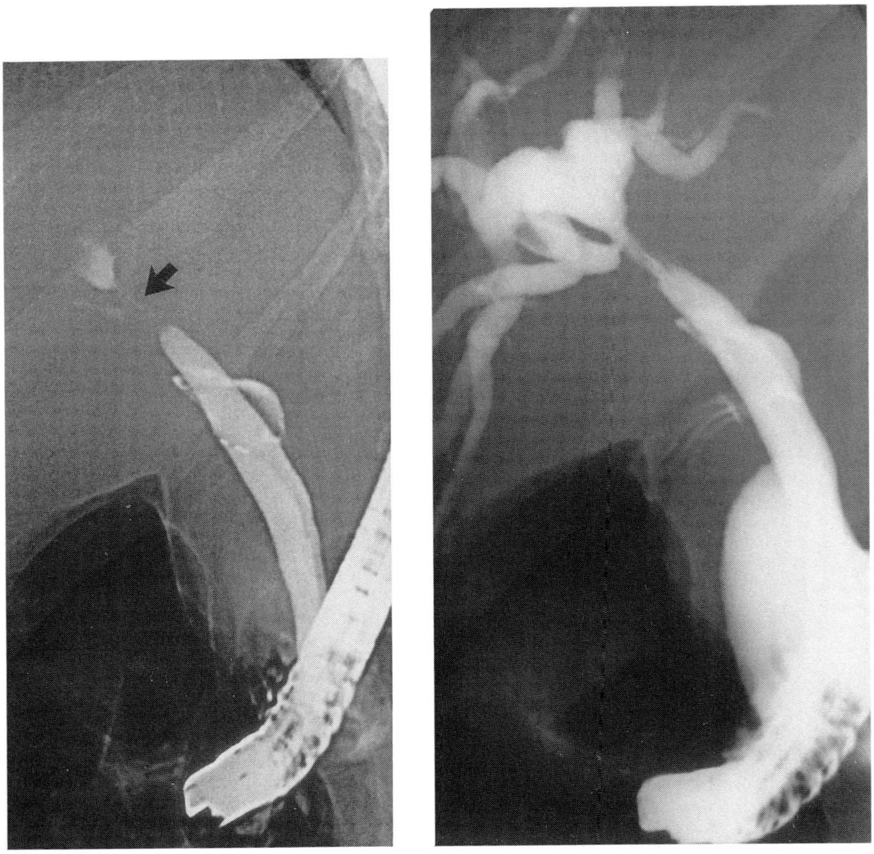

(A) (B)

Figure 12. Plastic biliary stent. (A) Cholangiogram demonstrating a common hepatic duct stricture (arrow) due to cholangiocarcinoma. A small amount of contrast can be seen just proximal to the stricture. (B) By traversing the stricture with the cannula the marked intrahepatic duct dilatation is identified. (C) A plastic stent has been inserted (arrows) (next page). (D) Endoscopic view of the stent extending from the major papilla (next page).

of which 26 were malignant (21 extrinsic/5 intrinsic). The sensitivity of ENA for extrinsic cancers was superior to brush cytology.

Retrograde choledochoscopy allows direct visualization of intrinsic lesions, providing a sensitivity near 100% for cholangiocarcinoma (70), but the expertise required, lack of availability, and additional procedural time and expense make this impractical in most cases. Lee et al. (64) examined 149 patients with biliary strictures (74 malignant/75 benign) and found that the clinical diagnosis based on ERCP findings, history, and physical exam were much more sensitive than brush cytology (88 versus 37%) but less specific (77 versus 100%).

In summary, tissue sampling should always be obtained when ERCP demonstrates a biliary stricture. Endobiliary brush cytology, biopsy, and ENA have a

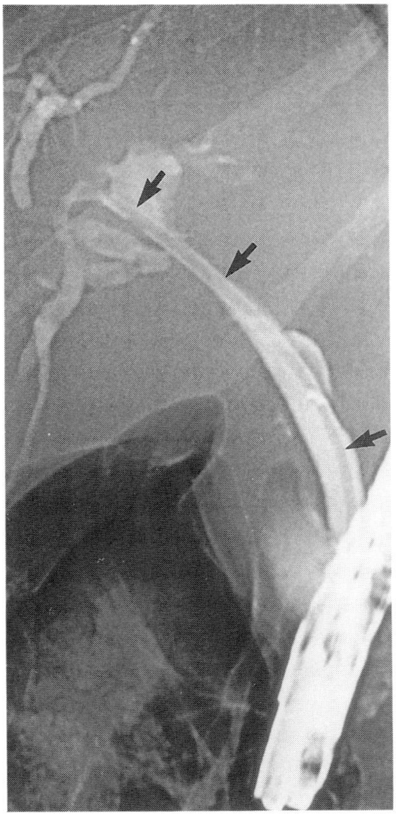

(C)

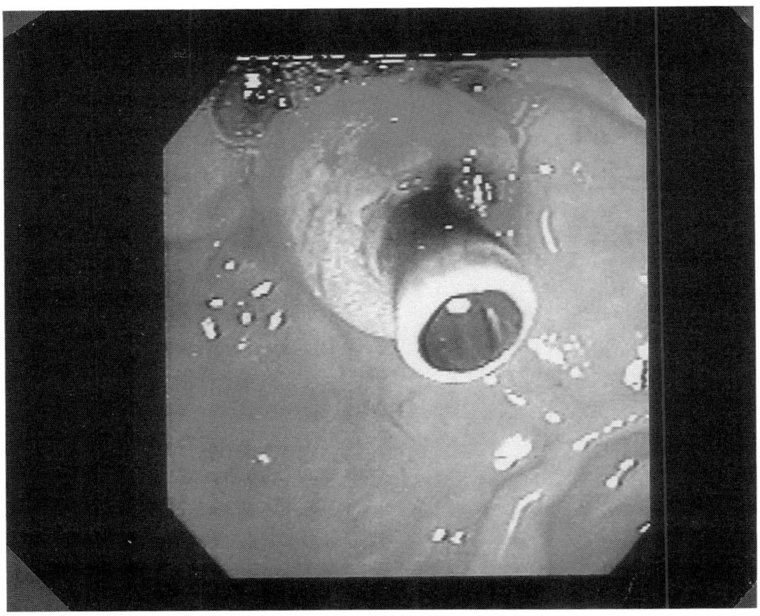

(D)

Figure 12. *(Continued)*

Table 3. Palliation of malignant biliary obstruction: randomized trials comparing endoscopic biliary decompression to percutaneous biliary decompression or operative bypass[a]

Study	Procedure Type	No. Patients	Technical Success	Relief of Jaundice	Complications	Median Hospital Stay (days)	30-day Mortality	Median Survival (days)
Speer et al. (72)	E	39	89%	81%[b]	19%[b]	NA	15%[b]	159
	P	36	76%	61%	67%	NA	33%	113
Shephard et al. (73)	E	27	82%	91%[b]	30%[b]	5[b]	9%[b]	152
	S	25	92%	92%	56%	13	20%	124
Anderson et al. (74)[c]	E	30	100%	NA	NA	No difference	20%	81
	S	19	NA	NA	NA		24%	108
Smith et al. (75)	E	100	95%	92%	11%[b]	19[b]	8%	147
	S	101	93%	91%	29%	26	15%	182

[a]E, endoscopic biliary stent; P, percutaneous drainage; S, surgical bypass; NA, data not available.
[b]$p < .05$.
[c]Fifty patients initially randomized, 25 E/25 S, but 5 randomized to S refused and then underwent E. All figures in table are based on treatment groups. No significant differences existed when calculated for randomization groups as well.

limited sensitivity but have a very low morbidity and a very high specificity. Sensitivity can be enhanced by using all three methods.

Endoscopic Decompression of Malignant Biliary Obstruction

In the setting of biliary obstruction, ERCP is performed to obtain diagnostic information from both the cholangiographic appearance of the stricture and actual endoscopic tissue sampling. Once the biliary system has been breached by instrumentation a decompressive procedure should be done to avoid cholangitis. Soehendra and Reynders-Frederix (71) introduced endoscopic placement of biliary stents in 1979. Several well controlled studies have since documented their safety and efficacy in the palliation of malignant biliary obstruction (Fig. 12) when compared with surgical and transhepatic approaches (Table 3) (72–75).

Although curative resection of pancreatobiliary cancers is the ultimate goal, realistically, the majority of patients require only palliation. Biliary stenting for obstructive jaundice has been prospectively shown to reduce anorexia, improve appetite, and enhance quality of life (76, 77). Naggar et al. (78) reviewed eight publications that cited 856 cases comparing endoscopic stenting to percutaneous decompression or surgical bypass in both open and randomized trials. Endoscopic insertion of endoprosthesis was successful in 90% of cases and had a related mortality of 1.3% and a 30-day mortality of 12%. Complications including fever, hemorrhage, and cholangitis occurred in 20% of cases. Overall survival was not affected by type of therapy. When compared with transhepatic drainage there were fewer complications and lower associated mortality. Likewise when compared with surgical bypass there were fewer early complications and shorter required hospitalizations. Unfortunately, stent occlusion resulting in cholangitis in the follow-up period was a significant problem. The inability to insert a stent endoscopically in approximately 10% of cases stems primarily from either not being able to place a guide wire proximal to the stricture or simply not being able to cannulate the CBD freely. The development of low-friction guide wires (Glidewire, Microvasive and Tracerwire, Wilson Cook Inc.) has improved our ability to traverse tight strictures and cannulate difficult papillae. The use of the precut technique utilizing a "needle knife" to unroof the intraduodenal segment of the CBD has also enhanced our abilities to cannulate the bile duct freely. When these measures fail the endoscopist should consider a combined approach with radiology.

The combined approach is best undertaken immediately after ERCP if a cholangiogram has been performed, because the contrast in the proximal biliary system will assist the radiologist. Improved leverage with a percutaneous approach will usually enable anterograde passage of a guide wire through a tight stricture. Once the guide wire is in the duodenum the endoscopist can utilize it to pass successive dilators and finally insert a stent. This technique is safer than percutaneous drainage because the transhepatic tract need not be dilated. Dowsett et al. (79), using the combined approach, successfully inserted stents in 60 of 72 patients where endoscopic approach alone was difficult. Using the "slippery" wires, precut technique, and a combined approach where necessary provides success in greater than 95% of cases.

The location of a stricture (proximal versus distal) to some extent dictates the likelihood of success with endoscopically placed stents. Advanced pancreatic and duodenal cancers may not allow intubation of the descending duodenum owing to stricture or mass effect. Boender et al. (80) correlated failure of stent insertion with increasing size of a pancreatic head tumor and/or extrinsic invasion of the papilla.

Hilar strictures have also been more difficult to manage endoscopically, and some authors suggest percutaneous drainage for these cases (81). The difficulty lies in providing adequate drainage to avoid cholangitis. Deviere et al. (82) reduced the incidence of cholangitis from 28 to 17% by inserting a second stent to insure drainage of both the left and right lobes. Polydorou et al. (83) found that only 5% of hilar lesions required placement of a second stent.

Clearly the endoscopic approach for decompression of malignant biliary obstruction is preferable. In the past few years there has been intensified research into maintaining stent patency. The rate of occlusion with plastic stents is related to stent size, and thus a stent 10 French or greater should always be utilized (84). Larger stent diameters may prolong patency but an endoscopic instrument channel will not accommodate a stent larger than 12 French. Unfortunately, most stents clog within 4 months. The development of metal-mesh expandable stents (Wallstent, Schneider, Gianturco Z stent, Wilson Cook Inc., Endocoil, InStent) that can be inserted using a small-diameter delivery system and expand to diameters as high as 30 French have been met with guarded enthusiasm (Fig. 13). Four prospective randomized trials have compared endoscopic plastic stents to metal stents (85–88). Each study demonstrated that metal stents remain patent longer and that they are cost effective (Table 4). Notably, 50% of the patients randomized to receive plastic stents died prior to a need for stent exchange.

Metal stents are not without problems because they are expensive and may eventually occlude owing to tumor ingrowth. Once deployed they can not be removed or repositioned. Tumor ingrowth can be treated with diathermal cleaning, balloon catheter trawling, or insertion of another metal stent or a plastic stent (89). Because of their high cost, metal stents should not be used in patients with limited life expectancy (<6 months). A recent retrospective analysis of data from 154 patients who received Wallstents showed that 32% died within 3 months. Factors associated with longer life-span were the absence of liver metastases, a bilirubin <3.2 mg %, distal location, and short length (≤2 cm) of the malignant stricture (90).

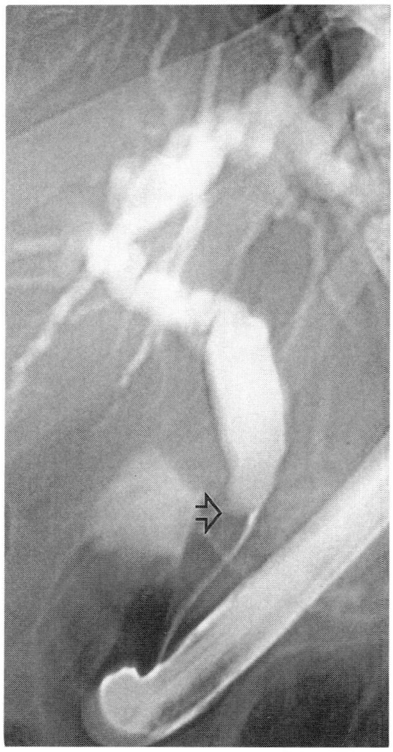

(A)

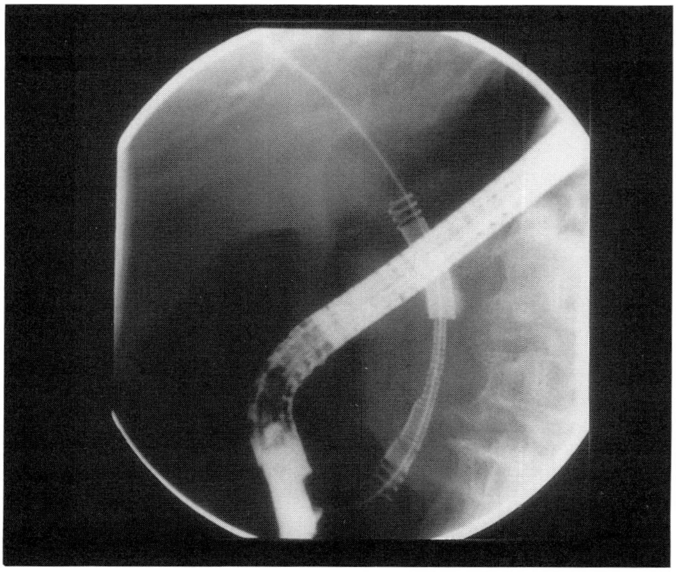

(B)

Figure 13. Self-expanding metal stent. Patient presented with a mass in the head of the pancreas. (A) This cholangiogram demonstrates the distal and rather abrupt nature of the stricture (open arrow). Proximal biliary dilatation is noted. (B) An Endocoil® is seen partially deployed upon the introducer catheter. (C) The stent is now fully deployed with an internal diameter of 10 mm (next page). (D) Endoscopic view of the Endocoil® (next page).

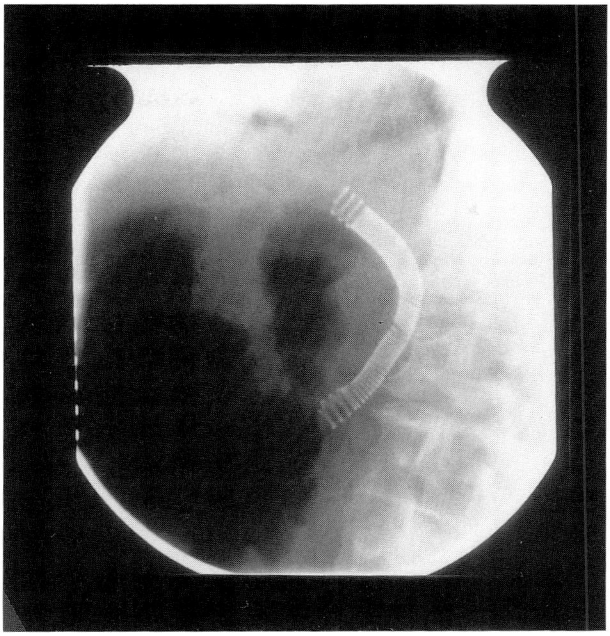

(C)

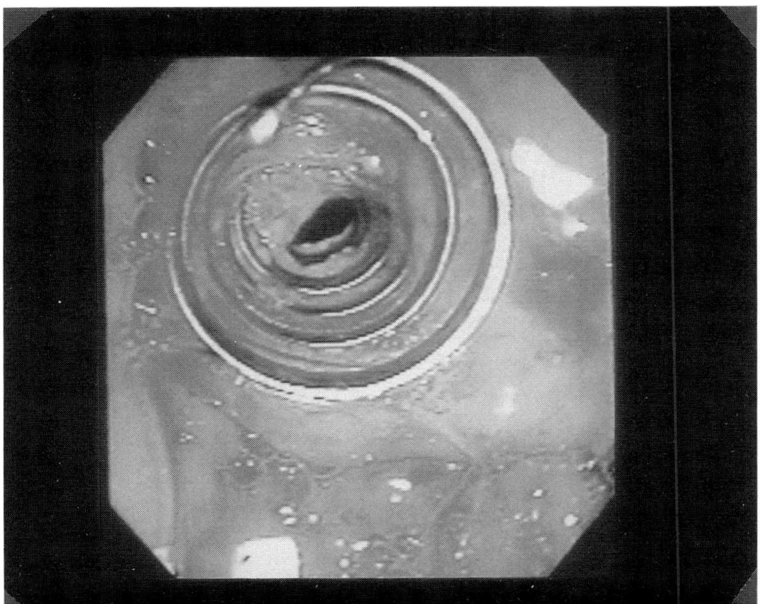

(D)

Figure 13. *(Continued)*

Table 4. Expandable metal stents versus plastic stents for malignant biliary strictures[a]

Study	Stent Type	No. Patients	Cholangitis	Stent Occlusion	More Cost-Effective
Neuhaus et al. (85)†	P	92	9%[b]	39%[b] at 6 months based on actuarial life table	Metal
	M	61	0%		
Davids et al. (86)	P	56	41%[b]	54%[b] at median 126 days[b]	Metal
	M	49	25%	33% at median 273 days	
Carr-Locke et al. (87)	P	78	NA	13% at median 62 days[b]	Metal
	M	86	NA	13% at median 111 days	
Knyrim et al. (88)	P	28	36%[b]	43%[b] at median 138 days ± 21	Metal
	M	27	15%	22% at mean 186 days ± 57	

[a] Technical success of stent placement was similar for all series (plastic = 98%, metal = 99%). No difference in survival seen in all series. P, plastic; M, metal; NA, data not available.
[a] $p < .05$. †Comparative study. All others were prospective and randomized.

Another approach to improving stent patency is to eliminate side holes. Studies have demonstrated that side holes are primary targets for early clogging. Two studies using stents without side holes have been reported. In a randomized study comparing conventional plastic stents with and without holes patency rates were similar (79). But in an open study using a 10-French Teflon stent (Tannenbaum) improved patency rates (55 patients/median patency = 64 weeks) were seen (80). Currently, a randomized controlled multicenter trial is being done in the United States comparing the Tannenbaum to conventional plastic stents.

BENIGN BILIARY STRICTURES

Benign biliary strictures, owing to their associated sequelae of cholestasis, cholangitis, choledocholithiasis, and secondary biliary cirrhosis, remain clinically challenging to surgeons, radiologists, and gastroenterologists. Advancements in endoscopic technology including dilating devices and stents, both plastic and self-expanding metal, have made nonsurgical management of these strictures an attractive option. Management choices often reflect only the local level of expertise, but clinicians managing biliary strictures should consider the stricture's etiology and anatomy, the patient's overall condition and prognosis, and the expected likelihood of success, in both short-term and long-term measures. Endoscopic approaches are highly successful at providing immediate decompression of an obstructed biliary tree. When compared to surgery, endoscopy is less invasive and less expensive.

The most common cause of benign biliary stricture is operative trauma. Operative bile duct injuries resulting in strictures, simple leaks, fistulas, and complete transection are discussed below. The second most common cause of benign biliary stricture is pancreatitis and its sequelae. Other less frequent causes of strictures or bile duct obstruction are listed in Table 5. Diseases associated with diffuse cholangiopathy and secondary diffuse stricture formation are considered below.

Strictures Due to Benign Pancreatic Disease

Bile duct obstruction due to pancreatic disease is caused by the passage of the distal CBD through the posterior surface of the pancreas just prior to entering the

Table 5. Causes of bile duct obstruction

Intrinsic Causes	*Extrinsic Causes*
Stones (primary obstruction and Mirizzi syndrome)	Tumors - lymphoma, hepatoma, adenopathy, etc.
Tumors	Pancreatitis: acute and chronic, pseudocyst, abscess
Malignant	Retroperitoneal fibrosis
Primary cholangiocarcinoma and ampullary carcinoma	Vascular lesions
Metastatic: gallbladder carcinoma, hepatoma, lymphoma, adenocarcinoma, etc.	Cystic liver disease
Benign	Duodenal disorders
Adenomas	Peptic ulcer disease
Mesenchymal tumors	Crohn's disease
Hamartomas	Eosinophilic gastroenteritis
Granular cell tumors	Periampullary diverticula
Localized benign strictures	Villous adenoma
Papillary stenosis	Annular pancreas
Trauma (postoperative and penetrating abdominal)	Sarcoidosis
Chronic pancreatitis (fibrosis)	
Necrotizing cholangitis	
Cystic fibrosis	
Parasitic infection	
Fungal infection (*Candida*)	
Tuberculosis	
Diffuse benign strictures	
Sclerosing cholangitis	
Hepatic artery infusion cholangiopathy	
AIDS cholangiopathy (*cryptosporidium*, cytomegalovirus, etc.)	
Hemobilia	
Biliary atresia	
Biliary cysts	

duodenum. Both acute and chronic pancreatitis can result in stenosis, although obstruction is usually more permanent with chronic pancreatitis due to associated fibrosis. The prevalence of CBD stricture due to chronic alcoholic pancreatitis ranges from 4 to 10% (93). Benign CBD obstruction may also occur with pancreatic pseudocyst, abscess, and benign pancreatic tumors.

ERCP is valuable in the evaluation of these patients because it defines any associated pancreatic abnormalities that may warrant surgical intervention. The typical cholangiographic appearance of a CBD stricture due to pancreatic inflammatory disease is a gradual, smooth narrowing. Common bile duct displacement away from the duodenum is commonly seen although nonspecific. Endoscopic tissue sampling (see malignant bile duct strictures) should always be obtained in an attempt to rule out malignancy. Endosonography may be helpful in this setting.

Endoscopic Management of Strictures Due to Benign Pancreatic Disease

Beyond the diagnostic utility of ERCP, the rationale for endoscopic intervention (biliary decompression) in the setting of chronic pancreatitis is fivefold (94). These include (1) treatment of symptoms of cholestasis (for example, itching and nausea), (2) drainage of infected bile if present, (3) allowing time for reversible pancreatic inflammatory component to regress (that is, allowing bile duct narrowing to regress), (4) preventing secondary biliary cirrhosis, and (5) differentiation of pain of cholestasis from that of pancreatitis.

Distal CBD narrowing typically extends 2–4 cm, making sphincterotomy alone inadequate for management. Endoscopic management with the placement of plastic biliary stents has not been encouraging. This technique is highly successful in providing clinical relief of symptoms via immediate decompression, especially when cholangitis is present. But persistence of strictures and associated complications, including stent migration and inevitable occlusion, requiring periodic exchange makes this an unattractive option for long-term management. Deviere et al. (95) inserted one or two plastic stents in 25 patients with chronic pancreatitis (23 endoscopically/2 percutaneously). All patients had cholestasis, 19 had jaundice, and 7 had cholangitis. There were no early complications and all cholangitis and cholestasis resolved. Unfortunately, 18 patients later developed complications related to stent migration (10) or stent occlusion (8), and of the 21 patients available for long-term follow-up, only 3 (14%) remain asymptomatic without stents.

Stenting of a biliary stricture due to chronic pancreatitis may assist in the diagnosis of chronic abdominal pain. Meier et al. (96) placed stents in eight patients with chronic pancreatitis, CBD strictures, and chronic abdominal pain. Seven of these patients had resolution of their pain and five of these seven continued to have pain relief after a surgical biliary drainage procedure, without a pancreatic drainage procedure. This diagnostic utility has not been reproduced by other investigators.

Endoscopically placed expandable metallic stents for benign biliary strictures have been infrequently used. This stems primarily from the inability to remove most of these stents after placement and the concern over long-term occlusion as occurs with malignant disease. The internal diameter of these stents far exceeds that of multiple plastic stents and early migration has not been reported to be a problem. Based on their poor experience with plastic stents, Deviere et al. (97) treated 20 patients with symptomatic CBD stricture due to chronic pancreatitis. At a mean follow-up of 33 months (range 24–42), 18 patients (90%) remained asymptomatic with patent stents. Two patients developed epithelial hyperplasia within the stent resulting in obstruction within 6 months of placement. Membrane-coated stents may prevent this complication in the future.

Rare Causes of Focal Bile Duct Obstruction

Benign tumors of the bile duct including adenomas, mesenchymal tumors, hamartomas, and granular cell tumors have been reported to cause biliary obstruction (55). Although all of these tumors may result in abnormal cholangiograms, there are no distinguishing features to offer specific diagnosis. Tuberculosis, candidiasis, bile duct parasites, and hemobilia can all result in intrinsic bile duct obstruction. Cystic fibrosis and primary sclerosing cholangitis can each present with extrahepatic stricture formation (98, 99). Biliary cysts and atresia can result in biliary obstruction. Extrinsic bile duct compression can result from numerous causes including adenopathy, retroperitoneal fibrosis, vascular lesions (100, 101), nonparasitic hepatic cysts

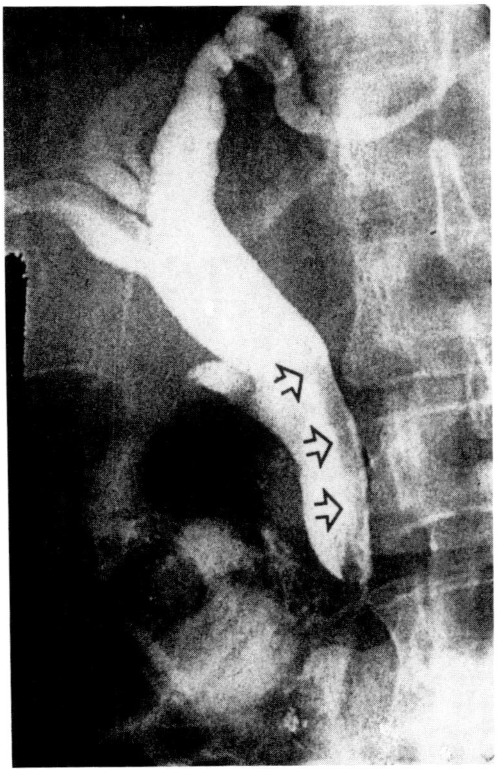

Figure 14. Biliary ascariasis. Cholangiogram demonstrating a linear filling defect (open arrows) in the distal common bile duct.

(102), annular pancreas (103), duodenal ulcer disease (104), eosinophilic gastroenteritis (105), and even periampullary duodenal diverticula (106).

Bile duct parasites including *Ascaris, Clonorchis, Opisthorchis,* and *Fasciola* can all cause biliary obstruction. Adult ascarids can be visualized endoscopically when extruding from the papilla or as a distinct filling defect when cholangiography is performed (Fig. 14). Flukes can also often be seen with cholangiography as 1–2 cm filling defects. *Clonorchis* has long been associated with Oriental cholangiohepatitis, and biliary helminth infestations of all types may result in cholangitis, choledocholithiasis, stricture formation, and even carcinoma.

OPERATIVE BILE DUCT INJURY

Operative injury to the bile duct is most often associated with cholecystectomy, but may also occur with hepatic resection or transplantation, or any procedure involving the pancreas, stomach, duodenum, or portal vein. More than 85% of cholecystectomies are now done laparoscopically. Although this technique has clearly reduced the overall associated morbidity and cost, one clear tradeoff has

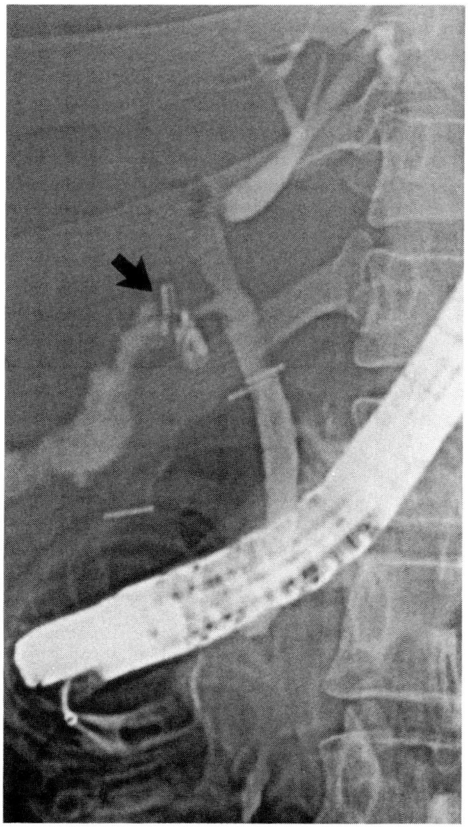

Figure 15. Biliary leak. This patient presented with abdominal pain and leukocytosis 3 days postlaparoscopic cholecystectomy. Cholangiogram demonstrates extravasation of contrast (arrow) at the cystic duct stump site.

been the increased risk of bile duct injury. Major bile duct injuries include complete bile duct transection, strictures, and leaks leading to fistulas, bilomas, bile ascites, or bile peritonitis. The incidence of major bile duct injury after open cholecystectomy is 0.2 to 0.3% (107). Rates of bile duct injury reported with laparoscopic cholecystectomy vary greatly, but the largest series estimate the incidence to be 0.4 to 0.8% (108–110). Early in the experience of individual surgeons, rates as high as 2% have been noted with laparoscopic technique (110).

The most common location for a bile leak is the cystic duct stump (Fig. 15). This is usually due to inadequate clip ligation, a tear in the remnant proximal to the clip, or a necrotic duct remnant that fails to close because of an ongoing necroinflammatory response. Common duct injuries may be a consequence of errant clip placement, excessive cautery, excessive dissection, excessive traction, or the misidentification of the common duct for the cystic duct with inadvertent transection ("classic injury") (111–113). Many of these injuries are not immediately recognized, with the majority of patients presenting several days later with malaise, abdominal pain, nausea, vomiting, fever, and/or jaundice. Whenever rapid recovery does not occur following laparoscopic cholecystectomy, the physician should suspect a bile duct injury. Additionally, strictures may occur at the site of previous T-tube placement or at the biliary–enteric anastomotic site in previously repaired bile duct injuries. A small minority of these injuries, especially strictures, may not become clinically evident for months to years, presenting with episodic cholangitis, painless jaundice, or only after complications related to secondary biliary cirrhosis are manifest.

Strictures are most often defined by the Bismuth (114) grading system (see Chapter 12, Table 1): Type I strictures are more than 2 cm from the confluence of the left and right hepatic ducts, Type II strictures are less than 2 cm from the confluence but still have remnant common hepatic duct, Type III strictures are flush with the confluence, Type IV strictures involve the confluence of the right and left hepatic ducts, and Type V strictures involve the right hepatic duct and may or may not involve the common hepatic duct.

Bile duct complications occur in 7–38% of patients after orthotopic liver transplant (OLT), the majority of which are strictures and leaks (115). The most common biliary anastomosis is choledochocholedochal, with choledochojejunal occurring in most other cases. Leaks most often occur at the T-tube site following removal or at the actual anastomotic site. Stricture location varies depending on the underlying etiology. Anastomotic strictures are the most common and are usually technical in nature related to poor local blood supply (116). Nonanastomotic strictures or leaks occur most often because of hepatic artery occlusion but may also result from extended graft preservation times, the use of ABO blood group incompatible grafts, or chronic ductopenic rejection. Additionally, intrahepatic and nonanastomotic extrahepatic biliary strictures are significantly more common in patients who have liver transplantation for primary sclerosing cholangitis than in patients who receive allografts for other end-stage liver diseases (117).

Endoscopic retrograde cholangiopancreatography is the most useful test for the definitive diagnosis of major bile duct complications (112, 118). Endoscopic retrograde cholangiopancreatography detects retained calculi, strictures, biliary leaks or fistulas, complete obstruction, and previously unsuspected cancers. Although cholescintigraphy has been reported to have an 83–87% accuracy in predicting the presence of postoperative biliary leaks (119), cholangiography is essential in defining the exact location of the leak and its possible relationship to downstream strictures or calculi. Cholestasis in the post-OLT patient has many potential etiologies with early ERCP and liver biopsy frequently allowing a rapid diagnosis and treatment. Historically, bile duct injuries have been managed surgically, but with the advent of advanced endoscopic techniques many of these complications may now be managed endoscopically.

Endoscopic Management of Postoperative Bile Leakage

Cystic duct leakage can be managed successfully by temporary placement of a nasobiliary drain (120), endoscopic sphincterotomy, and/or the placement of a biliary stent (121–127). The goal of therapy is to reduce the biliary–duodenal pressure gradient, normally about 8 mm H_2O, to induce preferential flow toward the duodenum, away from the leak or fistula. A sphincterotomy must adequately cut the sphincteric muscle to be effective, whereas stent placement essentially equalizes biliary and duodenal pressures. Stent size does not appear to be important in determining success and removal can usually be achieved in 2 to 4 weeks.

Common duct leaks, especially those with distal strictures, are probably best managed with biliary stents. When obstruction to bile flow distal to a leak exists owing to retained calculus or stricture, concurrent endoscopic stone extraction and/or stricture dilation is also needed. Some have suggested that concurrent dilation of a stricture with the placement of a stent is rarely indicated because many strictures are inflammatory or due to adjacent biloma formation (111). When large or symptomatic bilomas exist, percutaneous drainage should be obtained.

Fouch et al. (121), treated 23 of 23 patients with postoperative biliary leaks successfully with endoscopic placement of biliary stents plus percutaneous biloma drainage in a subset. Liguory et al. (122) treated 52 patients with postoperative fistulas, using sphincterotomy alone in 37, stent placement in eight, and percutaneous drainage in seven. Fistula closure was achieved in 40 of 52 (77%) patients. Twenty-four of these patients had retained calculi and were treated with sphincterotomy alone, resulting in closure of the fistula in 21 patients. In a series containing 14 patients with persistent postoperative fistula (>2 months) without distal obstruction Feretis et al. (123) achieved 100% closure with a combination of endoscopic therapy including sphincterotomy, nasobiliary drainage, and/or stent placement. Ponchon et al. (124) used sphincterotomy, stenting, or a combination to treat 24 patients with either postoperative or spontaneous fistula, achieving rapid closure in two-thirds of these patients. Failure cases were associated with large leaks and/or intrahepatic locations. Branum et al. (125) reviewed 50 cases of postlaparoscopic biliary injury, focusing on type of injury and management. Twelve of these patients had biliary leaks that were initially treated with sphincterotomy or endoprosthesis, with 10 (83%) resolving within 10 days. In another recent report, Kozarek et al. (126) reported on endoscopic management of biliary injuries incurred with laparoscopic cholecystectomy. Twenty-nine patients had bile leakage and/or stricture (five cystic duct leak, eight fistula, nine leak and stricture, seven stricture) and were managed with a combination of sphincterotomy, endoprosthesis, and percutaneous biloma drainage. Nineteen of 22 (86%) patients had resolution of bile leakage. In the largest series to date, Davids et al. (127) treated 54 patients with biliary leaks. Five of these patients had complete transections (classic injury) resulting in surgical referral, whereas successful endoscopic drainage was possible in 48 of the 49 remaining patients with resultant fistula closure in 43 (90%) patients.

Most reported series have demonstrated that sphincerotomy alone will result in prompt resolution of simple cystic duct stump leaks, but some endoscopists rather prefer the transient placement of an endoprosthesis, thus retaining long-term sphicteric function. In contrast, a recent report by Libby et al. (128) described three patients that developed postoperative bile leakage from the cystic duct stump, despite having undergone sphincterotomy prior to surgery. All three of these patients' leaks responded to biliary stenting.

Biliary leakage that occurs early on following OLT is most often handled surgically or by interventional radiology owing to the high risk for infection in these patients and the often associated hepatic artery occlusion. Leaks that occur later, for instance, at the time of elective T-tube removal, can often be managed endoscopically. O'Conner et al. (129) reported on successful endoscopic management of such leaks in 12 of 13 (92%) patients.

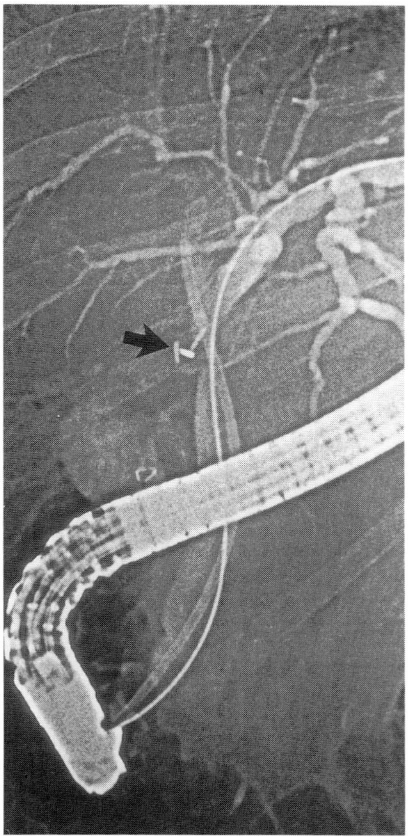

Figure 16. Surgical bile duct injury. This patient presented with jaundice 5 days after laparascopic cholecystectomy. A surgical clip (arrow) is often noted at the stricture site.

Endoscopic Management of Postoperative Biliary Strictures

Endoscopic techniques utilized in successful management of postoperative strictures are similar to those used involving most other types of strictures (see malignant strictures). Diagnostic ERC is critical in defining the possible presence of leaks or retained calculi, the length of the stricture and the possible presence and location of surgical clips (Fig. 16). Surgical clips near the stricture site often indicate a poorer response to endoscopic therapy. Endoscopic sphincterotomy is often helpful because these patients often require repeat procedures involving multiple cannulations.

One distinct difference in management when compared with malignant strictures is the degree of need for stent placement following dilation. If an ERCP is being performed for an elevated alkaline phosphatase or mild cholestasis, hydrostatic balloon dilation (Fig. 17) may suffice if balloon waist ablation is achieved and the follow-up cholangiogram shows no persistent stricture. Otherwise, if the patient presents with jaundice, proximal calculi, or cholangitis or following dilation has a persistent stricture, then one or two large-caliber (at least 10-French) stents should be inserted. Owing to inevitable stent occlusion resulting from bacterial biofilm, it

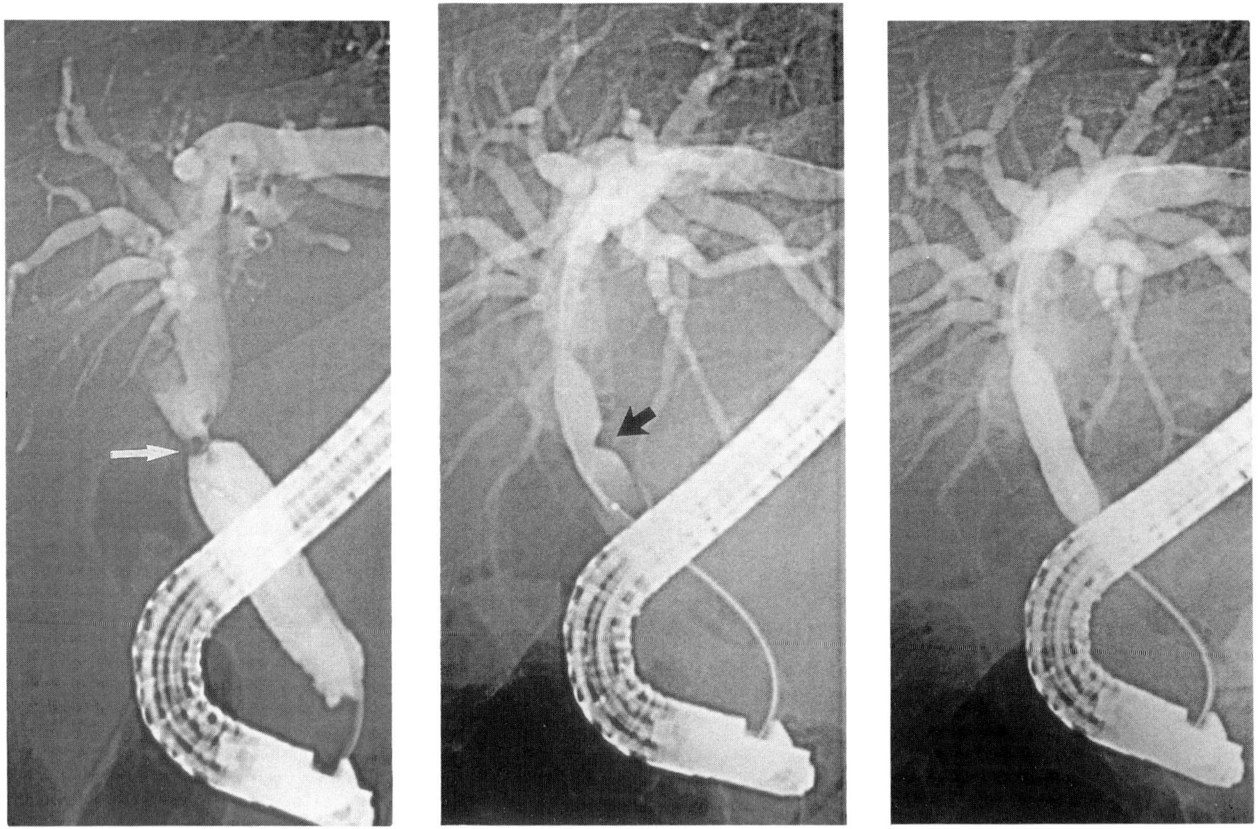

(A) (B) (C)

Figure 17. Hydrostatic balloon dilation of a benign biliary stricture. (A) Cholangiogram demonstrates a Bismuth Type I stricture (arrow). (B) An 8-mm hydrostatic balloon is positioned over a guide wire. The balloon waist (arrow) is noted at the tightest point of the stricture. (C) Nearly complete waist ablation has been achieved.

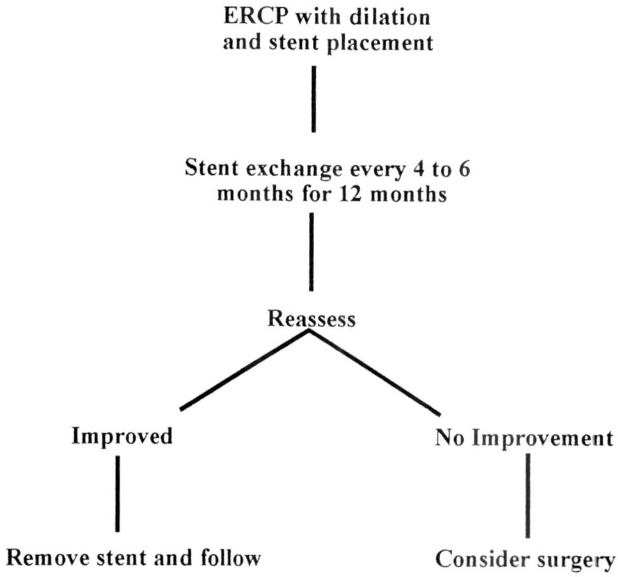

Figure 18. Approach to the management of patients with postoperative strictures.

is generally recommended that routine stent exchange (and repeat balloon dilation) be performed every 3 to 4 months for up to 1 year or more (Fig. 18). Final stent removal depends on the cholangiographic appearance at the time of follow-up exams. Strictures that persist for greater than 1 year despite aggressive endoscopic therapy may require surgical repair. Routine interval monitoring of liver-associated enzymes, symptoms, and when indicated, ultrasound imaging are all necessary following final stent removal because recurrent stenosis has been noted up to 7 years later (130).

Several large series have now documented the efficacy of endoscopic management of postoperative (both cholecystectomy and OLT) biliary strictures (Table 6) (126, 131–133). Geenen et al. (131) attempted endoscopic therapy in 25 patients with benign biliary strictures, of which 18 were postoperative. Twenty-three underwent balloon dilation followed by stent insertion in 18 with periodic exchange for up to 2 years. Eighteen of the 23 patients had good results based on clinical symptoms, liver enzyme levels, proximal biliary duct diameter, and biliary drainage times with a mean follow-up time (after stent removal) of 4 ± 0.3 years. Berkelhammer et al. (132) attempted stent placement (20% required initial balloon dilation) in 29 patients with postoperative biliary strictures (five with concomitant fistula). Stent insertion was successful in 25 (86%) with a mean stenting duration of 162 days (range of 24 to 780 days). At a mean follow-up of 19 months 74% of patients had a good-to-excellent clinical result. Notably, patients that presented within 3 months of their surgical injury had a more favorable response to therapy. This finding has not been demonstrated in any other reports. An extended follow-up report (134) shows no redevelopment of symptoms at 6.5 years. In the series by Kozarek et al. (126), 16 of 29 patients with postoperative bile duct injury had strictures that were

Table 6. Endoscopic management of postoperative biliary strictures[a]

Study	Number of Patients	Associated Biliary Leak	Technical Success (%)	Treatment Method	Mean Period of Stenting (months)	Long-term Resolution (%)	Mean Follow-up Period (months)[d]
Geenen et al. (131)[b]	25 (9)[c]	NA	92	BD, 23 S, 18	17 ± 5	78	48 ± 4
Berkelhammer et al. (132)	29 (5)	5 (17%)	86	BD, 6 S, 29	5 (R-1–26)	74	19 (R-2–42)
Kozarek et al. (126)	16 (NA)	9 (56%)	100	BD, 0 S, 16	≤12	81	≥12
Davids et al. (133)	70 (27)	20 (29%)	94	BD, 15 S, 66	12 (R-3–24)	83	42 (R-4–99)

[a] NA, data not available; BD, balloon dilation; S, stent; R, range.
[b] All benign strictures but only 18 were postoperative.
[c] Number in parentheses represents patients that had previously attempted surgical repair of bile duct injury.
[d] Follow-up period after stent removal.

managed with stent insertion (no balloon dilation). Thirteen of 16 (81%) were free of biliary symptoms, ductal dilatation, and abnormal liver enzymes at a minimum follow-up of 1 year. In the largest series reported to date, Davids et al. (133) successfully placed two 10-French stents in 66 of 70 patients with postoperative strictures. Of the 46 patients available for long-term follow-up (mean of 42 months), 83% were asymptomatic without stents and had normal liver enzymes and 17% redeveloped strictures.

Strictures occurring after OLT have also been successfully treated with endoscopic management. O'Connor et al. (129) reported successful endoscopic management utilizing sphincterotomy, balloon dilation, and stent placement, in 9 of 14 patients with biliary strictures. Likewise, Bourgeois et al. (135) successfully treated 10 of 11 patients with post-OLT biliary stricture using bougie dilation and stent placement. Patients presenting with strictures within 3 months of transplant responded to short-term (3 months) stenting whereas those presenting later required prolonged stenting and periodic exchange.

Many operative bile duct injuries are amenable to endoscopic therapy. Injuries involving multiple ducts, large leaks, short tight strictures due to clip misplacement, or long strictures due to ischemic injury are less likely to respond to nonoperative management. In these situations, ERCP provides valuable diagnostic information and often converts an urgent surgical intervention into an elective and controlled one (111).

CHOLANGIOPATHIES

Sclerosing cholangitis refers to bile duct fibrosis or sclerosis that may be idiopathic or caused by infective, inflammatory, ischemic, or direct chemical or toxic processes. It is considered secondary when caused by AIDS, stones, postoperative, or toxic agents.

Primary Sclerosing Cholangitis

Primary sclerosing cholangitis (PSC) is a nonbacterial inflammatory disease of unknown etiology that is characterized by chronic inflammatory fibrosis of either or

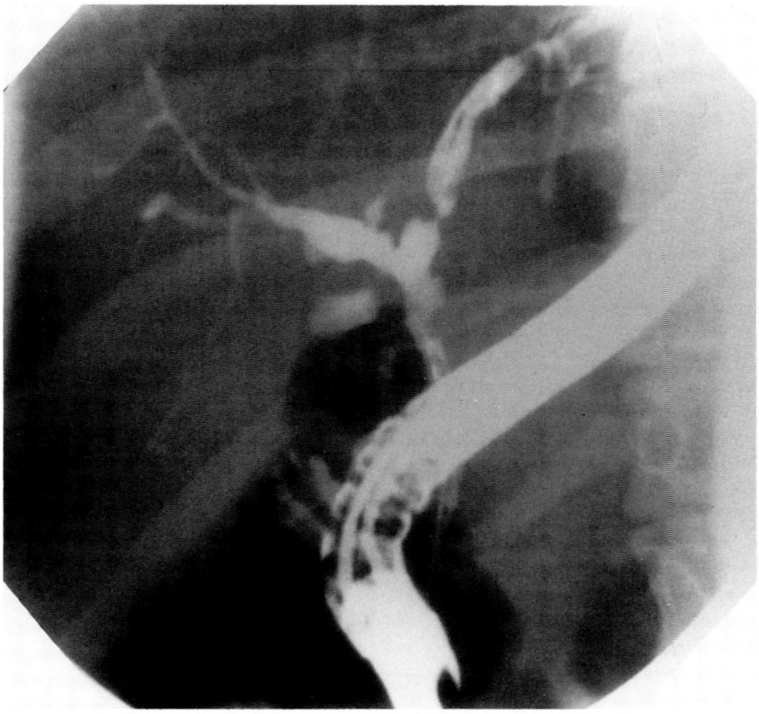

Figure 19. Primary sclerosing cholangitis. Cholangiogram demonstrating typical features of PSC: short band-like strictures, ductal ectasia, and diminished arborization.

both the intrahepatic and extrahepatic biliary duct systems (136). Primary sclerosing cholangitis is associated with many disorders, of which ulcerative colitis is by far the most common (50–75% of cases) (137). The male to female ratio is 2:1, and two-third of the patients are younger than 45 years of age (136). The diagnosis is established by a combination of clinical, biochemical, histological, and most of all radiological criteria. Patients typically present with progressive fatigue, cholestasis, and finally jaundice (136, 137). Alkaline phosphatase concentrations are elevated in 95–98% of cases (138, 139). Clinical criteria should exclude conditions known to cause sclerosing cholangitis.

Cholangiography is considered the "gold standard" for diagnosis (136, 138, 140). Endoscopic retrograde cholangiopancreatography provides detailed anatomic information that may have an impact on both immediate therapy and long-term prognosis (141). Primary sclerosing cholangitis almost always involves the intrahepatic ducts and in the majority of cases, also the extrahepatic ducts (139, 140, 142, 143). Cholangiographic features include short band-like strictures, ductal ectasia, diminished arborization or pruning, and mural irregularities that may be shaggy or nodular (Fig. 19). Occasionally there may be diverticula or sacculations, long strictures, and even major duct obliteration (142). The gallbladder, cystic duct, and pancreatic duct are involved in a minority of patients (142). Cholangiographic images typically remain stable for years; the process is slowly progressive. Chen and Goldberg

(143) classified cholangiographic findings of PSC based on distribution and severity of involvement.

Differentiating cholangiocarcinoma from PSC can be very difficult because 10% of bile duct carcinomas present are diffuse and sclerosing, mimicking PSC (142). Likewise, the incidence of cholangiocarcinoma is 7–15% in patients with PSC (136, 144). Cholangiocarcinoma complicating PSC should be considered when there is rapid clinical deterioration with jaundice, weight loss, and abdominal discomfort (145). Cholangiographic findings suggestive of malignant degeneration include intraductal polypoid masses greater than 1 cm, marked ductal dilatation, or rapidly progressive stricture formation or proximal dilatation (145, 146).

Complications of PSC aside from cholangiocarcinoma include cholestasis resulting in pruritus and fat-soluble vitamin deficiencies, cholangitis, dominant strictures, and duct stone formation (137). Endoscopic retrograde cholangiopancreatography should be performed to rule out dominant strictures and/or choledocholithiasis whenever there is rapid worsening of symptoms or the hepatic biochemical profile. Although choledocholithiasis can result in secondary PSC it may also occur as a complication of PSC (140). Endoscopic stone extraction utilizing balloon dilation and sphincterotomy when indicated is highly successful (140). Dominant strictures may be dilated with balloons or dilating catheters. When dilation is insufficient, endoscopic placement of stents may be successful. Several case series of PSC managed endoscopically have now been reported (147–150) (Table 7). In summary, endoscopic therapy is often an effective means of palliation for symptomatic dominant strictures in PSC, but liver transplantation is the treatment of choice in patients with progressive deterioration of liver function.

Secondary Sclerosing Cholangitis

Long-standing biliary obstruction with resultant chronic or recurrent cholangitis and direct toxic injury can lead to ductal fibrosis and stricturing and eventual secondary sclerosing cholangitis. Cholangiographic findings like those of PSC have been reported in metastatic cancer, lymphoma, polycystic liver, cirrhosis, previous

Table 7. Endoscopic management of symptomatic primary sclerosing cholangitis[a]

Study	Number of Patients	Technical Success (%)	Treatment Method	Clinical Improvement	Mean Follow-up Period (months)
Craig et al. (147)	23	83	D, 3 D and S, 16	8 (6)[b]/14	26 (R-2–58)
Lombard et al. (148)	6	100	D and S, 6	5 (4)/6	25 (R-12–49)
Johnson et al. (149)	35	100	D, 24 D and S, 11	Yes[c]	24

[a] D, dilation; S, stent; R, range.
[b] Number in parentheses represents patients that have had their stents removed.
[c] Average number of hospitalizations decreased from 2.3/year to 0.4/year. There was also a significant fall in bilirubin and improved radiographic scores.

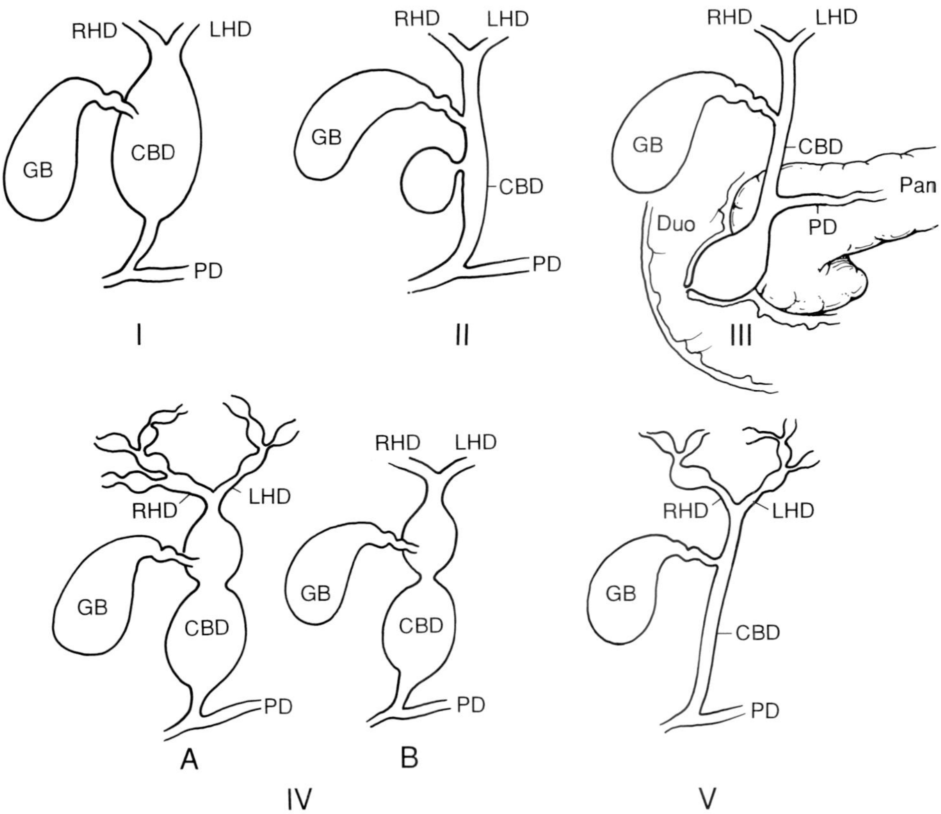

Figure 20. Classification of choledochal cysts. Type I: fusiform or cystic dilatation of the extrahepatic biliary tree. In some instances the hepatic duct proximal to the cyst is normal. Type II: a diverticular outpouching of the CBD that looks like a gallbladder. Type III (choledochocele): a small saccular dilatation of the distal CBD that typically protrudes into the duodenal lumen adjacent to the ampulla. Type IVA: multiple cystic dilations of both the intrahepatic and extrahepatic biliary tree. Type IVB: multiple cystic dilatations of the extrahepatic biliary tree. Type V: multiple cysts involving only the intrahepatic biliary tree (Caroli's disease).

biliary tract surgery, choledocholithiasis, AIDS, drug-related conditions, and histiocytosis (151). Despite similarities, certain conditions have typical cholangiographic patterns.

Hepatic Artery Infusion Cholangiopathy

Direct infusion of fluorodeoxyuridine (FUDR) into the hepatic artery results in a sclerosing pattern of bile duct injury in 7% of patients (152). Direct toxic injury or ischemia have been proposed as the pathological mechanisms leading to fibrosis and stricture (152–154). The cholangiographic appearance of FUDR-induced cholangiopathy is difficult to differentiate from PSC (152). Strictures localized to the right–left hepatic duct confluence, an increase in cystic duct and gallbladder lesions,

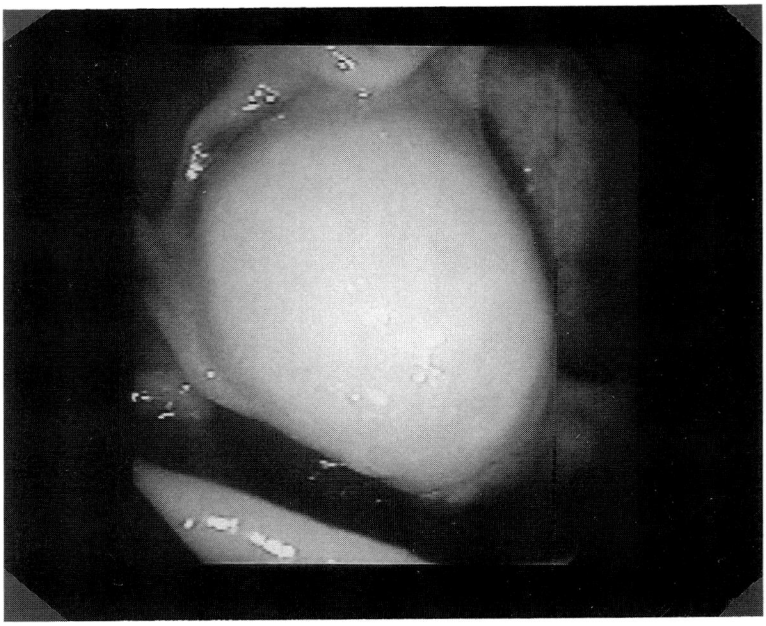

Figure 21. Type III choledochal cyst (choledochocele). Endoscopic view showing a prominent periampullary protrusion by the CBD.

and decreased involvement of intrahepatic ducts and distal common bile duct have been reported more frequently with hepatic artery infusion cholangiopathy (155).

Another iatrogenic cause for secondary sclerosing cholangitis is the injection of scolicidal solution (2% formaldehyde, 20% sodium chloride or alcohol) for the treatment of hydatid disease (156). The part of the biliary tree with direct contact to the therapy is affected owing to toxic injury of the bile duct epithelium.

AIDS-Related Cholangiopathy

AIDS-related cholangiopathy is defined by a combination of right upper quadrant abdominal pain, elevation of the serum alkaline phosphatase level, and morphological anomalies in the biliary tract (157). The serum bilirubin is usually normal or slightly elevated (158). Infection with *Cryptosporidium,* cytomegalovirus, and Microsporida have been frequently associated with biliary disease but a direct cause-and-effect relationship has been difficult to prove owing to the common frequency with which these organisms are found with advanced AIDS, regardless of biliary disease, and their lack of clinical response to medical therapy (157). Ultrasound demonstrates dilated intrahepatic or extrahepatic ducts (158). AIDS patients with pain and dilated ducts should undergo ERCP for diagnostic and therapeutic indications.

Cello (158) reviewed 40 cases of AIDS-related cholangiopathy and described four different patterns of cholangiopathy: papillary stenosis, sclerosing cholangitis, combined papillary stenosis with intrahepatic and extrahepatic sclerosing cholangitis, and long, extrahepatic bile duct strictures (>1–2 cm). A "beaded" appearance

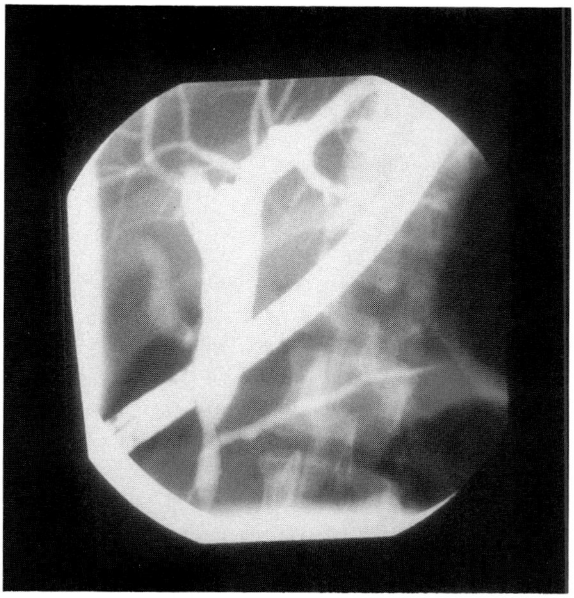

(A)

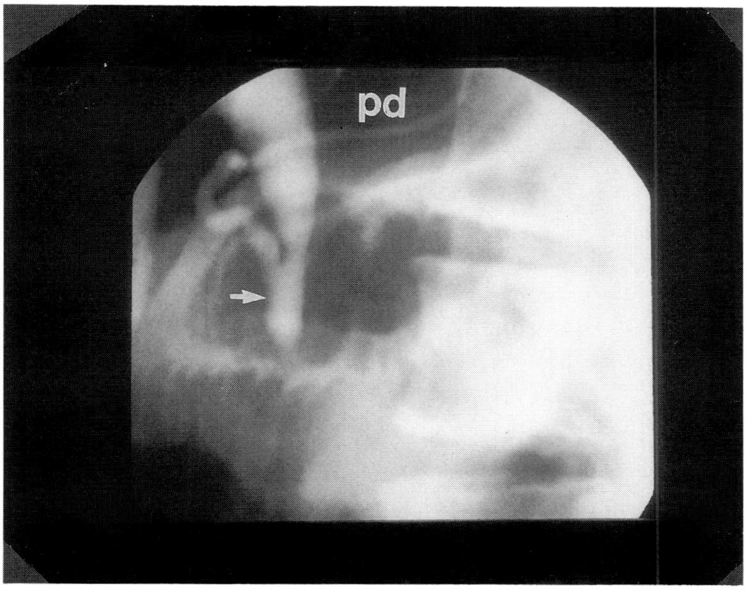

(B)

Figure 22. Type I choledochal cyst. (A) Cholangiogram showing cystic dilatation of the extrahepatic biliary tree. (B) cholangiogram demonstrating an anomalous pancreatobiliary junction with a long common channel (arrow).

suggesting intramural submucosal infiltration and edema helps to differentiate it from PSC. Patients with papillary stenosis and pain have been shown to respond (86–100%) to ES (158, 159). Survival is not affected by endoscopic intervention but ES is often helpful with pain management. In the setting of AIDS, other potential causes of biliary obstruction should be entertained including lymphoma, Kaposi's sarcoma, and even choledocholithiasis.

Recurrent Pyogenic Cholangitis

Recurrent pyogenic cholangitis is commonly referred to as Oriental cholangiohepatitis owing to its prevalence in Southeast Asian populations. This syndrome includes chronic or recurrent cholangitis, choledocholithiasis (pigment stones), and frequent association with biliary parasites including *Ascaris, Clonorchis,* and other liver flukes (160). Chronic inflammation results in stricture, fistula, abscess, and cirrhosis. This condition may predispose to cholangiocarcinoma (161).

Endoscopic retrograde cholangiopancreatography is required to confirm the diagnosis and will provide potential for therapeutic intervention. Marked dilatation of extrahepatic ducts, beyond that seen with other types of chronic cholangitis, is typical (2). Stones, sludge, and inflammatory debris may be seen throughout the biliary tree. Significant biliary strictures are found in 35% of patients (162). Hilar strictures involving the left hepatic duct are found most frequently (163).

Chronic disease may lead to cirrhosis with severe attenuation of the intrahepatic ducts. Surgical therapy has been the traditional approach, but ERCP with ES, stone extraction, and the placement of biliary stents, when appropriate to ensure drainage, may be effective (164, 165). Regression of cholangiographic findings has been noted when the above is achieved in conjunction with appropriate treatment of infection (166).

CHOLEDOCHAL CYSTS

Biliary cysts can involve any part of the biliary tree (167) and are classified into five types (Fig. 20). Ultrasound and CT are helpful in evaluating patients with suspected biliary cysts. However, cholangiography provides better detail of biliary anatomy. In Type III (choledochocele) patients ERCP demonstrates a periampullary protrusion (Fig. 21). The cholangiogram demonstrates protrusion of the distal CBD into the duodenal lumen. In Type I patients ERCP shows cystic dilatation of the extrahepatic biliary tree (Fig. 22A) and may demonstrate an anomalous pancreatobiliary junction with a long common channel (Fig. 22B). In expert hands ERCP is preferable to percutaneous cholangiography because it can provide temporary management with stent placement for patients with cholangitis or more permanent management with sphincterotomy in patients with choledochocele. In some patients both a percutaneous and a retrograde approach may be needed to define the biliary tree further prior to surgical intervention.

REFERENCES

1. Kawai K, Akasaka Y, Murakami K, et al. Endoscopic sphincterotomy of the ampulla of Vater. *Gastrointest Endosc.* 1974;20:148–151.

2. Lim JH. Oriental cholangiohepatitis: pathologic, clinical, and radiologic features. *AJR.* 1991;157:1–8.
3. Kennedy RH, Thompson MH. Are duodenal diverticula associated with choledocholithiasis. *Gut.* 1988;29:1003–1006.
4. Homans J. Gall-stones formed around silk sutures, twenty months after recovery from cholecystotomy. *Ann Surg.* 1987;26:114–116.
5. Martinez J, Combs W, Brady PG. Surgical clips as a nidus for biliary stone formation: diagnosis and therapy. *Am J Gastroenterol.* 1995;90:1521–1524.
6. GenVesten L, Berci G. The current status of biliary tract surgery: an international study of 1,072 consecutive patients. *World J Surg.* 1986;10:116–122.
7. Morgenstern L, Wong L, Berci G. Twelve hundred open cholecystectomies before the laparoscopic era: a standard for comparison. *Arch Surg.* 1992;127:400–403.
8. McSherry CK. Open cholecystectomy. *Am J Surg.* 1993;165:435–439.
9. Erickson RA, Carlson B. The role of endoscopic retrograde cholangiopancreatography in patients with laparoscopic cholecystectomies. *Gastroenterology.* 1995;109:252–263.
10. Hawasli A, Lloyd L, Pozios V, et al. The role of endoscopic retrograde cholangiopancreaticogram in laparoscopic cholecystectomy. *Am Surg.* 1993;59:285–288.
11. Rieger R, Wolfgang W. Yield of prospective, noninvasive evaluation of the common bile duct combined with selective ERCP/sphincterotomy in 1390 consecutive laparoscopic cholecystectomy patients. *Gastrointeset Endosc.* 1995;42:6–12.
12. Elfant AB, Bourke MJ, Alhalel R, et al. Success and complications of 294 ERCP's in Billroth-II patients: a 5-year review [abstract]. *Gastrointest Endosc.* 1995;41:A395.
13. Osnes M, Rosseland AR, Aabakken L. Endoscopic retrograde cholangiography and endoscopic papillotomy in patients with a previous Billroth II resection. *Gut.* 1986;27:1193–1198.
14. Huibregste K, Katon RM, Tytgat GNJ. Precut papillotomy via the needle knife papillotome: A safe and effective technique. *Gastrointest Endosc.* 1986;32:403–405.
15. Dowsett JF, Polydorou AA, Vaira D, et al. Needle knife papillotomy: how safe and how effective? *Gut.* 1990;31:905.
16. Foutch PG. A prospective assessment of results for needle knife papillotomy and standard endoscopic sphincterotomy. *Gastrointest Endosc.* 1995;41:25–32.
17. Brodisch RJ, Fink AS. ERCP, cholangiography and laparoscopic cholecystectomy. Soc of Am Gastrointest Endoscoping Surgeons (SAGES) opinion survey. *Surg Endosc.* 1993;7:3–8.
18. Cotton PB, Chung SC, Davis WZ, et al. Issues in cholecystectomy and management of duct stones. *Am J Gastrointerol.* 1994;89:S169–176.
19. Abboud PC, Malet PF, Berlin JA, et al. Predicting common bile duct stones before cholecytectomy: a meta-analysis [abstract]. *Gastroenterology.* 1995;108:A403.
20. Hauer-Jensen M, Garesen R, Nygaard K, et al. Prospective randomized study of routine intraoperative cholangiography during open cholecystectomy: long-term follow-up and multivariant analysis of predictors of choledocholithiasis. *Surgery.* 1993;113:318–323.
21. Neoptplemos JP, London NJ, Carr-Locke DL. Controlled trial of urgent endoscopic retrograde sphincterotomy versus conservative treatment for acute pancreatitis due to cholelithiasis. *Lancet.* 1988;2:979–983.
22. Fan ST, Lai ECS, Mok FPT, et al. Early treatment of acute biliary pancreatitis by endoscopic papillotomy, *New Engl J Med.* 1993;328:228–232.
23. Miller RE, Kimmelstiel FM, Winkler WP. Management of common bile duct stones in the era of laparoscopic cholecystectomy. *Am J Surg.* 1995;169:273–276.

24. Cisek PL, Greaney GC. The role of endoscopic retrograde cholangiopancreatography with laparoscopic cholecystectomy in the management of choledocholithiasis. *Am Surg* 1994;60:772–776.

25. Saltzstein EC, Peacock JB, Thomas MD. Preoperative bilirubin, alkaline phosphatase, and amylase levels as predictors of common duct stones. *Surg Gynecol Obstet.* 1982;154:381–384.

26. Reiss R, Deutsch AA, Nudelman I, et al. Statistical value of various clinical parameters in predicting the presence of choledochal stones. *Surg Gynecol Obstet.* 1984;159:273–276.

27. Stave R, Osnes M. Endoscopic gallstone extraction following hydrostatic balloon dilation of a stricture in the common bile duct. *Endoscopy.* 1985;17:159–160.

28. May GR, Cotton PB, Edmunds SEJ, Chong W. Removal of stones from the bile duct at ERCP without sphincterotomy. *Gastrointest Endosc.* 1993;39:749–954.

29. MacMathuna P, White P, Clarke E, et al. Endoscopic sphincteroplasty: a novel and safe alternative to papillotomy in the management of bile duct stones. *Gut.* 1994;35:127–129.

30. Bergman JJGHM, Rauws EAJ, Tytgat GNJ, Huibregts K. A prospective randomized trial comparing endoscopic sphincterotomy (EST) with endoscopic balloon dilation (EBD) for removal of common bile duct stones (CBDS); initial report [abstract]. *Gastrointest Endosc.* 1994;40:99.

31. Hawes RH, Sherman S. Choledocholithiasis. In: Bockus, ed. *Gastroenterology,* 5th ed. Philadelphia: Saunders, 1995.

32. Chen YK, Foliente RL, Santoro MJ, et al. Endoscopic sphincterotomy-induced pancreatitis: Increased risk associated with nondilated bile ducts and sphincter of oddi dysfunction. *Am J Gastroenterol.* 1994;89:327–333.

33. Binnie NR, Nixon SJ, Palmer KR. Mirizzi syndrome managed by endoscopic stenting and laparoscopic cholecystectomy. *Br J Surg.* 1992;79:647.

34. Binmoeller KF, Thonke F, Soehendra N. Endoscopic treatment of Mirizzi's syndrome. *Gastrointest Endosc.* 1993;39:532–536.

35. Leese T, Neoptolemos JP, Baker AR, et al. The management of acute cholangitis and the impact of endoscopic sphincterotomy. *Br J Surg.* 1986;73:988–992.

36. Leung JWC, Song JJY, Chung SCS, et al. Urgent endoscopic drainage in acute suppurative cholangitis. *Lancet.* 1989;1:1307–1309.

37. Lai ECS, Mok FPT, Tan ESY, et al. Endoscopic biliary drainage for severe acute cholangitis. *N Engl J Med.* 1992;326:1582–1586.

38. Jamidar PA, Beck GJ, Hoffman BJ, et al. Endoscopic retrograde cholangiopancreatography in pregnancy. *Am J Gastroenterol.* 1995;90:1263–1267.

39. Baillie J, Cairns SR, Putnam WS, et al. Endoscopic management of choledocholithiasis during pregnancy. *Surg Gynecol Obstet.* 1990;171:1–4.

40. Axelrad AM, Fleischer DE, Strack LL, et al. Performance of ERCP for symptomatic choledocholithiasis during pregnancy: techniques to increase safety and improve patient management. *Am J Gastroenterol.* 1994;89:109–112.

41. Sherman S, Hawes R, Lehman JG. Management of bile duct stones. *Semin Liver Dis.* 1990;10:205–221.

42. Foutch PG. A prospective assessment of results for needle-knife papillotomy and standard endoscopic sphincterotomy. *Gastrointest Endosc.* 1995;41:25–32.

43. Lauri A, Horton RC, Davidson BR, et al. Endoscopic extraction of bile duct stones: management related to stone size. *Gut.* 1993;34:1718–1721.

44. Siegel JH, Ben-Zvi JS, Pullano WE. Endoscopic electrohydraulic lithotripsy. *Gastrointest Endosc.* 1990;36:134–136.

45. Cotton PB, Kozarek RA, Schapiro RH, et al. Endoscopic laser lithotripsy of large bile duct stones. *Gastroenterology* 1990;22:1128–1133.
46. Palmer KR, Hoffman AF. Intraductal mono-octanoin for the direct dissolution of bile duct stones: experiences in 343 patients. *Gut.* 1986;27:196–202.
47. Neoptolemos JP, Hall C, O'Connor HJ, et al. Methyl-tert-butyl ether for treating bile duct stones: the British experience. *Br J Surg.* 1990;77:32–35.
48. Bergman JJGHM, Rauws EAJ, Tijssen JGP, Tytgat GNJ, Huibregtse K. Biliary endoprostheses in elderly patients with endoscopically irretrievable common bile duct stones: report of 117 patients. *Gastrointest Endosc.* 1995;42:195–201.
49. Navicharern P, Rhodes M, Flook D, Lawrie B. Endoscopic retrograde cholangiopancreatography (ERCP) and stent placement in the management of large common bile duct stones. *Austral N Z J Surg.* 1994;64:840–842.
50. Bar-Meir S, Halpern H, Bardan E, et al. Frequency of papillary dysfunction among cholecystectomized patients. *Hepatology.* 1984;4:328–330.
51. Dodds WJ. Biliary tract motility and its relationship to clinical disorders. *AJR.* 1990;155:247–258.
52. Geenen JE, Hogan WJ, Dodds WJ, et al. The efficacy of endoscopic sphincterotomy after cholecystectomy in patients with sphincter-of-Oddi dysfunction. *N Engl J Med.* 1989;320:82–87.
53. Rolny P, Geenen JE, Hogan WJ. Postcholecystectomy patients with "objective signs" of partial bile outflow obstruction: clinical characteristics, sphincter of Oddi manometry findings, and results of therapy. *Gastrointest Endosc.* 1993;39:778–781.
54. Botoman VA, Kozarek RA, Novell LA, et al. Long-term outcome after endoscopic sphincterotomy in patients with biliary colic and suspected sphincter of Oddi dysfunction. *Gastrointest Endosc.* 1994;40:165–170.
55. Ansel HJ. Malignant conditions of the bile ducts. In: Silvis SE, Rohrmann CA Jr, Ansel HJ, eds. *Text and Atlas of Endoscopic Retrograde Cholangiopancreatography.* New York: AGAKU-SHOIN; 1995:245–272.
56. Plumley TF, Rohrmann CA, Freeny PC, et al. Double duct sign: reassessed significance in ERCP. *AJR.* 1982;138:31–35.
57. Foutch PG, Kerr DM, Harlan JR, Kummet TD. A prospective controlled analysis of endoscopic cytotechniques for diagnosis of malignant biliary strictures. *Am J Gastroenterol.* 1991;86:577–580.
58. Monhandas KM, Swaroop S, Gullar SU, et al. Diagnosis of malignant obstructive jaundice by bile cytology: results improved by dilating the bile duct strictures. *Gastrointest Endosc.* 1994;40:150–154.
59. Pescatore P, Heubner C, Heine M, Manegold BC. The value of histological analysis of occluded biliary endoprosthesis. *Endoscopy.* 1995;27:597–600.
60. Foutch PG, Ker DM, Harlan JR, Kummet TD. A prospective, controlled analysis of endoscopic cytotechniques for diagnosis of malignant biliary strictures. *Am J Gastroenterol.* 1991;86:577–580.
61. Foutch PG. Diagnosis of cancer by cytologic methods performed during ERCP. *Gastrointest Endosc.* 1994;40:249–252.
62. Pugliese V, Conio M, Nicolo G, et al. Endoscopic retrograde forceps biopsy and brush cytology of biliary strictures: a prospective study. *Gastrointest Endosc.* 1995;42:520–526.
63. Ponchon T, Gagnon P, Berger F, et al. Value of endobiliary brush cytology and biopsies for the diagnosis of malignant bile duct stenosis: results of a prospective study. *Gastrointeste Endosc.* 1995;42:565–572.

64. Lee JG, Leung JW, Baillie J, et al. Benign, dysplastic, or malignant—making sense of endoscopic bile duct brush cytology: results in 149 consecutive patients. *Am J Gastroenterol.* 1995;90:722–726.

65. Sugiyama M, Atomi Y, Wada N, et al. Endoscopic transpapillary bile duct biopsy without sphincterotomy for diagnosing biliary strictures: a prospective comparative study with bile and brush cytology. *Am J Gastroenterol.* 1996;91:465–467.

66. Cunningham JT, Tarnasky PR, Hawes RH, et al. Biliary stricture sampling by three methods: a prospective comparison [abstract]. *Gastrointest Endosc.* 1995;41:394.

67. Sherman JS, Esber EJ, Pezzi JS, et al. Yield of ERCP tissue sampling of biliary strictures by brush, forceps and needle aspiration methods [abstract]. *Gastrointest Endosc.* 1995;41:415.

68. Foutch GP. Diagnosis of cancer by cytologic methods performed during ERCP. *Gastrointest Endosc.* 1994;40:249–252.

69. Howell DA, Beveridge RP, Bosco, Jones M. Endoscopic needle aspiration in the diagnosis of biliary strictures. *Gastrointest Endosc.* 1992;38:531–535.

70. Ponchon T, Chavaillon A, Ayela P, Lambert R. Retrograde biliary ultrathin endoscopy enhances biopsy of stenoses and lithotripsy. *Gastrointest Endosc.* 1989;35:292–297.

71. Soehendra N, Reynders-Frederix V. Palliative Gallengangdrainage. *Dtsch Med Wochenschr.* 1979;104:206–209.

72. Speer AG, Cotton PB, Russel RCG, et al. Randomized trial of endoscopic versus percutaneous stent insertion in malignant obstructive jaundice. *Lancet.* 1987;2:57–62.

73. Shephard HA, Royle G, Ross APR, et al. Endoscopic biliary endoprosthesis in the palliation of malignant obstruction of the distal common bile duct: A randomized trial. *Br J Surg.* 1988;75:1166–1168.

74. Andersen JR, Sorensen SM, Kruse A, et al. Randomized trial of endoscopic endoprosthesis versus operative bypass in malignant obstructive jaundice. *Gut.* 1989;30:1132–1135.

75. Smith AC, Dowsett JF, Russell RCG, et al. Randomised trial of endoscopic stenting versus surgical bypass in malignant low bile duct obstruction. *Lancet.* 1994;344:1655–1660.

76. Ballinger AB, McHugh M, Catnach SM, et al. Symptom relief and quality of life after stenting for malignant bile duct obstruction. *Gut.* 1994;35:467–470.

77. Sherman S, Lehman G, Earle D, et al. Endoscopic palliation of malignant bile duct obstruction: improvement in quality of life [abstract]. *Gastrointest Endosc.* 1995;41:414.

78. Nagger E, Krag E, Matzen P. Endoscopically inserted biliary endoprosthesis in malignant obstructive jaundice: A survey of the literature. *Liver.* 1990;10:321–324.

79. Dowsett JF, Vaira D, Hatfield ARW, et al. Endoscopic biliary therapy using the combined percutaneous and endoscopic technique. *Gastroenterology.* 1989;96:1180–1186.

80. Boender J, Nix GAJJ, Schutte HE, et al. Malignant common bile duct obstruction: factors influencing the success rate of endoscopic drainage. *Endoscopy* 1990;22:259–262.

81. Cucreux M, Ligoury CL, Lefebvre JF, et al. Management of malignant hilar biliary obstruction by endoscopy: Results and prognostic factors. *Dig Dis Sci.* 1992;37:778–783.

82. Deviere J, Baize M, de Toeuf J, et al. Long-term follow-up of patients with hilar malignant stricture treated by endoscopic internal biliary drainage. *Gastrointest Endosc.* 1988;34:95–101.

83. Polydorou AA, Cairns SR, Dowsett JF, et al. Palliation of proximal malignant biliary obstruction by endoscopic endoprosthesis insertion. *Gut.* 1991;32:685–690.

84. Speer A, Cotton PB, MacRea K. Endoscopic management of malignant biliary obstruc-

tion: Stents of 10 French gauge are preferable to stents of 8 French gauge. *Gastrointest Endosc.* 1988;34:412–417.

85. Neuhaus H, Hagenmuller F, Griebel M, Classen M. Self expanding metal stents versus conventional plastic endoprostheses for malignant biliary obstruction [abstract]. *Gastrointest Endosc.* 1991;37:253.
86. Davids PHP, Groen AK, Rauws EAG, et al. Randomized trial of self-expanding metal stents versus polyethylene stents for distal malignant biliary obstruction. *Lancet.* 1992;340:1488–1492.
87. Carr-Locke DL, Ball TJ, Connors PJ, et al. Multicenter, randomized trial of Wallstent biliary endoprostheses versus plastic stents [abstract]. *Gastrointest Endosc.* 1993;39:310.
88. Knyrim K, Wagner HJ, Pausch J, Vakil. A prospective, randomized, controlled trial of metal stents for malignant obstruction of the common bile duct. *Endoscopy.* 1993;25:207–212.
89. Sherman S, Hawes RH, Lehman GA. Endoscopic biliary and pancreatic drainage procedures. In: Silvis SE, Rohrmann CA Jr, Ansel HJ, eds. *Text and Atlas of Endoscopic Retrograde Cholangiopancreatography.* New York: IGAKU-SHOIN; 1995:413–445.
90. Hoepffner N, Foerster, Eibing D, Domschke W. Prognostic factors for the palliative treatment of malignant biliary obstruction with Wallstents [abstract]. *Gastrointest Endosc.* 1995;42:399.
91. Sung JJY, Chung SCS, Tsui CP, et al. Omitting side-holes in biliary stents does not improve drainage of the obstructed biliary system: a prospective randomized trial. *Gastrointest Endosc.* 1994;40:321–325.
92. Binmoeller KF, Seifert US, Thonke F, et al. The Tannenbaum stent: a new plastic biliary stent without side holes. *Am J Gastroenterol.* 1995;90:1764–1768.
93. Aranha GV, Prinz RA, Freeark RJ, et al. The spectrum of biliary tract obstruction from chronic pancreatitis. *Arch Surg.* 1984;119:595–600.
94. Smith MT, Lehman GA. Endoscopic management of benign biliary strictures. In: Braasch JW, Thompkins RK, eds. *Surgical Disease of the Biliary Tract and Pancreas: Multidisciplinary Management.* St. Louis: CV Mosby; 1994:290–313.
95. Deviere J, Devaere S, Baize M, Cremer M. Endoscopic biliary drainage in chronic pancreatitis. *Gastrointest Endosc.* 1990;36:96–100.
96. Meier PB, Silvis SE, Daigle-Bjerke, Vennes JA. Nonoperative biliary drainage differentiates chronic pancreatitis (CP) from biliary pain in CP patients with benign bile duct strictures [abstract]. *Gastrointest Endosc.* 1991;37:250.
97. Deviere J, Cremer M, Baize M, et al. Management of common bile duct stricture caused by chronic pancreatitis with metal mesh self expandable stents. *Gut.* 1994;35:122–126.
98. Gaskin KJ, Waters DLM, Howman-Giles R, et al. Liver disease and common bile duct stenosis in cystic fibrosis. *N Engl J Med.* 1988;318:340–346.
99. Oren R, Goldin E, Harats N, et al. Localized primary sclerosing cholangitis mimicking a cholecystectomy stricture relieved by an endoprosthesis. *Postgrad Med J.* 1991;67:482–484.
100. Sharara AI, Le TH, Suhocki P, Jowell PS. Extrahepatic biliary obstruction resulting from a pancreatic pseudoaneurysm. *Gastrointest Endosc.* 1995;42:176–177.
101. Bayraktar Y, Balkanci F, Kayhan B, et al. Bile duct varices or "pseudo-cholangiocarcinoma sign" in portal hypertension due to cavernous transformation of the portal vein. *Am J Gastroenterol.* 1992;87:1801–1806.
102. Byrne J, Balasubramanian K, Garberoglio C. A nonparasitic liver cyst presenting as a Klatskin tumor. *Endoscopy.* 1994;26:269.

103. Baggott BB, Long WB. Annular pancreas as a cause of extrahepatic biliary obstruction. *Am J Gastroenterol.* 1991;86:224–226.

104. Kim CH, Farrugia G, Farnell MB. High-grade obstruction of the proximal extrahepatic bile duct: An unusual complication of duodenal ulcer disease. *Am J Gastroenterol.* 1991;86:1826–1828.

105. Farahvash MJ, Bastani B, Farahvash MR, Irvanlou G. Eosinophilic gastroenteritis presenting with biliary and partial duodenal obstruction. *Am J Gastroenterol.* 1990;85:1022–1024.

106. Buse PE, Edmundowicz SA. Proximal common bile duct obstruction secondary to a periampullary duodenal diverticulum: successful treatment with endoscopic stenting. *Gastrointest Endosc.* 1991;37:635–637.

107. Garden OJ. Iatrogenic injury to the bile duct. *Br J Surg.* 1991;78:1412–1413.

108. Deveney KE. The early experience with laparoscopic cholecystectomy in Oregon. *Arch Surg.* 1993;128:627–632.

109. Orlando R, Russell JC, Lynch J, et al. Laparoscopic cholecystectomy: a statewide experience. *Arch Surg.* 1993;128:494–499.

110. Southern Surgeons Club: A prospective analysis of 1518 laparascopic cholecystectomies. *N Engl J Med.* 1991;324:1073–1078.

111. Kozarek RA. Endoscopic techniques in management of biliary tract injuries. *Surg Clin North Am.* 1994;74:883–893.

112. Branum G, Schmitt C, Baillie J, et al. Management of major biliary complications after laparoscopic cholecystectomy. *Ann Surg.* 1993;217:532–541.

113. Davidoff AM, Pappas TN, Murray EA, et al. Mechanisms of major biliary complications after laparoscopic cholecystectomy. *Ann Surg.* 1992;215:196–202.

114. Bismuth H. Postoperative strictures of the biliary tract. In: Blumgart LH, ed. *The Biliary Tract. Clinical Surgery International, v.* Edinburgh: Churchill Livingstone; 1983;209–218.

115. Borgeois N, Deviere J, Yeaton P, et al. Diagnostic and therapeutic endoscopic retrograde cholangiography after liver transplantation. *Gastrointest Endosc.* 1995;42:527–534.

116. Lewis WD, Jenkins RL. Biliary strictures after liver transplantation. *Surg Clin North Am.* 1994;74:967–978.

117. Sheng R, Zajkok B, Campbell WL, AbuElmagd K. Biliary strictures in hepatic transplants: Prevalence and types in patients with primary sclerosing cholangitis vs those with other liver diseases. *AJR.* 1993;161:297–300.

118. Vitale GC, Stephens SG, Wieman TJ, et al. Use of endoscopic retrograde cholangiopancreatography in the management of biliary complications after laparoscopic cholecystectomy. *Surgery.* 1993;114:806–814.

119. Brugge WR, Rosenberg DJ, Alavi A. Diagnosis of postoperative bile leaks. *Am J Gastroenterol.* 1994;89:2178–2183.

120. Howell DA, Bosco JJ, Sampson LN, Bula V. Endoscopic management of cystic duct fistulas after laparoscopic cholecystectomy. *Endoscopy.* 1992;24:796–798.

121. Foutch PG, Harlan JR, Hoefer M. Endoscopic therapy for patients with a post-operative biliary leak. *Gastrointest Endosc.* 1993;39:416–421.

122. Liguory C, Vitale GC, Lefebre JF, et al. Endoscopic treatment of postoperative fistulae. *Surgery.* 1991;110:179–184.

123. Feretis C, Kekis B, Bliouras N, et al. Postoperative external and internal biliary fistulas, unassociated with distal bile duct obstruction: endoscopic treatment. *Endoscopy.* 1990;22:211–213.

124. Ponchon T, Gallez J-F, Coleman J, et al. Endoscopic treatment of biliary tract fistulas. *Gastrointest Endosc.* 1989;35:490–498.

125. Branum G, Schmitt C, Baillie J, et al. Management of major biliary complications after laparoscopic cholecystectomy. *Ann Surg.* 1993;217:532–541.

126. Kozarek RA, Ball TJ, Patterson DJ, et al. Endoscopic treatment of biliary injury in the era of laparoscopic cholecystectomy. *Gastrointest Endosc.* 1994;40:10–16.

127. Davids PHP, Rauws EAJ, Tytgat GNJ, Huibregtse K. Postoperative bile leakage: endoscopic management. *Gut.* 1992;33:1118–1122.

128. Libby ED, Branch MS, Cotton PB. Cystic duct leak after laparoscopic cholecystectomy despite preoperative sphincterotomy. *Gastrointest Endosc.* 1995;41:511–514.

129. O'Conner TP, Lewis D, Jenkins RL. Biliary tract complications after liver transplantation. *Arch Surg.* 1995;130:312–317.

130. Pitt HA, Kaufman SL, Coleman J, et al. Benign postoperative biliary strictures. Operate or dilate. *Ann Surg.* 1989;210:417–427.

131. Geenen DJ, Geenen JE, Hogan WJ, et al. Endoscopic therapy for benign bile duct strictures. *Gastrointest Endosc.* 1989;35:367–371.

132. Berkelhammer C, Kortan P, Haber GB. Endoscopic biliary prostheses as treatment for benign postoperative bile duct strictures. *Gastrointest Endosc.* 1989;35:95–101.

133. Davids PHP, Rauws EAJ, Coene PPLO, et al. Endoscopic stenting for post-operative biliary strictures. *Gastrointest Endosc.* 1992;38:12–18.

134. Walden D, Raijman L, Fuchs E, et al. Long term follow-up of endoscopic stenting (ES) for benign postoperative bile duct strictures (BPBDS) [abstract]. *Gastrointest Endosc.* 1993;39:335.

135. Bourgeois N, Deviere J, Yeaton P, et al. Diagnostic and therapeutic endoscopic retrograde cholangiography after liver transplantation. *Gastrointest Endosc.* 1995;42:527–534.

136. LaRusso NF, Wiesner RH, Ludwig J, et al. Primary sclerosing cholangitis. *N Engl J Med.* 1984;310:899–903.

137. Lindor KD, Wiesner RH, La Russo NF. Recent advances in the management of primary sclerosing cholangitis. *Semin Liver Dis* 1987;7:322.

138. Helzberg JH, Petersen JM, Boyer JL. Improved survival with primary sclerosing cholangitis. *Gastroenterology.* 1987;92:1869–1875.

139. Cameron JL, Gayler BW, Sanfey H, et al. Sclerosing cholangitis. Anatomical distribution of obstructive lesions. *Ann Surg.* 1984;200:54.

140. Kaw M, Silverman WB, Rabinovitz M, Schade RR. Biliary tract calculi in primary sclerosing cholangitis. *Am J Gastroenterol.* 1995;90:72–75.

141. Craig DA, Mac Carty RL, Wienser RH, et al. Primary sclerosing cholangitis: value of cholangiography in determining the prognosis. *AJR.* 1991;157:959–964.

142. Mac Carty RL, LaRusso NF, Wiesner RH, et al. Primary sclerosing cholangitis: findings on cholangiography and pancreatography. *Radiology.* 1983;149:39–44.

143. Chen LY, Goldberg HI. Sclerosing cholangitis: broad spectrum of radiographic features. *Gastrointest Radiol.* 1984;9:39–47.

144. Mir-Madjlessi SH, Farmer RG, Sivak Jr, MV. Bile duct carcinoma in patients with ulcerative colitis. Relationship to sclerosing cholangitis: report of six cases and review of the literature. *Dig Dis Sci.* 1987;32:145.

145. Rosen CB, Nagorney DM, Wiesner RH, et al. Cholangiocarcinoma complicating primary sclerosing cholangitis. *Ann Surg.* 1991;213:21–25.

146. MacCarty RL, La Russo NF, May GR, et al. Cholangiocarcinoma complicating primary sclerosing cholangitis: cholangiographic appearance. *Radiology.* 1985;156:43–46.

147. Craig PI, Williams SJ, Hatfield ARW et al. Endoscopic therapy in the management of

primary sclerosing cholangitis assessment of clinical response. *Gastroenterology.* 1991;100:A732.

148. Lombard M, Farrant M, Karani J, et al. Improving biliary-enteric drainage in primary sclerosing cholangitis: Experience with endoscopic methods. *Gut.* 1991;32:1364–1368.
149. Johnson GK, Geenen JE, Venu RP, et al. Endoscopic treatment of biliary tract strictures in sclerosing cholangitis: a larger series and recommendations for treatment. *Gastrointest Endosc.* 1991;37:38–43.
150. Cotton PB, Nickl N. Endoscopic and radiologic approaches to therapy in primary sclerosing cholangitis. *Semin Liver Dis.* 1991;11:40–48.
151. Terada T, Nakanuma Y. Intrahepatic cholangiographic appearance simulating primary sclerosing cholangitis in several hepatobiliary diseases: A postmortem cholangiographic and histopathological study in 154 livers at autopsy. *Hepatology.* 1995;22:75–81.
152. Botet JF, Watson RC, Kemeny N, et al. Cholangitis complicating intraarterial chemotherapy in liver metastasis. *Radiology.* 1985;156:335–337.
153. Pien EH, Zeman RK, Benjamin SB, et al. Iatrogenic sclerosing cholangitis following hepatic arterial chemotherapy infusion. *Radiology* 1985;156:329–330.
154. Ludwig J, Kim CH, Wiesner RH, et al. Floxuridine-induced sclerosing cholangitis: an ischemic cholangiopathy? *Hepatology.* 1989;9:215–218.
155. Clark RA, Gallant TE. Bile duct strictures associated with heaptic arterial infusion chemotherapy. *Gastrointest Radiol.* 1987;12:148–151.
156. Belghiti J, Benhamou J-P, Houry S, et al. Caustic sclerosing cholangitis. A complication of the surgical treatment of hydatid disease of the liver. *Arch Surg.* 1986;121:1162–1165.
157. Benhamou Y, Caumes E, Gerosa Y, et al. AIDS-related cholangiopathy. Critical analysis of a prospective series of 26 patients. *Dig Dis Sci* 1993;38:1113–1118.
158. Cello JP. Human immunodeficiency virus-associated biliary tract disease. *Semin Liver Dis.* 1992;12:213–218.
159. Bouche H, Housset C, Dumont J-L, et al. AIDS-related cholangitis: diagnostic features and course in 15 patients. *J Hepatol.* 1993;17:34–39.
160. Yellin AE, Donovan AJ. Biliary lithiasis and helminthiasis. *Am J Surg.* 1981; 142:128–136.
161. Ona FV, Dytoc JNT. Clonorchis-associated cholangiocarcinoma: A report of two cases with unusual manifestations. *Gastroenterology.* 1991;101:831–839.
162. Van Sonnenberg E, Casola G, Cubberley DA, et al. Oriental cholangiohepatitis: Diagnostic imaging and interventional management. *AJR.* 1986;146:327–331.
163. Nakayama F, Soloway RD, Nakama T, et al. Hepatolithiasis in East Asia. Retrospective study. *Dig Dis Sci.* 1986;31:21–26.
164. Lam SK: A study of endoscopic sphincterotomy in recurrent pyogenic cholangitis. *Br J Surg.* 1984;71:262–266.
165. Choi TK, Wong J. Endoscopic retrograde cholangiopancreatography and endoscopic papillotomy in recurrent pyogenic cholangitis. *Clin Gastroenterol.* 196;15:393–415.
166. Khuroo MS, Dar MY, Yattoo GN, et al. Serial cholangiographic appearances in recurrent pyogenic cholangitis. *Gastrointest Endosc.* 1993;39:675–679.
167. Lipsett PA, Kalloo AN, Scott JS, Pitt HA. Biliary Cysts. In: Pitt HA, Carr-Locke DL, Ferrucci JT, eds. *Hepatobiliary and Pancreatic Disease.* Boston: Little, Brown; 1995:173–184.

14

SURGICAL SUMMARY: BILIARY TREE

Ravi S. Chari, M.D.
The University of Toronto
Toronto, Ontario

Theodore N. Pappas, M.D.
Duke University Medical Center
Durham, North Carolina

In the preceding chapters, various diagnostic modalities designed for investigating biliary tract pathology have been discussed in detail. Although each has merits and disadvantages, none is complete in its delineation of biliary tract disease; as such, several diagnostic strategies are used in concert to effect an accurate diagnosis, and in some instances achieve a therapeutic goal. In this chapter, an overall approach to biliary tract disease and the role of various radiological interventions designed to aid efficiently in preoperative diagnosis and operative decisions is discussed.

OVERVIEW

The most common presenting sign of biliary tract disease is jaundice. As stated in Chapter 7, ultrasound is the initial screening modality of choice for evaluating the biliary tree. It is sensitive and accurate, and cost effectively provides a comprehensive examination of the entire abdomen. The finding of biliary tree dilatation is specific for biliary tract obstruction. Features used to distinguish dilated intrahepatic ducts from portal veins are discussed in detail in Chapter 7; dilated intrahepatic ducts are typically a manifestation of extrahepatic duct obstruction (pathological entities causing intrahepatic duct dilatation alone are discussed below). Several points about dilated hepatic ducts should be reemphasized: (1) Ultrasound findings of intrahepatic bile duct dilatation are specific, but not equally sensitive; up to 23% of patients with biliary obstruction do not have ductal dilatation. (2) The degree

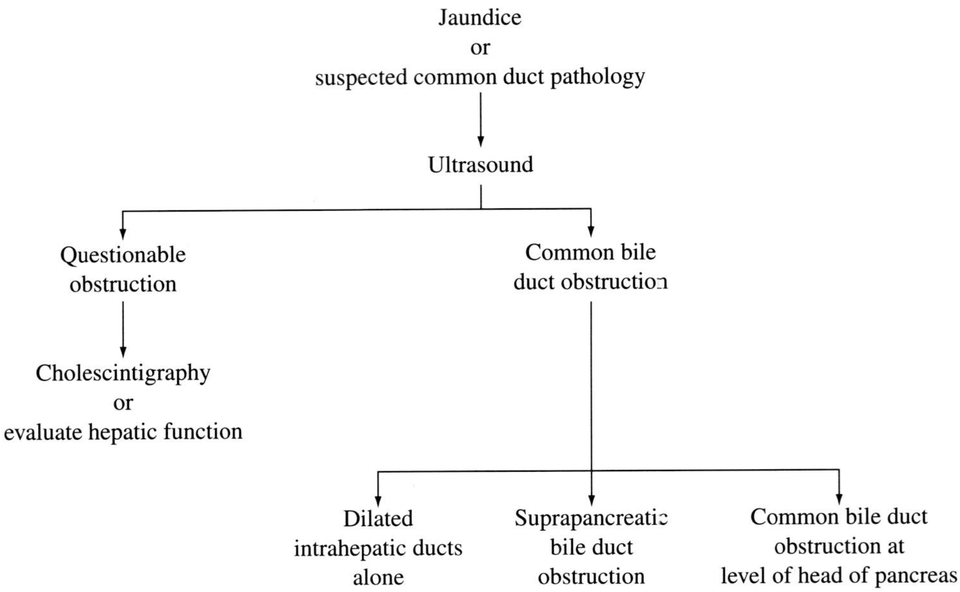

Figure 1. Algorithm: overview of approach to biliary pathology.

of hyperbilirubinemia and duration of jaundice do not correlate with the presence or absence of intrahepatic biliary dilatation (1). A patient with obstructive jaundice caused by cholangitis, partial obstruction, or intermittent obstruction from choledocholithiasis may not manifest duct dilatation. Conversely, the presence of ductal dilatation is not always accompanied with an increase in serum bilirubin. In those patients with questionable biliary obstruction, cholescintigraphy is useful in demonstrating early, nondilated common bile duct (CBD) obstruction (Chapter 9). In patients with anicteric dilatation, such as that seen in patients with chronic pancreatitis, elevations in the alkaline phosphatase may be more sensitive than the serum bilirubin (2). The caliber of the CBD ranges from 4 to 8 mm and the normal CBD increases in diameter with advancing age (3) and following cholecystectomy (4–6). In accordance with Laplace's law, the extrahepatic ducts dilate preferentially. Biliary obstruction is suggested if there is a common hepatic duct greater than or equal to 8 mm (7). In addition to determining the presence or absence of biliary obstruction, ultrasound may also be able to determine the cause and level of obstruction. With current technology, the level and cause of biliary obstruction can be determined in 92 and 71% of cases, respectively (8). The level of the obstruction can be divided into three areas of the extrahepatic biliary tree: porta hepatis, suprapancreatic CBD, and intrapancreatic CBD (Fig. 1). Based on these three zones, further investigations can be undertaken to define the specific pathology.

PORTA HEPATIS OBSTRUCTION

The sonographic features of porta hepatis obstruction are characterized by intrahepatic duct dilatation (Fig. 2) with a relatively normal caliber CBD; depending on

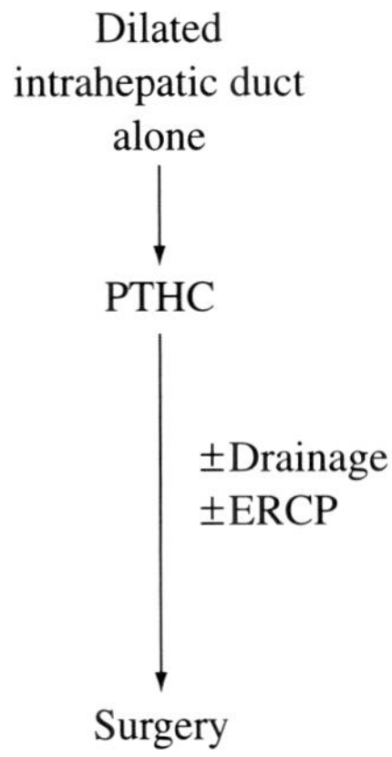

Figure 2. Algorithm: approach to obstruction at the level of the portal hilum.

the level of obstruction, the cystic duct and gallbladder may be involved. Focal intrahepatic duct dilatation may be seen if only the right or left hepatic duct is involved. Most commonly, these obstructions arise from primary or secondary neoplasms (including adenopathy).

CHOLANGIOCARCINOMA

Bile duct cancer is classified according to its location within the ductal system. Sixty percent of the tumors are located in the upper third (Klatskin tumors) (9). Upper-third tumors, or hilar tumors, are further classified into four types, as described by Bismuth and Corlette (10): Type I involves the common hepatic duct, Type II extends to the confluence of the right and left hepatic ducts, type III extends into either the right (Type IIIa) or left (Type IIIb), and Type IV extends into both the right and left hepatic ducts.

When biliary obstruction is confirmed by ultrasound or computed tomography (CT), further visualization is necessary using either percutaneous transhepatic cholangiography (PTHC) or endosopic retrograde cholangiopancreatography (ERCP). The latter is advantageous for lower lesions and brushings, for cytological diagnosis can be performed concomitantly, whereas PTHC is preferred for proximal lesions of the biliary tree. Percutaneous biliary drainage is indicated for palliation of pruritus and treatment of cholangitis in patients with upper-third tumors or in those for whom ERCP is not feasible (11, 12). Additionally, preoperative biliary drainage is indicated in selected patients with resectable cholangiocarcinomas to facilitate definition of operative anatomy (13). Abdominal CT should be performed prior to percutaneous biliary drainage, because it is helpful in planning the approach if bile duct dilatation is limited to only one hepatic lobe. Cross-sectional imaging also permits planing a suitable percutaneous tract to avoid potentially necrotic or hemorrhagic intrahepatic masses. Vascular invasion precludes surgical resection, and determination of this should be ascertained with selective celiac angiography. More recently, magnetic resonance cholangiopancreatography (MRCP), based on the principle that the biliary and pancreatic secretions within the ductal system have markedly prolonged T2 values (see Chapter 10), has been used to define ductal anatomy (14). Magnetic resonance imaging (MRI) has the added advantage of defining cross-sectional anatomy like CT; it also has the ability to detect vascular anatomy (magnetic resonance angiography, MRA). The exact role of MRCP has yet to be determined, however.

PRIMARY SCLEROSING CHOLANGITIS

Primary sclerosing cholangitis (PSC) is an idiopathic cholestatic disease characterized by inflammatory, fibrous strictures of the intrahepatic and extrahepatic bile ducts. The causes of PSC are unknown. The diagnosis can be suspected from the clinical picture (intermittent jaundice, which begins insidiously in the third to fifth decades; right upper quadrant pain, fever, weight loss, and fatigue; the disease is characterized by remissions and exacerbations) and fluctuating elevations of the serum alkaline phosphatase and serum bilirubin. The alkaline phosphatase is usually elevated out of proportion to the serum bilirubin. The diagnosis is confirmed by cholangiography: multiple dilatations and strictures (beading). Endoscopic retrograde cholangiopancreatography is the preferred procedure because of the difficulties in cannulation of the intrahepatic ducts by PTHC because they are nondilated and fibrous. No specific therapy is available for PSC. A multicenter review of nonoperative percutaneous dilatation of dominant strictures in patients with PSC found that only 42% of patients had successful long-term results (15). More favorable results were reported with endoscopic stenting (16). There is a progressive nature of the disease and an aggressive surgical approach has been advocated for those patients who experience symptoms. There are two primary surgical options: biliary tract resection and long-term stenting, or hepatic transplantation. Overall, in patients with symptomatic PSC without cirrhosis and primary hilar or extrahepatic strictures, resection of the hepatic bifurcation and long-term transhepatic stenting are acceptable (17). In patients with primarily intrahepatic disease or with advanced cirrhosis, liver transplantation is the preferred treatment.

SUPRAPANCREATIC COMMON BILE DUCT OBSTRUCTION

These obstructions occur above the pancreas but below the porta (Fig. 3). Although malignancy is the most common cause, this also is the region of many benign biliary strictures, especially postoperative biliary strictures (18).

BENIGN BILIARY STRICTURES

Benign biliary strictures represent one of the most difficult challenges than a surgeon faces; significant advances in minimally invasive techniques have aided dramatically in their diagnosis and treatment. If strictures are unrecognized or treated improperly, life-threatening complications such as biliary cirrhosis (19), cholangitis, and portal

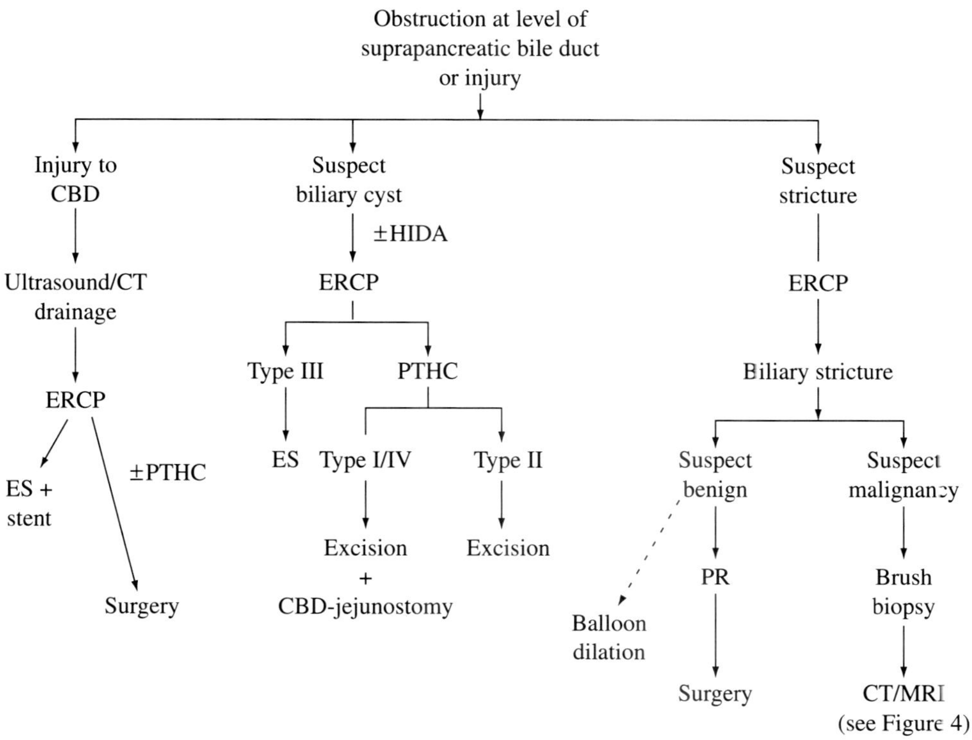

Figure 3. Algorithm: approach to biliary obstruction at the level of the suprapancreatic bile duct.

hypertension can occur. To avoid these potential complications, every biliary stricture should be treated with the goal of relieving the obstruction and reestablishing bile flow. Most biliary strictures occur after primary operations on the gallbladder or biliary tree. There has been an increased frequency of biliary tree injuries with the advent of laparoscopic cholecystectomy. Injury during nonbiliary procedures and trauma can also result in stricture formation. The location of a bile duct stricture is of primary importance in dictating management and predicting outcome; to this end, a classification of benign bile duct strictures based on anatomic pattern of involvement has been developed (20). Most patients with benign postoperative biliary strictures present early after their initial operation; after open cholecystectomy, 10% present within the first week, 70% within 6 months, and 80% within 1 year of surgery (21). Those suspected of having a stricture within days of surgery present in one of two ways: (1) progressive elevation of alkaline phosphatase and total bilirubin, and (2) bile draining from operative drains or the wound itself. In patients with injured ducts and bile leak after laparoscopic cholecystectomy, bile peritonitis is a frequent early presentation. In patients who present late, the usual presentation is that of cholangitis. Radiological evaluation in patients with benign postoperative biliary injury plays a central role. Ultrasound should be the first investigation; the presence of a biliary fluid collection in the face of sepsis should prompt the placement of a percutaneous drain. Nuclear medicine scan with iminodiacetic acid can be used to confirm a leak; however, most often this is not indicated. The standard for patients with bile duct strictures is cholangiography (22). Endoscopic retrograde cholangiopancreatography is most often the initial route of cholangiography because the biliary tree is often not dilated; it is also therapeutic in those cases of cystic duct stump leak: endoscopic sphincterotomy (ES) alone or ES with stent placement (23–25) provides a low resistance path for bile flow, diverting it away from the open cystic duct. The leak usually resolves within 2–4 weeks in 80–90% of patients (26–28). Common duct leaks are best managed with biliary stents (Chapter 13). Percutaneous transhepatic cholangiography is technically more difficult in this setting because the intrahepatic biliary tree is nondilated (Chapter 12). When the duct is injured or transected, the information obtained from ERCP is often limited in that the discontinuity of the extrahepatic bile duct usually prevents adequate filling of the proximal biliary tree. Percutaneous transhepatic cholangiography is more useful because it defines the anatomy of the proximal biliary tree, and with the placement of transhepatic catheters, surgical reconstruction can be facilatated (29).

In those patients who present late after cholecystectomy, the possibility of malignancy should be excluded. Computed tomography (Chapter 8) scan or MRI (Chapter 10) should be performed to rule out the presence of a pancreatic mass. If there is no evidence of a mass or hilar adenopathy to account for a duct stricture, cholangiography should be performed. Endoscopic retrograde cholangiopancreatography should be attempted first; PTHC is indicated if ERCP is unsuccessful or if Roux-en-Y bypass makes ERCP unfeasible.

Once the diagnosis of a postoperative biliary stricture has been made, there are several therapeutic options available: operative repair, ERCP balloon dilation, or percutaneous balloon dilation. In Chapter 12, the merits and indications of percutaneous drainage are discussed, and those of ERCP are similarly elucidated in Chapter 13. Several general comments can be made summarizing these chapters regarding the role of minimally invasive management of benign biliary strictures: (1) injuries involving multiple ducts, large leaks, short tight strictures due to clip misplacement, long strictures due to ischemic injury (common after laparoscopic cholecystectomy) are less likely to respond to nonoperative management; (2) patients who are in good medical condition achieve the most durable result following surgical repair (30); (3) results of dilational techniques are improving (Chapter 13). Currently, surgical repair should be offered to all patients with benign biliary strictures and balloon dilation should be reserved for patients who are at high risk for reconstructive procedures. As centers of excellence gain experience with indication and techniques, the role of nonoperative dilation as a therapeutic option may be expanded.

INTRAPANCREATIC COMMON BILE DUCT OBSTRUCTION

The most common level of CBD obstruction is at the level of the pancreatic head. Common bile duct stones, neoplasms, and inflammatory strictures are the most common etiologies (Fig. 4).

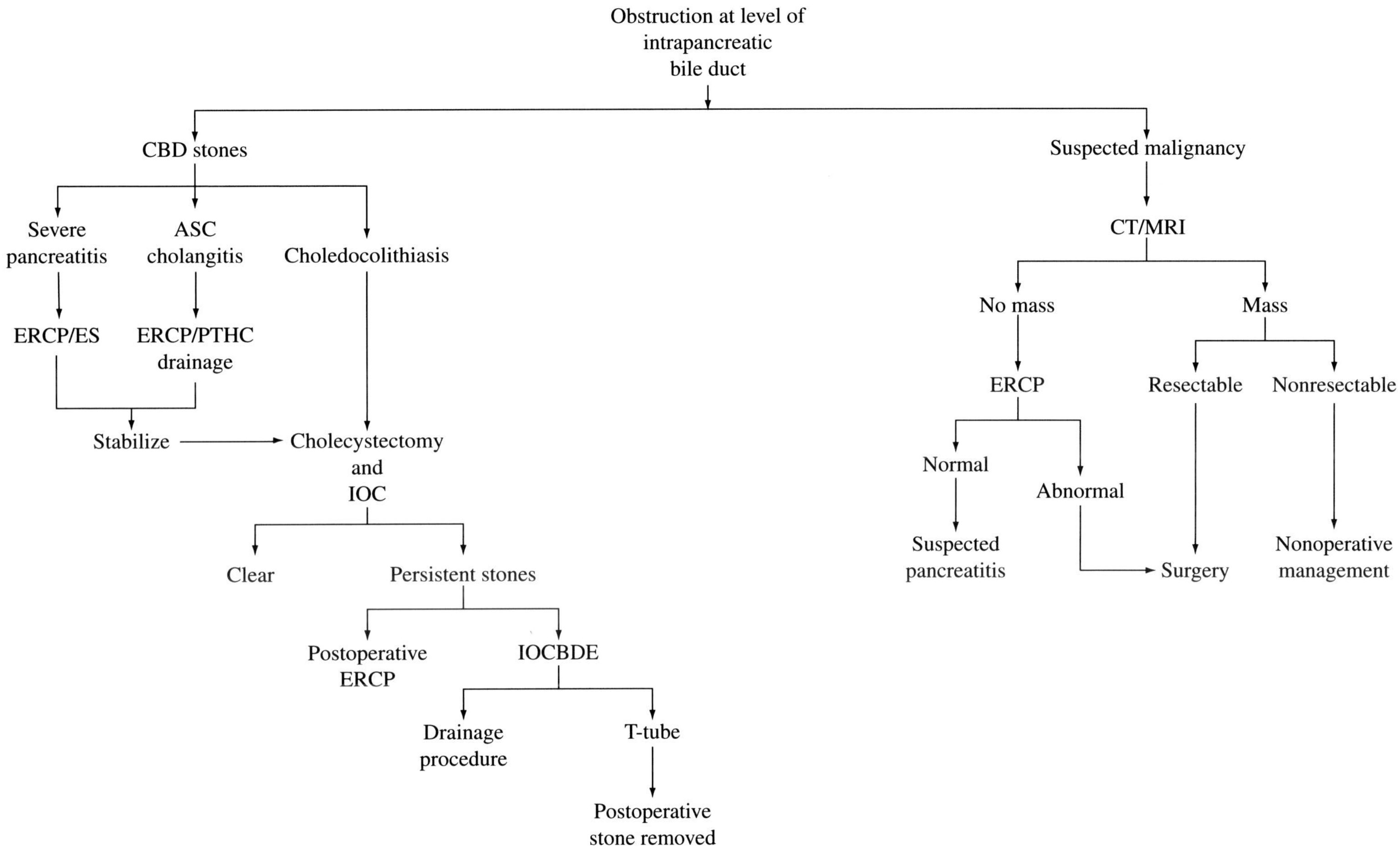

Figure 4. Algorithm: approach to biliary obstruction at the level of the intrapancreatic bile duct.

CHOLEDOCHOLITHIASIS

Common duct stones usually cause symptoms when they create obstruction; the clinical presentation depends on the level and the degree of obstruction and on the presence or absence of biliary infection. Simple obstruction results in right upper quadrant pain and jaundice. Typically, jaundice due to common duct stones is more transient or intermittent than when biliary obstruction is due to malignancy. Pancreatitis is an associated finding in 4–8% of patients with choledocholithiasis (31, 32).

Although abnormal laboratory test results may be suggestive, the most reliable means of detecting CBD stones is cholangiography; the morbidity associated with invasive cholangiography, however, precludes its routine use. Ultrasound is 97% accurate in diagnosing stones in the gallbladder, and at present ultrasound visualization of choledocholithiasis is successful in at least 70% of patients (7, 33). Other series report sensitivities of 15–30%. The true sensitivity is probably somewhere between these. Computed tomography is reported to be more accurate than ultrasound in the detection of choledocholithiasis (75–90%) (34, 35). The role of MRCP is currently under investigation, but appears promising. Cholangiography (ERCP) remains the standard.

Prior to the advent of laparoscopic cholecystectomy, the management strategy of choledocholithiasis was cholecystectomy, intraoperative cholangiography (IOC) (Chapter 11), and common duct exploration (CBDE) if warranted. Clinical criteria useful in predicting the presence of common duct stones are outlined and discussed in Chapter 11; clearly, a policy of selective IOC should be advocated. Initial experience with intraoperative laparoscopic ultrasound has been reported (36), but widespread use and acceptance are still lacking. When laparoscopic cholecystectomy became common, unfamiliarity with the complexity of laparoscopic CBDE increased the utilization of both preoperative ERCP to clear the duct (obviating the need for IOC), and postoperative ERCP after laparoscopic IOC demonstrated the presence of stones. The latter is currently the most preferred management strategy (37); when there is high likelihood of preoperative choledocholithiasis, selective preoperative ERCP and duct clearance is an equivalent strategy. Endoscopic retrograde cholangiopancreatography can successfully manage stones in 90% of cases (38) (Chapter 13). Preoperative ERCP should be reserved for patients with severe pancreatitis (39, 40) ascending cholangitis (41, 42), or jaundice. Preoperative ascending cholangitis should be managed with preoperative duct decompression (ERCP preferred to PTHC), and stabilization of the patient prior to definitive operative management.

CHOLEDOCHAL CYSTS

Cystic lesions of the biliary tract are uncommon problems that appear in various forms and combinations. Nonbiliary hepatic cysts are not considered in this section; they can be distinguished from biliary cysts by a combination of noninvasive imaging and cholangiography. Choledochal cysts are localized dilatations of the bile duct, and the most popular classification (38) describes five variations. Type I, or cystic dilation of the common bile duct, is by far the most common variety, constituting

65–90% of reported cases. Type I cysts can be further classified into those that are saccular (Ia), localized (Ib), or fusiform (Ic). Type II are isolated diverticula of the common bile duct; these are rare and make up less than 3% of all cases. Type III cysts, also known as choledochoceles, are characterized by dilatation of the intraduodenal portion of the common bile duct. Types IV and V were added to the above classification in 1977 (43). Type IV consists of multiple cysts, either intrahepatic and extrahepatic (IVa) or extrahepatic only (IVb), whereas type V forms (Caroli's disease) of the anomaly are single or multiple intrahepatic cysts only. Like other biliary tract pathology, the most common presentation is jaundice (43). Patients with type III cysts may present with recurrent acute pancreatitis, biliary colic, cholangitis, or duodenal obstruction with nausea and vomiting (44, 45). Ultrasound is the most helpful initial screening technique. Once a thick-walled cyst in the right upper quadrant is demonstrated by ultrasound, further investigation with cholangiography should be undertaken. Computed tomography and MRI (with MRCP) can complement the ultrasound findings particularly when the diagnosis is in doubt, and it may also detect mass lesions, such as cholangiocarcinoma. Nuclear biliary studies with an iminodiacetic acid derivative should be obtained in patients presenting with acute symptoms to exclude acute cholecystitis. Accurate delineation of the biliary tree should be performed with ERCP or PTHC; these two studies are complementary, with ERCP more accurately visualizing the distal duct, and PTHC the proximal duct. In the future MRCP may be able to supplant these two studies for diagnosing choledochocysts. Cholangiograms are useful to exclude other causes of dilated CBD (stricture, tumor, choledocholithiasis) and to establish the anatomic relations necessary to formulate an operative plan. Endoscopic retrograde cholangiopancreatography is usually performed first because it visualizes the ampulla, allowing demonstration of a choledochocele, and it also defines the abnormalities of the pancreatobiliary junction (46); ERCP/ES is the treatment of choice for Type III choledochal cysts. Percutaneous transhepatic cholangiography not only defines the upper biliary tract anatomy, but well-placed catheters can aid in intraoperative dissection and visualization. Using these various imaging modalities, preoperative diagnosis of choledochal cysts has increased from fewer than 40% in the 1970s to greater than 80% in the 1990s (47, 48).

HEAD OF PANCREAS PATHOLOGY

For those patients with head of pancreas cancer, the most common presenting sign is weight loss (92%) followed by jaundice (82%) (49). The most frequent investigation after routine blood work is ultrasound. Following the demonstration of dilated extrahepatic or intrahepatic ducts, CT is usually ordered next. Although ultrasound is reported to be as sensitive as CT in detecting pancreatic head masses (50), CT is superior to ultrasound in detecting local invasion, vascular involvement, and lymph node metastases, and determining resectability (51). Magnetic resonance imaging performs similarly and in one study was superior to helical CT for identifying pancreatic head masses (52). Endoscopic retrograde cholangiopancreatography should be used judiciously, because of cost, complexity, and potential risk. In the setting of pancreatic cancer, based on clinical presentation and initial ultrasound and CT/MRI, ERCP should be used primarily in two groups of patients: (1) patients in whom cross-sectional imaging has revealed dilatation of the biliary duct and/or pancreatic duct, but no mass is detected. A subset of this group includes patients who have gallstones and bile duct dilatation by ultrasound and no mass by CT/MRI; ERCP may be necessary to distinguish choledocholithiasis from pancreatic cancer, especially in elderly patients with an antecedent history of weight loss. (2) The second group in whom ERCP is indicated is those with a mass in the head of the pancreas and either clinical or cross-sectional imaging signs of chronic pancreatitis; ERCP, particularly when combined with cytological examination of the pancreatic juice, may help distinguish chronic pancreatitis from carcinoma. Overall, ERCP has a 90% sensitivity and specificity of diagnosing pancreatic cancer (53). This selective approach to the use of ERCP in the diagnosis of pancreatic cancer was endorsed in a review designed to assess the value of various diagnostic tests in 126 patients with pancreatic cancer (54).

SUMMARY

Ultrasound is by far the most cost-effective, efficient modality for surveying the biliary anatomy. Further definition of anatomic or pathological variants should be used on a selective basis. Although ERCP and PTHC are highly informative, their uniform application to the investigation of biliary tract disease is unnecessary, and furthermore dangerous. Computed tomography and MRI play a key role in the determination of concomitant malignancy. Cholescintigraphy has a limited role in the work-up of common duct disease, and should be reserved for cases of early duct obstruction and cases in which acute cholecystitis is in the differential diagnosis. Magnetic resonance imaging with MRCP is a new emerging technology combining the anatomic capabilities of both CT and cholangiography; the exact role in the delineation of common duct pathology is not fully defined. Finally, while limited in indication in this era, IOC (and IO ultrasound) is an important technique for the surgeon to master and use in selected cases.

REFERENCES

1. Sample WF, Sarti DA, Goldstein R, et al. Gray-scale ultrasonography of the jaundiced patient. *Radiology.* 1980;128:719.
2. Zeman RK, Taylor KJW, Burrell MI, et al. Ultrasound demonstration of anicteric dilation of the biliary tree. *Radiology.* 1980;134:689.
3. Wu CC, Ho YH, Chen CY. Effect of aging on common bile duct diameter: a real-time ultrasonographic study. *J Clin Ultrasound.* 1984;12:473.
4. Grahm MF, Cooperberg PL, Cohen MM, et al. The size of the normal common hepatic duct following cholecystectomy: an ultrasonograpic study. *Radiology.* 1980;135:137.
5. Mueller PR, Ferucci JT, Simeone JF, et al. Postcholycystectomy bile duct dilation: myth or reality. *AJR.* 1981;136:355.
6. Niederau C, Muller J, Sonnenberg A, et al. Extrahepatic bile duct in healthy subjects, in patients with cholelithiasis, and in postcholecytstectomy patients: a prospective ultrasonic study. *J Clin Ultrasound.* 1983;11:23.
7. Laing FC. The gallbladder and bile ducts in diagnostic ultrasound. In: Rumack CM,

Wilson SR, Charboneau JW, eds. *Diagnostic Ultrasound.* St. Louis: Mosby Year Book; 1991:106–144.

8. Laing FC, Jeffrey RB, Wing VW. Biliary dilatation: defining the level and cause by real time ultrasound. *Radiology.* 1986;160:39.
9. Klastskin G. Adenocarcinoma of the hepatic duct at its bifurcation within the porta hepatis. *Am J Med.* 1965;38:241.
10. Bismuth H, Nakache R, Diamond T. Management strategies in resection for hilar cholangiocarcinoma. *Ann Surg.* 1992;215:31.
11. Ferrucci JT, Mueller PR, Harbin WP. Percutaneous transhepatic biliary drainage: technique, results and applications. *Radiology.* 1980;135:1.
12. Berquist TJ, May GR, Johnson CM, Adson MA, Thistle JL. Percutaneous biliary decompression: internal and external drainage in 50 patients. *AJR.* 1981;136:901.
13. Crist DW, Kadir S, Cameron JL. The value of preoperatively placed percutaneous biliary catheters in reconstruction of the proximal part of the biliary tree. *Surg Obstet Gynecol.* 1987;165:421.
14. Outwater EK, Gordon SG. Imaging pancreatic and biliary ducts with MR. *Radiology.* 1994;192:19.
15. Mueller PR, van Sonnenberg E, Ferrucci JT, et al. Biliary stricture dilation: multicenter review of clinical management in 73 patients. *Radiology.* 1986;160:17.
16. Johnson GK, Gechen JE, Venu RS, et al. Partial hepatectomy for intrahepatic stones. *Gastrointest Endosc.* 1991;37:38.
17. Cameron JL, Pitt HA, Zinner MJ, et al. Resection of hepatic duct bifurcation and transhepatic stenting for sclerosing cholangitis. *Ann Surg.* 1988;207:614.
18. Lillemoe KD, Pitt HA, Cameron JL. Current management of benign bile duct strictures. *Adv Surg.* 1992;25:119.
19. Way LW, Bernholt RA, Thomas MJ. Biliary stricture. *Surg Clin North Am.* 1981;61:963.
20. Bismuth H. Postoperative strictures of the bile duct. In: Blumgart LH, ed. *The Biliary Tract.* Edinburgh: Churchill Livingstone; 1982:209.
21. Pitt HA, Miyamoto T, Parapatis SK, et al. Factors influencing outcome in patients with postoperative biliary strictures. *Am J Surg.* 1982;144:14.
22. Branum GD, Schmitt C, Baillie J, et al. Management of major biliary complications after laparoscopic cholecystectomy. *Ann Surg.* 1993;17:547.
23. Foutch PG, Harlan JR, Hoefer M. Endoscopic therapy for patients with postoperative biliary leak. *Gastrointest Endosc.* 1993;39:416.
24. Libby ED, Branch MS, Cotton PB. Cystic duct leak after laparoscopic cholecystectomy. *Gastrointest Endosc.* 1995;41:511.
25. Liguory C, Vitale GC, Lefebre JF, et al. Endoscopic treatment of postoperative fistulae. *Surgery.* 1991;110:179.
26. Feretis C, Kekis B, Bliouras N, et al. Postoperative external and internal biliary fistulas, unassociated with distal bile duct obstruction: endoscopic treatment. *Endoscopy.* 1990;22:211.
27. Kozarek RA, Ball TJ, Patterson DJ, et al. Endoscopic treatment of biliary injury in the era of laparoscopic cholecystectomy. *Gastrointest Endosc.* 1994;40:10.
28. Davids PHP, Rauws EAJ, Tytgat GNJ, Huibregtse K. Postoperative bile leak: endoscopic management. *Gut.* 1992;33:1118.
29. Crist DW, Kadir S, Cameron JL. The value of preoperatively placed percutaneous biliary catheters reconstruction of the proximal part of the biliary tract. *Surg Gynecol Obstet.* 1987;38:1013.

30. Pitt HA, Kaufman SL, Coleman J, White RI, Cameron JL, Benign postoperative biliary strictures: operate or dilate. *Ann Surg.* 1989;210:417.
31. Patti MG, Pellegrini CA. Gallstone pancreatitis. *Surg Clin North Am.* 1990;70:1277.
32. Armstrong CP, Taylor TV, Jeacock J. The biliary tract in patients with acute gallstone pancreatitis. *Br J Surg.* 1985;72:551.
33. Laing FC. Ultrasound diagnosis of choledocholithiasis. *Semin. Ultrasound CT MR.* 1987;8:103.
34. Baron RL, Stanley RJ, Lee KTJ, Koehler RE, Levitt RG. Computed tomography features of biliary obstruction. *AJR.* 1983;140:1179.
35. Jeffrey RB, Federle MP, Laing FC, Wall S, Rego J, Moss AA. Computed tomography of choledocholithiasis. *AJR.* 1983;140:1179.
36. Ascher SM, Evans SRT, Zeman RK. Laparoscopic cholecystectomy: ultrasound of the extrahepatic biliary tree and the natural history of postoperative transabdominal ultrasound findings. *Semin Ultrasound CT MR.* 1993;14:331.
37. Brodish RJ, Fink AS. ERCP, cholangiography and laparoscopic cholecystectomy. Soc of Am Gastrointest Endoscoping Surgeons (SAGES) opinion survey. *Surg Endosc.* 1993; 7:3.
38. Hawasli A, Lloyd L, Pozios V, et al. The role of endoscopic retrograde cholangiopanceatogram in laparoscopic cholecystectomy. *Am Surg.* 1993;59:252.
39. Neoptplemos JP, London NJ, Carr-Locke DL. Controlled trial of urgent endoscopic retrograde spincterotomy versus conservative treatment for acute pancreatitis due to cholelithiasis. *Lancet.* 1988;ii:979.
40. Fan ST, Lai ECS, Mok FPT, et al. Early treatment of acute biliary pancreatitis by endoscopic papillotomy. *N Engl J Med.* 1993;328:228.
41. Leese T, Neoptplemos JP, Baker AR, et al. The management of acute cholangitis and the impact of endoscopic sphincterotomy. *Br J Surg.* 1986;79:647.
42. Leung JWC, Song JJY, Chung SCS, et al. Urgent endoscopic drainage in acute suppurative cholangitis. *Lancet.* 1989;i:1307.
43. Chijiwa K, Koga A. Surgical management and long term results in the treatment of choledochal cysts. *Am J Surg.* 1993;165:238.
44. Venu RP, Geenen JE, Hogan WJ, et al. Role of endoscopic retrograde cholangiopoancreatography on the diagnosis and treatment of choledochocele. *Gastroenterology.* 1984;87:1144.
45. Martin RF, Biber BP, Bosco JJ, Howell DA. Symptomatic choledochoceles in adults: endoscopic retrograde cholangiopancreatography recognition and management. *Arch Surg.* 1992;127:536.
46. Weidmeyer DA, Stewart ET, Dodds WV, et al. Choledochal cysts: findings on cholangiopancratography with emphasis on ectasia of the common channel. *AJR.* 1989;153: 969.
47. Flanigan DP. Biliary cysts. *Ann Surg.* 1975;182:635.
48. Lopez RR, Penson CW, Campbell JR, Harrison M, Katon RM. Variation in management based on type of choledochal cyst. *Am J Surg.* 1991;161:612.
49. Howard JM, Jordan GL, Jr. Cancer of the pancreas. *Curr Probl Cancer.* 1977;2:5.
50. Maringhini A, Ciambra M, Raimondo M, et al. Clinical presentation and ultrasonography in the diagnosis of pancreatic cancer. *Pancreas.* 1993;8:146.
51. Gulliver DJ, Baker ME, Cheng CA, Meyers WC, Pappas TM. Malignant biliary obstruction: efficacy of thin-section dynamic CT in determining resectability. *AJR.* 1992;159: 503.

52. Semecka RC, Kelekis NL, Molina P, et al. Pancreatic masses with inconclusive findings of spiral CT; is this a role for MRI? *JMRI.* 1776;6:585–588.
53. DiMagno EP, Malegelada JR, Taylor WF, Go VLW. A prospective comparison of current diagnostic diagnostic tests for pancreatic carcinoma. *N Engl J Med.* 1977;297:737.
54. Alvarez C, Livingston EH, Ashley SW, Schwartz M, Reber HA. Cost-benefit analysis of the work-up for pancreatic cancer. *Am J Surg.* 1993;165:53.

III

LIVER

15

ULTRASOUND OF THE LIVER

Steven C. Horii, M.D.
University of Pennsylvania Medical Center
Philadelphia, Pennsylvania

The use of diagnostic ultrasound (US) for examination of the liver is one of the earliest uses of the technique. Shortly after the end of World War II (1), the realization that sound penetrated the liver well and that the reflected sound could be used to assess the anatomic structure of the liver was quickly realized by the researchers developing ultrasound equipment. By today's standards, the equipment was certainly crude and, without gray-scale images, relied on distortions of the normal bright reflectors (portal venous and biliary tree branches) or overall size to provide diagnostic information. Owing to technological advancement, however, the quality of the images improved rapidly. Today's equipment not only provides images with shades of gray showing the liver, but can image blood flow as well, on some machines as a color overlay over vessels.

This chapter is concerned with ultrasound (the term ultrasound here means diagnostic ultrasound) of the adult liver, describing transabdominal ultrasound of the liver, that is, studies done through the intact abdominal wall, as well as intraoperative ultrasound of the liver, done as an adjunct to abdominal surgical procedures. Equipment, techniques, and the more common diseases and imaging situations encountered in both types of ultrasound are discussed.

EQUIPMENT FOR TRANSABDOMINAL ULTRASOUND

Transabdominal ultrasound of the liver is most commonly performed with real-time equipment using sector- or curved-array ultrasound transducers. The sector-shaped image is preferred for liver scanning because it affords a large angle of view despite what may be a small acoustic "window" through which to scan. Transducer frequencies used range from about 3 to 7 MHz. Some of the newer equipment uses "broad-band" transducers that can be tuned over a range of frequencies. Most of the current machines use phased-array technology in the construction and operation of the transducers themselves. This spin-off from military radar systems (2) results in nonmechanical transducers that, despite their absence of moving parts, generate swept-beam, sector-shaped images in real time. The phased-array technology also allows variable focusing of the ultrasound beam in real time. The rate at which images can be obtained, the "frame rate" of the machine, is not "real time" in the sense that the image is updated at intervals and does not represent continuous motion. This frame rate depends completely on the physics of the imaging process and is limited by the finite speed of sound (about 1540 m/sec) in soft tissue. Because the ultrasound imaging process is basically a pulse-echo system, the transducer has to "listen" for at least the time it takes for the sound pulse to travel into the organ being imaged and return. It is this waiting time that determines how fast a new image frame can be created. The liver, being one of the larger organs in the body, requires a bit longer for sound pulses to traverse than for smaller organs. Thus frame rates for liver imaging are lower than for, say, cardiac imaging. The importance of this to the person doing the imaging is that rapid motion of the liver during scanning results in blurred images. To the sonographer or person watching the scan in progress, however, the image does not flicker despite frame rates that can be lower than 10 frames/sec. The reason for this is also a feature of modern ultrasound equipment. Whatever the frame rate at which the images are actually generated, circuitry displays them at video rates. For example, for a frame rate of 10 frames/sec it would show the first frame three times, the second frame three times, and so on, each for 1/30 sec. If image frames are acquired more quickly, proportionally fewer repeats are shown by the video display circuitry. This conversion circuitry also allows for recording of the video on standard video cassette recorders for a repeatable record of the acquired images.

Color flow Doppler-capable machines allow visualization of blood flow. This type of equipment uses the Doppler frequency shift of moving blood to show structures with blood flow. The changes in Doppler shift are shown as changes in the shade or intensity of a color and changes in flow direction result in complete changes in color. Typically, several color display maps are available and the selection of which color represents flow toward the transducer is arbitrary; this means that the color of a vessel alone does not distinguish between arterial and venous flow. Increasingly, color flow Doppler is being used as an adjunct to gray-scale imaging of the liver.

TECHNIQUES OF TRANSABDOMINAL ULTRASOUND

Patient preparation for scanning the liver is chiefly to have the patient fast for at least 4–6 hr prior to the scans. The reason for this is twofold; first, keeping the patient fasting avoids contracting the gallbladder, and second, fasting reduces bowel gas content. If the patient has to take oral medications, they can be taken with water or other clear liquids. If the liver alone is of interest in scanning, fasting may be dispensed with, though the risk of obviating the subcostal scanning approaches due to bowel gas is increased.

As noted, the sector-type transducer is beneficial in scanning the liver because it helps reduce the limits to acoustic access. Unfortunately, the physics of ultrasound propagation means that air, other gases, and bone are very effective barriers to sound of the frequencies used for imaging. The lungs above the liver prevent an approach from above and bowel inferior to the liver is often partially gas-filled, resulting in another acoustic barrier.

One approach to imaging the liver involves having the patient inspire deeply, resulting in the diaphragm displacing the liver inferiorly. A scan done from the subcostal area and angled cephalad will then usually show the liver. Another method is to scan between the ribs (themselves acoustic barriers). A third is to place the patient rolled into an oblique position with the right side up (about 30–45°). Combining this position with deep inspiration usually allows visualization of the high right and left lobes of the liver. Also, this position (called right anterior oblique, or RAO) is valuable for visualizing the main portal vein and common bile duct longitudinally and provides a good view of the gallbladder. Figure 1 shows examples of the liver visualized using supine transverse (subcostal) and RAO (also subcostal) scanning.

Saggital scans of the liver are usually obtained through both left and right lobes, extending from the midline to the left as far as liver is seen and to the right past the right kidney. Transverse scans are obtained usually by subcostal scanning angled cephalad. The most cephalad scans are usually at the level of the hepatic veins and the most inferior at the tip of the right lobe. Additional scans are those obtained to show the portal venous and biliary anatomy, plus the gallbladder. If there is an interest in the blood flow in the liver, scans directed at the vessels are done with color flow Doppler imaging, often supplanted with duplex Doppler flow wave forms.

If the ultrasound is being done for correlation with computed tomography (CT) or magnetic resonance (MR) imaging, it is often best to scan the patient supine, because the liver position will be better correlated with the other imaging. In this circumstance, scanning through the intercostal spaces may provide the correlation needed because this technique can be used to generate true transverse scan planes (difficult with subcostal scanning).

Though this chapter emphasizes imaging of the liver, most ultrasound examinations include other abdominal organs as well. The pancreas, kidneys, spleen, and great vessels are usually included in a complete study of the abdomen.

DETECTION OF LIVER DISEASE

The chief means by which transabdominal ultrasound of the liver shows diseases is through alterations in anatomic structure, sonographic liver texture, or blood flow patterns. For subtle disease presentations, the ultrasound findings may be correspondingly minimal and therefore difficult to detect.

It is the vascular anatomy of the liver that is used to divide it into segments that are important for surgery. The definition developed by Couinaud (3) is typically used. In this system, the three hepatic veins provide the three major vertical dividing planes (or scissurae) resulting in four vertical sections. A horizontal plane defined by the main pedicles of the right and left portal vein branches divides these into eight segments with the caudate lobe forming an additional segment. The importance of this method of dividing the liver is that it follows functional anatomy; each segment has its own arterial supply, venous drainage, portal circulation, and biliary and lymphatic drainage. In Couinaud's description, segment I is the caudate lobe, II

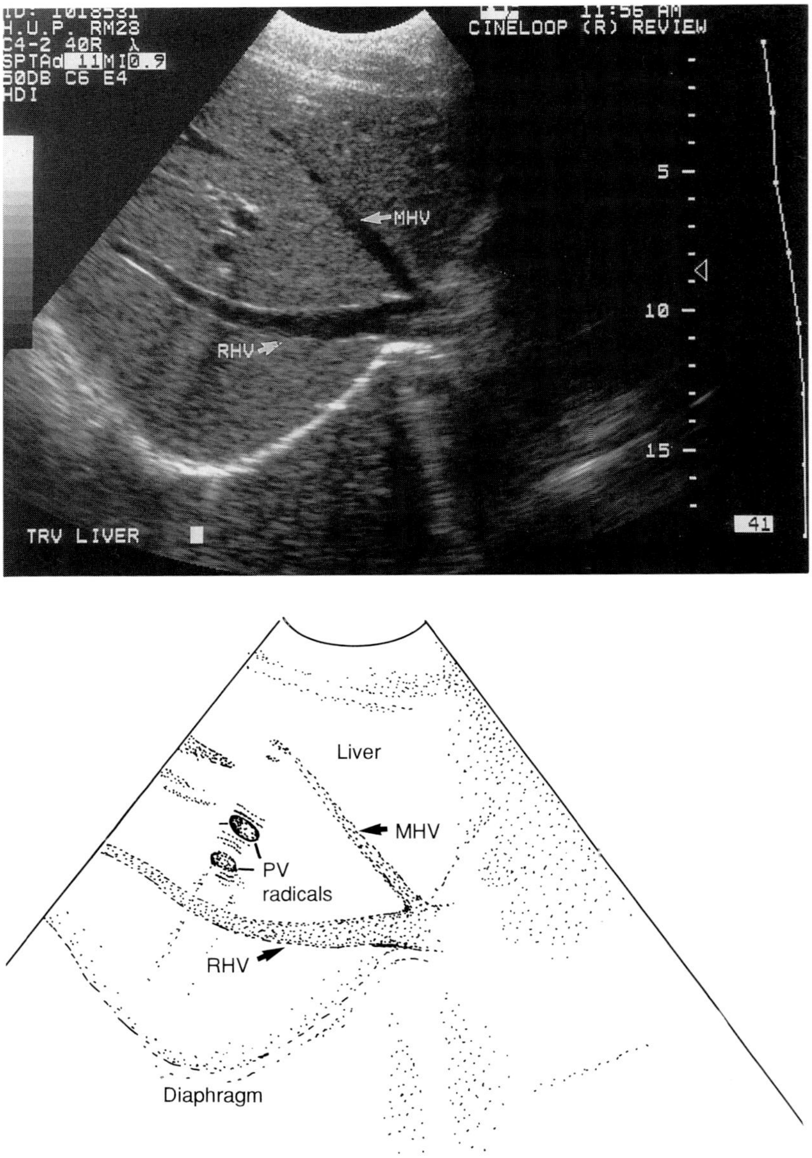

(A)

Figure 1. Supine transverse scans of a normal liver (22-year-old female). (A) Right (RHV) and middle (MHV) hepatic veins. The round structures between the two hepatic veins are portal vein (PV) radicles. (B) Scan done angled more towards the patient's left showing the middle (MHV) and left (LHV) hepatic veins (next page). (C) is an oblique scan through the liver with the patient in the right anterior oblique (RAO) position. The curved arrow shows the main portal vein. The small arrow points out the right branch of the hepatic artery. The arrowhead and open arrow show the common hepatic and common bile duct, respectively. The large straight arrow points to the inferior vena cava (next page). Note in this and other parts of this figure the overall relatively homogeneous echo texture of the liver parenchyma.

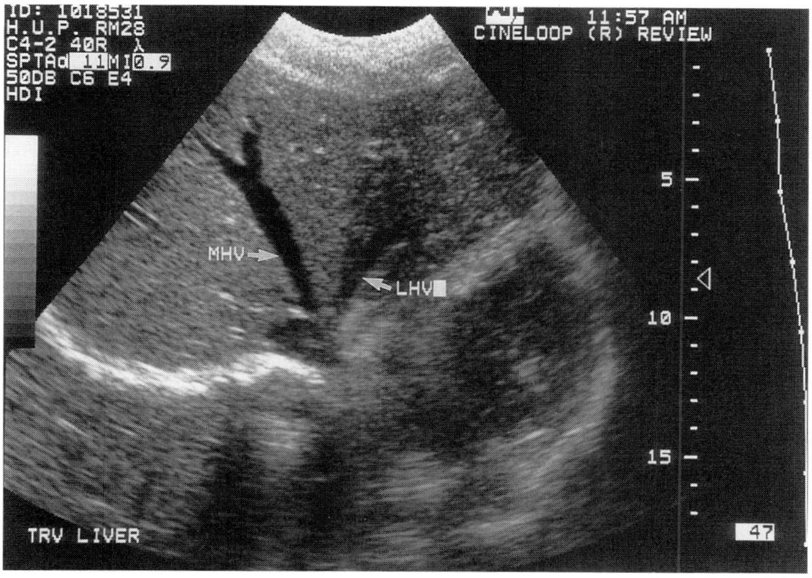

(B)

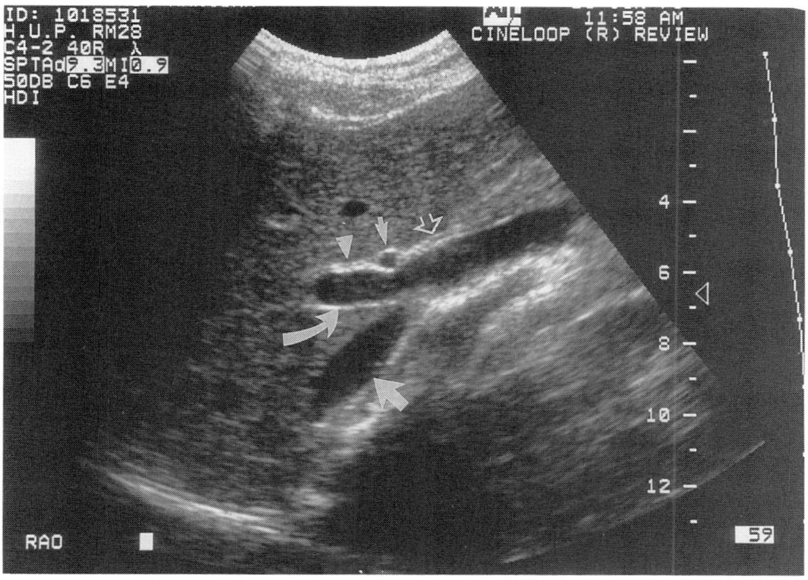

(C)

Figure 1. *(Continued)*

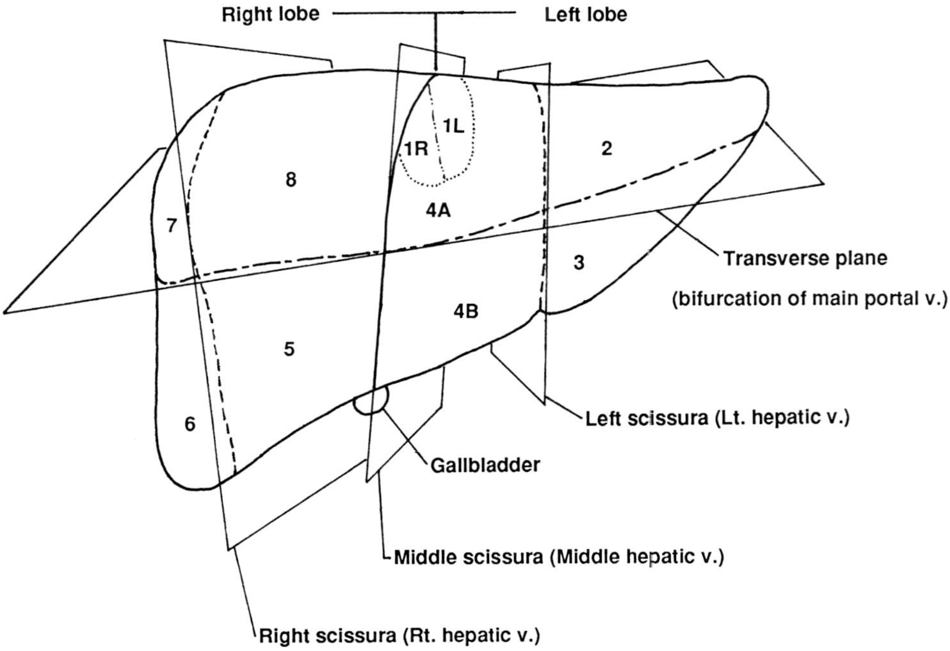

Figure 2. A schematic of the anatomic segments of the liver after Couinaud. The three vertical planes or scissurae are defined by the main hepatic vein branches. The horizontal plane is defined by the bifurcation of the main portal vein. Segments 1R and 1L are the right and left aspects of the caudate lobe (shown with a dotted outline). Segments 2 and 3 are the superior and inferior lateral portions of the left lobe. Segments 4A and 4B are the superior and inferior medial portions of the left lobe. Segments 5 and 6 are the inferior medial and lateral divisions of the right lobe. Segments 7 and 8 are the superior lateral and medial portions of the right lobe (adapted from References 3 and 106).

and III are the superior lateral and inferior lateral segments of the left lobe, IV is the medial segment of the left lobe (subdivided into IVa and IVb for superior and inferior to the left main portal branch, respectively), V and VI represent the inferior medial and lateral segments of the right lobe, and VII and VIII the superior lateral and medial segments of the right lobe. Figure 2 is a schematic illustration of these divisions of the liver.

A more general description of locations in the liver identifies position in the right or left lobes. The main lobar fissure, in which the middle hepatic vein courses, divides the anterior segment of the right lobe from the medial segment of the left. An imaginary plane running in the craniocaudal direction and extending from the gallbladder fossa through the inferior vena cava is a landmark for dividing the right and left lobes. However, when the locations of focal lesions are being described for the surgeon, the Couinaud description will be more informative. At the least, the location of any focal lesion relative to adjacent known portal venous, hepatic arterial or venous, or biliary branches will be of value, particularly if intraoperative ultrasound is contemplated (as discussed below).

The hepatic vasculature and biliary tree are readily visualized by ultrasound. Hepatic veins typically have very thin, often sonographically invisible, walls. Portal veins, biliary ducts, and hepatic artery branches, on the other hand, have readily identifiable walls. Distinguishing portal venous, biliary, and hepatic arterial structures is usually accomplished through familiarity with the anatomy. Color flow Doppler imaging is useful when there is any question because the flow direction and pulsatility distinguishes portal and arterial branches and absence of flow helps identify biliary ducts.

The upper normal limit of hepatic size, measuring from the dome to the tip of the right lobe at the midhepatic line, has been described as 15.5 cm (4). Such longitudinal measurements may be difficult with real-time ultrasound equipment because the field of view of these machines may not encompass the entire liver on a single image, and combining images is difficult at best.

CONGENITAL AND DEVELOPMENTAL ANOMALIES

Agenesis of parts of the liver has been reported (5, 6), though this is usually an incidental discovery because the remainder of the liver hypertrophies and liver function tests are usually normal. Complete situs inversus results in a mirror image of the usual anatomy with the bulk of the liver on the left (and a right-sided aorta, spleen, and descending colon).

Occasionally, diaphragmatic slips indent the hepatic dome and give the appearance of supernumerary hepatic fissures. True accessory fissures are uncommon.

Variants in hepatic arterial supply are well-known. The main hepatic artery itself, instead of arising from the celiac axis (about 45% have such variation), may arise from the superior mesenteric artery (about 2.5%). This is less common than the variants in which the right hepatic artery arises from the superior mesenteric artery or the left hepatic artery arises from the left gastric artery (about 11 and 10%, respectively) (7).

The hepatic veins are subject to considerable variation, with differences in branching and accessory veins seen fairly commonly (8). Some 30% of the general population have an accessory vein that drains Couinaud's segment VIII (the superoanterior segment of the right lobe) and empties into the middle hepatic vein or, occasionally, the right hepatic vein. Other accessory veins, some draining directly into the inferior vena cava, have also been described.

Variants of the portal venous system are the least common of hepatic vascular alterations. Absence of the right portal vein or of segments of the left portal vein is usually accompanied by altered branching of the portal vein on the affected side (9).

True hepatic cysts are assumed to be congenital in origin. Unlike cysts resulting from infection or trauma, true cysts have no such etiology and are epithelium-lined. Cysts in the liver have the "classic" appearance for ultrasound: a thin-walled, anechoic, round structure with posterior acoustic enhancement. Figure 3 shows a hepatic cyst. In my experience, it is not unusual for hepatic cysts to be "minimally complex," to borrow terminology from a description of renal cystic masses (10). Probably as a result of hemorrhage into these cysts, they have thin septations or are slightly irregular in outline. Any cystic mass that has a very thick wall, an irregularly thickened wall, thick septations, or numerous internal echoes should be viewed with suspicion of other etiologies. Estimates are that true hepatic cysts have

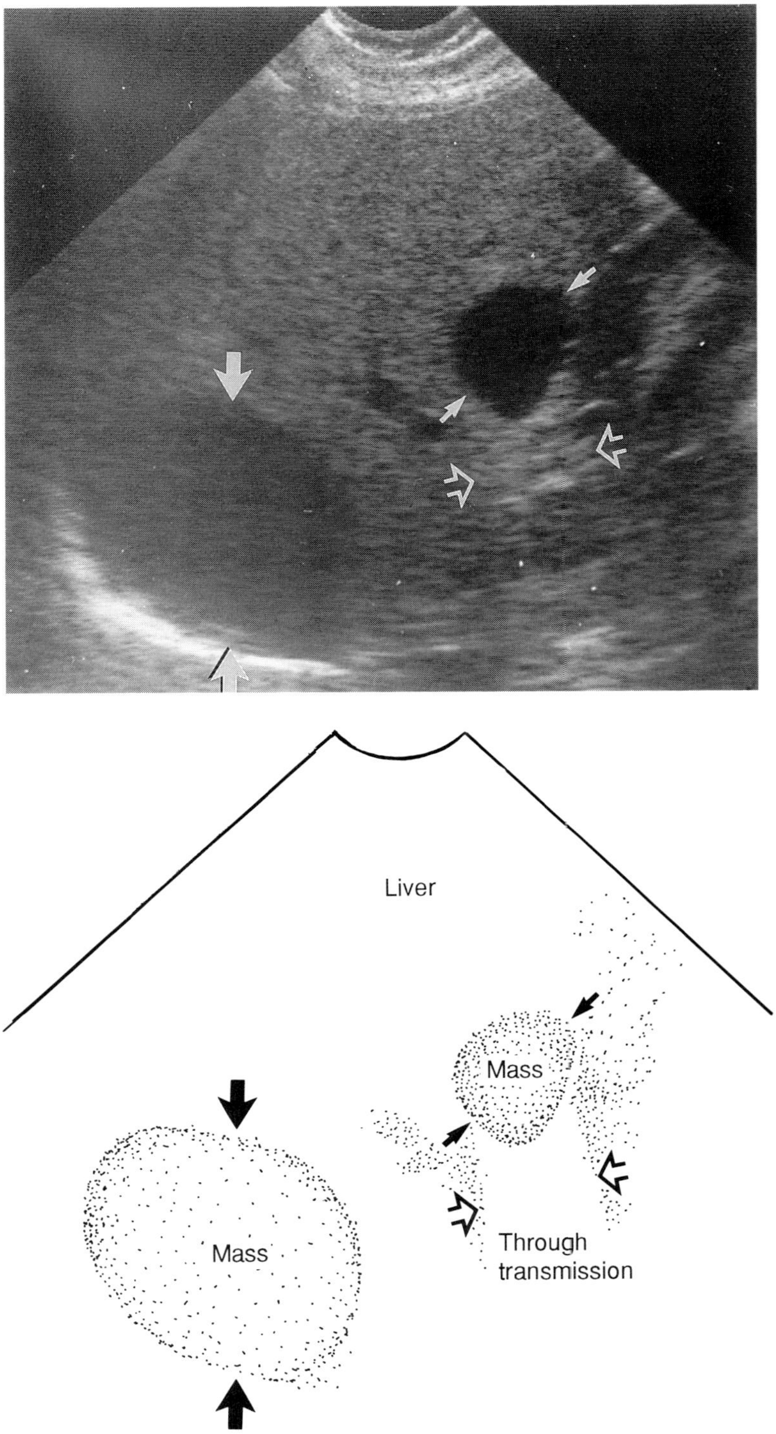

(A)

Figure 3.

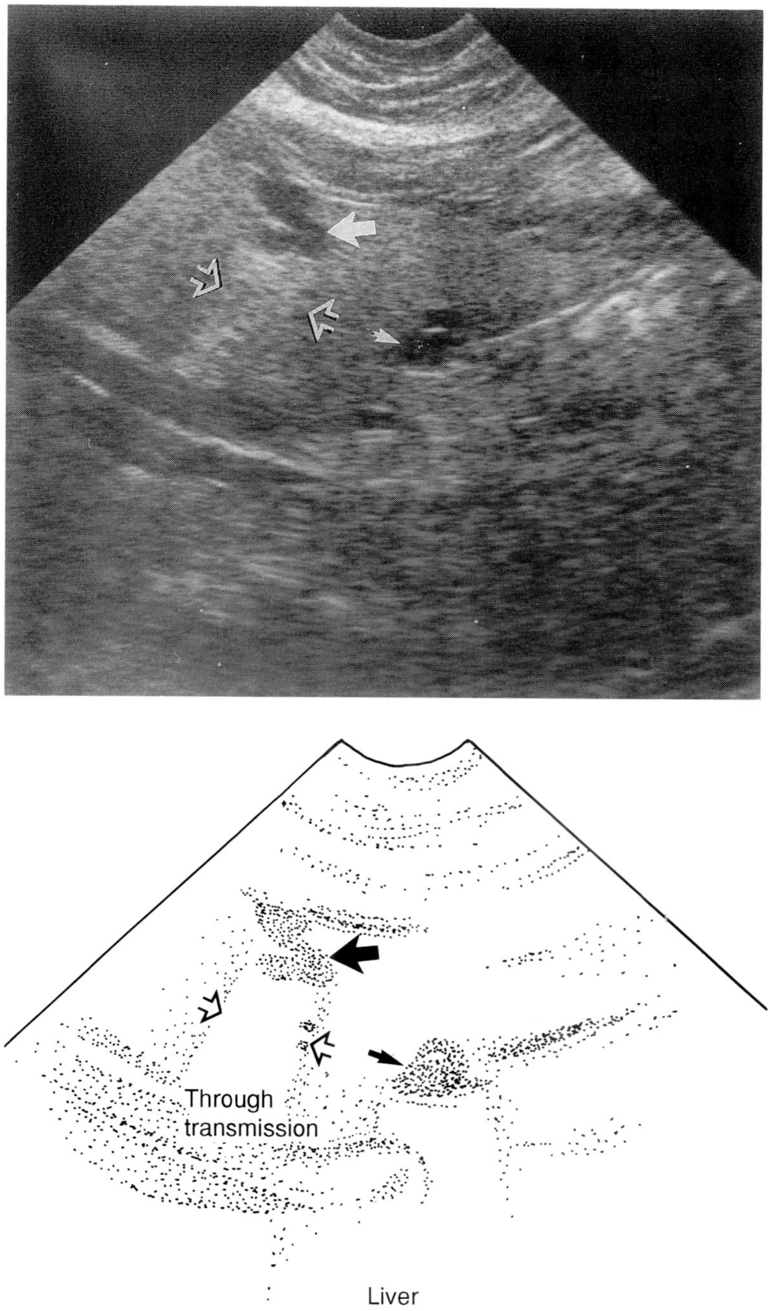

(B)

Figure 3. A patient (67-year-old male) in whom liver lesions were incidentally noted on a CT examination of the spine. (A) Two hypoechoic, well-demarcated lesions (solid large and small arrows) (previous page). (B) Two additional lesions in the same patient. These are not completely anechoic (small arrow) or smooth in outline (large arrow). In both (A) and (B) note the increased brightness of echoes behind these cysts (open arrows in both illustrations). This is known as "enhanced through transmission" and results from the lower attenuation of the ultrasound by the fluid in the masses compared to the surrounding parenchyma.

a general prevalence of about 2.5% but increase with age to about 7% in those over 80 years old (11).

True hepatic cysts also occur along with adult polycystic kidney disease (autosomal dominant form). Some 57–74% of patients who have this form of polycystic disease have associated hepatic cysts (12, 13)

DIFFUSE LIVER ABNORMALITIES

The appearance of the ultrasound texture of the liver can be an indicator of diffuse disease. Unfortunately, human perception is not an especially good discriminator of textures when the differences in texture are the result of "higher-order" statistical properties and textures are not adjacent to each other. Another problem is that too high or low a gain setting of the ultrasound machine can make the liver texture appear diffusely abnormal. Some research has shown, however, that there are texture features of diffuse diseases that computer processing of ultrasound images can detect (14). In the literature, reports of overall sensitivity of ultrasound for detection of diffuse liver disease range from 27% with a specificity of 96% (15) to a sensitivity of 60% and specificity of 92% (16). Differences in such reports could easily result from differences in patient populations. Note that the specificities are similar, indicating that if a finding of diffuse disease is made by ultrasound, it is likely to reflect a real abnormality.

Hepatitis

Hepatitis is an example of an infectious process that generally alters the texture of the liver, decreasing the normal echogenicity during an acute phase (presumably the result of edema and cellular inflammatory infiltration) and increasing it if there is resulting fatty change or fibrosis. The decreased echogenicity of the liver may be very hard to perceive, though a comparison with the spleen is useful because that organ is usually less echogenic than the liver. One sign that has been described (17) is an unusual prominence of the portal complexes (portal veins and bile ducts) because the normal echogenicity of their walls makes them stand out in a liver with a diffuse decreased echogenicity.

Fatty Infiltration

A common diffuse liver abnormality is fatty infiltration. This condition, resulting from accumulation of increased amounts of triglycerides in the hepatocytes, is often reversible and may be focal or have "spared" areas. Figure 4 shows examples of fatty infiltration of the liver. Usually, the hepatocyte-increased triglyceride storage does not result in abnormal liver function tests unless the etiology of the fatty change itself results in liver chemistry alterations. The literature has a large list of etiologies of fatty infiltration (or fatty change) (18), the most common being obesity. Alcohol intake, fasting, hyperlipidemia, excess steroids (endogenous or exogenous), diabetes, total parenteral nutrition, severe hepatitis, intestinal bypass procedures for obesity control, glycogen storage disease, cystic fibrosis, congenital generalized lipodystrophy, and toxic agents (chemotherapeutic and chemical) are all reported

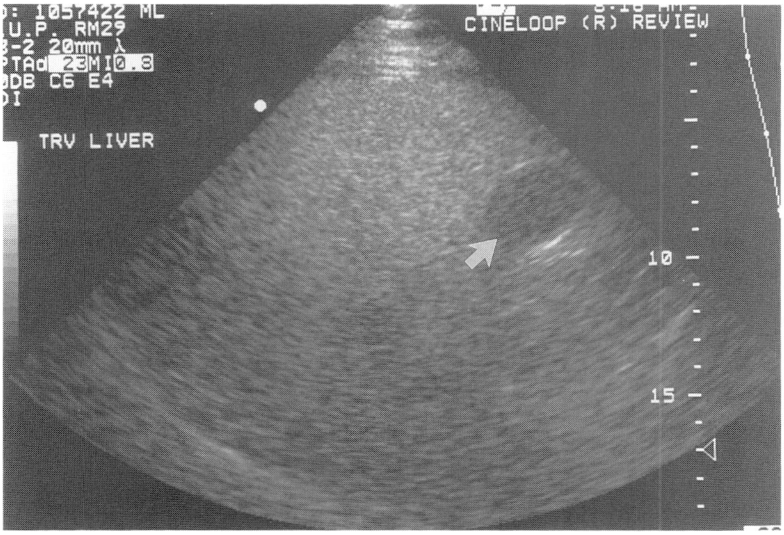

(A)

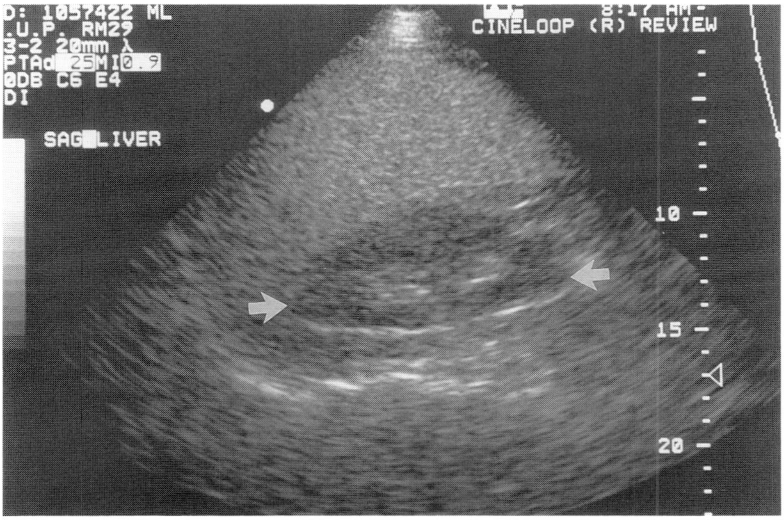

(B)

Figure 4. A 42-year-old male with mild liver function test abnormalities. (A) Diffuse increase in echogenicity of the liver parenchyma as well as increased attenuation (evidenced by the darker posterior aspect of the liver). These changes represent diffuse fatty infiltration. The arrow points out the gallbladder. (B) Contrast between the abnormally echogenic liver and the cortex of the normal right kidney (arrows). Note that the normal portal vein branches with their echogenic walls are not evident in the parenchyma; this is due to the vastly increased echogenicity of the liver.

etiologies. Unlike decreased echogenicity, the increased echogenicity of fatty liver is usually easier to recognize. Mild, moderate, and severe grades have been described (19). In the mild grades, the increased echogenicity may be hard to perceive for the inexperienced sonographer; the portal venous borders are still seen and the diaphragm is readily visualized. The abnormality may be that it is difficult to set the ultrasound machine depth-gain compensation to achieve a uniform display of the liver texture. In the severe form, the echogenic portal vein borders blend into the parenchyma, making them look more like hepatic veins. Smaller portal vessels are nearly completely masked by the increased echogenicity. The attenuation is so high that it is difficult to see the normally echogenic diaphragm. An important caveat in fatty infiltration is that it may mask small focal lesions, and if metastatic or other focal masses are suspected alternative liver imaging (CT or MRI) should be considered.

Cirrhosis

Cirrhosis from varied causes (alcoholic or post-infectious) results in the same ultrasound appearance of the liver because the pathological process of liver fibrosis and resulting nodularity is an end point. The nodularity is due to a combination of hepatocyte death, fibrotic changes, and regeneration. In its micronodular form, the nodules are on the order of 1 mm to 1 cm in size. The macronodular form, in contrast, has a larger variation of nodule sizes up to 5 cm (20). The ultrasound appearance of the liver is one of diffuse heterogeneity. Because the use of low-frequency transducers can produce spuriously coarse-looking liver texture, practitioners must learn to recognize how their equipment shows normal liver. Switching to a higher-frequency transducer may also be helpful, though some depth penetration in large or obese patients will then be sacrificed. If the patient has ascites around the liver, an irregular liver surface is good evidence of cirrhosis (though extensive metastatic disease can also produce the finding; clinical grounds should help differentiate these etiologies). Figure 5 shows an example of a cirrhotic liver. In severe cirrhosis, the inferior surface of the liver will appear irregular even without ascites to outline it. In acute cirrhosis, the entire liver may be enlarged, but as the disease progresses, the left lobe and caudate lobe tend to remain normal sized (or enlarge) as the right lobe diminishes in size (21). Finally, it may be possible to identify regenerating nodules to assist in diagnosis. However, the possible occurrence of hepatocellular carcinoma (including the multifocal variety) in patients with cirrhosis from chronic hepatitis should make the practitioner cautious about assuming that discrete nodular hepatic masses seen on ultrasound are regenerating nodules. Biopsy to confirm or reject this possibility is often necessary.

Storage Diseases

The storage diseases, glycogen and iron, diffusely alter the appearance of the liver. Glycogen-storage disease (type I—renal and hepatic involvement) has an ultrasound appearance indistinguishable from fatty infiltration: diffusely increased echogenicity. In the nonpediatric age group who have glycogen-storage disease, an increased occurrence of liver cell adenomas and, to a lesser extent, hepatocellular

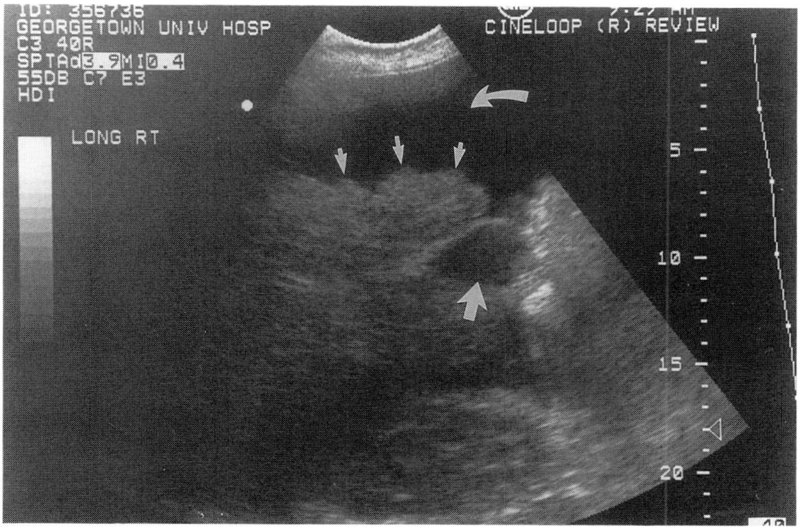

Figure 5. A longitudinal view of the liver in a patient with advanced cirrhosis (54-year-old female). The small arrows show the irregular liver edge. The curved arrow points out the ascites. The large arrow shows the gallbladder.

carcinomas has been described (22). The finding of focal masses in such patients should raise the suspicion of these neoplasms.

Disorders of iron metabolism can result in increased stores of iron in the liver. Hemochromatosis is a term usually reserved for the hereditary form of the disease of excessive iron uptake. Other causes including the iron-loading anemias (such as β-thalassemia, sideroblastic anemia, and pyruvate kinase deficiency), congenital atransferrinemia, increased oral intake of iron, and parenteral iron administration (23) can all result in increases of hepatic iron stores. Increased hepatic iron in chronic liver disease, in contrast, is usually reticuloendothelial rather than hepatic parenchymal. The increased iron content of the hepatocytes results in liver parenchyma of very high ultrasound attenuation. I have seen this manifested by the inability to image the deep portions of the liver fully in an individual whose body habitus is thin. In late iron-storage diseases, especially hemochromatosis, the liver becomes cirrhotic. Ultrasound is not the imaging study of choice for iron-storage diseases, but should be considered in the patient with abnormal liver function tests whose liver is very difficult to penetrate despite the use of high output settings and low-frequency transducers.

Diffuse Metastatic Disease

Occasionally, metastatic diseases may result in diffuse infiltration of the liver. On the basis of ultrasound imaging alone, this can be very difficult to distinguish from cirrhosis. The clinical history should help distinguish the etiologies. Breast and lung carcinomas and melanoma are among the nonhematologic neoplasms that can produce diffuse liver metastases (24). Diffuse liver involvement from the leukemias and lymphomas is also a common pattern. Figure 6 is an example of diffuse liver involvement by lymphoma. Because distinguishing a primary source from the liver ultrasound appearance alone is nearly impossible, biopsy is usually indicated.

Infectious Processes

Diffuse infectious processes of the liver include the viral hepatitides and bacterial or parasitic diseases. Hepatitis was discussed above. Although most bacterial infections do not result in diffuse hepatic involvement, in the patient who is immunocompromised for any reason, atypical infections are likely. Of the bacterial diseases, infection by *Mycobacterium avium intracellulare* (MAI) is known to cause diffuse liver disease. Among viral illnesses in immunocompromised patients, cytomegalovirus may cause a diffuse hepatic infiltration. In both these infections, the result has a very similar ultrasound appearance of innumerable small echogenic foci scattered throughout the liver (25, 26). Figure 7 shows an example of diffuse hepatic involvement by MAI in an AIDS patient.

Immunocompromised patients may also become infected with the protozoan *Pneumocystis carinii*. This organism, if it involves the liver, can result in an ultrasound appearance indistinguishable from that of MAI or cytomegalovirus infection (26). Diffuse fungal infection, chiefly from *Candida*, is another infectious process that affects the immunocompromised host. Unlike MAI, cytomegalovirus, or *Pneumocystis carinii* infection, however, diffuse hepatic candidiasis most often produces a diffuse, coarse hypoechoic pattern, though late scarring can produce calcifications (24). I have seen diffuse hepatic candidiasis produce an appearance sonographically indistinguishable from extensive metastatic disease with innumerable hypoechoic masses in the liver.

Schistosomiasis can also produce diffuse changes in the liver, though what is usually seen is the end result of the infection with an appearance of cirrhosis and portal hypertension. The infectious process results in chronic periportal inflammation with resultant scarring and rise in resistance to portal venous flow.

FOCAL LIVER ABNORMALITIES

A search for focal liver abnormalities is one of the more common reasons for performing a diagnostic ultrasound examination. Focal liver lesions encompass a large number of etiologies; those described here are either common or illustrative. Ultrasound has a much higher sensitivity for detection of focal liver abnormalities than for diffuse disease, but the sensitivity varies with the etiology.

Benign

Focal Fatty Infiltration. In addition to the more common diffuse pattern of fatty infiltration, this entity may involve focal regions of the liver, producing irregularly bordered echogenic areas. Occasionally, these may follow an anatomic plane, giving rise to a more sharply demarcated edge. Focal fatty change has also been known to produce rounded lesions that can be difficult to distinguish from other focal liver abnormalities.

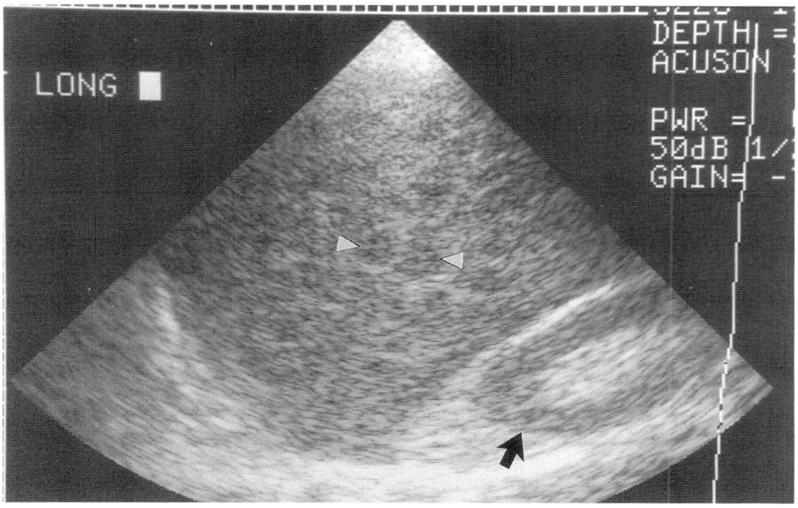

(A)

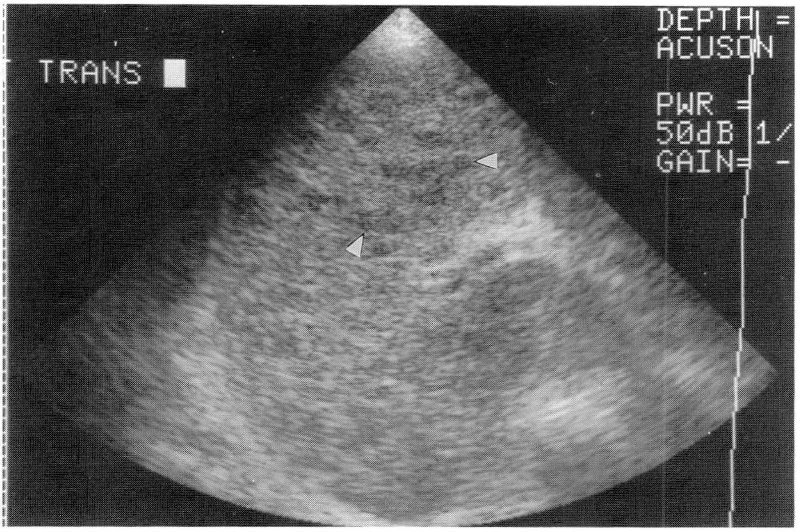

(B)

Figure 6. Biopsy proved diffuse hepatic involvement by lymphoma (mixed cell) in a 50-year-old male. (A) An overall very heterogeneous liver in longitudinal view. The arrowheads point to two of the numerous masses in the liver. The arrow shows the right kidney. (B) More of the many small lesions in a transverse view. The arrowheads again show two of the more readily visible masses.

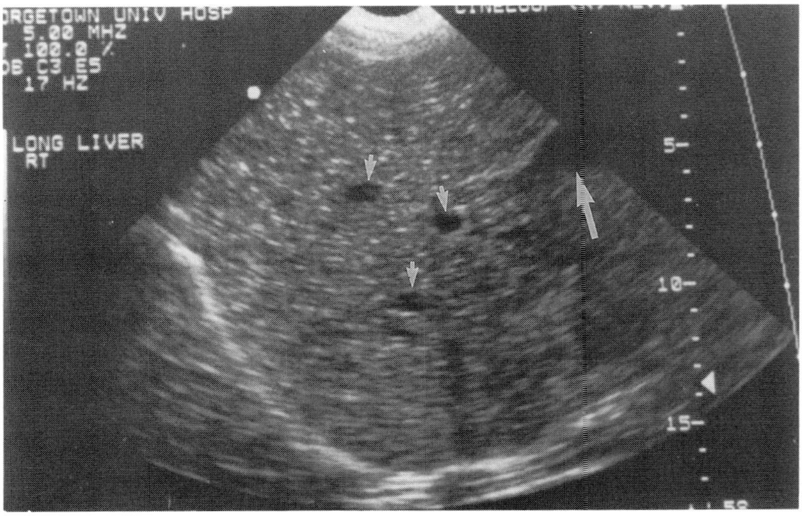

(A)

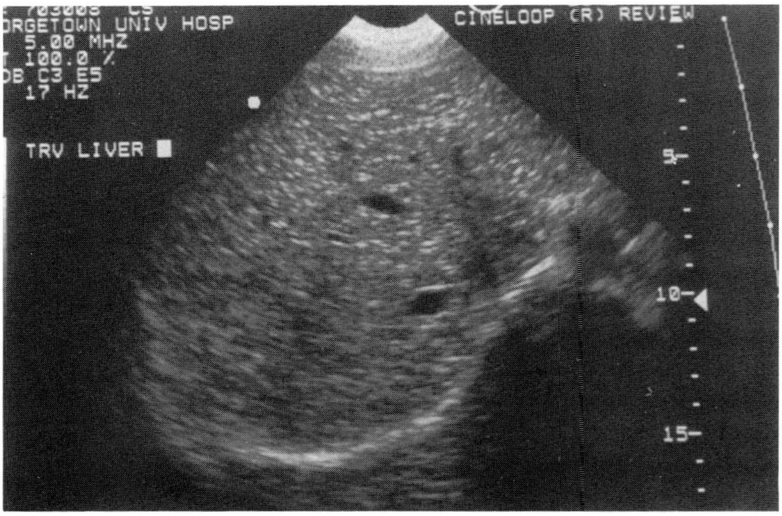

(B)

Figure 7. A 37-year-old male AIDS patient with disseminated MAI. (A) Longitudinal and (B) lateral view of the liver showing widespread punctate echogenic foci representing hepatic involvement by MAI. In (A) the small arrows show portal vein branches. The large arrow points to the neck of the gallbladder.

An important differential diagnostic point is that focal fatty infiltration does not result in any mass effect. Hence hepatic vessels and biliary ducts pass through these regions with no displacement or narrowing (24). This is not true of most of the other focal liver lesions described in this section.

In the situation of diffuse fatty infiltration, the opposite phenomenon of focal infiltration may occur. This is focal sparing; it results in relatively hypoechoic areas in the background of an overall increase in hepatic echogenicity. Figure 8 is an example of focal sparing in fatty infiltration.

Hepatic Hemangioma. Another common benign liver lesion is the hepatic cavernous hemangioma, occurring in some 4% of the general population and showing a distinct female preponderance (about 5:1) (27). These lesions have a characteristic ultrasound appearance of a well-circumscribed, round, homogeneous, echogenic mass. They may be multiple, though a multiplicity of lesions should increase the suspicion of a metastatic etiology. Figure 9 shows a hemangioma. Atypical appearances of hemangiomata are not common, but do occur. Large hemangiomata may have irregular borders and be slightly to moderately heterogeneous. Occasionally, they are hypoechoic relative to the rest of the liver, especially in fatty infiltration.

Unfortunately, despite the vascular nature of these lesions, Doppler and even color flow Doppler imaging is not very useful in confirming their nature because of the very slow blood flow in them. High flow on Doppler studies, in fact, should raise the suspicion that the lesion is not a hemangioma. Confirmation that a lesion is a hemangioma is through the use of radionuclide-labeled red cell single photon emission CT (SPECT) scans or an MR examination. Although CT specifically done to evaluate a suspected hemangioma is also effective, both radiolabeled red cell SPECT and MR are more so, with MR particularly advantageous for small lesions (28–31).

Liver Cell Adenoma and Focal Nodular Hyperplasia. Liver cell adenomas and focal nodular hyperplasia (FNH) are two benign liver conditions that result in hepatic masses. These entities are often impossible to distinguish on the basis of ultrasound findings alone. In both cases, the masses may be solitary or multiple, though liver cell adenomas are much more likely to be single lesions. Differentiating between adenomas and FNH is often based on radionuclide or angiographic examination, though biopsy is often needed for definitive diagnosis. On the basis of ultrasound and other noninvasive examinations, percutaneous biopsy has been recommended if FNH is suspected and operative biopsy if adenoma is more favored (32). This recommendation is based in part on the tendency of adenomas to bleed. Spontaneous hemorrhage from hepatic adenoma is uncommon, but strongly suggests adenoma over FNH if it occurs. Differentiation is important because hepatic adenomas have a malignant transformation potential as well as a risk of hemorrhage (33). The ultrasound appearance of both hepatic adenomas and FNH can be hypoechoic, echogenic, mixed, or nearly isoechoic compared to normal liver (24). Figure 10 shows an example of a large liver cell adenoma. Recent reports of the use of color flow Doppler ultrasound suggest that some of the angiographic features characteristic of FNH, the central avascular area (or "scar") with abundant peripheral flow and some radial vessels, can be visualized with this technique and may help differentiate FNH from other liver lesions (34–36).

Liver Abscess. Infectious liver processes that result in focal lesions include both bacterial and fungal etiologies. Most bacterial liver abscesses are the result of direct extension from infected biliary radicles (24) in patients with infectious cholangitis and cholecystitis. Other routes for bacterial infection of the liver include the portal venous system, especially in patients with bacterial infections of the bowel, and the

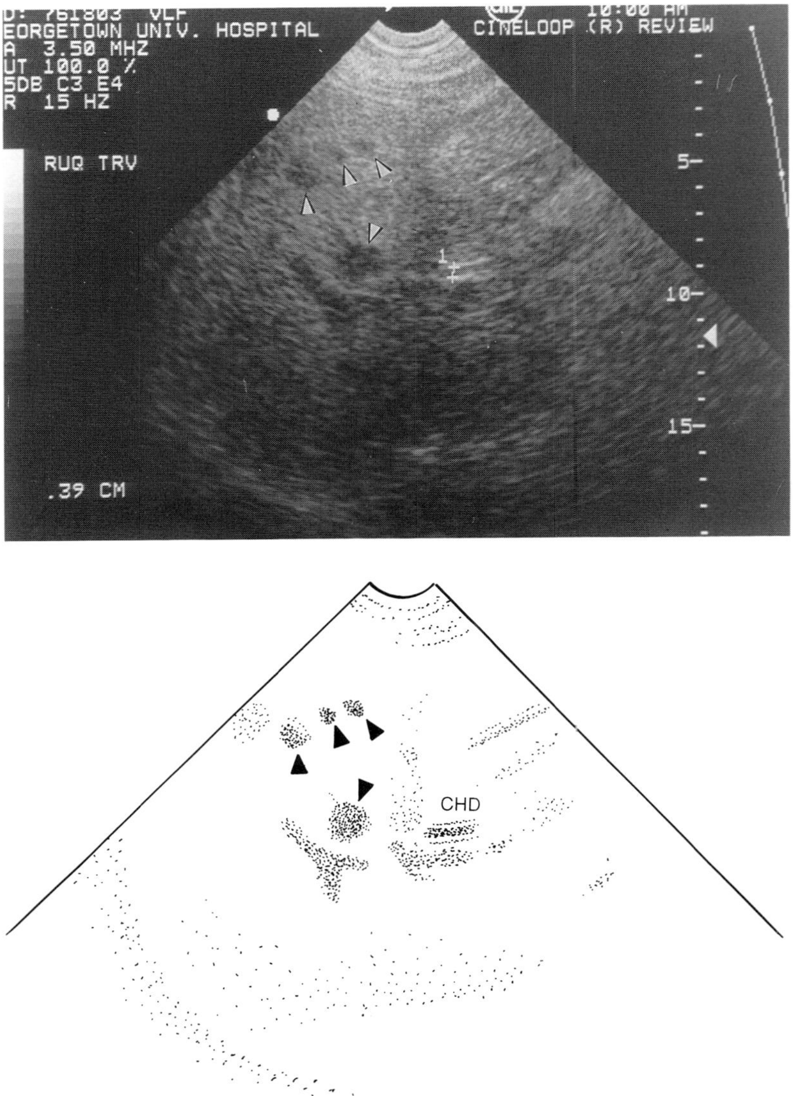

(A)

Figure 8. This patient (a 45-year-old male) has diffuse fatty infiltration of the liver. In the longitudinal view (A), arrowheads point to focal hypoechoic "lesions." These represent areas of focal sparing of the liver from the fatty change. The "hypoechoic" appearance of these areas in part represents normal liver texture surrounded by much more echogenic parenchyma. The cross-shaped cursors are measuring the common hepatic duct (0.39 cm—normal). (B) Similar regions (arrowheads) adjacent to the gallbladder (curved arrow) (next page).

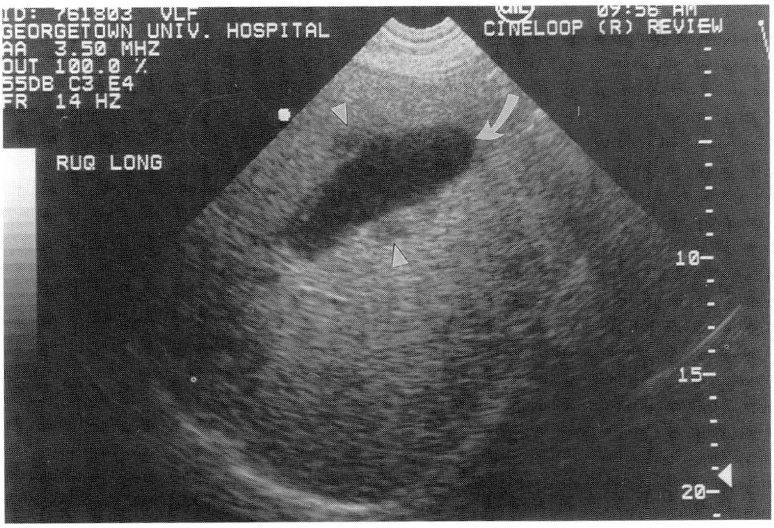

(B)

Figure 8. *(Continued)*

hepatic arteries in patients with systemic bacteremia from a variety of causes. Direct puncture wounds of the liver in cases of penetrating abdominal trauma can introduce bacteria into the liver parenchyma.

The appearance of bacterial hepatic abscesses varies to some degree according to when the scans are performed relative to the onset of infection. In very early infection, before there is much necrosis and pus formation, the affected area or areas may be barely distinguishable from the unaffected surrounding liver. There may be a slight decrease in normal echogenicity in the infected area, but the difference can be obscured in obese patients whose livers are difficult to penetrate and in those with preexisting diffuse liver disease. As the abscess is established it is more readily seen. The sonographic character of abscesses can range from nearly solid to cystic. Those that consist largely of purulent material are often nearly cystic in appearance, though fine internal echoes or a fluid-fluid level may be seen. The border of the abscess can range from a well-defined, often thick, wall to an ill-defined transition to normal liver. Color flow Doppler may show increased flow around an abscess corresponding to hyperemia. If the infecting agent is a gas-producing bacterium, gas bubbles may be present in the abscess. These may be trapped in the debris within, producing bright foci in the abscess associated with ill-defined ("dirty") shadowing. If the internal consistency is largely liquefied, the gas bubbles rise to the least dependent portion of the collection, producing bright echoes in that portion also with "dirty" shadowing behind. Particularly with an arterial hematogenous source, liver abscesses may be multiple.

The efficacy of ultrasound for diagnosis of hepatic abscesses is high but compared to CT, has been reported as both superior (37), with a 93% detection rate compared with 87% for CT, and inferior (38), with a 79% detection rated compared with 97%

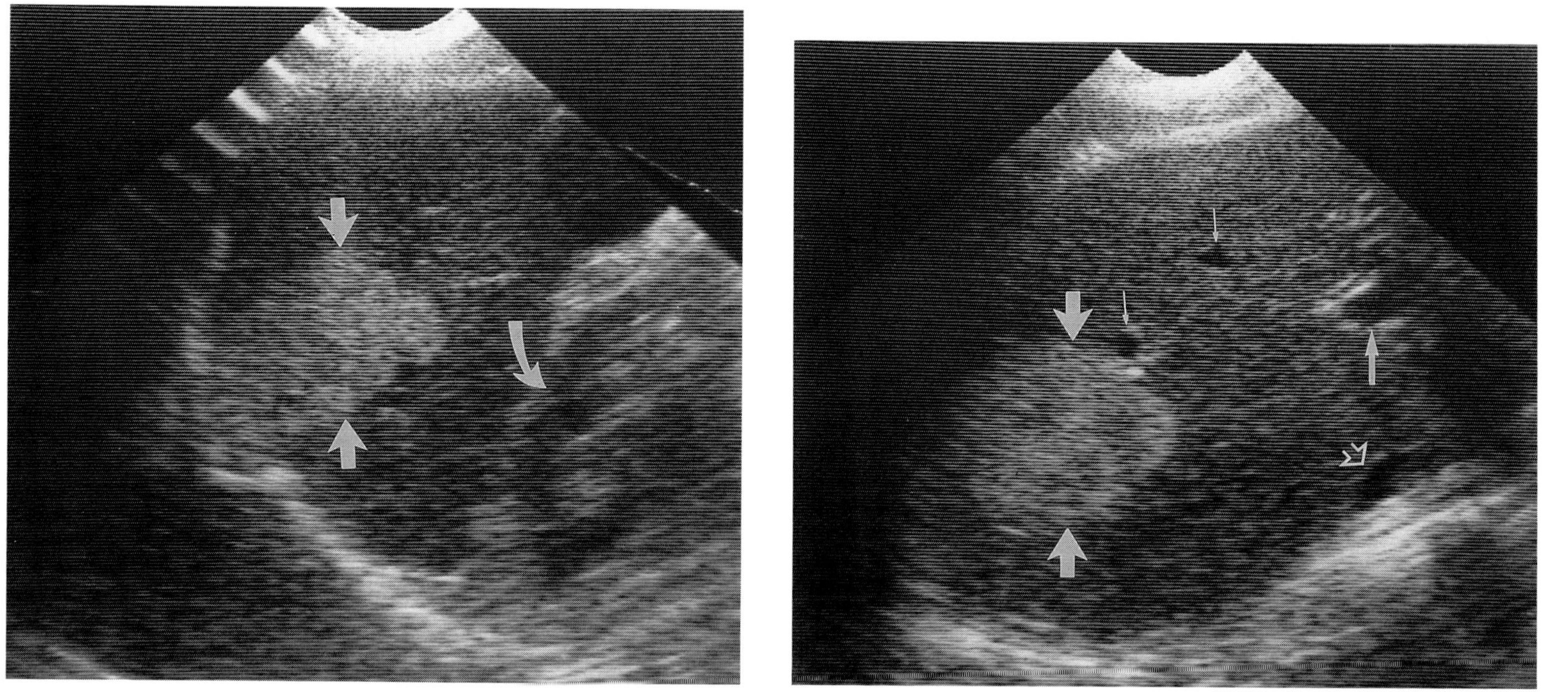

(A) (B)

Figure 9. Longitudinal (A) and transverse (B) scans of the liver in an 80-year-old male. This patient had colon carcinoma, but the echogenic mass shown (arrows) was noted to be unchanged in size or ultrasound character for more than a year following a previous ultrasound study. In addition, liver function tests were normal. This mass represents a hemangioma. Note the well-circumscribed appearance. The slight heterogeneity of the mass is not unusual in larger hemangiomata and usually represents thrombosed portions of the hemangioma. The curved arrow in (A) shows the right kidney. The small arrow in (B) points out the main portal vein and the open arrow shows the inferior vena cava. The two very small arrows show portal vein branches.

for CT. Halvorsen and colleagues (38) noted the reasons for the failures of both imaging methods to detect the lesions missed. In CT, the missed cases had a diffuse low-attenuation pattern throughout the liver. For ultrasound, false negatives were due to the location of the abscess high in the dome of the liver, the small size of the abscess, and large but very early abscesses.

Though the clinical history usually helps differentiate a hepatic abscess from other causes of focal liver lesions, based on ultrasound appearance the differential diagnosis for hepatic abscesses includes hemorrhagic hepatic cysts, hepatic hematomas, and necrotic metastases. Parasitic infections (discussed in the next section), particularly amebic, can produce liver lesions indistinguishable from pyogenic abscesses on the basis of ultrasound alone.

Parasitic Diseases. Included in the category of hepatic abscesses is the lesion caused by the parasitic amoeba *Entamoeba histolytica*. This protozoan parasite infects the colon and, if it penetrates the colonic mucosa, can enter the draining veins of the colon and so gain access to the portal venous system. This is the mechanism of hepatic infection. If established in the liver, the amebic abscess has features that are very similar to pyogenic abscesses. It is usually hypoechoic with an ill-defined wall. Internally, there are numerous fine echoes (Fig. 11). Both shape (round or ovoid more commonly than in pyogenic abscesses) and the ultrasound texture (fine internal echoes more commonly than in pyogenic abscesses) (39) may be of value in distinguishing the two etiologies. A positive result from a serum hemagglutinin test for amebiasis is considered confirmatory of the diagnosis (40).

Infection by the parasitic agent *Echinococcus granulosus* (the most common etiologic agent in humans) may result in liver involvement. This parasite, a tapeworm in the primary host, causes hydatid disease in humans, a secondary host (24). The "classic" lesion on ultrasound is usually a solitary complex cystic mass in the right lobe of the liver. It may reach a large size and have a variable internal appearance. The simplest in appearance have internal debris and the most complex have multiple "daughter cysts." Echinococcal cysts may also occur in other organs besides the liver, and identifying a liver lesion should prompt thorough evaluation of other abdominal organs, and possibly the central nervous system. Figure 12 illustrates hepatic echinococcal disease. Treatment of hepatic echinococcal disease is chiefly surgical, though percutaneous drainage and medical therapy have also been used (24).

Malignant

Metastases. Metastases to the liver, whether from other viscera that have portal venous drainage or from distant primary malignancies, are unfortunately common. That the liver has both a large portal and systemic blood flow would certainly account for this high incidence. Autopsy series of patients with primary neoplasms have shown liver metastases in some 38–41.4% (41). Of metastases, nearly half (48%) are from viscera with portal venous drainage. However, breast and lung malignancies are the next highest in frequency of liver metastases (42). Note that these data are for patient populations in the United States. In some Southeast Asian and South African countries, the incidence of hepatocellular carcinoma is much higher than in the United States and Europe.

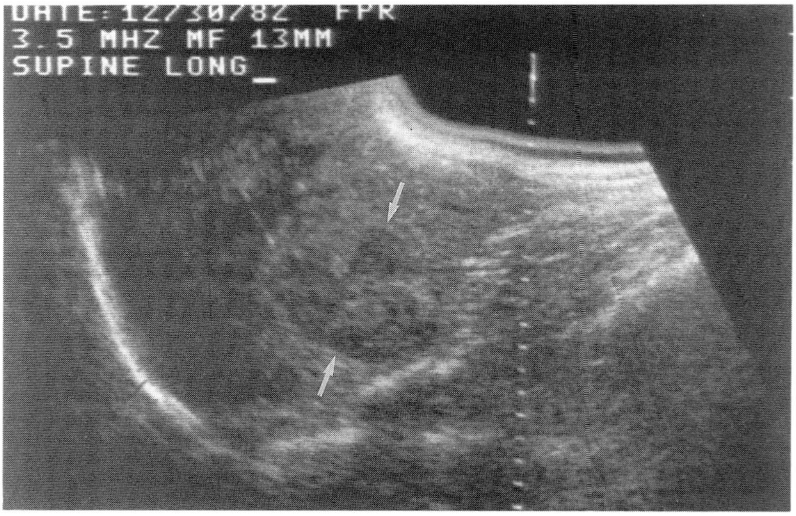

(A)

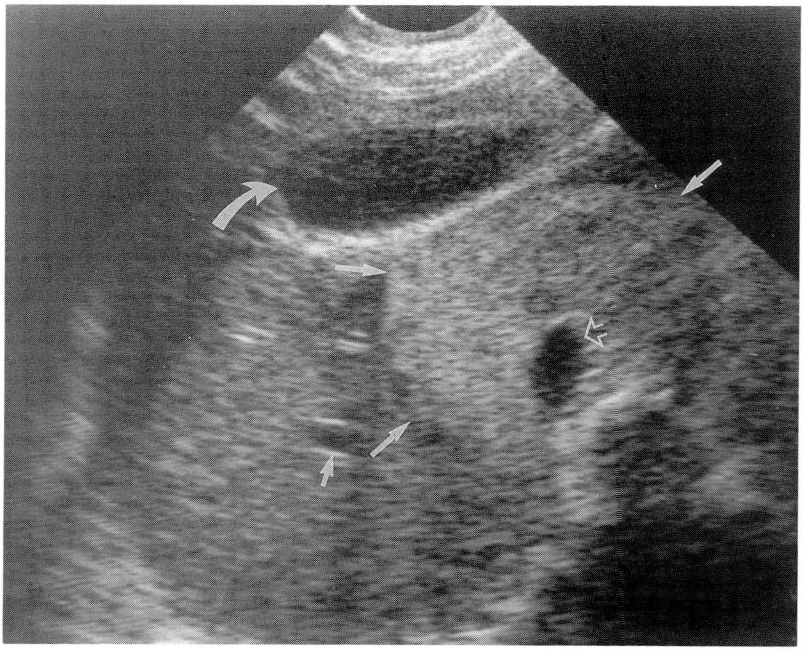

(B)

Figure 10. These scans are from a young woman (28 years old) who presented with "irritable bowel" and mild liver function test abnormalities. (A) is a saggital articulated-arm scan of the liver (an older piece of ultrasound equipment now rarely used). The arrows show a portion of a large, irregular liver mass. (B) Real-time transverse scan of the liver. The small arrows show a portion of the mass surrounding the inferior vena cava (open arrow). The short small arrow points out the right branch of the portal vein. The curved arrow shows the gallbladder. (C) CT scan of the liver. Note that the mass (low attenuation area; small arrows) appears much larger than on the ultrasound study. This is in part an artifact owing to the ultrasound scan being angled cephalad and thus not through the same portion of the liver as shown on the CT. The curved arrow shows the gallbladder. The long straight arrow points out the portal vein. The inferior vena cava is shown by the open arrow (next page).

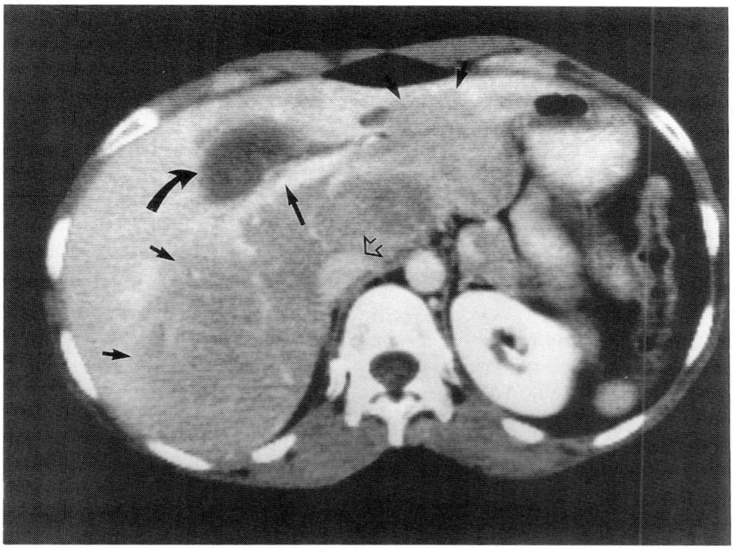

(C)

Figure 10. *(Continued).*

Ultrasound has proved to be sensitive and specific for the detection of metastatic disease, but not usually specific for the primary malignant etiology. Sensitivity appears to be lower for lymphomatous liver involvement (43) than for other metastases. For colon carcinoma metastatic to the liver, sensitivity as high as 100% has been reported (44).

The ultrasound appearance of metastatic lesions is variable. Size, echogenicity relative to normal liver, borders, interior texture, and presence of internal blood flow by color flow Doppler all vary and, unfortunately, do not do so with any regularity with respect to the primary tumor. Figure 13 shows an example of extensive metastatic disease. There are, however, some tendencies that can help narrow a differential diagnosis or direct a search for a primary lesion (24).

Metastases that are hypoechoic relative to normal liver are generally associated with hypovascular pathology. Lymphomas of both the Hodgkin's and non-Hodgkin's type should be considered when hypoechoic metastases are seen. This is especially true in primary non-Hodgkin's lymphoma of the liver or in AIDS-associated lymphoma (45, 46). Lymphomatous involvement of the liver is otherwise more likely to be a diffuse process.

Echogenic metastases are more likely to have hypervascular pathology. Metastases from gastrointestinal and hepatocellular primaries are more likely to be echogenic, though they are not always hypervascular. See Figure 14 for an example of an echogenic metastasis very similar to a hemangioma in appearance. Highly vascular primary tumors such as pancreatic islet cell carcinoma, renal cell carcinoma, choriocarcinoma, and carcinoid, when metastatic to the liver often result in echogenic metastases.

Cystic metastases are not common, though primary tumors that have a cystic component, such as mucinous carcinoma of the large bowel and cystadenocarcinoma

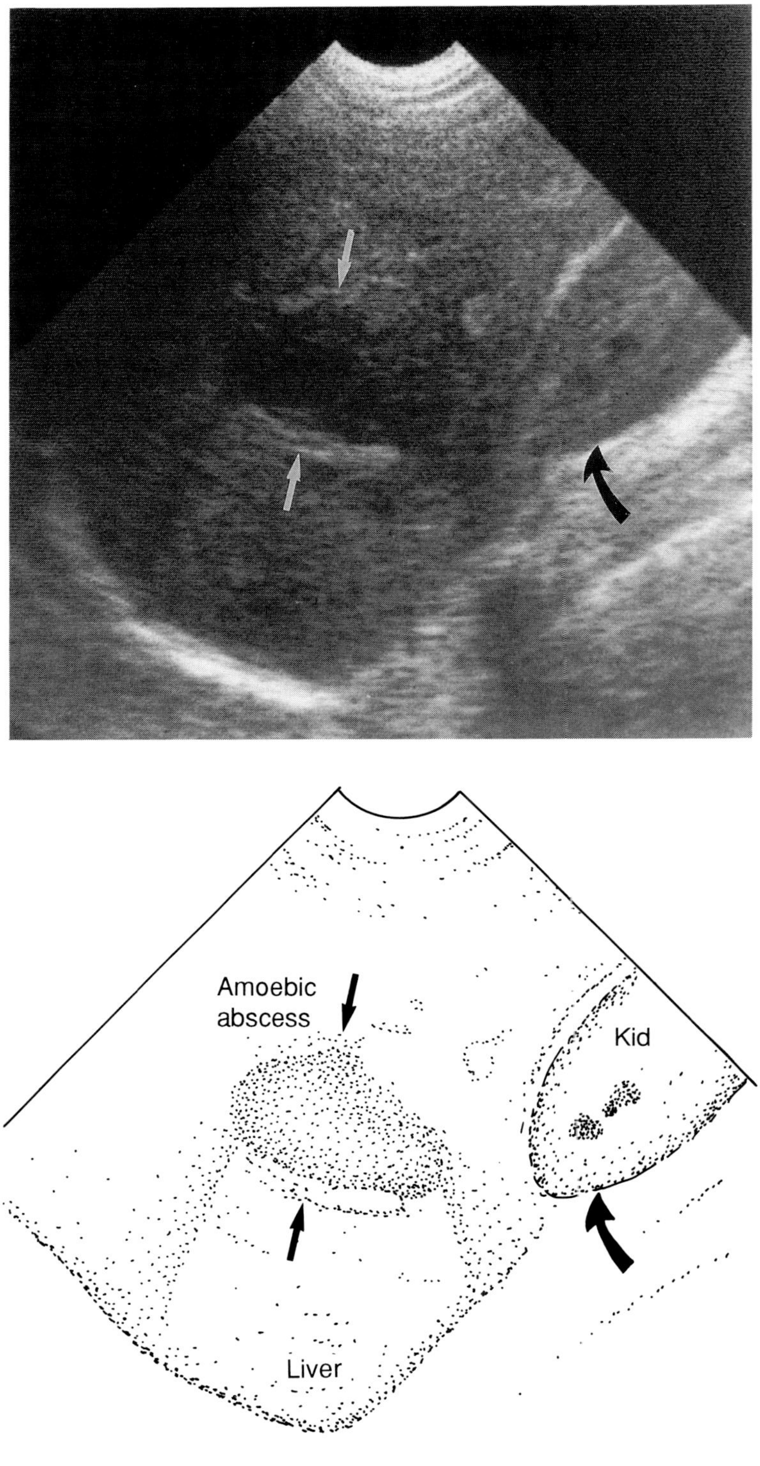

Figure 11. An amebic liver abscess in a 38-year-old woman who had had several bouts of amebic dysentery in the past. The scan is transverse through the liver and the abscess is shown by the arrows. The curved arrow points out the right kidney.

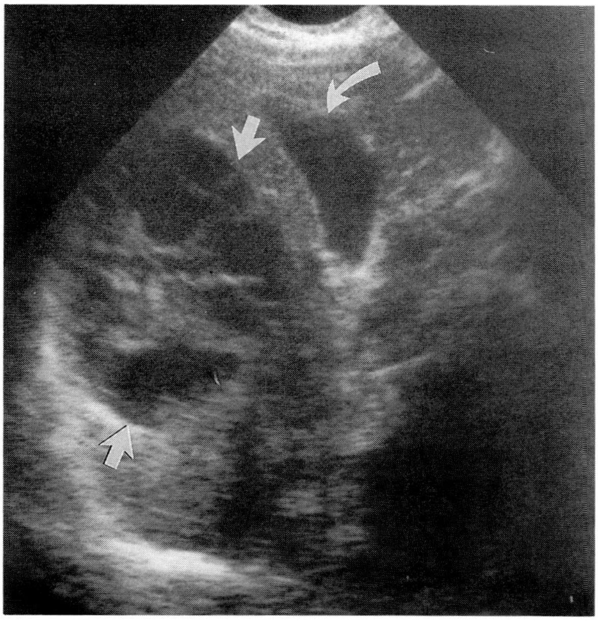

(A)

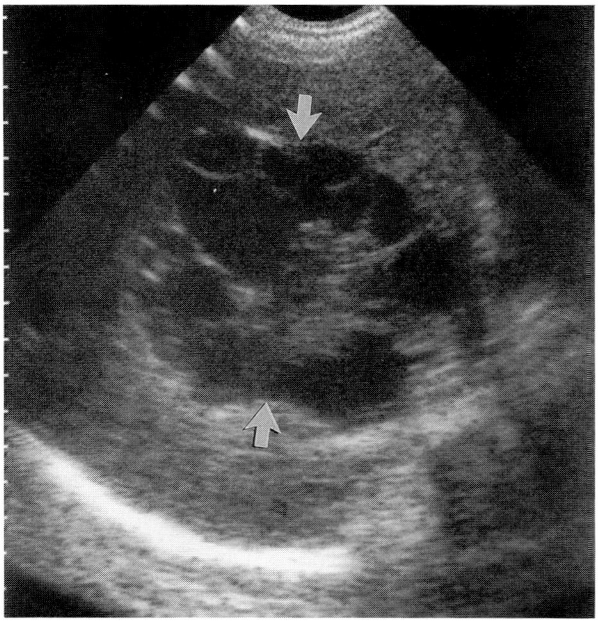

(B)

Figure 12. Saggital (A) and transverse (B) scans of the liver in an 83-year-old woman showing an incidentally discovered complex liver mass (arrows). This represents an echinococcal cyst. In (A) the curved arrow shows the gallbladder with some mass effect on its superior aspect secondary to the mass

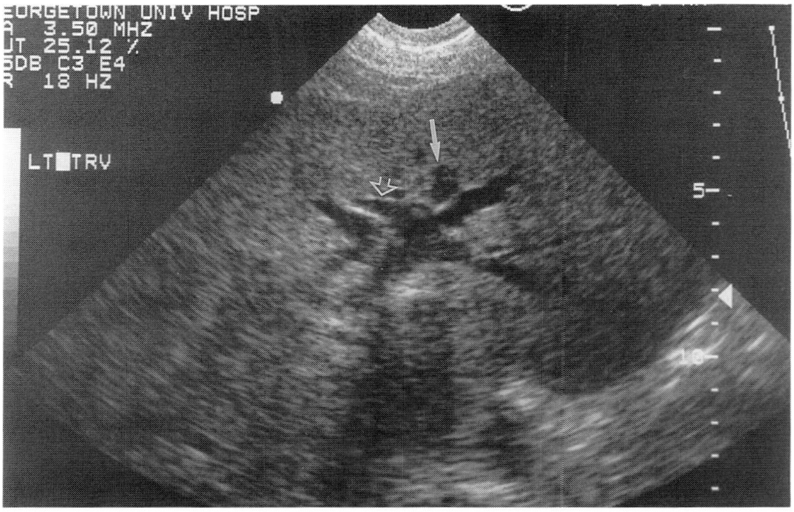

Figure 13. Transverse scan through the left lobe of the liver in a 49-year-old woman with weight loss and jaundice. The patient had multiple hypoechoic liver metastases, one of which is shown by the arrow. The open arrow points to a dilated bile duct, part of the more widespread biliary ductal dilatation due to metastases obstructing the biliary tree at the porta hepatis. The lesions were poorly differentiated and the primary was unknown, though both a gallbladder and gynecologic neoplasm were possibilities.

of the pancreas and ovary, may produce cystic lesions when metastatic to the liver. These lesions, however, are usually not confused with simple hepatic cysts because they have thick walls, mural nodules, thick septations, and complex fluid content. The mural nodules and thick septations, if present, may also show flow in them on color flow Doppler. The thin septations that may be seen in hepatic cysts should not show any flow within them. A solid metastatic lesion that has become necrotic may develop a cystic appearance, though this is also usually easily differentiated from a simple cyst because the borders are irregular or the walls thick. Metastases from primary sarcomas are somewhat more likely to have necrosis.

Some metastases have a so-called "bull's-eye" or "target" appearance. These metastases have a hypoechoic rim with an echogenic center (see Fig. 25). They are not characteristic of any particular primary tumor, though when bronchogenic carcinoma is metastatic to the liver it is more likely to produce this pattern. The etiology of the hypoechoic region is attributed differently in autopsy studies. Wernecke and colleagues (47) concluded that, in the population studied, the hypoechoic halo was due in a majority of cases to a region of proliferating tumor in the periphery of the lesion. In a pathological–sonographic series by Marchal and colleagues (48) a different conclusion was reached; the halo is extratumoral and the result of compression of peritumoral liver parenchyma in a majority of cases. The discrepancies between these two sets of contradictory findings could readily be explained by differences in the primary tumor incidence mix between the two patient populations. What is certain is that the phenomenon has more than one cause.

Some primary tumors develop liver metastases with calcifications within the masses. In this circumstance, the lesions have focal areas of high echogenicity associated with acoustic shadowing (see Fig. 23). If the calcifications are small and

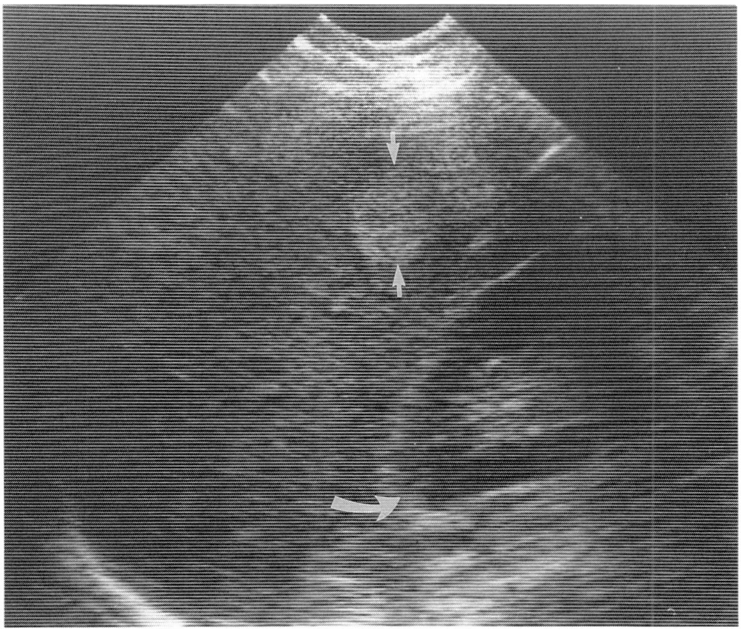

(A)

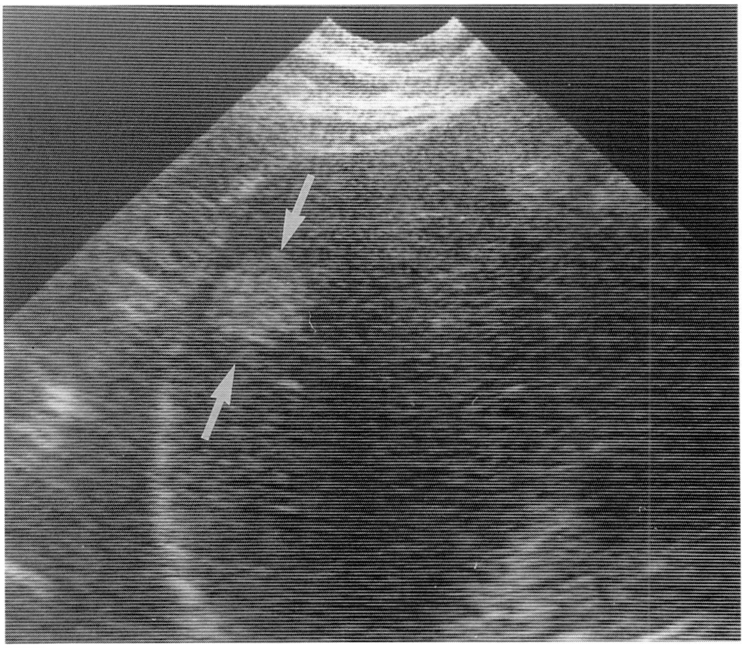

(B)

Figure 14. Two images showing two different lesions in the same patient, a 65-year-old female with colon carcinoma. The echogenic mass shown by the arrows in (A) proved to be a hemangioma by radionuclide-labeled red cell single photon emission CT scanning. The curved arrow in (A) shows the kidney. The echogenic mass in (B) (arrows) proved to be a metastasis. Note that the upper pole of the kidney is not seen on this transverse scan, which would be the case if this were the same lesion imaged in (A).

diffusely scattered, the entire lesion may be echogenic and the shadowing may be so pronounced that only the anterior aspect of the mass is seen. There is a sizable list of primary neoplasms that can result in calcified metastases. The most common is mucinous adenocarcinoma of the colon. Other primary malignancies that are known to produce calcified metastases include pancreatic endocrine tumors, leiomyosarcomas, gastric adenocarcinoma, osteogenic sarcoma, chondrosarcoma, neuroblastoma, and ovarian cystadenocarcinoma and teratocarcinoma (49).

A pattern of liver metastases that is particularly difficult to detect and, if detected, hard to distinguish from cirrhosis on the basis of the ultrasound alone, is seen with diffuse metastatic disease. Typically, the overall liver texture is very coarsened, and if an examination is done with a high-frequency transducer for the portion of the liver that can be visualized, innumerable small masses may be evident. Withers and Wilson (24) attribute such a pattern most commonly to metastatic lung carcinoma and malignant melanoma.

Primary Hepatic Malignancies. Of the primary malignant tumors of the liver, the most common is hepatocellular carcinoma (HCC). As noted earlier, the incidence of HCC has a wide variation with geographic location. In the United States and Europe, incidence is typically fewer than five cases per 100,000 population per year. In areas of high incidence, the incidence can be more than four times higher, at more than 20 cases per 100,000 population per year (42). The primary etiologic agents for HCC fall into three categories: infectious, chemical, and cirrhotic.

The infectious etiology is an increased risk of HCC in people with hepatitis B or C. For hepatitis B, the risk seems to be high in those who develop a carrier state. The risk in hepatitis C is somewhat different in that HCC tends to develop in chronic hepatitis C after the disease has resulted in cirrhosis (42).

The one chemical agent known to increase risk of HCC is aflatoxin B_1. This by-product of the metabolism of *Aspergillus flavus* appears to be associated with a mutation in the tumor suppressor gene p53. Epidemiologic studies have connected the ingestion of foods contaminated with aflatoxin B_1 with higher than expected rates of HCC (42).

Cirrhosis is the most common etiologic factor in the United States and Europe. Estimates of the lifetime risk of developing HCC in the setting of cirrhosis is 15%. Unfortunately, it appears that halting alcohol consumption once cirrhosis is established does not reduce the risk of HCC (42).

The ultrasound appearance of HCC varies with the gross pathological appearance of the tumor. Solitary lesions may range from echogenic (mimicking a hemangioma) to hypoechoic (Fig. 15). Borders may be well-defined or irregular. The latter would raise suspicion of an aggressive lesion. Early, small HCCs tend to be hypoechoic because there is little in the way of necrosis at this stage (50). Larger tumors tend to have areas of necrosis and fibrosis making their ultrasound appearance heterogeneous. Multifocal hepatoma and a pattern of diffuse liver involvement by HCC can be very difficult to distinguish from metastatic disease because they result in multiple masses and diffusely heterogeneous liver texture, respectively. One tendency of HCC that can be of diagnostic value is the propensity of the tumor to invade the portal veins. Metastases can also do this, but in my experience this is less common than with HCC.

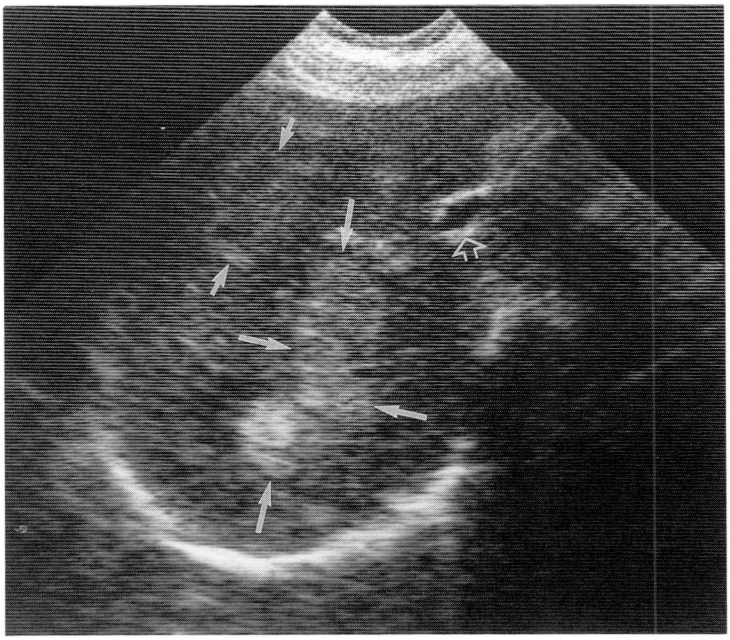

(A)

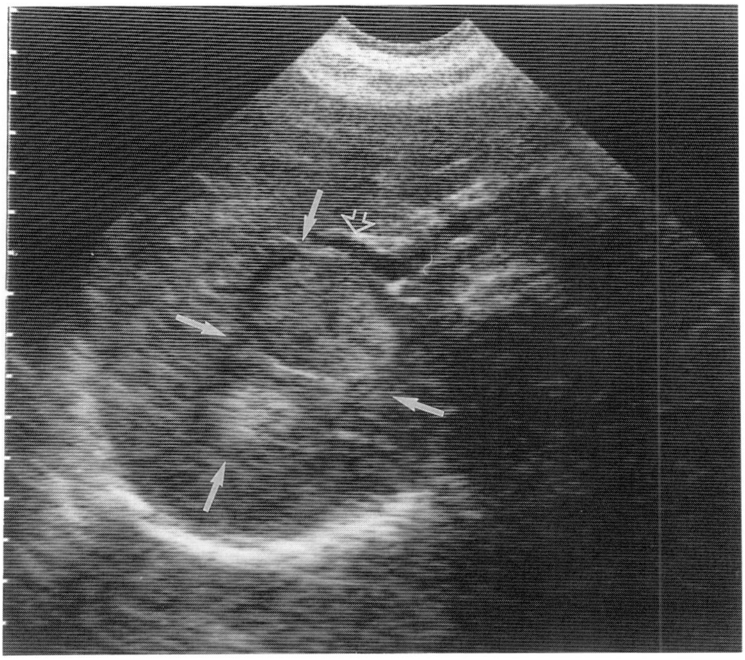

(B)

Figure 15. A hepatocellular carcinoma with metastases in a 62-year-old Asian woman. She had a history of long-standing chronic active hepatitis. In (A) the long arrows show the primary mass and the short arrows point out a metastasis. The open arrow points to the left portal vein. (B) A more caudal view of the tumor (arrows). The open arrow shows the right portal vein draped over the mass.

A variant of HCC has been described that has a distinctly different incidence (younger patients), absence of other etiologic factors for HCC, no elevation of serum alpha-fetoprotein, and, most importantly, better prognosis than the other forms of HCC (42). This form, known as fibrolamellar carcinoma, is more often a solitary lesion. The ultrasound appearance is also variable as for HCC, but the histology often has fibrous bands that course through the tumor and there may also be small calcifications. These features can result in the appearance of a central echogenic scar and calcifications in the mass, findings that are not common in HCC and help to distinguish between the two (51).

Angiosarcoma of the liver is a rare lesion that has a distinct carcinogenic etiology (42). Thorotrast, a long-abandoned radiographic contrast agent containing radioactive thorium dioxide, was avidly taken up by the reticuloendothelial cells of the liver. Patients who received this contrast agent (from the 1920s to the 1950s) have hepatic angiosarcoma (and HCC as well) at a higher incidence than expected. Radium salts, used to provide phosphorescent instrument markers and watch dials (and long ago replaced by nonradioactive replacements) are another radioactive substance associated with an increased incidence of angiosarcoma in exposed individuals. Most of those workers exposed to radium, however, developed bone neoplasms. Vinyl chloride is an industrial chemical widely used in the production of plastics. Exposure to this agent is another known etiologic factor in the development of angiosarcoma. Other chemical agents, including forms of arsenic, copper, and phenylethylhydrazine, also have an association. The ultrasound appearance of angiosarcomas is that of a (usually) large mass with a heterogeneous appearance (24, 52, 53). Unfortunately, there are no features that distinguish angiosarcomas from solitary metastases or HCC. The history of exposure to one of the etiologic agents, though, should raise the suspicion when a liver mass is found.

Another vascular malignant liver lesion is the hemangioendothelioma (also called a hepatic epithelioid hemangioendothelioma). Some reports have indicated an increased incidence in patients with a history of vinyl chloride exposure as for angiosarcomas. Unlike angiosarcoma, however, hemangioendothelioma has a better prognosis, so attempts to differentiate it from other hepatic malignancies are warranted (54, 55). The ultrasound appearance apparently varies with how long the tumor has been developing in the liver. Initially, the appearance is of multiple focal hypoechoic lesions that can be readily mistaken for metastases (56). As the disease progresses and the lesions enlarge, they coalesce, forming larger, irregular hypoechoic masses (57).

In the pediatric patient, other hepatic primary tumors, including hepatoblastoma, infantile hemangioendothelioma, and embryonal sarcoma produce lesions readily detected by ultrasound. Figure 16 is an example of a rare embryonal sarcoma in an adolescent. The primary tumors arising in the biliary tree are considered in other chapters of this book.

DOPPLER AND COLOR FLOW DOPPLER IMAGING

The development of low-cost, high-speed digital signal processing hardware has made possible the development of ultrasound machines that can process whole areas of the image for detection and quantitation of blood flow. These technical

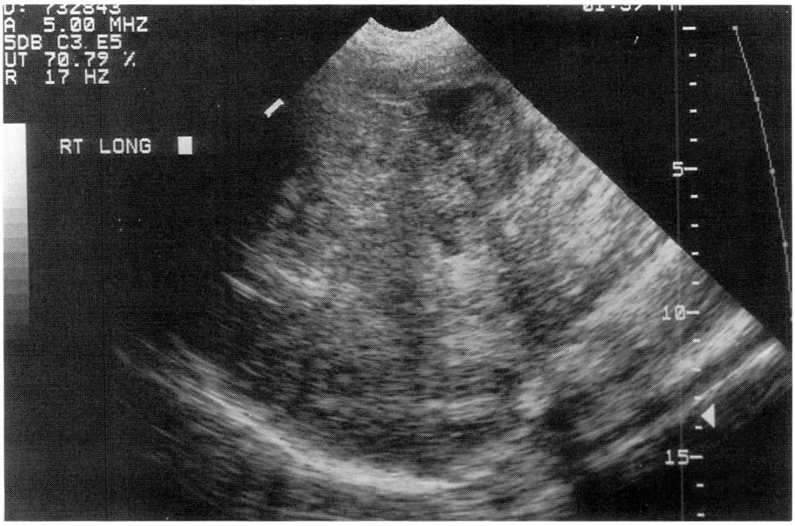

Figure 16. This longitudinal (A) image of the liver in a 15-year-old girl demonstrate a diffuse tumor so extensive that it was difficult to find normal liver on any images. Extensive work-up eventually showed this to be an embryonal cell sarcoma, a rare tumor in this age group.

advances have also improved pulsed Doppler (also referred to as duplex Doppler) systems. The end result is an ultrasound machine that can show blood flow in organs in a qualitative fashion and allow for specific quantitative measurements. For example, determining patency and flow direction of the hepatic and portal veins can be accomplished in a very short time using color flow Doppler imaging. If quantitative information, such as volume flow or flow velocity, is needed, the color flow imaging can be used to guide the placement of a sample volume for pulsed Doppler evaluation.

Disturbances of Blood Flow in the Liver

Systemic Circulation. The hepatic arteries and veins are readily visualized with color flow Doppler (CFD) imaging. The variations in both arterial and venous anatomy are well-known and may be imaged with CFD. Arterial occlusion is readily identified by an absence of color flow signal in the common hepatic artery or its branches. Some care should be taken in that CFD systems have multiple imaging parameters that can be adjusted, and artifactual absence or presence of a flow signal is not an uncommon problem. The experienced sonographer understands the sources of these artifacts and can help distinguish true pathological states from these nonpathological situations.

Doppler imaging of the celiac artery and common hepatic artery may help demonstrate arterial stenoses. The presence of abnormally high velocity wave forms with evidence of flow turbulence is indicative of Doppler measurement just at or past a stenotic area (58). The normal progression of Doppler wave forms from a high resistance pattern in the proximal celiac axis (low diastolic flow) to low resistance (high diastolic flow) in the common hepatic artery may also be altered. The hepatic artery and branches may be involved with aneurysmal or pseudoaneurysmal changes as a result of connective tissue diseases, infection, pancreatitis, and trauma (58). Gray-scale imaging may not be able to distinguish readily between cystic structures adjacent to the arteries and aneurysm or pseudoaneurysm. Color flow Doppler imaging, however, readily shows the flow within the structures, allowing the proper diagnosis to be made.

Doppler examination of the hepatic veins has been shown to be useful in evaluation for possible Budd–Chiari syndrome, but its value in hepatic veno-occlusive disease is less apparent (59). This is likely due to the nature of hepatic veno-occlusive disease with its obstructive effect on the centrilobular or sublobular veins without occluding the large veins (60). Doppler wave forms in the hepatic veins are useful in evaluating liver disease with indirect effects on the venous blood flow. Normal hepatic venous Doppler wave forms show a triphasic appearance with a to-and-fro flow direction (Fig. 17). This results from the hepatofugal flow in diastole reversed briefly by the right atrial contraction in systole. In evaluation of liver transplants, acute rejection is associated with an abnormal alteration of these wave forms; the normal excursion is damped with loss of the reversed phase (61). Cirrhosis may show similar effects on the hepatic venous Doppler wave form, depending on the severity of the disease (62). In congestive heart failure, alterations of both the hepatic and portal venous Doppler wave forms have been observed. In the hepatic veins, the normal systolic reversed flow is increased in extent and the portal veins show an increase in pulsatility (58, 63).

Shapiro and colleagues (64) have noted that some caution may be indicated in interpretation of the hepatic venous Doppler wave forms; in their study of 75 patients with no hepatic or cardiac disease, seven patients had abnormal flattened wave forms. In four of these seven patients, normal triphasic patterns were seen in the hepatic veins upon prolonged inspiration. Because such Doppler studies are not usually used as a screening test for diffuse liver disease, the problem of false positives is likely minimal.

Portal Circulation. The great value of CFD and duplex Doppler in imaging of the liver is the evaluation of the hemodynamic state of the portal venous system (Fig. 18). Both readily detect absent or reversed flow, and duplex Doppler wave forms can give some insight into the extent of disease. In addition, both CFD and duplex Doppler are useful in evaluation of treatments for portal hypertension and cirrhosis, from surgically created portosystemic shunts to liver transplants.

Cirrhosis and attendant portal hypertension have a variety of findings on ultrasound. The imaging characteristics are described above. Much of what is seen regarding the hemodynamic state of the portal system relies on real-time imaging combined with CFD and duplex Doppler. Color flow Doppler imaging readily shows portal flow that may be reversed (hepatofugal), have a pulsatile instead of steady or slowly varying flow velocity, show a diminished response to deep inspiration, and communicate with collateral veins (58). Varices in the splenic hilum and esophagogastric junction can sometimes be seen with gray-scale and CFD imaging. A patent paraumbilical vein resulting from portal hypertension is also sometimes seen, and if seen, is specific for portal hypertension (65). Figure 19 shows abnormal portal flow in cirrhosis and Figure 20 shows a spontaneous portosystemic shunt from the portal system to a thoracic vein.

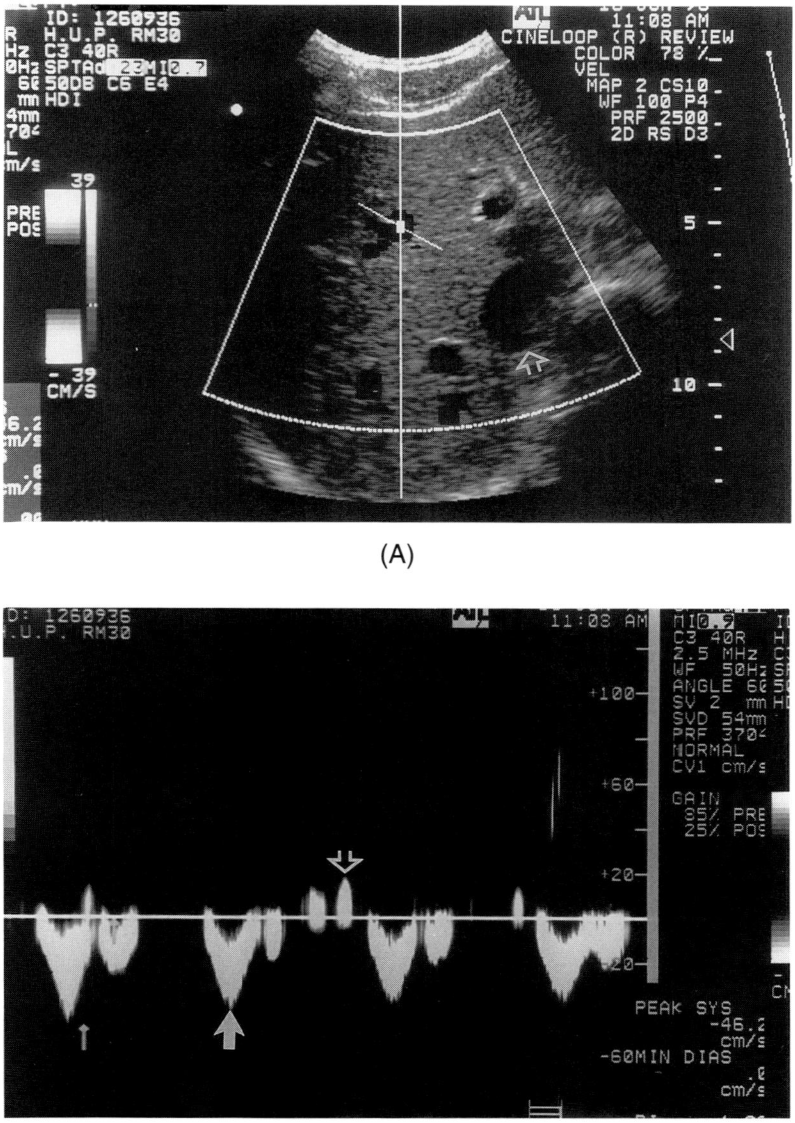

(A)

(B)

Figure 17. This is the same patient as in Figure 1. (A) Doppler sample volume (the small white rectangle on the vertical line with an angled line through it) placed within the middle hepatic vein (MHV). The sector-shaped white line is the color flow Doppler area. (B) Doppler tracing from the MHV. The large solid arrow shows the normal flow away from the liver. The vertical scale at the right shows velocity; the negative value indicates flow away from the direction of the ultrasound Doppler beam shown by the vertical white line in (A). The open arrow in (A) shows the inferior vena cava. The open arrow in (B) shows the normal reversed flow in the MHV during systole as the right atrium contracts.

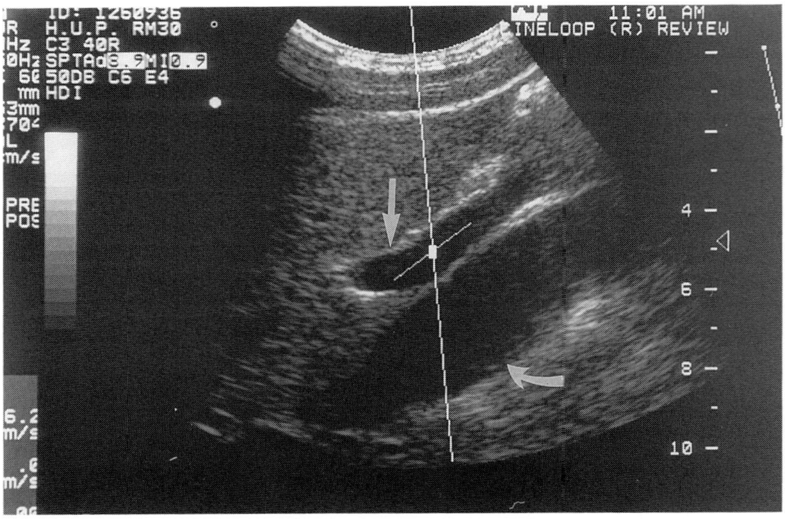

(A)

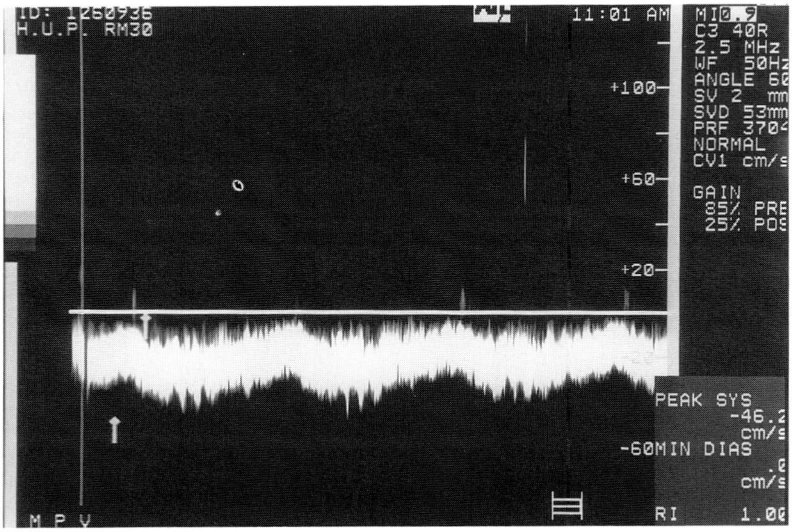

(B)

Figure 18. Also the same patient as in Figure 1. (A) Doppler sample volume placed in the main portal vein (MPV; arrow). The curved arrow points to the inferior vena cava. Its large size is usually normal in young individuals. (B) Doppler tracing of normal portal venous flow. Note that from the Doppler beam direction defined in (A) normal hepatopetal portal flow has a negative velocity. The slight variation in velocity with time is a result of patient respiration.

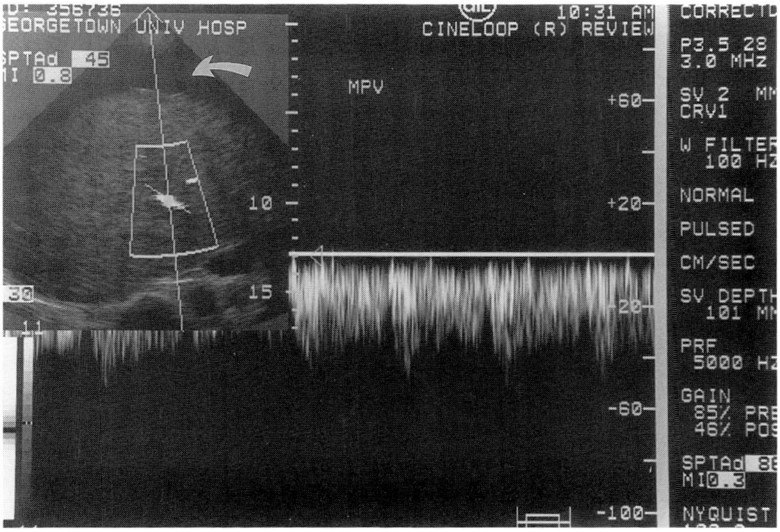

(A)

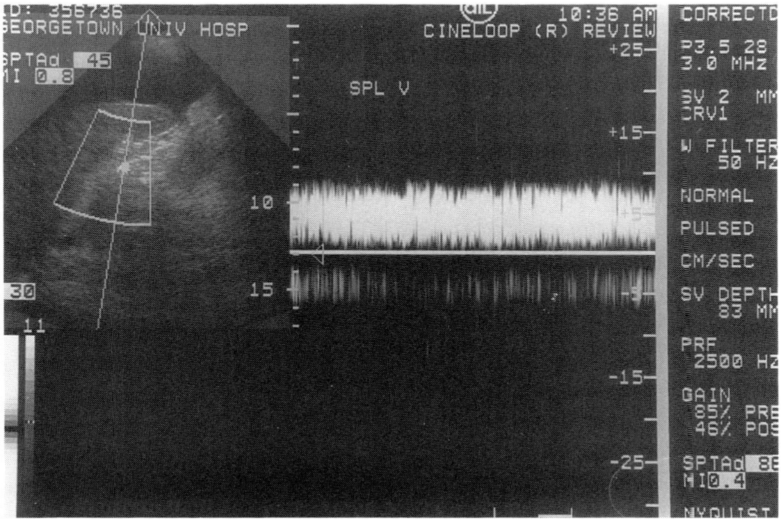

(B)

Figure 19. The same patient as in Figure 5. (A) Doppler sample volume has been placed in the main portal vein. For this beam angle, normal flow should have a positive velocity. In this case, the flow is reversed and so has a negative velocity. As in Figure 17, the white sector shows a color flow Doppler area. The curved arrow shows the ascites. (B) Doppler sample volume is in the splenic vein (SPL V). For this beam angle, normal flow should be away from the spleen (negative velocity). The flow here is abnormal and reversed, flowing toward the spleen with a resultant positive velocity (note the velocity scale on the right side of the image).

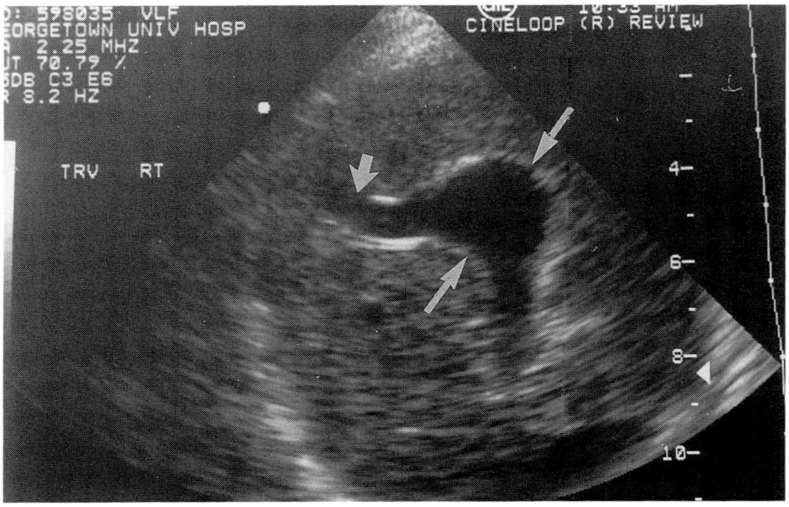

(A)

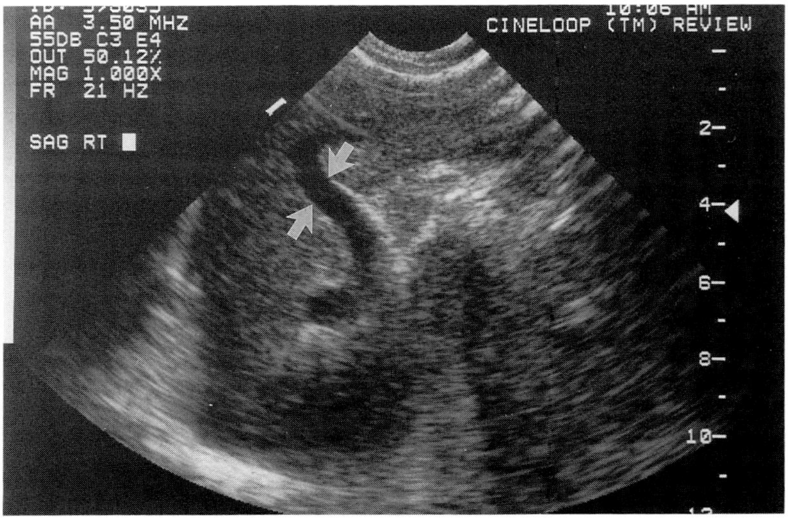

(B)

Figure 20. A 56-year-old male with cirrhosis. The arrows in (A) point to the very large bifurcation of the right portal vein branch. An unusual vein was seen connecting to the right portal at this location (large arrow). On a saggital view (B), the arrows show this vein coursing anteriorly and superiorly from the portal vein. Doppler studies showed flow away from the portal vein in this spontaneous portosystemic shunt. This proved to be a connection to a thoracic vein and is shown in (C) on a CT examination (arrows, next page). Other scans showed that this vein could be followed to the anterior thorax.

Blood Flow Imaging in Radiological and Surgical Interventions. The development of the transjugular approach to creating portosystemic shunts (66, 67) has permitted a less invasive approach to portosystemic shunting. However, CFD and duplex Doppler imaging are nearly a requirement prior to transjugular intrahepatic portosystemic (TIPS) shunts. The ultrasound studies are useful for demonstrating the patency of the hepatic and portal veins and establishing the directions and

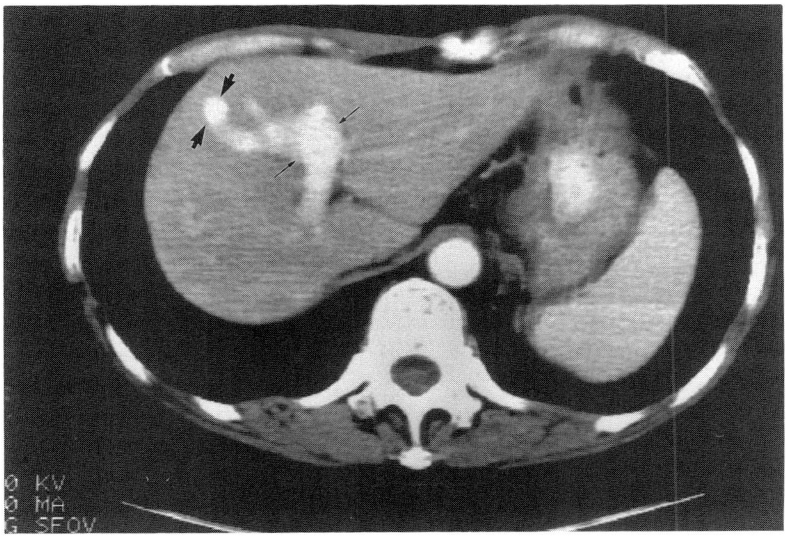

(C)

Figure 20. *(Continued).*

magnitude of blood flow in the vessels to be shunted (68). After placement of a TIPS shunt, CFD and duplex Doppler are useful for follow-up. Immediate post-shunt complications (shunt occlusion) are readily demonstrated. In the longer term, the study by Haskal and colleagues (69) showed a significant degree of stenoses developing more slowly in about 32% of their study population. These data would support the idea of the ultrasound follow-up for TIPS shunts that has become a routine part of the care of the patients who have them (70).

Ultrasound has long been used for the guidance of fine-needle and core biopsies of the liver. The addition of CFD allows lesions to be evaluated for vascularity prior to biopsy. It also allows visualization of major arterial and venous branches in the liver prior to biopsy for diffuse disease.

Gray-scale ultrasound augmented by CFD and duplex Doppler has also proved to be useful both before and after liver transplantation (71, 72). Prior to transplantation, ultrasound can be used to assess the circulatory aspects of the patient's liver and, in cases of metastases and primary tumors, whether resection or transplantation is indicated. Ultrasound is also used to evaluate the patient for other conditions that would preclude transplantation, such as other severe diseases or widespread metastases.

After liver transplantation, evaluation for possible rejection was noted above. In addition, any fluid collections in the region of the liver can be evaluated for any blood flow that would suggest pseudoaneurysm formation. Gray-scale ultrasound is useful in excluding postoperative biliary obstruction and abscess formation.

INTRAOPERATIVE ULTRASOUND

Diagnostic ultrasound equipment has an advantage over other medical imaging devices in that it can be made small enough to be readily portable. Owing to both the physics and engineering of ultrasound imaging, contemporary ultrasound systems offer a wide range of imaging capability in a relatively small and low-cost package. These characteristics, plus the noninvasive nature of ultrasound itself, make ultrasound imaging an excellent tool for use during surgery. The absence of significant bioeffects (73) means that the use of ultrasound during surgery poses minimal added risk to the patient or surgeon.

Ultrasound has proved a valuable adjunct to many types of surgical procedures, with use in neurosurgery (74) and abdominal surgery (75) predominant. There is also a considerable role that ultrasound plays in minimally invasive surgical treatments and interventional radiology, but the focus here is on the abdominal surgical use for examination of the liver.

The equipment and techniques used for intraoperative ultrasound are described, as well as typical applications and example images. The particular application described here is for intraoperative liver ultrasound, but the equipment and techniques are more generally applicable in surgery.

Equipment

There are typically two general classes of equipment used for intraoperative ultrasound (IOUS) of the liver. One class is the ultrasound equipment used in radiology or other imaging departments as discussed above. The other class is machines designed specifically for use in an operating room. The equipment used in medical imaging departments is usually large, with machine weights often 400–800 pounds (180–360 kg). However, these machines provide very high image quality and, because they are used for multiple types of examinations, great flexibility in functions. For example, most current machines include conventional and color flow Doppler capability and M-mode displays and accept a wide range of transducer types. A type of machine designed for portable use is often at the low end of the weight range and usually has fewer capabilities. Modern electronics, however, has allowed for order-of-magnitude reductions in the size of the internal components, so that even such small systems often include color flow imaging. It is important to note that the systems used in medical imaging departments, or even for portable (bedside) examinations, are usually not safe to use in the presence of flammable anesthetic agents.

Ultrasound systems designed specifically for use in the operating room fall in the range of the smaller end of in-department machines to purpose-built devices that are very small, with weights less than 100 pounds (45 kg). These have both a small "footprint" to fit better in an operating room, and a low weight so as to be readily movable. There is usually a compromise made for this compactness, however, in that many of these machines support only a limited range of transducers and do not have color flow or conventional Doppler capability. Depending on the manufacturer, these machines may or may not be safe for use in the presence of flammable anesthetics.

Both types of machines are designed to meet electrical safety requirements, but the operating room environment often has a large number of electrically operated devices. Provided the grounding is done correctly and that the equipment is properly maintained, risk from electrical shock should be no greater than for other equipment.

It may be useful, however, to have the hospital biomedical engineers check the grounding.

The "business end" of an ultrasound machine is the transducer. This part of the equipment sends and receives the ultrasound signals and so is a critical part of the system. There are very good descriptions of how these transducers are constructed and operate (76, 77) so these topics are not described in detail here. However, transducers used intraoperatively have some requirements that their conventional diagnostic counterparts do not. Certainly they must be capable of being either sterilized or used in a manner that allows only a sterile surface to come in contact with the patient or surgical field. Figure 21 shows examples of transducers designed to be completely sterilized, typically by gas sterilization and sometimes by immersion. Transducers that are completely sterilized provide some advantages for the surgeon or radiologist in that there need be no concern about any of the transducer parts coming in contact with the sterile field. A disadvantage is that the transducer has to undergo a sterilization cycle before it can be used again, so some provision has to be made for this when the equipment may be needed for multiple cases.

Providing a barrier between the transducer and the sterile field is another approach used. In this method, a sterile cover is put over the transducer. Figure 22 shows an ultrasound transducer that must be covered for intraoperative use. So long as the outside surface is not contaminated or the cover broken, the transducer is isolated from the sterile environment. Ultrasound gel is placed inside the cover to couple the sound from the transducer to the sterile surface of the cover. This technique allows for quick transition from case to case in that sterilization of the transducer is not needed; a new cover is placed on the transducer for each use. This method also allows transducers used for general imaging to be used in intraoperative applications. The disadvantage of this method is that it is more cumbersome to perform, and if the barrier is broken, sterility is compromised.

Because the distance between the ultrasound machine and the patient may be larger than is usual in the non-intraoperative scanning scenario, a common characteristic of ultrasound transducers designed for intraoperative use is a long connecting cable. Compared to their conventional scanning counterparts, intraoperative transducers may have cables 3 ft (1 m) longer, for a total length of 6–9 ft (2–3 m). This does pose some problems for transducer designers because the longer cables can make for increased losses in the generating pulse and received signal. Also, longer cables are more subject to the pickup of electrical noise.

The transducers themselves are typically of two types, those that use a mechanical method to generate the scan and those that scan electronically. The latter type have nearly completely replaced the former. The all-electronic transducer is usually either a linear array (see the caption for Fig. 1) or a phased array. Linear arrays produce rectangular images whereas phased arrays yield sector-shaped images. There are no clear advantages of one type of transducer over another; the application generally determines which is better. For example, if only a small surgical window is available, the phased array with its wider angle of coverage may do a better job, but the linear array is often capable of higher spatial resolution. Because scans are being performed in direct contact with the liver rather than through the anatomic structures of the abdominal wall, there is no attenuation of the sound beam before it gets to the liver. This allows the use of higher-frequency transducers, typically in the 5–10 MHz range, than are used for nonoperative sonography. The higher-

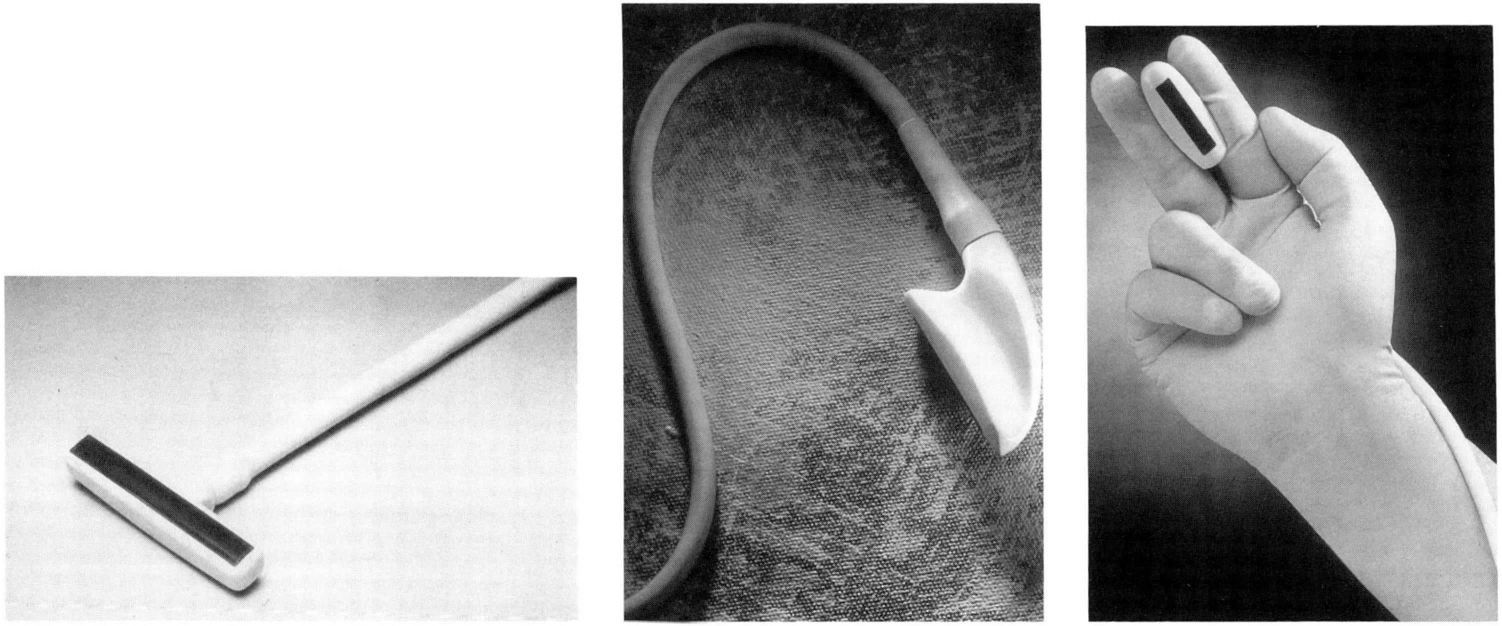

(A) (B) (C)

Figure 21. (A) Intraoperative linear array transducer. The dark rectangular area represents the active transducer surface that is held against the organ to be imaged. The transducer is approximately 50 mm long. This particular unit images perpendicular to the operators' fingers (which would hold the transducer parallel to the cable). The entire transducer is sterilizable. Courtesy of Aloka, Wallingford, CT. (B) This is another type of intraoperative linear array transducer. The entire unit may be sterilized. Note how readily the cable bends, a desirable characteristic for intraoperative transducers because this avoids constraints in moving inside a small space. The transducer has contoured finger grips along the sides. Courtesy of ATL Ultrasound, Bothell, WA. (C) This is the same transducer as in (B), demonstrating how it is held. Note that this transducer images parallel to the operator's fingers in contrast to the unit in (A). This transducer has a smaller active surface than that in (A), but the entire unit is also smaller as a result. Courtesy of ATL Ultrasound, Bothell, WA.

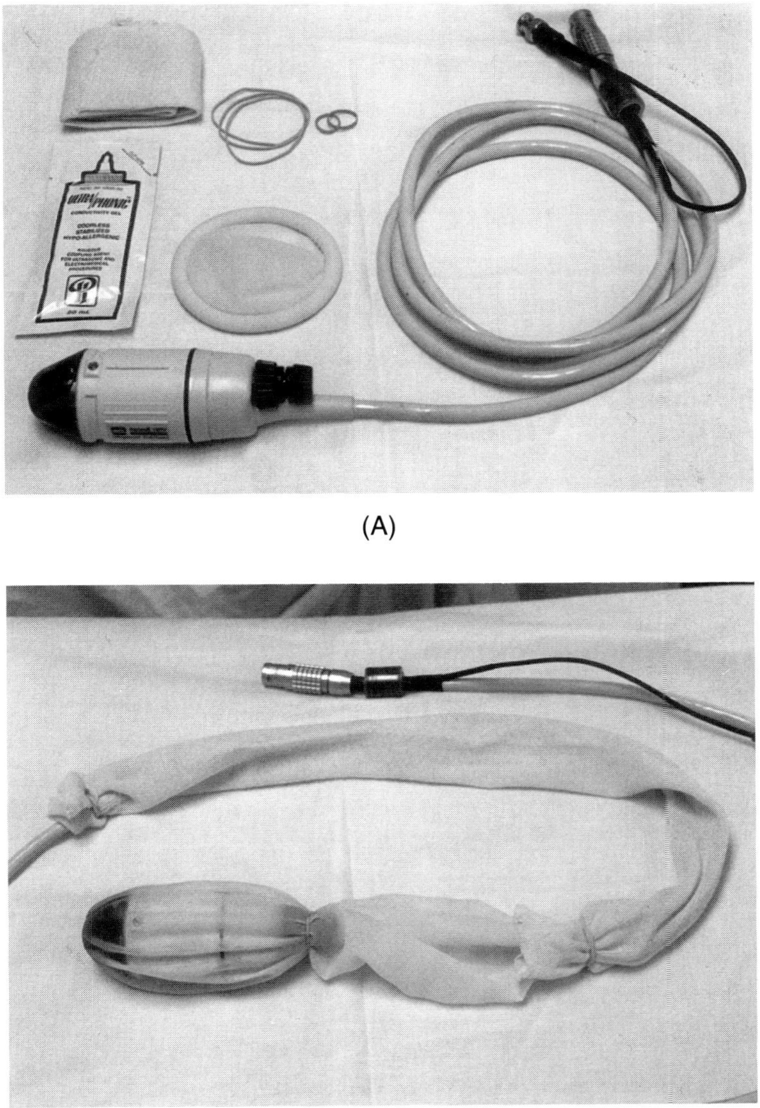

(A)

(B)

Figure 22. (A) An ultrasound transducer of the type that is not readily sterilizable. This is a mechanical scanner that produces a sector-shaped image (ATL Ultrasound, Bothell, WA). The transducer is the pointed device at the bottom left of the photograph. Shown with the transducer are the probe cover, sterile gel (used either inside the probe cover, or for scanning on intact, but prepped, skin—it is NOT used intraoperatively), a stockinette cord cover, and rubber bands to hold the cord cover in place. All of the items except the transducer are normally sterilized and contained in a pouch. (B) The same transducer in (A) with the covers applied. In surgical use, the entire covered surface to the end of the stockinette would be considered sterile (provided proper technique had been used in preparing the transducer).

frequency transducers yield better spatial resolution. For IOUS of the liver, the size of the organ often requires the use of transducers in the lower end of the frequency range (5–7 MHz).

Some transducers can be fitted with attachments that will hold a biopsy needle at a specific angle. The ultrasound machine then displays a guide line superimposed on the image that shows the potential needle path. This allows the physician performing the biopsy to have a much greater degree of certainty about hitting the intended structure.

Techniques

One of the first considerations for intraoperative ultrasound of the liver is who performs the scans. This varies to some extent from institution to institution, but sometimes individual surgeons determine the answer. Even if the surgeon personally does the scans, it is usually advisable to have a radiologist familiar with ultrasound imaging present. For those not familiar with ultrasound imaging, it is easy to become disoriented, a problem exacerbated by the unconventional scan planes used intraoperatively. If the surgeon scans, the radiologist and technologist typically assist by preparing the transducer, either by placing it in its sterile cover or connecting the nonsterile end to the machine. The technologist usually operates the machine and makes any permanent image records (on videotape, film, or a paper printer) and the radiologist keeps up a dialogue with the surgeon about what is being imaged.

If the radiologist scans, he or she puts on operating room scrub attire, goes through the usual surgical scrub procedure, and puts on gown and gloves. Effectively, the radiologist becomes a member of the surgical team, following sterile procedures. In this case, the assistance of a technologist is mandatory because the radiologist is not able to operate the machine and scan simultaneously.

The choice of who scans is often determined on a case-by-case basis. The surgeon scanning has the advantage of correlating what he or she feels (say, an alteration of the texture of the liver surface) with what the image shows. The radiologist often has a better established understanding of the appearance of different lesions.

If the surgeon scans, the radiologist often directs the surgeon to scan over hepatic landmarks that are visible or palpable and from which the radiologist can help determine the location of any lesions and their relationship to nearby anatomic structures. Typical examples are the gallbladder, falciform ligament, and main portal vein. The vascular structures, in particular, are useful because they also provide benchmarks for the segmentation of the liver (78) and are readily followed during scanning. The surgeon also scans over areas of suspected abnormality based on appearance or palpation. The radiologist may direct scanning to areas seen to be abnormal on other imaging studies such as CT or MR scans. Such studies are usually also made available in the operating room for reference during the procedure.

If the radiologist scans, the surgeon provides a brief orientation to the operative field, and may also help position the liver for scanning. In this instance, the surgeon usually articulates the particular abnormality being sought or ruled out. The radiologist usually stops over abnormalities, shows the surgeon where they are, and the surgeon usually then examines the area to determine if the abnormality is palpable and may mark the location of abnormalities on the liver capsule. This is usually accomplished with a brief pulse from the coagulation forceps. The radiologist will usually have reviewed other imaging studies beforehand so that a targeted study is done, supplemented by a general survey for other abnormalities.

Irrespective of who scans, the surgeon and radiologist work together as a team and constant, concise communication is a must. The technologist operates the ultrasound machine and makes a permanent record of the imaging findings. The radiologist goes on to generate a report of the procedure and findings for the medical record.

APPLICATIONS OF INTRAOPERATIVE ULTRASOUND

Detection and Localization of Liver Masses

Table I provides a listing of typical applications of IOUS of the liver with references to published articles in the surgical and radiological literature. The chief use of IOUS of the liver is in identification of liver masses whether believed to be metastatic lesions (79–86) or primary hepatocellular carcinomas (87, 88). The sensitivity in this application, particularly for small lesions, has been reported as high as 96–98% (83, 89). This is often compared to preoperative CT with various contrast enhancement techniques, which have a lower reported sensitivity of 50–91% (the latter with CT done during arterial portography) (79, 83). Figures 23, 24, and 25 show IOUS images of metastatic colon cancer lesions in the liver. Detection of lesions as small as 3 mm in diameter with intraoperative ultrasound has been described (90). Figure 24 includes images of small lesions, illustrating that the claim of detecting such small lesions is not an exaggeration. Characterizing liver masses once detected is difficult for ultrasound. Many etiologies of liver masses result in ultrasound findings that are similar, as described above. Metastases, for example, tend to have a similar appearance despite the origin (most have an echogenicity greater than normal liver). Hemangiomas may be multiple and very difficult to differentiate from metastases. A report from Choji and colleagues (91) at Hokkaido University in Japan, however, suggests that IOUS of the liver may have an advantage over nonoperative ultrasound in that mechanical compression of hemangiomas during intraoperative scanning results in reducing their echogenicity, whereas this finding was not seen with intraoperative compression of other liver masses.

The use of IOUS of the liver as a screening tool has also been described for colorectal cancer (92, 93) and in cirrhotic livers (94) in part because of the better sensitivity of IOUS of the liver at detecting masses than preoperative imaging studies. In the references cited, lesions not apparent on preoperative studies were detected at surgery during IOUS of the liver, prompting biopsy or an alteration of the surgery.

Detection of Gallbladder and Biliary Calculi

The value of nonoperative ultrasound of the liver is well established for gallbladder calculi (95), with sensitivity and specificity, even in difficult patients, typically 91 and 100%, respectively (96). For use in detecting choledocholithiasis, however, nonoperative ultrasound is less sensitive, ranging from 36% (97) to 90% (98) with specificities similar to those for cholecystolithiasis. Intraoperative liver ultrasound

Table 1. Representative application and value of intraoperative ultrasound[a]

Application	Summary	Reference
Detection of metastases	IOUS was found superior to both delayed CT and bolus-contrast enhanced CT (82% sensitivity for IOUS and palpation vs. 50–54% for the CT studies)	Knol JA, Marn CS, Francis IR, et al. Comparisons of dynamic infusion and delayed computed tomography, intraoperative ultrasound, and palpation in the detection of liver metastases. *Am J Surg.* 1993;165:81–88
Detection of liver masses	IOUS was found to provide more information about the nature of liver masses than preoperative CT or intraoperative palpation. Types of masses included metastases, hepatocellular carcinomas, and hemangiomas	Boggs RR, Rouch CA, Chua GT. Intraoperative ultrasound of hepatic tumors. *Indiana Med.* 1992;85:496–498
Localization of liver masses	A method of correlating lesions identified at IOUS with anatomic segments is based on the anatomy of the hepatic veins and branches	Solomon MJ, Stephen MS, White GH, Eyers AA. A new classification of hepatic territories using intraoperative ultrasound. *Am J Surg.* 1992;163:336–338
Contrast examination of malignant liver masses	An experimental polysaccharide (SU 454) ultrasound contrast agent was injected into the portal venous or biliary system and increased the detectability of small liver lesions by increasing the echogenicity of the surrounding liver	el Mouaaouy A, Naruhn M, Becker HD, Schlief R. Intraoperative echo-contrast ultrasound examination of malignant liver neoplasms—initial clinical experience. *Surg Endosc (Germany).* 1991;5: 214–218
Surgical decision making	In 12% of patients undergoing abdominal surgery for liver or other pathological processes, the surgical approach and management were altered as a result of the IOUS examination	Rifkin MD, Rosato FE, Branch HM, et al. Intraoperative ultrasound of the liver: An important adjunctive tool for decision making in the operating room. *Ann Surg.* 1987;205: 466–472
Detection of choledocholithiasis	IOUS was shown to be sensitive for detection of biliary ductal calculi compared to intraoperative cholangiography, but was thought to be more technically demanding and necessitated considerable training and experience	Buckley AR, Scudamore CH, Becker CD, Cooperberg PL. Intraoperative imaging of the biliary tree: sonography vs. operative cholangiography. *J Ultrasound Med.* 1987;6: 589–595
Identification of liver neoplasms in cirrhotic livers	IOUS found 7 cases of small (2–3 cm) hepatocellular carcinomas in patients with cirrhotic livers. This led to subsegmental resections. The authors also reported other uses of IOUS and emphasized the utility in finding, localizing, and guiding the biopsy of (when necessary) small liver masses	Gozzetti G, Mazziotti A, Bolondi L, et al. Intraoperative ultrasonography in surgery for liver tumors. *Surgery.* 1986;99:523–530
Screening of patients during surgery for colorectal cancer	IOUS was used to screen the entire liver in patients undergoing surgery for colorectal carcinomas. In 11.9% of the operations, IOUS identified a total of 14 metastases not detected preoperatively. These masses were all less than 2 cm in diameter. The sensitivity of IOUS was found to be significantly higher than preoperative CT and ultrasound while retaining a similar specificity	Machi J, Isomoto H, Yamashita Y, et al. Intraoperative ultrasonography in screening for liver metastases from colorectal cancer: comparative accuracy with traditional procedures. *Surgery.* 1987;101:678–684
An adjunct to other intraoperative procedures	IOUS was found to be valuable in the intraoperative biopsy of deep-seated liver masses (Castaing et al.) and for guidance for fluid aspiration, agent injection, catheter placement, surgical tissue dissection for incision, resection, and extraction of stones and foreign bodies (Machi et al.)	Castaing D, Emond J, Kunstlinger F, Bismuth H. Utility of operative ultrasound in the surgical management of liver tumors. *Ann Surg.* 1986;204: 600–605 Machi J, Sigel B, Kurohiji T, et al. Operative ultrasound guidance for various surgical procedures. *Ultrasound Med Biol.* 1990;16:37–42

[a]IOUS = intraoperative ultrasound.

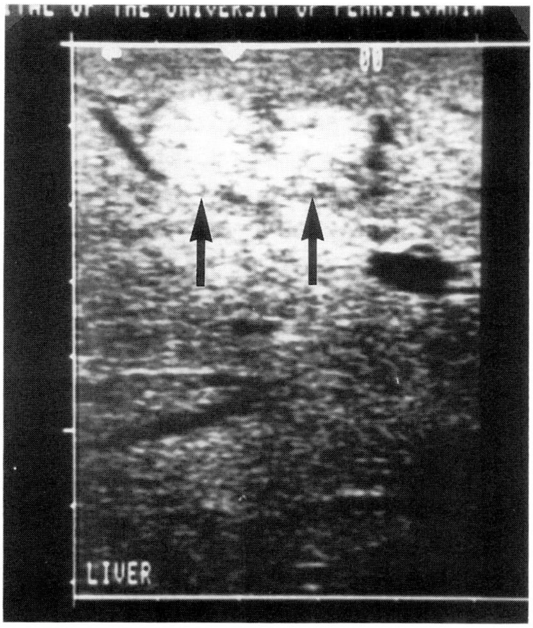

(A)

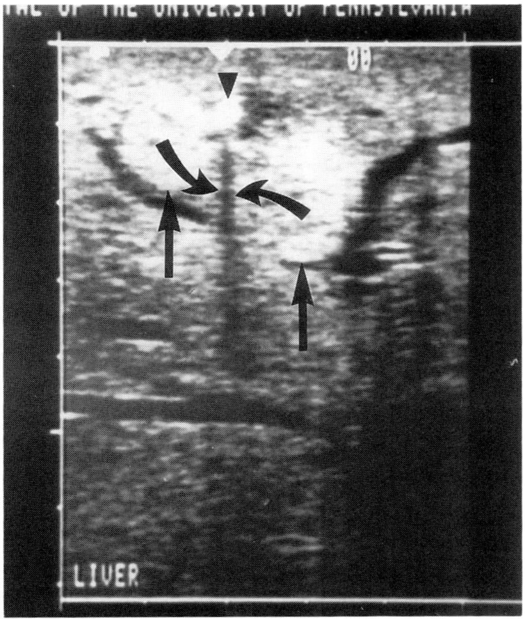

(B)

Figure 23. (A) Intraoperative ultrasound image of the liver showing two adjacent liver masses (arrows). Note that they are more echogenic than the surrounding liver parenchyma. These represent liver metastases from colon carcinoma. These lesions are approximately 13 mm in greatest diameter. The transducer is a 7.5-MHz linear array (Johnson & Johnson, Warren, NJ). (B) A different view of the same two liver masses (arrows). A calcification (arrowhead) is also seen. Note the acoustic shadowing posterior to the calcification (curved arrows). Such shadowing is characteristic of calcifications.

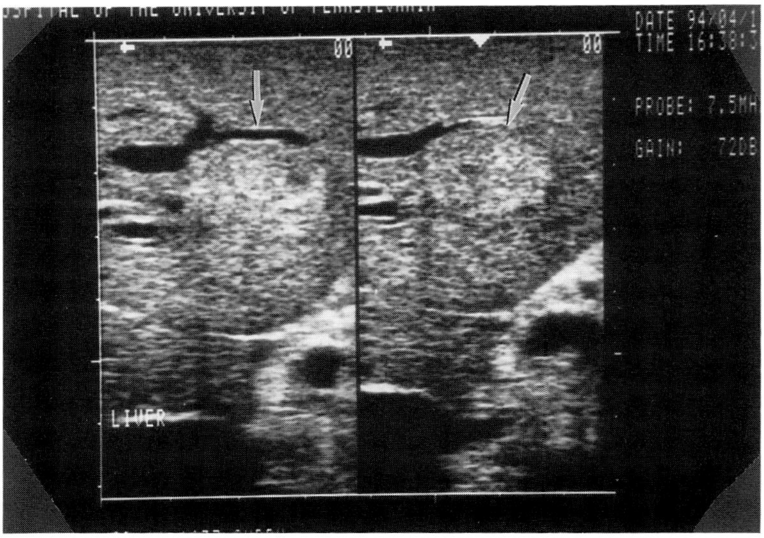

(A)

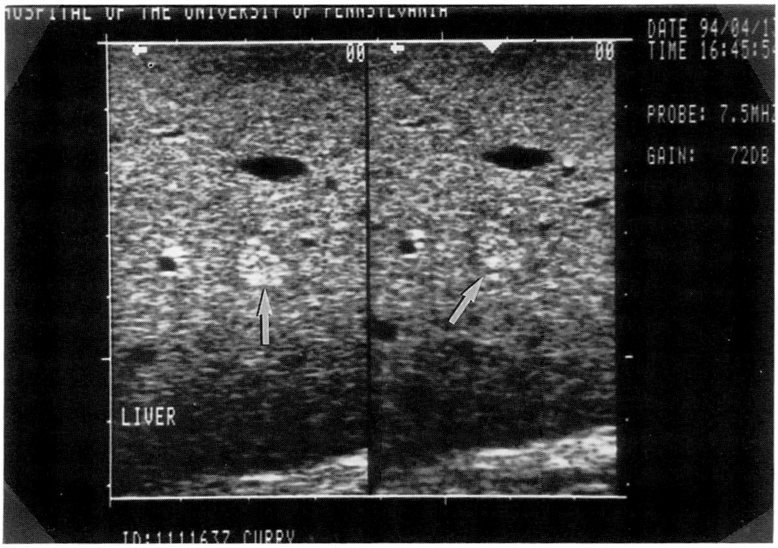

(B)

Figure 24. (A) A liver metastasis (colon primary) showing displacement of a hepatic vein branch (arrows). This image (and subsequent ones) consists of two views of the same mass from slightly different scanning positions, a capability of the particular machine used (Johnson & Johnson, Warren, NJ). (B) and (C, next page). The same patient as in (A) showing two other small metastases. The lesion in (B) (arrows) is approximately 9 mm in greatest diameter. The lesion in (C) is about 6 mm in greatest diameter. The lesion in (C) was not seen on preoperative CT or ultrasound imaging. This illustrates the small size of lesions detectable by IOUS of the liver.

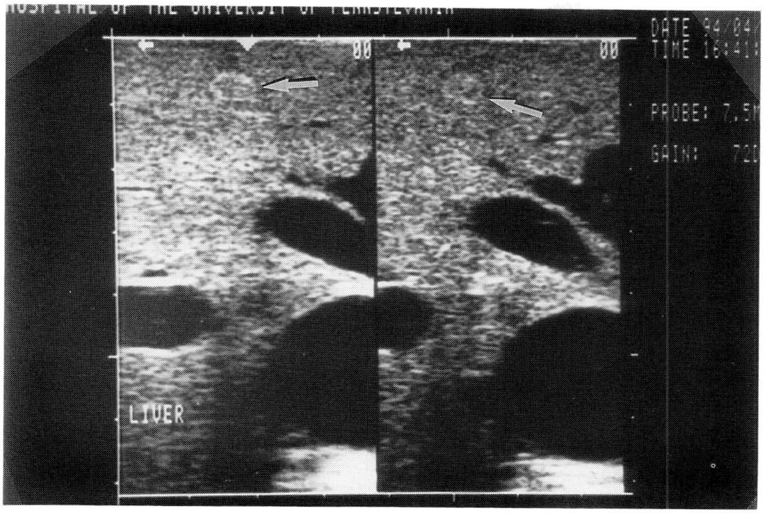

(C)

Figure 24. *(Continued)*

can also be used with some success to identify choledocholithiasis much as intraoperative cholangiography is currently used, though this use reportedly requires considerable operator experience and skill (99). A new ultrasound method, employing a catheter-sized transducer developed for intravascular use, promises improved sensitivity when used intraoperatively to examine the biliary tree for calculi (100, 101). Important to note for this technique is that the catheter-sized transducer can be introduced through standard surgical laparoscopes and that the transducer (in these papers) was placed alongside the bile ducts, not inserted into them.

Guidance for Operative Procedures

Another application for which IOUS of the liver is well suited is for intraoperative guidance. Aside from the identification of masses, IOUS of the liver can be used with success to direct intraoperative biopsies of deep-seated small lesions that would be very difficult to hit without some guidance (102). Such lesions may be difficult or impossible to palpate. Machi and colleagues (93) have also described extensive experience with the use of IOUS. They report that IOUS was valuable for biopsy guidance and also for aspiration of fluid collections, placement of catheters, identification of dissection planes, resections, and extraction of stones and foreign bodies. In the latter category, the U.S. Army has noted that IOUS may be valuable in detecting and localizing types of shrapnel fragments that are non-radioopaque (103).

Intraoperative Assessment of Blood Flow

The increased capability of ultrasound machines has made possible the use of spectral and color flow Doppler during intraoperative scans. This requires larger

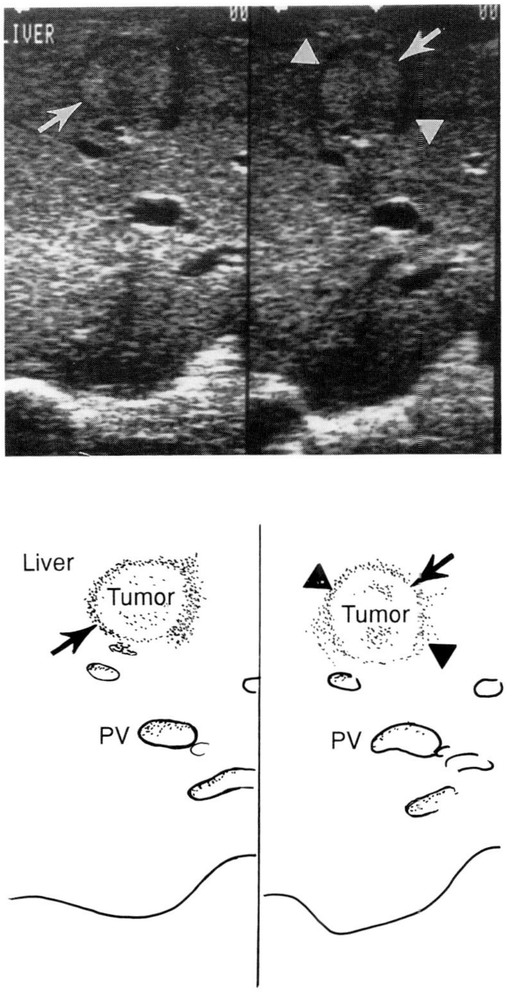

Figure 25. A metastatic lesion in the liver (colon primary) (arrows) showing a peripheral ring of decreased echogenicity (arrowheads). This finding is sometimes seen with metastases and helps make them more conspicuous. It is not a reliable indicator of the type of primary tumor.

or more costly systems at present, but the size and cost of such systems is generally decreasing. A report of the use of Doppler techniques to measure portal blood flow during partial hepatic resections indicated that the resulting measurements were useful in establishing a base line for subsequent postoperative evaluation (104). Undoubtedly, as blood flow measurement and corresponding physiological correlation become more readily available, the use of these ultrasound augmentations is sure to increase.

DISCUSSION

Ultrasound of the liver has proved over several decades of use to be a valuable and cost-effective method for the diagnosis of diseases affecting the organ. Its use in detecting most focal and many diffuse forms of liver disease is well known. The use of color flow and duplex Doppler has further expanded the diagnostic range of ultrasound, allowing both qualitative and quantitative determinations of blood flow in normal and pathological systemic and portal vessels. In many cases, coupled with clinical and laboratory information about the patient, ultrasound either supports the clinical diagnosis or actually makes it. The examination is readily performed, even at the patient's bedside, and has not been shown to have any signficant biologic effects.

Though CT and MRI may have better spatial resolution than ultrasound, and the use of contrast agents with both allows determination of some vascular parameters, neither CT nor MRI operate (yet) in real time. To anyone who performs ultrasound examinations regularly, the additional information conveyed by the real-time imaging process cannot be overstated.

The limitations to transabdominal imaging of the liver are mostly in having to penetrate the structures of the abdominal wall and having normal anatomy (ribs, lung, and bowel) prevent ready access to all parts of the liver. To a great extent, these disadvantages are overcome when the ultrasound system is used intraoperatively.

Advances in electronics have made possible the development of ultrasound systems small enough to be used readily during surgery. The superiority of IOUS of the liver for detection and localization of even very small liver lesions has been demonstrated. The use of the technique with resulting identification of preoperatively unsuspected liver masses is one good indicator of the effectiveness of the technique (93, 94). As has also been reported (105) IOUS of the liver results in decisions to change surgical approaches or techniques in a significant proportion of patients in whom it is used. This also supports the effectiveness argument. There is little, in fact, to argue against effectiveness. However, whether the effectiveness improves patient outcomes or reduces costs is less clear from the literature. Certainly, resection of unsuspected liver metastases or primary lesions would suggest improved cancer survival rates and the changes in surgical management during the surgical procedure would support cost effectiveness by reducing operating time and postoperative complications. Long-term outcomes studies and detailed examinations of costs, however, have not been yet reported (to my knowledge). Nonetheless, the absence of added significant risk, the simplicity of the IOUS technique, and the widespread use in intraoperative evaluation of the liver with the demonstration of potential to change surgical approaches and treatment plans certainly support the continued use of IOUS.

ACKNOWLEDGMENT

I would like to express my thanks to the ultrasound technologists at Georgetown University Medical Center and the University of Pennsylvania Medical Center for helping to obtain some of the images used in the figures. Harvey Nisenbaum, M.D., F.A.C.R. of the Department of Radiology, University of Pennsylvania Medical Center, provided the intraoperative ultrasound images.

REFERENCES

1. Ludwig GD, Struthers FW. Considerations underlying the use of ultrasound to detect gallstones and foreign bodies in tissues. *Naval Med Res Inst Rep.* Project #004 001; June 1949: Report No. 4.

2. Stimson GW. *Introduction to Airborne Radar.* El Segundo, CA: Hughes Aircraft Company; 1983.
3. Couinaud C. Le foie. In: *Etudes anatomiques et chirugicales.* Paris: Masson et Cie; 1957.
4. Gosink BB, Leymaster CE. Ultrasonic determination of hepatomegaly. *J Clin Ultrasound.* 1981;9:37–41.
5. Belton R, Van Zandt TF. Congenital absence of the left lobe of the liver. *Radiology.* 1983;147:184.
6. Radin DR, Colletti PM, Ralls PW, et al. Agenesis of the right lobe of the liver. *Radiology.* 1987;164:639–642.
7. Michels NA. Newer anatomy of the liver: variant blood supply and collateral circulation. *JAMA.* 1960;172:125–132.
8. Cosgrove DO, Arger PH, Coleman BG. Ultrasonic anatomy of the hepatic veins. *J Clin Ultrasound.* 1987;15:231–235.
9. Fraser-Hill MA, Atri M, Bret PM, et al. Intrahepatic portal venous system; variations demonstrated with duplex and color duplex and color Doppler. *Radiology.* 1990; 177:523–526.
10. Bosniak MA. The current radiological approach to renal cysts. *Radiology.* 1986;158: 1–10.
11. Gaines PA, Sampson MA. The prevalence and characterization of simple hepatic cysts by ultrasound examination. *Br J Radiol.* 1989;62:335–337.
12. Segal AJ, Spataro RF. Computed tomography of adult polycystic disease. *J Comput Assist Tomogr.* 1982;6:777–780.
13. Levine E, Cook LT, Granthem JJ. Liver cysts in autosomal dominant polycystic kidney disease: clinical and computed tomographic study. *AJR.* 1985;145:229–233.
14. Garra BS, Insana MF, Shawker TH, et al. Quantitative estimation of liver attenuation and echogenicity: normal state versus diffuse liver disease. *Radiology.* 1987;162:61–67.
15. Maharaj B, Bhoora IG, Patel A, et al. Ultrasonography and scintigraphy in liver disease in developing countries: a retrospective survey. *Lancet.* 1989;2:853–856.
16. Henriksson L, Kelter U. Ultrasonography and scintigraphy of the liver in focal and diffuse disease. *Acta Radiol.* 1987;28:165–168.
17. Kurtz AB, Rubin CS, Cooper HS, et al. Ultrasound findings in hepatitis. *Radiology.* 1980;136:717–723.
18. Zakim D. Metabolism of glucose and fatty acids by the liver. In Zakim D, Boyer TD, eds. *Hepatology: A Textbook of Liver Disease.* Philadelphia: WB Saunders Co; 1982:76–109.
19. Scatarige JC, Scott WW, Donovan PJ, et al. Fatty infiltration of the liver: ultrasonographic and computed tomographic correlation. *J Ultrasound Med.* 1984;3:9–14.
20. Anthony PP. The morphology of cirrhosis: definition, nomenclature, and classification. *Bull WHO.* 1977;55:521.
21. Harbin WP, Robert NJ, Ferrucci JT Jr. Diagnosis of cirrhosis based on regional changes in hepatic morphology. *Radiology.* 1980;135:273–283.
22. Grossman H, Ram PC, Coleman RA, et al. Hepatic ultrasonography in type I glycogen storage disease (von Gierke disease): Detection of hepatic adenoma and carcinoma. *Radiology.* 1981;141:753–756.
23. Bacon BR, Brown KE. Iron metabolism and disorders of iron overload. In: Kaplowitz N, ed. *Liver and Biliary Diseases.* Baltimore: Williams and Wilkins; 1996:350–351.
24. Withers CE, Wilson SR. The Liver. In: Rumack CM, Wilson SR, Charboneau JW, eds. *Diagnostic Ultrasound.* St. Louis: Mosby Yearbook; 1991:45–86.
25. Wetton CW, McCarty M, Tomlinson D, et al. Ultrasound findings in hepatic mycobacte-

rial infections in patients with acquired immune deficiency syndrome (AIDS). *Clin Radiol.* 1993;47:36–38.

26. Towers MJ, Withers CE, Hamilton PA, et al. Visceral calcification in AIDS may not always be due to *Pneumocystis carinii. AJR.* 1991;156:745–747.
27. Edmondson HA. Tumors of the liver and intrahepatic bile ducts. In: *Atlas of Tumor Pathology, Fascicle 25.* Washington, DC: Armed Forces Institute of Pathology 1958. Section VII: 113.
28. Freeney PC, Marks WM. Hepatic hemangioma: dynamic bolus computed tomography. *AJR.* 1986;147:711–719.
29. Brunetti JC, Van Heertum RL, Yudd AP, et al. The value of SPECT in the diagnosis of hepatic hemangioma. *Clin Nucl Med.* 1988;13:800–804.
30. Birnbaum BA, Weinreb JC, Megibow AJ, et al. Definitive diagnosis of hepatic hemangiomas: magnetic resonance imaging versus Tc-99m-labeled red blood cell SPECT. *Radiology.* 1990;176:95–101.
31. Birnbaum BA, Noz ME, Chapnick J, et al. Hepatic hemangiomas: diagnosis with fusion of MR, CT, and Tc-99m-labeled red blood cell SPECT images. *Radiology.* 1991; 181:469–474.
32. Lowe V, Khangure MS. Hepatic adenoma and focal nodular hyperplasia; a diagnostic dilemma. *Australas Radiol.* 1990;34:124–130.
33. Kerlin P, Davis GL, McGill DB, et al. Hepatic adenoma and focal nodular hyperplasia: clinical pathologic and radiologic features. *Gastroenterology.* 1983;84:994–1002.
34. Yamamoto H, Yamanaka T, Yoshida Y, Miyata M. Detection of focal nodular hyperplasia of the liver with color Doppler ultrasonography. *Gastroenterol Japan.* 1993;28: 924–930.
35. Golli M, Mathieu D, Anglade MC, et al. Focal nodular hyperplasia of the liver: value of color Doppler US in association with MR imaging. *Radiology.* 1993;187:113–117.
36. Maresca G, Barbaro B, Summaria V, et al. Color Doppler sonography in the differential diagnosis of focal hepatic lesions. The SH U508A (Levovist) experience. *Radiol Med (Italy).* 1994;87(5 suppl 1):41–49.
37. Klatchko BA, Schwartz SI. Diagnostic and therapeutic approaches to pyogenic abscesses of the liver. *Surg Gynecol Obstet.* 1989;168:332–336.
38. Halvorsen RA, Foster WL Jr, Wilkinson RH Jr., et al. Hepatic abscess: sensitivity of imaging tests and clinical findings. *Gastrointest Radiol.* 1989;14:364.
39. Ralls PW, Barnes PF, Radin DR. Sonographic features of amoebic and pyogenic liver abscesses: a blinded comparison. *AJR.* 1987;149:499–501.
40. Donovan AJ, Yellin AE, Ralls PW. Hepatic abscesses. *World J Surg.* 1991;15:162–169.
41. Craig JR, Peters RL, Edmondson RA. Tumors of the liver and intrahepatic bile ducts. In: *Atlas of Tumor Pathology, Second Series, Fasicle 26.* Washington, DC: Armed Forces Institute of Pathology; 1989.
42. La Brecque DR: Neoplasia of the liver. In: Kaplowitz N, ed. *Liver and Biliary Diseases.* Baltimore: Williams and Wilkins; 1996:391–436.
43. Scholmerich J, Volk BA, Gerok W. Value and limitations of abdominal ultrasound in tumour staging—liver metastasis and lymphoma. *Eur J Radiol.* 1987;7:243–245.
44. Tempero MA, Williams CA, Anderson JC. The value of hepatic ultrasound and biochemical tests in screening for liver metastases. *J Clin Oncol.* 1986;4:1074–1078.
45. Sanders LM, Botet JF, Straus DJ, et al. Computed tomography of primary lymphoma of the liver. *AJR.* 1989;152:973–976.
46. Townsend RR, Laing FC, Jeffrey RB, et al. Abdominal lymphoma in AIDS; evaluation with ultrasound. *Radiology.* 1989;171:719–724.

47. Wernecke K, Henke L, Vassallo P, et al. Pathologic explanation for hypoechoic halo seen on sonograms of malignant liver tumors: an in vitro correlative study. *AJR*. 1992;159:1011–1016.
48. Marchal GJ, Pylyser K, Tshibwabwa-Tumba EA, et al. Anechoic halo in solid liver tumors: sonographic, microangiographic, and histologic correlation. *Radiology*. 1985; 156:479–483.
49. Bruneton JN, Ladree D, Caramella E, et al. Ultrasonographic study of calcified hepatic metastases: a report of 13 cases. *Gastrointest Radiol*. 1982;7:61–63.
50. Sheu JC, Chen DS, Sung DL, et al. Hepatocellular carcinoma: ultrasound evolution in the early stage. *Radiology*. 1985;155:463–467.
51. Friedman AC, Lichtenstein JE, Goodman Z, et al. Fibrolamellar hepatocellular carcinoma. *Radiology*. 1985;157:583–587.
52. Buelow PC, Buck JL, Ros PR, Goodman ZD. Malignant vascular tumors of the liver: radiologic-pathologic correlation. *Radiographics*. 1994;14:153–166.
53. Fitzgerald EJ, Griffiths TM. Computed tomography of vinyl chloride-induced angiosarcoma of the liver. *Br J Radiol*. 1987;60:593–595.
54. Scoazec JY, Lamy P, Degott C, et al. Epithelioid hemangioendothelioma of the liver. Diagnostic features and role of liver transplantation. *Gastroenterology*. 1988;94:1447–1453.
55. Pichlmayr R, Weimann A, Ringe B. Indications for liver transplantation in hepatobiliary malignancy. *Hepatology*. 1994;20(1 pt 2):33S–40S.
56. Banerjee B, Rennison A. Epithelioid haemangioendothelioma of liver: a vascular tumor easily mistaken for metastatic carcinoma on ultrasound imaging. *Br J Radiol*. 1992; 65:611–613.
57. Furui S, Itai Y, et al. Hepatic epithelioid hemangioendothelioma: report of five cases. *Radiology*. 1989;171:63–68.
58. Koslin DB, Mulligan SA, Berland LL. Duplex assessment of the portal venous system and the splanchnic vasculature. In: Zweibel WJ, ed. *Introduction to Vascular Ultrasonography,* 3rd ed. Philadelphia: WB Saunders; 1992:367–385.
59. Hosoki T, Kuroda C, Tokunaga K, et al. Hepatic venous outflow obstruction: evaluation with pulsed duplex sonography. *Radiology*. 1989;170:733–737.
60. Bacon BR, Joshi SN, Granger DN. Ischemia, congestive failure, Budd–Chiari Syndrome, and veno-occlusive disease. In: Kaplowitz N, ed. *Liver and Biliary Diseases*. Baltimore: Williams and Wilkins; 1996:478–479.
61. Coulden RA, Britton PD, Farman P, et al. Preliminary report: hepatic vein Doppler in the early diagnosis of acute liver transplant rejection. *Lancet*. 1990;336:273–275.
62. Bolondi L, Li Bassi S, Gaiani S, et al. Liver cirrhosis: changes of Doppler waveform of hepatic veins. *Radiology*. 1991;178:513–516.
63. Lomas DJ, Britton PD, Summerton CB, Seymour CA. Duplex Doppler measurements of the portal vein in portal hypertension. *Clin Radiol*. 1993;48:311–315.
64. Shapiro RS, Winsberg F, Maldjian C, Stancato-Pasik A. Variability of hepatic vein Doppler tracings in normal subjects. *J Ultrasound Med*. 1993:12:701–703.
65. Morin C, Lafortune M, Pomier G, et al. Patent paraumbilical vein: anatomic and hemodynamic variants and their clinical importance. *Radiology*. 1992;185:253–256.
66. Burgener FA, Gutierrez OH. Production of a nonsurgical intrahepatic portacaval shunt in portal hypertension using a Gruntzig balloon dilatation catheter. *J Radiol (France)*. 1985;66:7–11.
67. Richter GM, Palmaz JC, Noldge G, et al. The transjugular intrahepatic portosystemic

stent-shunt. A new nonsurgical percutaneous method. *Radiologe (Germany)*. 1989; 29:406–411.

68. Ferral H, Foshager MC, Bjarnason H, et al. Early sonographic evaluation of the transjugular intrahepatic portosystemic shunt (TIPS). *Cardiovasc Intervent Radiol.* 1993; 16:275–279.
69. Haskal ZJ, Pentecost MJ, Soulen MC, et al. Transjugular intrahepatic portosystemic shunt stenosis and revision: early and midterm results. *AJR.* 1994;163:439–444.
70. Longo JM, Bilbao JI, Rousseau HP, et al. Transjugular intrahepatic portosystemic shunt: evaluation with Doppler sonography. *Radiology.* 1993;186:529–534.
71. Longley DG, Skolnick ML, Zajko AB, Bron KM. Duplex Doppler sonography in the evaluation of adult patients before and after liver transplantation. *AJR.* 1988; 151:687–696.
72. Oliver JH 3rd, Federle MP, Campbell WL, Zajko A. Imaging the hepatic transplant. *Radiol Clin North Am.* 1991;29:1285–1298.
73. Williams RA. *Ultrasound: Biological Effects and Potential Hazards.* London: Academic Press; 1983.
74. Naidich TP, Quencer RM, eds. *Ultrasound of the Central Nervous System.* Berlin: Springer-Verlag; 1987.
75. Mack LA, Lee RA, Nyberg DA. Intraoperative sonography of the abdomen. In: Rumack CR, Wilson SR, Charboneau JW, eds. *Diagnostic Ultrasound, I.* St. Louis: Mosby Year Book; 1991:492–504.
76. Wolbarst AB. *Physics of Radiology.* Norwalk, CT: Appleton & Lange; 1993.
77. Powis RL, Powis WJ. *A Thinker's Guide to Ultrasonic Imaging.* Baltimore: Urban & Schwarzenberg; 1984.
78. Solomon MJ, Stephen MS, White GH, Eyers AA. A new classification of hepatic territories using intraoperative ultrasound. *Am J Surg.* 1992;163:336–338.
79. Knol JA, Marn CS, Francis IR, et al. Comparisons of dynamic infusion and delayed computed tomography, intraoperative ultrasound, and palpation on the diagnosis of liver metastases. *Am J Surg.* 1993;165:81–88.
80. Brower ST, Dumitrescu O, Rubinoff S, et al. Operative ultrasound establishes resectability of metastases by major hepatic resection. *World J Surg.* 1989;13:649–657.
81. Ravikumar TS, Kane R, Cady B, et al. Hepatic cryosurgery with intraoperative ultrasound monitoring for metastatic colon carcinoma. *Arch Surg.* 1987;122:403–409.
82. Stewart PJ, Chu JM, Kos SC, et al. Intra-operative ultrasound for the detection of hepatic metastases from colorectal cancer. *Aust NZ J Surg.* 1993;63:530–534.
83. Soyer P, Levesque M, Elias D, et al. Detection of liver metastases from colorectal cancer: comparison of intraoperative US and CT during arterial portography. *Radiology.* 1992;183:541–544.
84. Boldrini G, de Gaetano AM, Giovannini I, et al. The systemic use of operative ultrasound for detection of liver metastases during colorectal surgery. *World J Surg.* 1987; 11:622–627.
85. Oudkerk M, van Ooijen B, Mali SP, et al. Liver metastases from colorectal carcinoma: detection with continuous CT angiography. *Radiology.* 1992;185:157–161.
86. Vogel SB, Drane WE, Ros PR, et al. Prediction of surgical resectability in patients with hepatic colorectal metastases. *Ann Surg.* 1994;219:508–514.
87. Hayashi N, Yamamoto K, Tamaki N, et al. Metastatic nodules of hepatocellular carcinoma: detection with angiography, CT, and US. *Radiology.* 1987;165:61–63.
88. Belghiti J, Panis Y, Farges O. Intrahepatic recurrence after resection of hepatocellular carcinoma complicating cirrhosis. *Ann Surg.* 1991;214:114–117.

89. Parker GA, Lawrence W Jr., Horsley JS, 3rd, et al. Intraoperative ultrasound of the liver affects operative decision making. *Ann Surg.* 1989;209:569–577.

90. Clouse ME. Current diagnostic imaging modalities of the liver. *Surg Clin North Am.* 1989;69:193–234.

91. Choji K, Shinohara M, Nojima T, et al. Significant reduction of the echogenicity of the compressed cavernous hemangioma. *Acta Radiol.* 1988 29:317–320.

92. Vogel SB, Drane WE, Ros PR, et al. Prediction of surgical resectability in patients with hepatic colorectal metastases. *Ann Surg.* 1994;219 508–516.

93. Machi J, Isomoto H, Yamashita Y, et al. Intraoperative ultrasonography in screening for liver metastases from colorectal cancer: comparative accuracy with traditional procedures. *Surgery.* 1987;101:678–684.

94. Gozzetti G, Mazziotti A, Bolondi L, et al. Intraoperative ultrasonography in surgery for liver tumors. *Surgery.* 1986;99:523–530.

95. Glassman AB. Hepatobiliary imaging: imaging modalities. *Ann Clin Lab Sci.* 1990; 20:56–59.

96. Silidker MS, Cronan JJ, Scola FH, et al. Ultrasound evaluation of cholelithiasis in the morbidly obese. *Gastrointest Radiol.* 1988;13:345–346.

97. Stott MA, Farrands PA, Guyer PB, et al. Ultrasound of the common bile duct in patients undergoing cholecystectomy. *J Clin Ultrasound.* 1991;19:73–76.

98. Thornton JR, Lobo AJ, Lintott DJ, Axon AT. Value of ultrasound and liver function tests in determining the need for endoscopic retrograde cholangiopancreatography in unexplained abdominal pain. *Gut.* 1992;33:1559–1561.

99. Buckley AR, Scudamore CH, Becker CD, Cooperberg PL. Intraoperative imaging of the biliary tree: Sonography vs. operative cholangiography. *J Ultrasound Med.* 1987; 6:589–595.

100. Ascher SM, Evans SR, Goldberg JA, et al. Intraoperative bile duct sonography during laparoscopic cholecystectomy: experience with a 12.5-MHz catheter-based US probe. *Radiology.* 1992;185:493–496.

101. Ascher SM, Evans SR, Zeman RK. Laparoscopic cholecystectomy: intraoperative ultrasound of the biliary tree and the natural history of postoperative ultrasound findings. *Semin Ultrasound CT MR.* 1993;14:331–337.

102. Castaing D, Emond J, Kunstlinger F, Bismuth H. Utility of operative ultrasound in the surgical management of liver tumors. *Ann Surg.* 1986;204:600–605.

103. Goeringer F. Imaging systems for combat casualty care. Presented First International Conference on Image Management and Communication in Patient Care; June 6, 1989; Washington, DC.

104. Kawasaki T, Moriyasu F, Kimura T, et al. Changes in portal blood flow consequent to partial hepatectomy: Doppler estimation. *Radiology.* 1991;180:373–377.

105. Rifkin MD, Rosato FE, Branch HM, et al. Intraoperative ultrasound of the liver: An important adjunctive tool for decision making in the operating room. *Ann Surg.* 1987:205:466–472.

106. Netter FH. *Atlas of Human Anatomy.* Summit, NJ: Ciba-Geigy Pharmaceuticals; 1989: Plate 272.

16

COMPUTED TOMOGRAPHY OF LIVER DISEASE

Sean M. Mahan, M.D., Paul M. Silverman, M.D., Cirrelda Cooper, M.D., and Susan M. Ascher, M.D.

Georgetown University Medical Center
Washington, DC

Robert K. Zeman, M.D.

University of Vermont College of Medicine
Burlington, VT

The liver is the largest organ in the abdomen and is functionally complex in its involvement in metabolism and detoxification. Not surprisingly, it is also a target of a wide range of inflammatory, neoplastic, and vascular abnormalities. For many of these processes, computed tomography (CT) is the imaging modality of choice. Its role in the detection of hepatic disease has been well established, and methods for optimizing visualization of various disease processes are well documented (1). With the adjunctive use of iodinated contrast agents, focal hepatic diseases can be detected by differences in attenuation between normal and pathological tissues. In order to maximize these attenuation differences, it is important to scan the liver during the time that normal hepatic enhancement is at a maximum, causing most abnormalities to appear as relatively low-density lesions. To accomplish this, the contrast must be given using dynamic techniques that control for the timing between contrast administration and the actual scan. Careful adherence to these technical factors allows maximization of lesion conspicuity.

Scanning during different phases of contrast enhancement allows for lesion enhancement patterns to be recognized. This provides useful information in characterizing pathology and thereby improves the specificity of these studies. Careful evaluation of enhancement patterns can narrow the list of differential diagnostic possibilities and in some cases provide a specific diagnosis, such as with benign hemangiomas.

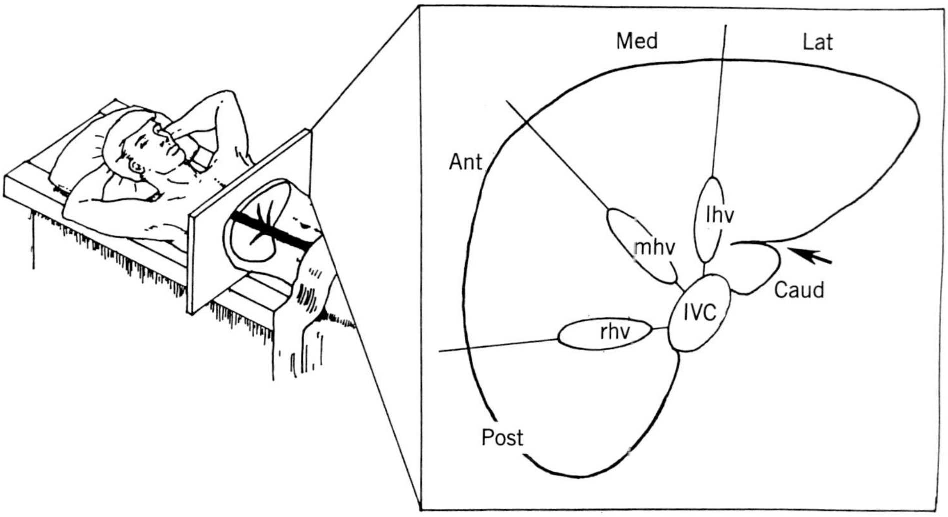

Figure 1. The segmental anatomy of the liver. This diagram illustrates a typical axial section through the liver. The liver is divided into segments by the hepatic veins (rhv = right hepatic vein, mhv = middle hepatic vein, lhv = left hepatic vein). The left lobe of the liver is divided into the lateral segment (lat) and the medial segment (med), and the right lobe of the liver s divided into the anterior segment (ant) and the posterior segment (post). The caudate lobe (caud) is bound by the fissure for the ligamentum teres (arrow) and the inferior vena cava (ivc).

Recently, helical (spiral) CT technology has been introduced and proved useful in improving examination of the liver. Unlike conventional CT, helical CT allows scanning the entire liver during a single breath held during peak contrast enhancement. In addition, by eliminating patient breathing during the scan, it alleviates problems with patient motion, as well as misregistration of axial slice selections, which can vary from breath to breath. These factors have made helical scanning a useful asset in improving the sensitivity of hepatic imaging and aiding in the detection of small lesions (2).

ANATOMY

The vascular anatomy that defines the surgical approach to hepatic resections is also relevant in hepatic imaging (Fig. 1) (3). Hepatic vascular territories define the liver into three lobes. The right and left lobes are separated by the major lobar fissure, which is defined by the middle hepatic vein superiorly, and by a line drawn from the vena cava through the gallbladder fossa inferiorly. The right lobe is further divided into anterior and posterior segments by the right intersegmental fissure, which is defined by the right hepatic vein. The left lobe is divided into medial and lateral segments by the left intersegmental fissure, which is defined by the left hepatic vein superiorly and the fissure for the ligamentum teres and falciform ligament inferiorly. The hepatic veins run in the interlobar and intersegmental fissures, whereas the portal triads, composed of the portal veins, hepatic arteries, and bile ducts, run in the intrasegmental parenchyma. The blood supply to the liver is dual: approximately three-fourths is supplied by the portal vein, while the remaining supply is from the hepatic artery. The caudate lobe is separated from the rest of the liver by the fissure for the ligamentum venosum anteriorly and the inferior vena cava posterolaterally. Its vascular supply varies, and receives hepatic arterial and portal venous supply from both the right and left branches. Its venous drainage is directly to the vena cava through multiple small veins. Knowledge of the appearance of these structures on CT allows for localization of lesions for possible resection and for assessment for changes on scans done at a later time.

DIFFUSE PARENCHYMAL DISEASE

Fatty Liver

Fatty infiltration of the liver is a common abnormality that results in an increase in the fat content of liver, and subsequently a decrease in attenuation radiographically. It is a nonspecific response by hepatocytes to varying etiologic factors. The most common cause is alcoholism; it has been shown that even small amounts of alcohol can increase hepatic fat content over a short period of time. Other etiologies include cirrhosis, diabetes, and chemotherapy. Nutritional deficiencies can also be a cause, such as malnutrition, hyperalimentation, and malabsorption associated with bypass surgery and inflammatory bowel disease (4). Fatty infiltration can occur with excessive steroids from either chronic therapy or Cushing's disease. There is also an acute form that may occur in the latter part of pregnancy.

In many cases it can be readily diagnosed by CT, and comes in three basic patterns: diffuse, focal, and multifocal. Diffuse fatty infiltration is the most common form and can be recognized by uniform decrease in attenuation of hepatic parenchymal tissue. Blood vessels run their course normally through the liver and after contrast administration they stand out as the rest of the liver appears less dense than usual. There is no evidence of mass effect, yet hepatomegaly is often present. The focal and multifocal forms typically appears as geographic regions of liver with low attenuation which are seen adjacent to regions of higher-density normal liver (Fig. 2). Again, there is no mass effect and vessels course normally through these regions. Furthermore, the margins of involved regions are typically angled, whereas neoplastic etiologies are often round. Careful evaluation of these signs can be used confidently to make the diagnosis of fatty infiltration without additional studies; however, in difficult cases, further evaluation with ultrasound and magnetic resonance imaging (MRI) can be helpful (5). Alternatively, follow-up CT scans can be done to assess for improvement upon withdrawal of the etiologic factor.

Cirrhosis

Cirrhosis represents chronic hepatic fibrosis that can result from a variety of causes. The most common causes include alcoholic liver disease and viral hepatitis. It is characterized by a chronic and progressive destruction of hepatocytes with a subsequent distortion in the hepatic architecture and deposition of fibrosis. Paren-

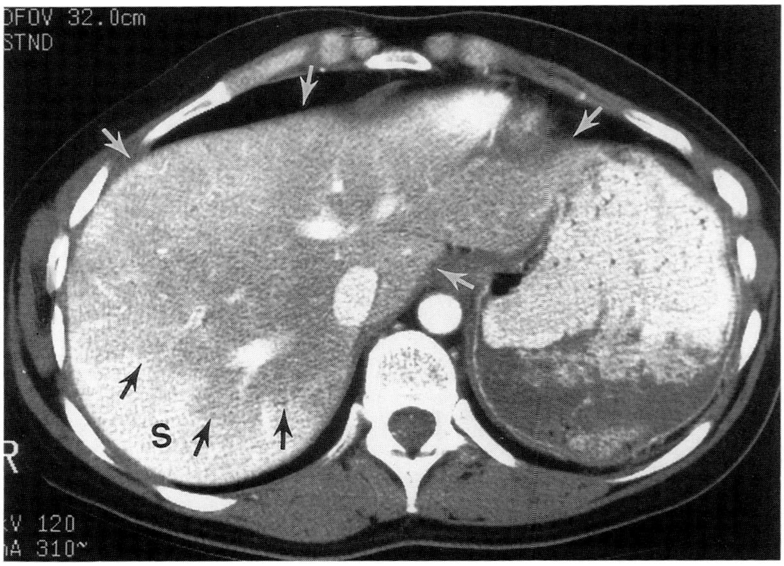

Figure 2. Fatty infiltration of the liver. The general diffuse hypodensity involving the left lobe, the anterior segment of the right lobe, and the caudate lobe represents areas of geographic fatty infiltration (arrows). Sparing is seen in the posterior segment of the right lobe (S).

chymal nodules develop from cell regeneration and scar formation. Portal hypertension, ascites, portosystemic shunts, and splenomegaly typically occur (6).

Characteristic imaging findings include fatty infiltration and hepatomegaly during early stages. With time, the liver develops an irregular contour due to alternating regions of atrophy and regenerating nodules. There is a characteristic decrease in the size of the right lobe and medial segment of the left lobe, with a compensatory enlargement of the lateral segment of the left lobe and the caudate lobe. In subtle cases, a ratio comparing the sizes of the caudate lobe and the right lobe can prove helpful. The caudate lobe should be measured transversely at the level of the main portal vein, and the right lobe should be measured transversely from the main portal vein to the lateral liver margin. A caudate-to-right lobe ratio greater than 0.65 suggests the diagnosis of cirrhosis with 96% confidence (5).

Other findings are due to the secondary portal hypertension that complicates the disease owing to the progressive fibrosis of the hepatic vascular bed. Ascites and splenomegaly develop. In addition, the portal vein, normally less than 13 mm in diameter, may be increased in size, or portal vein thrombosis may occur. This appears as a low-attenuation mass within the lumen of the vein does not enhance with contrast. Recognizing portosystemic collaterals can also help determine the presence of portal hypertension. These appear as brightly enhancing tubular structures, often tortuous, and occur at typical sites. Common locations include gastric and esophageal varices, recanalization of the paraumbilical veins, splenorenal shunts, paravertebral varices, and hemorrhoidal varices (Fig. 3). Note that the most important of these collaterals clinically are the esophageal varices, which present in 65% of patients with advanced cirrhosis and cause massive upper gastrointestinal hemorrhage and death in half of these patients (6).

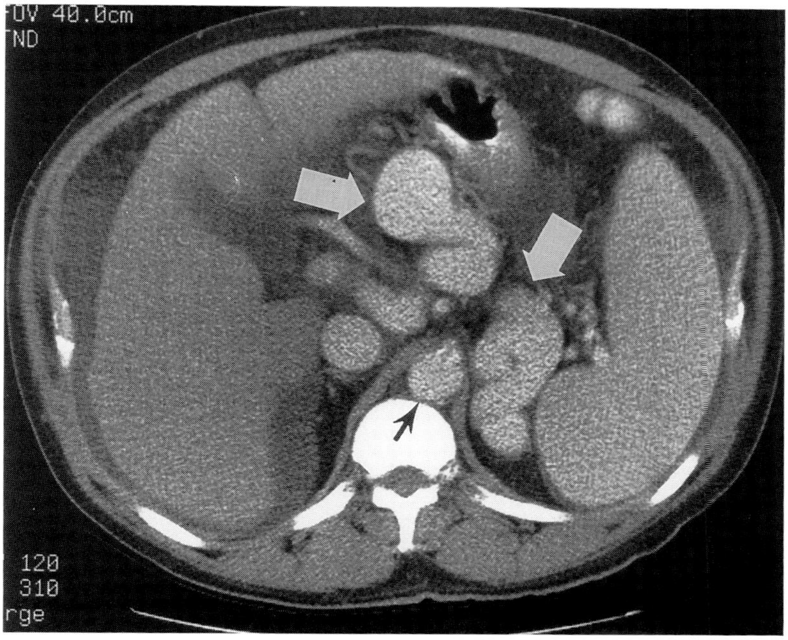

Figure 3. Abdominal and retroperitoneal varices. The large tubular-shaped masses (large arrows) enhance as much as the aorta (small arrow), indicating their vascular nature. They are enlarged esophageal and gastric varices that accompany portal venous hypertension. Irregular contours to the hepatic border, ascites, and splenomegaly are present in this patient with cirrhosis and portal hypertension.

Budd–Chiari Syndrome

Budd–Chiari syndrome results from occlusion of the hepatic venous drainage of the liver. This may result from a variety of etiologies, which include hypercoagulable states, neoplasm, and iatrogenic causes. Many cases are idiopathic (6). Computed tomography findings include nonopacification of the hepatic veins and heterogeneous enhancement of the liver parenchyma. Hepatomegaly is often present. In chronic cases, the caudate lobe compensatorily enlarges and brightly enhances relative to the affected lobes; this is due to the preservation of the normal venous drainage of the caudate, which does not drain into the hepatic venous system, but rather drains directly into the vena cava. Ascites may be an associated feature.

Hemochromatosis

Hemochromatosis is an uncommon disorder that results from excessive iron deposition within the liver. There are both primary and secondary forms of the disease. The primary disease is hereditary with an autosomal recessive pattern of inheritance. The secondary form is seen in patients with chronic anemias and erythroid hyperplasia, as well as those receiving multiple blood transfusions. High dietary iron may also cause secondary disease. With long-term disease there is an increased risk for cirrhosis and hepatocellular carcinoma. On CT, a diffuse increase in hepatic density can be seen due to the increased attenuation to X-rays by iron.

FOCAL HEPATIC MASSES

One of the primary goals in imaging lesions of the liver is being able to differentiate benign masses such as hemangiomas and cysts, which are both very common, from malignant neoplasms. Although cysts can be differentiated from solid masses with ultrasound, the sonographic appearance of solid lesions is often nonspecific. Computed tomography allows for discrimination of both benign cystic and solid masses, which are clinically insignificant, from their malignant counterparts. It is important to emphasize that adherence to dynamic contrast techniques is necessary to evaluate these processes accurately; by evaluating the various patterns of enhancement, benign lesions can often be identified, and unnecessary biopsies can be avoided. The features used to discern these lesions are addressed.

Benign Hepatic Tumors

Hemangioma. Hemangiomas are the most common benign tumor of the liver, and occur in 4–7% of patients in autopsy series. They are the second most common neoplasm, exceeded in frequency only by metastatic disease. Unfortunately, up to 10% of patients with hemangiomas have multiple lesions, and the diagnosis can easily be mistaken for metastases. The tumor consists of large, blood-filled vascular spaces that are lined by a thin wall of epithelium. Nearly all these lesions are asymptomatic when less than 5 cm in size, and only when they are larger do symptoms occur. These larger lesions can cause vague, right upper quadrant pain by either mass effect, hemorrhage, or arteriovenous shunting (7).

Blood flow through the large vascular spaces of the hemangioma is slow, which results in its classic imaging findings (8). On precontrast and very early post-contrast scans, hemangiomas appear as nonspecific well-defined hypodense masses. Shortly thereafter, delayed contrast enhancement occurs in a characteristic pattern of peripheral nodular enhancement that progresses to central enhancement centripetally on delayed exams (Fig. 4). In many cases the lesion becomes isodense with normal liver. When the classic enhancement pattern is present, the diagnosis of hemangioma can be made with confidence. Unfortunately, in atypical cases, differentiation of hemangioma from malignancy with a screening CT scan may not be possible. This diagnostic dilemma can be overcome by performing a dedicated CT scan tailored for characterization of a hemangioma (9). The technique involves administration of a dynamic bolus of intravenous contrast with subsequent CT scanning followed by reimaging over the course of minutes to characterize the enhancement pattern accurately (Table 1).

Atypical enhancement patterns are most often features of small (less than 1.5 cm) or very large (greater than 5 cm) hemangiomas. The small lesions may enhance rapidly, and the classic peripheral nodular appearance may not be seen. On the other hand, large lesions, which are called giant cavernous hemangiomas, secondarily thrombose and fibrose centrally. This central scar typically does not enhance completely. In cases where further work-up may be required, a tagged red blood cell nuclear medicine scan or dynamic contrast-enhanced MRI can be helpful. Biopsy should not be considered as a primary method of diagnosis because of the risk of hemorrhage, which can be severe and even fatal. However, in atypical cases where

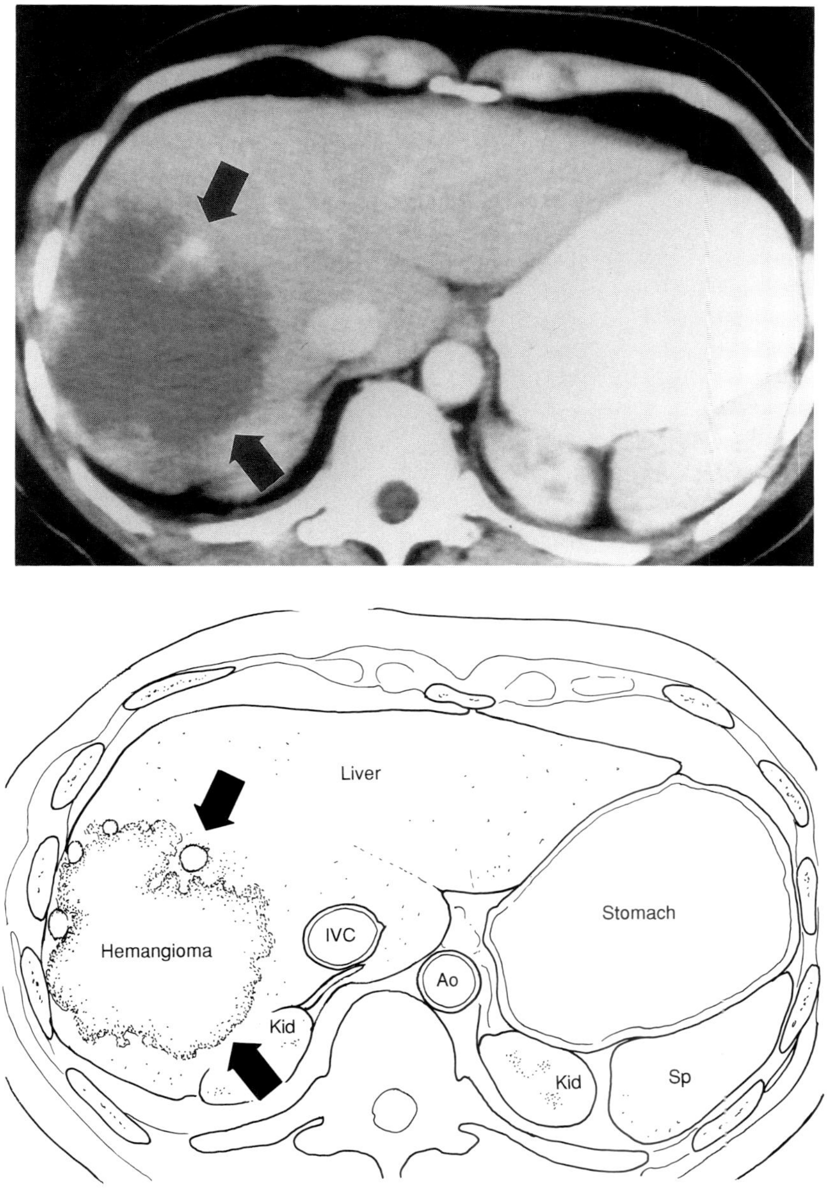

Figure 4. Cavernous hemangioma. A hypodense mass seen in the liver (arrows) has the characteristic puddling of contrast typically seen in hemangiomas. Note that in many cases complete enhancement can be seen, but is not necessary to make the diagnosis.

tissue diagnosis is required, a biopsy may be done safely with a small needle. Biopsy findings include normal epithelial cells without evidence of malignancy (10).

Focal Nodular Hyperplasia. This benign tumor, known as focal nodular hyperplasia (FNH), typically occurs in females (70–80% of all lesions) during the second and third decades, and is usually an asymptomatic incidental finding, although vague

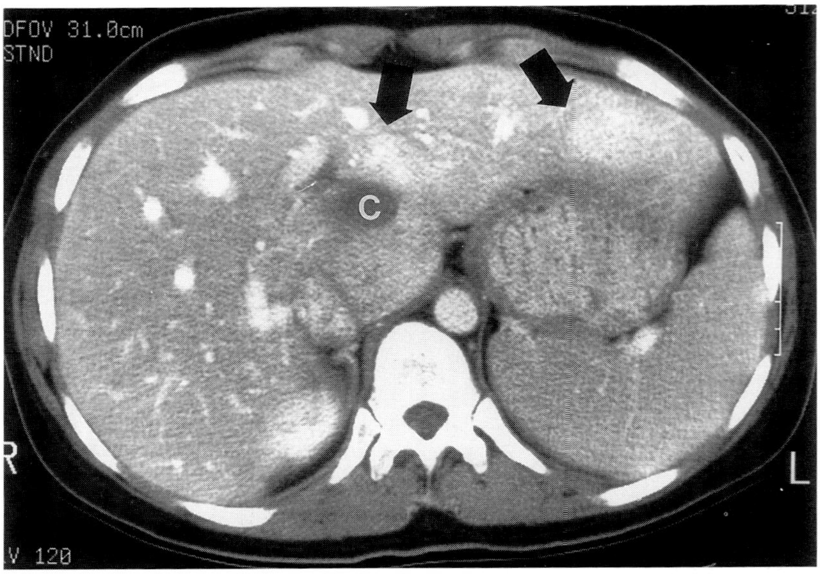

Figure 5. Focal nodular hyperplasia. This early-phase post-enhancement scan demonstrates focal brightly enhancing regions that are consistent with focal nodular hyperplasia (arrows). Also note the incidental hepatic cyst discovered (C).

right upper quadrant pain may occur. Focal nodular hyperplasia lesions contain all the histological elements of normal liver, including Kupffer cells, bile ducts, and hepatocytes, all abnormally arranged. They have no malignant potential, and are unlikely to hemorrhage. The significance in accurately diagnosing the lesion lies in differentiating it from other neoplasms that occur in the same patient population, particularly fibrolamellar hepatocellular carcinoma and hepatic adenoma (11).

Because of their prominent vascularity, FNH lesions demonstrate early enhancement pattern (Fig. 5). In addition, a central scar may be present. On delayed imaging, FNH is isodense to normal surrounding liver. These findings can also be seen with both fibrolamellar hepatocellular carcinoma and hepatic adenomas, and therefore a clear diagnosis cannot typically be made with CT scanning alone. Nuclear medicine sulfur colloid scans are often helpful and are recommended in cases where the diagnosis of FNH is considered. Because of the presence of Kupffer cells,

Table 1. Sensitivity and specificity for CT findings in the diagnosis of hepatic hemangiomas

CT Feature of Hemangioma	Sensitivity (%)	Specificity (%)
Nodular enhancement	76	90
Peripheral enhancement pattern	67	45
Isodense enhancement compared with aorta	77	97
Combination of two or three of the above findings	67–84	94–100

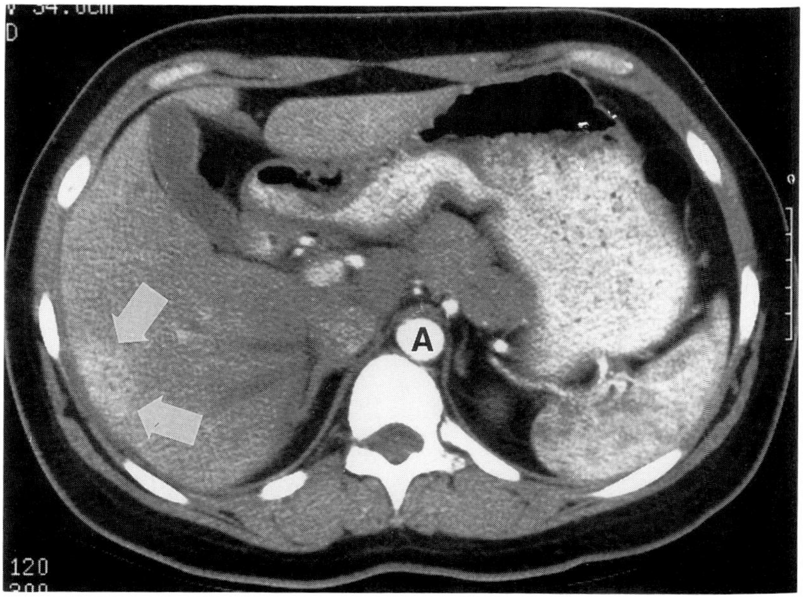

Figure 6. Hepatic adenoma. The dense mass in the right lobe of the liver demonstrates a classic early enhancement pattern of a hepatic adenoma (arrows). Note the early phase of the scan by the densely enhanced aorta (A).

60% of FNH lesions show normal homogeneous uptake of radiotracer; this, in conjunction with CT findings, is extremely suggestive of this diagnosis (11).

Hepatic Adenoma. Hepatic adenomas are rare, benign tumors that are significant because of their risk of major hemorrhage and small risk of malignant degeneration. In 95% of cases, these lesions occur in young adult women and are associated with the use of oral contraceptives, which increase both the risk of tumor growth and hemorrhage. Patients present because of abdominal mass, abdominal pain, or hemoperitoneum due to tumor rupture. Histologically, these lesions are composed entirely of abnormally arranged hepatocytes, and are completely devoid of Kupffer cells or bile duct tissue. As a result, they typically do not take up radiotracer on nuclear medicine sulfur colloid studies.

With dynamic enhanced CT, hepatic adenomas may appear as rounded intrahepatic lesions that demonstrate rapid and transient enhancement (Fig. 6). However, the enhancement pattern for this lesion is quite variable, and areas of central necrosis and hemorrhage are nearly always present. Central calcifications may be seen with larger lesions due to previous hemorrhage. In most cases, imaging findings are nonspecific.

Hepatic Cyst. Hepatic cysts are the second most common benign lesion of the liver, following hemangioma. They are typically solitary, although they may be multiple, especially in patients with polycystic kidney disease. In these patients, 50% have multiple hepatic cysts.

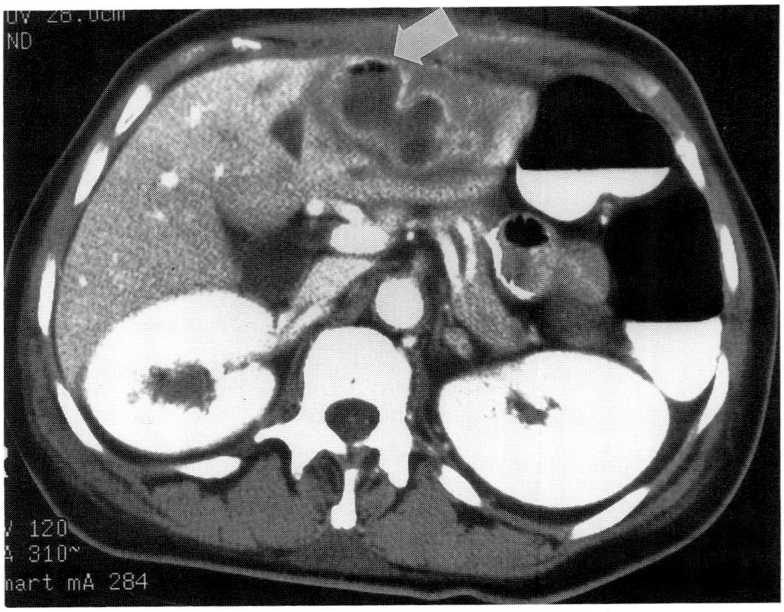

Figure 7. Pyogenic abscess. The irregular thick enhancing wall is classic for the appearance of a pyogenic abscess. Note the small black bubbles of gas that rest on the nondependent surface of the lesion (arrow). Gas is seen in 20% of such cases.

The criteria for the diagnosis of simple hepatic cyst include sharp margins with no definable wall (12). The CT density measurement is typically that of water (less than 20 Hounsfield units). They have no internal structure and demonstrate no enhancement on delayed imaging. When a lesion demonstrates these features, the diagnosis of hepatic cyst is made with confidence. Unlike cysts in the kidneys, hepatic cysts tend to possess lobulated margins. The differential diagnosis for cystic masses of the liver includes cystic metastases, pyogenic abscess, and biliary cystadenoma and cystadenocarcinoma. In these cases, differentiation can typically be made by adhering to the strict criteria for a simple hepatic cyst.

Hepatic abscess. Hepatic abscesses may be pyogenic, mycotic, or parisitic. Pyogenic or bacterial abscesses are focal collections of pus within the hepatic parenchyma, and most commonly occur as a sequela of ascending cholangitis, an ascending infection through the biliary pathway. Other causes include hematogenous spread, contiguous spread from an adjacent infection, and spread from secondary infection following surgery or trauma. Most commonly gram-negative organisms are involved, and patients present with typical symptoms that include nausea, vomiting, fever, chills, and right upper quadrant pain. Many patients have abnormal liver function tests, and jaundice may occur in up to one-third of patients. Patients typically appear septic, and without proper therapy rapid disease progression and death may occur.

Pyogenic abscesses are often solitary, but may be multifocal or multilocular (Fig. 7). Although they can appear cystic on unenhanced scans, contrast typically demonstrates thick enhancing walls. 20% of lesions contain gas, and air–fluid levels may be seen. Although metastatic disease can mimic the CT findings, the clinical picture is usually very different, and the combination of physical and CT findings can make a confident diagnosis. Needle aspiration can confirm the diagnosis, and treatment by percutaneous drainage may be done at the same time.

Amebic abscesses are rarely seen in the United States, but are common in other parts of the world, and may be seen in patients with recent travel history. The offending organism is Entamoeba histolytica; it is thought to infect the liver following colonic amebiasis via hematogenous spread through the portal vein. For this reason, the lesions are often peripheral in location. Patients usually present with abdominal pain, fever, weight loss, and symptoms due to colonic involvement; however, these patients are not typically septic. The CT appearance of these abscesses overlaps that of pyogenic abscesses, with a low-attenuation cystic appearance and thick enhancing walls. Gas is not typically present. Diagnosis can be confirmed by correlating imaging findings with history, clinical findings, and positive hemagglutination titers (13). Treatment is done medically with metronidazole.

Echinococcal infection of the liver can occur as a result of two organisms, Echinococcus granulosis and Echinococcus multilocularis. The former typically presents with large, encapsulated hepatic cysts, whereas the latter, more rare, is more often associated with disseminated disease. The parasite usually resides in the colon; extracolonic disease involves the liver in the majority of cases. Animals, typically dogs, are the definite chief hosts of the parasite, and humans become accidental hosts by ingesting food contaminated by ova from dog feces. The ingested eggs hatch in the accidental host's upper gastrointestinal tract, and subsequently spread to the liver via the portal system. In the liver, the parasite encysts, and the patient is usually asymptomatic until the cyst becomes large enough to cause abdominal pain. Computed tomography imaging of echinococcal abscesses typically demonstrates large cystic areas (Fig. 8). Calcifications may be present 50% of the time, and daughter cysts may be seen in 70% of patients. The presence of these additional finding scan suggest the diagnosis. Surgery is the treatment of choice for these lesions.

Mycotic abscesses of the liver may be seen typically in immunocompromised patients. They are usually suspected by elevated liver function tests in patients who are immunosuppressed. When they occur, they are typically multiple and are often accompanied by additional small abscesses within the spleen. The most common etiologic agent is Candida albicans. On CT, these mycotic abscesses appear as multiple small low-attenuation lesions with enhancing walls, and are often termed microabscesses because they appear as multiple small pyogenic abscesses (14) (Fig. 9). Correlation with CT findings and the proper clinical situation strongly suggests this diagnosis.

Malignant Hepatic Tumors

Metastatic Disease. Metastases are the most common malignant tumor of the liver, as well as the most common lesion overall. The primary tumor may be from almost any source; however, the most common lesions associated with hepatic metastases arise from the colon, stomach, pancreas, breast, and lung. In general, the presence of hepatic metastases is a grave prognostic indicator. However, with increasing interest in selective resection therapy for metastatic disease, the accurate diagnosis of the extent of liver involvement is critical.

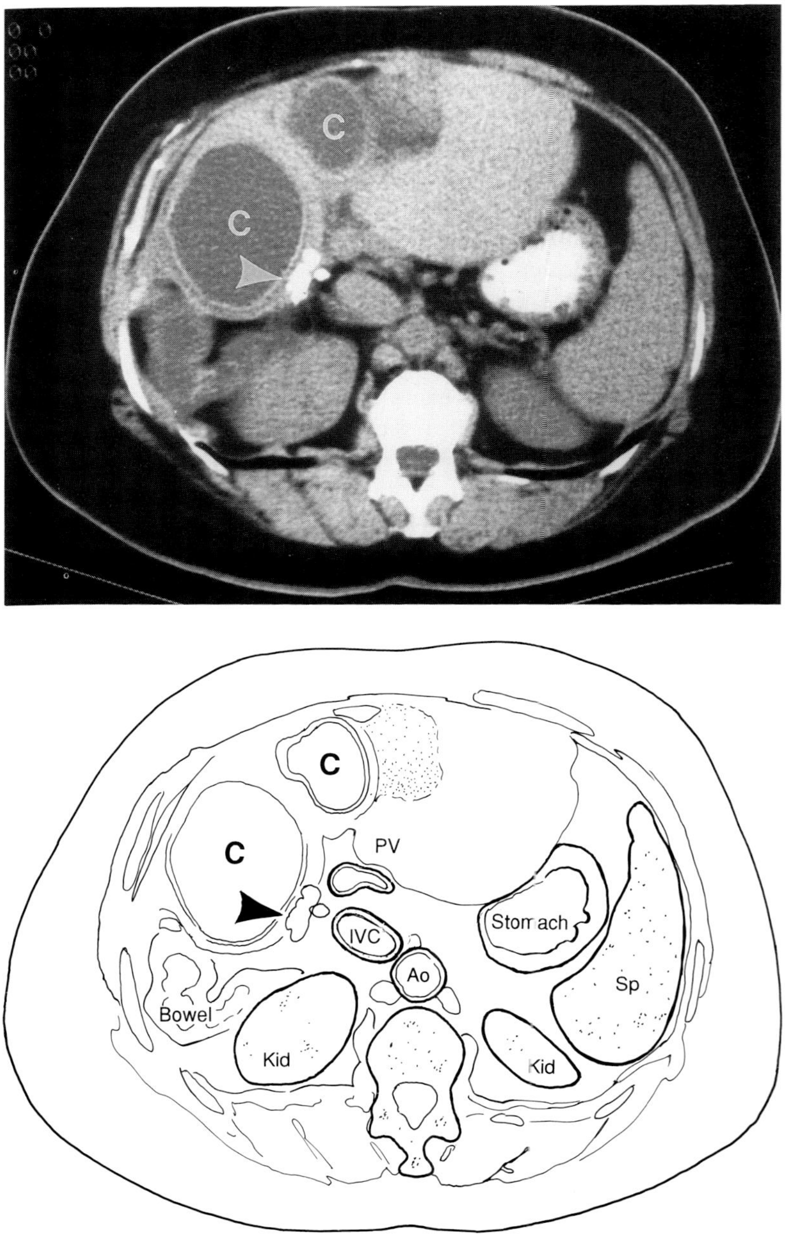

Figure 8. Echinococcal cysts. This patient demonstrates large hypodense cystic masses (C) with well-defined thick-walled capsules. Peripheral calcification (arrowhead) is observed.

Computed tomography findings of metastases include a wide spectrum of appearances. They may occur in any shape, size, or number. The lesions can be focal or diffuse, solitary or multiple. By far the most common appearance on CT is that of the low-attenuation lesion relative to surrounding normal liver; however, it is important to keep in mind that hyperdense and isodense lesions may also occur.

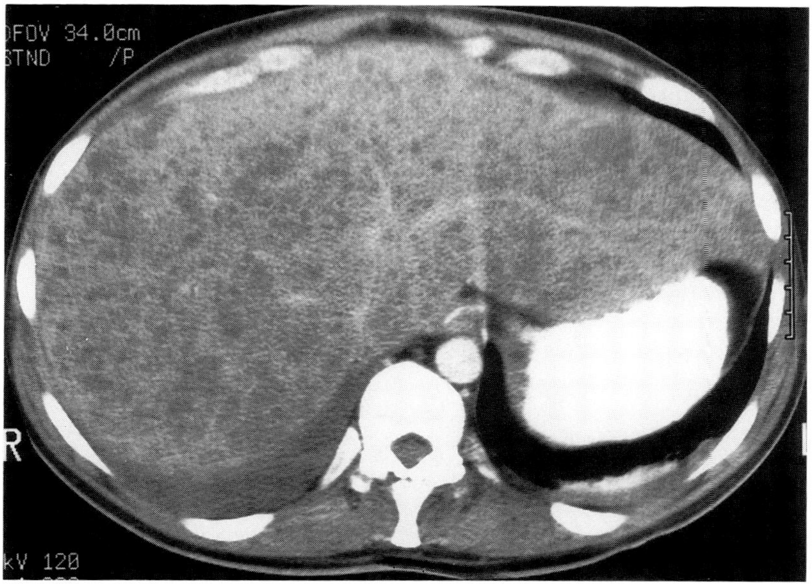

Figure 9. Candidiasis. Bone marrow transplant patient in whom the liver is diffusely involved by numerous small hypodense lesions that are microabscesses caused by Candida albicans.

They may be homogeneously solid, or they may have cystic, necrotic, or calcific regions within them (Fig. 10). In general, however, there is some degree of enhancement on contrast-enhanced scans. A diagnostic dilemma occurs in the case of the solitary metastatic lesion, as well as when the metastasis mimics another characteristic lesion such as the peripheral enhancement pattern of the hemangioma. Because of this possibility, metastatic disease must be considered in the differential of virtually any enhancing hepatic mass, and further evaluation with biopsy, dedicated dynamic scanning, or other imaging modality such as ultrasound or MRI is often necessary. Additionally, certain types of metastases, such as islet cell tumors, carcinoids, renal cell carcinomas, melanomas, and pheochromocytomas, are hypervascular in nature; subsequently, CT scanning done with the same protocol to detect colonic metastases can miss these hypervascular lesions, which may be isodense at the time of the scan. Therefore, either special dedicated protocols for these primary lesions should be utilized, or a precontrast study should be additionally done to evaluate for the presence of these lesions (15).

Another dilemma in the detection of metastatic disease lies in the limitations of the sensitivity of CT scanning. Although lesions as small as a few millimeters in size can be seen on CT, they are difficult to characterize when they are less than 8–10 mm in size. Of course, microscopic metastases will be missed, and follow-up studies must be done to exclude this possibility.

There is currently a growing interest in treating hepatic metastases with partial hepatic resection. Studies have shown that such therapy can improve survival of patients with certain tumors, such as hepatocellular carcinoma and colorectal carcinoma (16). To improve on the sensitivity of detection of metastatic deposits, the

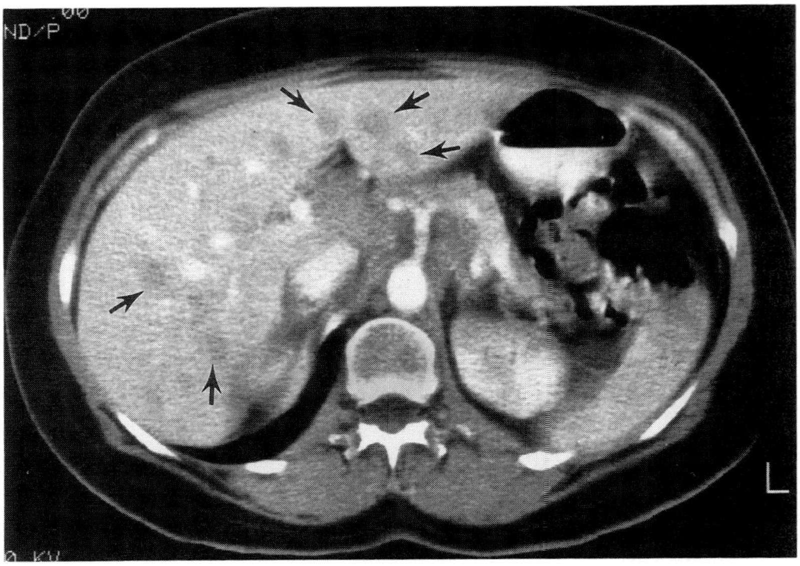

Figure 10. Metastatic disease. Patient with colon carcinoma and multiple intrahepatic lesions (arrows), many demonstrating the heterogeneous enhancement pattern of metastatic disease.

technique of CT arterial portography (CTAP) is being done to increase lesion conspicuity. The technique involves selective delivery of contrast into the portal system by angiographically catheterizing the splenic artery or the superior mesenteric artery, and then rapidly scanning the liver using dynamic technique. Because hepatic neoplasms are largely supplied by the hepatic arterial system, and the contrast is being selectively administered to the portal venous system, the result is an increase in the attenuation difference between the lesion and the normal liver parenchyma. Although the study is complex and requires both interventional and imaging modalities, reported sensitivity of CTAP in lesion detection is among the highest of radiological techniques. The reported sensitivities for CTAP for lesion detection range from 81 to 91%, and with helical CTAP the sensitivity improves to 94% (17).

Hepatocellular Carcinoma. Hepatocellular carcinoma, also known as hepatoma, is the most common visceral malignancy in the world, and represents 80–90% of primary liver malignancies. In the United States, the most common cause is cirrhosis, with 80% of these tumors arising in cirrhotic livers. Clinically, these patients present with pain, weight loss, and sometimes a palpable hepatic mass. Elevated serum alpha-fetoprotein suggests the diagnosis.

There are three classic patterns of tumor growth typically seen: solitary lesion (50%), diffuse infiltrative tumor (30%), and multifocal tumor (20%). These lesions are typically low-attenuation lesions that brightly enhance in a variable pattern. Enhancement is often bright but transient, and regions of tumor necrosis and hemorrhage are common, giving the lesions a heterogeneous appearance. Hepato-

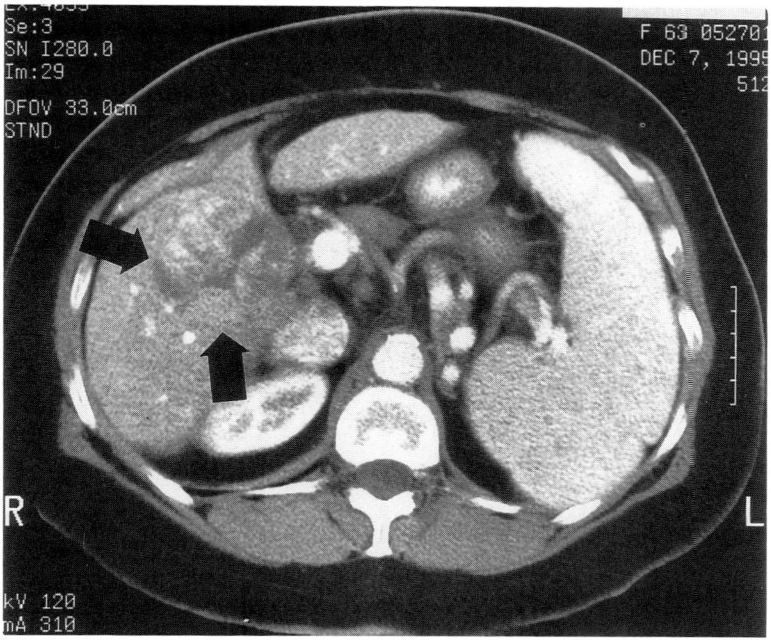

Figure 11. Hepatocellular carcinoma. CT section through the liver of a patient with cirrhosis and portal hypertension demonstrates a large heterogeneously enhancing hepatocellular carcinoma (arrows).

mas invade the portal vein in up to one-third of cases (12) (Fig. 11). This results in obstruction to the blood supply of the involved segment of liver, and as a result, wedge-shaped areas of decreased attenuation may be seen.

Fibrolamellar hepatocellular carcinoma is a distinctive subtype of hepatoma which occurs in younger patients, with a mean age of 20 years old. They typically occur in normal livers without underlying disease. Alpha-fetoprotein levels are typically not elevated, and the prognosis is typically better than with other hepatomas. On CT, these lesions appear as well-circumscribed masses that enhance uniformly. Sometimes a central scar can be seen, as with focal nodular hyperplasia and adenomas, which are in the differential diagnosis.

LIVER TRAUMA

In cases of blunt abdominal trauma, CT is the imaging modality of choice. With the administration of contrast, regions of hepatic injury can be identified as focal regions of decreased enhancement compared with normal liver parenchyma. Small regions of injury are typically classified as contusions, and are typically seen as low-density regions without associated hemoperitoneum. Lacerations represent larger lesions, and can be seen as linear or irregular low-density bands; they are commonly associated with intrahepatic hematomas and hemoperitoneum. When hematomas are subcapsular, they are typically seen as lentiform or crescent-shaped masses that lie on the periphery of the liver and are of low density compared to normal liver enhancement. Contrast within these areas of hematoma defines active ongoing hemorrhage, and urgent therapy may be required to prevent further morbidity and possible hypovolemic shock.

FUTURE DIRECTIONS

Improvements in both lesion detection and diagnosis can be expected as advancements in technology continue to be made. The advent of helical scanning provides faster scanning techniques, as well as greater flexibility in the acquisition of scans during varying phases of enhancement. As these changes continue to provide greater control in scan acquisition, improvements can be expected in hepatic enhancement, which is the major determinant of lesion conspicuity (2).

Newer technologies are also being made that link the timing of maximum contrast enhancement with the acquisition of the scan as it varies with the individual patient. These improvements will change the way CT scanning is done from a fixed delay, which may not be appropriate for every patient, to a variable delay based upon an individual patient's organ enhancement. This capability should further improve the detection of hepatic lesions, as well as eliminate suboptimal enhancement in patients with significant cardiovascular disease (18, 19).

REFERENCES

1. Burgener FA, Hamlin DJ. Contrast enhancement in abdominal CT: bolus vs. Infusion. *AJR.* 1981;137:351.
2. Zeman RK, Fox SH, Silverman PM, et al. Helical (spiral) CT of the abdomen. *AJR.* 1993;160:719–725.
3. Mukai JK, Stack CM, Turner DA, et al. Imaging of surgically relevant hepatic vascular and segmental anatomy. *AJR.* 1987;149:287–297.
4. Baker ME, Silverman PM. Nodular focal fatty infiltration of the liver: CT appearance, *AJR.* 1985;145:79–80.
5. Robbins SL, Coltran RS, Kumar V. *Pathologic Basis of Disease,* 3rd ed. Philadelphia: WB Saunders; 1984:884–942.
6. Harbin WP, Robert NJ, Ferrucci JT. Diagnosis of cirrhosis based on regional changes in hepatic morphology. *Radiology.* 1980;135:273–283.
7. Johnson CM, Sheedy PF II, Stanson AW, et al. Computed tomography and angiography of cavernous hemangiomas of the liver. *Radiology.* 1981;138:115–121.
8. Nelson RC, Chezmar JL. Diagnostic approach to hepatic hemangiomas. *Radiology.* 1990;176:11–13.
9. Freeny PC, Marks WM. Hepatic hemangioma: dynamic bolus CT. *AJR.* 1986;147: 711–719.
10. Birnbaum BA, Weinraub JC, Megibow AJ, et al. Definitive diagnosis of hepatic hemangiomas: MR imaging versus Tc-99m-labeled red blood cell SPECT. *Radiology.* 1990; 176:95–101.
11. Bluemke DA, Fishman EK. Spiral CT of the liver. *AJR.* 1993;160:787–792.

12. Murphy BJ, Casillas J, Ros PR, et al. The CT appearance of cystic masses of the liver. *Radiographics.* 1989;9:307–322.

13. Landay MJ, Setaiwan H, Hirsh G, et al. Hepatic and thoracic amoebiasis, *AJR* 1980;135:449–454.

14. Callen PW, Filly RA, Marcus FS. Ultrasonography and computed tomography in the evaluation of hepatic microabscesses in the immunocompromised patient. *Radiology.* 1980;136:433–434.

15. Bressler EL, Alpern MB, Glazer GM, et al. Hypervascular hepatic metastasis. *Radiology.* 1987;162:49–51.

16. Soyer P, Bluemke DA, Zeitoun G, et al. Detection of recurrent hepatic metastases after partial hepatectomy: value of CT combined with arterial portography. *AJR.* 1994; 162:1327.

17. Soyer P, Roche A, Gad M, et al. Preoperative segmental localization of hepatic metastases: utility of three-dimensional CT during arterial portography. *Radiology.* 1991; 180:653–658.

18. Silverman PM, Roberts SC, Ducic I, et al. Assessment of a technology that permits individualized scan delays on helical hepatic CT: a technique to improve efficiency in the use of contrast material. *AJR.* 1996;167:79–84.

19. Silverman PM, Roberts S, Tefft MC, et al. Helical (spiral) CT of the liver: value of an automated computer technique, smart prep, for obtaining images with optimal contrast enhancement. *AJR.* 1995;165:73–78.

17

NUCLEAR MEDICINE IN LIVER DISEASE

Harvey A. Ziessman, M.D.
Georgetown University Medical Center
Washington, DC

Many radiopharmaceuticals, each with unique mechanisms of uptake, have been used over the years to image benign and malignant tumors of the liver and to evaluate the cause of hepatic parenchymal dysfunction. This section on the liver highlights the fact that nuclear medicine is physiological imaging: the scintigraphic liver images represent not merely anatomy, but a specific hepatic function. An understanding of the radiopharmaceutical's mechanism of uptake allows one to make diagnoses based on pathophysiology. As an example, Tc 99m sulfur colloid (SC) has been used in the past for conventional liver and spleen imaging. Because its mechanism of uptake is phagocytosis by Kupffer cells in the liver, it can be used to differentiate focal nodular hyperplasia, which has Kupffer cells, from hepatic adenomas, which do not. This chapter discusses many other radiopharmaceuticals used for liver imaging with different mechanisms of uptake, that can be used to detect, diagnose, and follow patients with benign and malignant tumors of the liver, for example, Tc 99m IDA, Tc 99m MAA, xenon 133, gallium 67, Tc 99m sestamibi, and ^{18}F-fluorodeoxyglucose (Table 1).

PARENCHYMAL LIVER DISEASE

Technetium 99m sulfur colloid has been used over the years to evaluate various hepatic disorders. Although the mechanism of uptake of this radiopharmaceutical is due to the phagocytic function of the reticuloendothelial system, any diffuse process of the liver will be detected owing to the homogeneous distribution of Kupffer cells throughout the liver. The most common disease investigated by the method is cirrhosis. The resulting images depend to a large extent on the stage of cirrhosis. In early stages, hepatosplenomegaly, decreased hepatic uptake, and

Table 1. Radiopharmaceuticals used for liver tumor imaging

Radiopharmaceutical	Mechanism of Uptake	Tumor Diagnosis
Tc 99m SC	Kupffer cell	FNH
Tc 99m HIDA	Hepatocyte	FNH, hepatoma
Tc 99m RBC	Blood pool	Cavernous hemangioma
Tc 99m MAA	Blood flow	Intraarterial chemotherapy
Xenon 133	Lipid soluble	Fatty focal tumors
Gallium 67	Iron binding	Localized viable tumors
Thallium 201	ATPase transport	Nonspecific tumor imaging
Sestamibi	Mitochondrial	Nonspecific tumor imaging
F 18 FDG	Glycolysis	Nonspecific tumor imaging

increased bone marrow and splenic uptake are characteristic. As the disease advances, atrophy of the right lobe with compensatory hypertrophy of the left lobe often develops.

The Budd–Chiari syndrome is caused by obstruction of the hepatic venous outflow, in either the major hepatic veins or inferior vena cava. It is associated with hepatic malignancy, infection, and thrombotic disorders. If only a few hepatic veins are involved, radiocolloid uptake may be decreased in those segments. If most of the veins are involved a characteristic pattern is seen on Tc 99m SC scintigraphy, with uptake generally decreased; however, the caudate lobe is often spared owing to its drainage directly into the inferior vena cava, which appears as increased uptake in that area (1).

BENIGN LIVER TUMORS

Cavernous Hemangiomas of the Liver

Cavernous liver hemangiomas are the most common benign tumors of the liver. Histologically, these tumors are composed of endothelial-lined vascular channels of varying size separated by fibrous septa (2). Liver hemangiomas are usually single, although at least 10% of patients have multiple lesions. Pathologically, cavernous hemangiomas are not related to infantile capillary hemangiomas, angiodysplastic lesions, or hemangioendotheliomas.

Cavernous hemangiomas are usually asymptomatic and do not require specific therapy. Only very rarely do patients have symptoms due to thrombosis, infarction, hemorrhagic rupture, or massive hepatomegaly. Liver function tests are almost always normal. The tumors are usually discovered incidentally by CT or ultrasonography in the evaluation of patients with unrelated abdominal pain or in the work-up of patients with known cancer. The clinical problem is to determine whether these lesions represent malignant tumor. Because biopsy of a cavernous hemangioma has resulted in serious hemorrhage and death (3, 4), noninvasive diagnosis is preferable.

Noninvasive Diagnosis. Although characteristic findings have been described with ultrasonography (homogeneous, hyperechoic mass with well-defined margins and posterior acoustic enhancement), these findings are neither sensitive nor specific for making the diagnosis (5–7).

Contrast-enhanced computed tomography (CT) often cannot differentiate hemangiomas from other benign or malignant tumors. To achieve high specificity for the diagnosis of cavernous hemangioma, strict criteria must be used: (1) relative hypoattenuation before contrast injection, (2) early peripheral enhancement during the bolus dynamic phase, and (3) progressive opacification toward the center of the lesion with complete isodense fill-in by 30 min after contrast administration. If the study satisfies *all* the criteria, specificity can be as high as 85%. However, the sensitivity is only 55% (8); that is, 45% of patients have a nondiagnostic study. If one uses less strict criteria, the false positive rate rises substantially. Importantly, it is most difficult to assess multiple lesions at different CT slice levels.

With magnetic resonance imaging (MRI), cavernous hemangiomas have a characteristic pattern of high signal intensity on T2-weighted spin echo images ("lightbulb" sign). Studies suggest that the accuracy of MRI in differentiating hemangiomas and metastases is about 85% (9). Although MRI is more accurate than ultrasonography or CT, many benign and malignant tumors can have a similar appearance (5, 10, 11–13). Contrast enhancement does not improve the accuracy. A recent study using gadolinium-enhanced MRI found that a definite diagnosis of benign or malignant disease could be made in 84% of cases (14).

Technetium-labeled Red Blood Cells. Liver scintigraphy with Tc 99m-labeled red blood cells has proved to be both a sensitive and specific method for making the diagnosis of cavernous hemangiomas (15–18). Because cavernous hemangiomas of the liver are in reality large blood-filled cavities, one would expect them to accumulate a high concentration of the labeled red blood cells equivalent to the heart and greater than adjacent normal liver. Although this is true, it takes time for the patient's radiolabeled cells to equilibrate with the unlabeled cells in the large varix-like spaces. As a result, a classical three-phase pattern is seen on planar imaging. Blood flow to the lesion on the radionuclide angiogram phase is usually normal because these tumors are not hypervascular, but rather have an enlarged blood pool space. On immediate high-count imaging starting 60 sec after injection, no or minimal uptake is seen within the hemangioma. However, on delayed images taken at 1–2 hr, increased uptake can be seen (Fig. 1).

Many studies have now shown the superiority of single photon emission computed tomography (SPECT or nuclear CT) compared to planar two-dimensional imaging (Table 2) (17–22). The high target to background ratio (hemangioma/normal liver) improves detection of small, central, or multiple hemangiomas (Fig. 2), as well as those adjacent to the heart, spleen, and kidney, which can often be difficult to diagnose on planar imaging owing to overlapping activity. Few direct comparisons of Tc 99m red blood cell SPECT and MRI have been performed. However, one study using single-headed SPECT showed similar sensitivity for the two methods for lesions down to a size of 2 cm. Magnetic resonance imaging had a higher sensitivity for smaller lesions, especially when adjacent to large vessels (23), whereas SPECT had higher specificity. With present-day state of the art two- or three-headed SPECT cameras, sensitivity is significantly improved over single-headed SPECT (Table 3). It has been reported to be 100% for detecting hemangiomas down to a size of 1.4 cm (24). Hemangiomas as small as 0.5 cm can be detected,

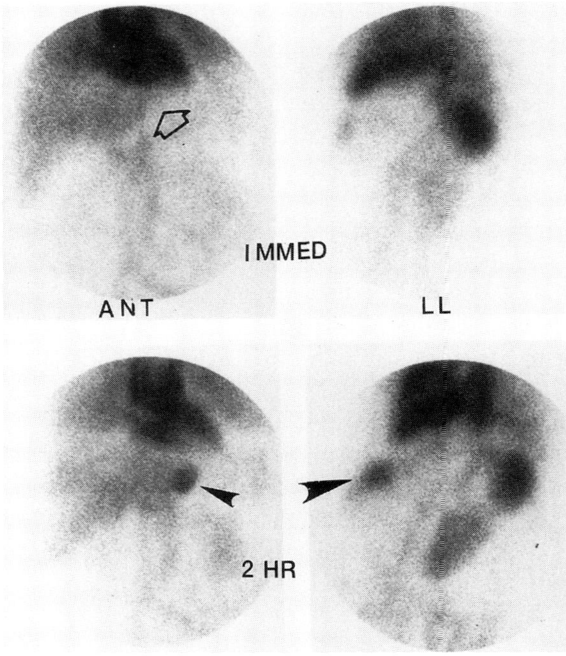

Figure 1. Two-phase Tc 99m RBC positive hemangioma study. Planar images obtained immediately (IMMED) after injection show a cold defect in the medial portion of the left lobe lesion (open arrowhead). Delayed images (2 HR) show increased uptake in the same left lobe location (closed arrowheads) that is equal in intensity to the heart. This is diagnostic of hemangioma.

but with somewhat lower sensitivity (Table 4). False positive SPECT studies are very rare (15, 18, 25).

Technetium-labeled Red Blood Cell Imaging Methodology. The patient's red blood cells are radiolabeled with 25 mCi of Tc 99m pertechnetate using a small

Table 2. TC 99m red blood cell scintigraphy for hemangioma sensitivity of planar versus SPECT

		Sensitivity (%)	
Study	Year	Planar	SPECT
Tumah et al. (19)	1987	43	100
Malik (21)	1987	77	100
Brodski et al. (17)	1987	44	78
Itenzo et al. (18)	1988	88	100
Brunetti (22)	1988	69	100
Kudo et al. (20)	1989	42	74
Ziessman et al. (24)	1991	30	71

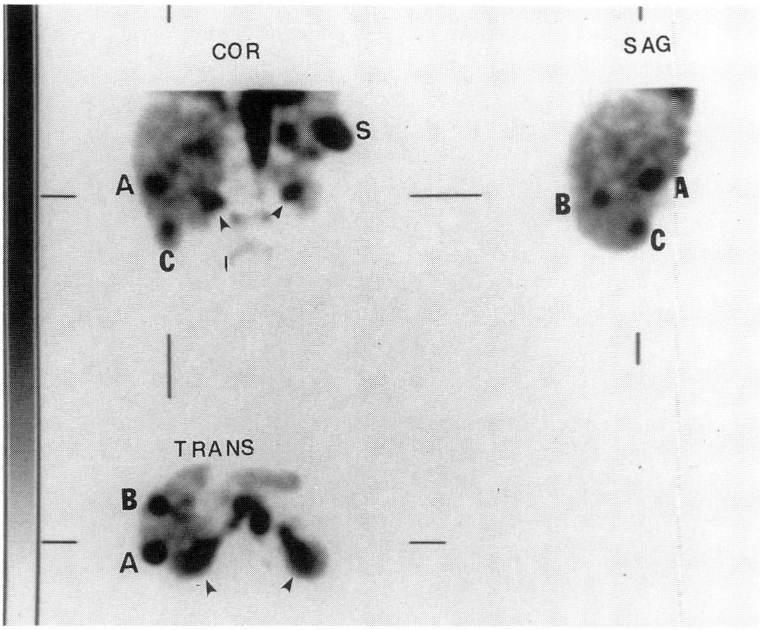

Figure 2. SPECT Tc 99m red blood cell study positive for three hemangiomas (A, B, C). This three-view computer display (transverse, coronal, and sagittal) illustrates the high-contrast resolution obtained with SPECT and its ability to image small and multiple hemangiomas. The three lesions measured 2.5 cm (A), 1.8 cm (B), and 1 cm (C) in size. Small arrowheads denote the kidneys.

volume of the patient's blood and a simple in-house kit labeling technique. With conventional planar imaging, a three-phase study is performed with the patient lying supine under the gamme camera. Following injection of the radiolabeled red blood cells, a rapid-acquisition (1- to 3-sec frames) blood flow study is acquired, followed by multiple immediate high-count images (approximately 2 min each) in different projections (for example, anterior, posterior, right lateral). Delayed images are acquired 2 hr after injection in the same views. Single photon emission CT should be routine. For SPECT the gamme camera acquires approximately 100

Table 3. Sensitivity for detecting hemangioma with single-headed versus triple-headed SPECT

	Sensitivity (%)	
Study	2–3 cm Lesion	1–2 cm Lesion
Single-headed SPECT		
Kudo et al. (20)	83	38
Birnbaum et al. (23)	92	58
Triple-headed SPECT		
Ziessman et al. (24)	100	65

Table 4. Sensitivity of triple-headed SPECT for detection of cavernous hemangioma based on lesion size

Lesion Size (cm)	Sensitivity (%)
>1.4	100
<1.3	91
1.0–2.0	65
0.9–1.3	33
0.5–0.9	20

sequential images at equal angles rotating 360° about the patient for a total study time of about 25 min. Reconstruction of cross-sectional images is then performed by computer using a mathematical algorithm similar to those used for CT. The study is interpreted by reviewing on computer screen a reconstructed three-dimensional rotating image and all cross-sectional sections (transverse, sagittal, coronal) (Fig. 2).

Focal Nodular Hyperplasia and Hepatic Adenoma

Focal nodular hyperplasia (FNH) and hepatic cell adenoma are both benign liver tumors that present as solid intrahepatic lesions in young and middle-aged women (26). It is important to distinguish between them because their natural history is quite different. They must also be distinguished from other liver tumors.

Hepatic adenomas often present with an abdominal crisis due to intraperitoneal hemorrhage, although sometimes abdominal pain or a mass may be the initial manifestation. This tumor has a strong association with contraceptive usage. Malignant transformation has been reported in an occasional case. Hepatic adenomas are typically 8–15 cm in size. Pathologically they are made up of sheets of hepatocytes without any substructure, with neither bile ducts nor Kupffer cells. Hemorrhage and necrosis are commonly seen.

Focal nodular hyperplasia, in contrast, has only a weak association with contraceptive use, is usually asymptomatic, and is discovered incidentally. Rarely it is associated with vague abdominal discomfort. The tumors are typically 3–7 cm in size. Pathologically, they have a stellate fibrous core and contain all three liver cell types, bile ducts, Kupffer cells, and hepatocytes.

Owing to their different natural history, these two benign tumors are treated very differently. Hepatic adenomas that can produce significant morbidity and even mortality require surgical removal, whereas specific therapy is usually not indicated for FNH.

Percutaneous biopsy is usually avoided owing to the increased risk of bleeding from these very vascular lesions and because the needle biopsy specimen is often too small for the pathologist to make a definitive diagnosis (27, 28). Instead, hepatic angiography or laparoscopic biopsy is often used to make the diagnosis. A noninvasive diagnosis could be very helpful in determining the appropriate work-up and therapy.

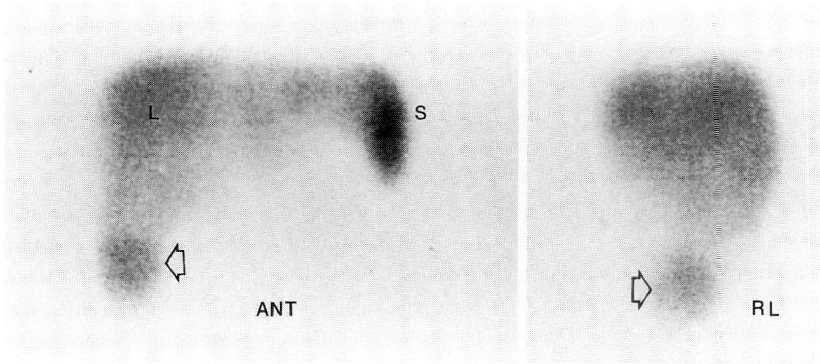

Figure 3. Focal nodular hyperplasia diagnosed with Tc 99m SC. The increased focal uptake at the inferior aspect of the right lobe (arrowheads) of the liver (L) is diagnostic of FNH. Anterior (ANT) and right lateral (RL) views. Spleen (S) is noted.

Ultrasonography, Computed Tomography, and Magnetic Resonance Imaging. The sonographic patterns seen with FNH and hepatic adenoma are nonspecific and varied and it is not usually feasible to differentiate the two (29, 30). Computed tomography is only moderately more specific than sonography (31–33); it can be of value in defining the site and extent of tumor. More specific patterns have been described with MRI; however, sensitivity and specificity data have not been reported (34–37).

Radionuclide Scintigraphy. Prior to the advent of CT, Tc 99m SC served for years as the primary method for imaging liver tumors. Although its role today is much more limited, this radiopharmaceutical can aid in the differential diagnosis of FNH and hepatic adenoma. Technetium 99m SC is extracted by the reticuloendothelial cells of the liver (Kupffer cells) (85%), spleen (10%), and bone marrow (5%). Because they lack Kupffer cells, benign and malignant tumors of the liver are seen as cold (photopenic) defects in an otherwise normal liver background. The one exception is FNH, which contains all three liver cell types, hepatocytes, bile ducts, and Kupffer cells. Approximately two-thirds of these tumors take up Tc 99m SC, one-third having increased uptake and one-third normal uptake (Fig. 3) (38). The remaining third are cold, presumably due to a relatively low number of Kupffer cells in these tumors. Therefore, the diagnosis of FNH can be made in two-thirds of cases where there is uptake. Hepatic adenomas are almost always cold, although one report has described some Tc 99m SC uptake in a minority of these tumors (39).

Because Tc 99m SC is rapidly extracted by the Kupffer cells of the liver, imaging can begin 15 min after injection. Multiple planar (traditional two-dimensional) views are obtained including the anterior, posterior, right and left lateral, and when needed, oblique views. Cross-sectional imaging with SPECT is now routinely performed in many laboratories. This three-dimensional imaging allows for detection of smaller and more central lesions compared to planar imaging owing to the improved contrast resolution. Single photon emission CT imaging with Tc 99m SC can detect most cold lesions 1.5 cm and greater in size. Smaller lesions can be seen if there is increased uptake.

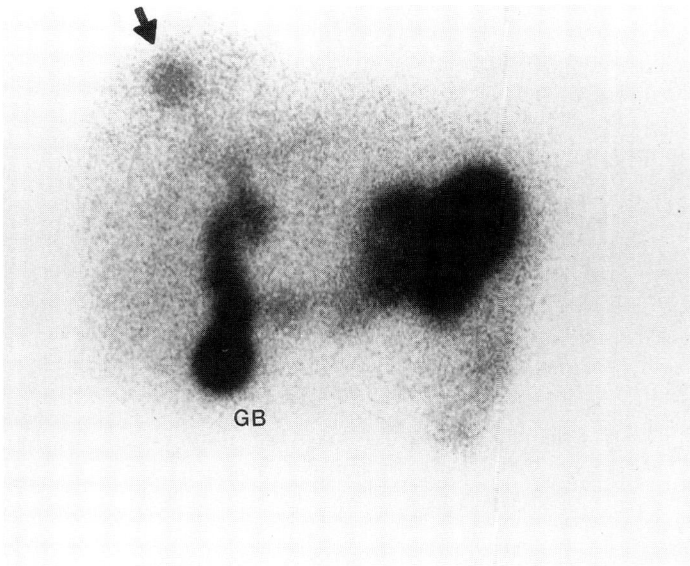

Figure 4. Focal nodular hyperplasia diagnosed by Tc 99m IDA. The focal increased uptake near the dome of the liver (arrow) is diagnostic of FNH. This uptake was seen on early images and became even more distinct on the later images (30–60 min) as the normal liver washed out. Gallbladder (GB) is noted.

Cholescintigraphy with Tc 99m IDA can also be helpful in the differential diagnosis of hepatic tumors. Because this radiopharmaceutical is extracted by hepatocytes, one would expect uptake in FNH, hepatic adenoma, and hepatocellular carcinoma. However, the pattern of uptake is very different in these three tumors. This section deals with its use in benign tumors, and hepatocellular carcinoma is discussed below under primary malignant tumors of the liver.

A characteristic diagnostic pattern is seen with FNH. This consists of increased blood flow, early normal or increased uptake, and delayed clearance ("hot spot") of the radiotracer within the tumor compared to normal liver washout (Fig. 4) (40). This pattern is quite specific. In a recent prospective study, increased uptake was seen in 23/25 lesions due to FNH (41). Its detectability was greater for cholescintigraphy (92%) than CT or MRI (84%). Although one might expect that hepatic adenomas would have a similar appearance, in fact, they usually have no uptake and are cold on Tc 99m IDA imaging (42, 43). The reason for this is uncertain.

Focal Fatty Infiltration

Focal fatty infiltration of the liver is seen as a low-attenuation lesion on CT that may be misinterpreted as a malignant metastasis. Ultrasonography is usually not helpful in differentiating the two. Radionuclide imaging with Tc 99m SC can usually suggest the diagnosis by demonstrating normal uptake (44); however, a cold defect is seen occasionally (45–48). Xenon 133, a radiopharmaceutical used most com-

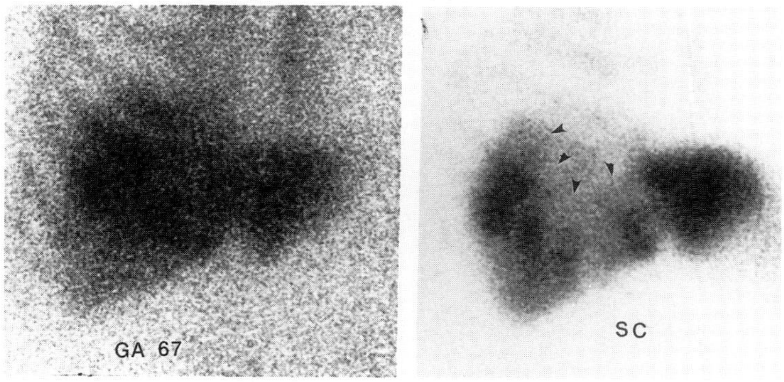

Figure 5. Gallium 67 study positive for hepatocellular carcinoma. The Ga 67 image on the left shows uptake within the tumor, which is seen as cold or relatively photopenic (small arrowheads) on Tc 99m SC image to the right.

monly for lung ventilation imaging, can be useful owing to its lipid solubility. Diffuse uptake in the liver is noted on ventilation studies in patients with fatty metamorphosis. This observation led to its use to confirm the diagnosis of focal fatty accumulations in the liver (49). Uptake with Xenon 133 in the area of the CT abnormality or cold Tc 99m SC lesion confirms fatty focal infiltration and distinguishes it from other space-occupying lesions of the liver such as abscess, hematoma, or primary or secondary neoplasm (50).

MALIGNANT LIVER TUMORS

Primary Tumors

Hepatocellular carcinoma (HCC) usually arises as a complication of liver cirrhosis, limiting the number of patients who can tolerate surgical resection and making initial recognition and differentiation from a regenerative nodule often difficult (51). Because survival rates are highest with early diagnosis, recognition of so-called minimal HCC is an important imaging challenge.

Although CT and MR are useful for detecting these tumors, the presence of regenerating nodules and fibrosis may obscure their detection and the specificity is poor (52). Nuclear scintigraphy can play an important noninvasive role when the diagnosis is in doubt and in the follow-up care of these patients.

Because up to 90% of hepatomas are gallium-avid, gallium 67 has been used to confirm the diagnosis and to differentiate it from regenerating liver nodules present in cirrhotic patients (53–56). Often Tc 99m SC is used in conjunction with gallium 67 to improve the accuracy for making this diagnosis (57) (Fig. 5). The dynamic flow portion of the Tc 99m SC study can demonstrate the increased vascularity of HCC. Regenerative nodules almost always have decreased flow. Images at 15–20 min show HCC to be cold (no uptake). In contrast, gallium 67 is avidly taken up by the tumor. No uptake is seen in regenerative nodules. Because

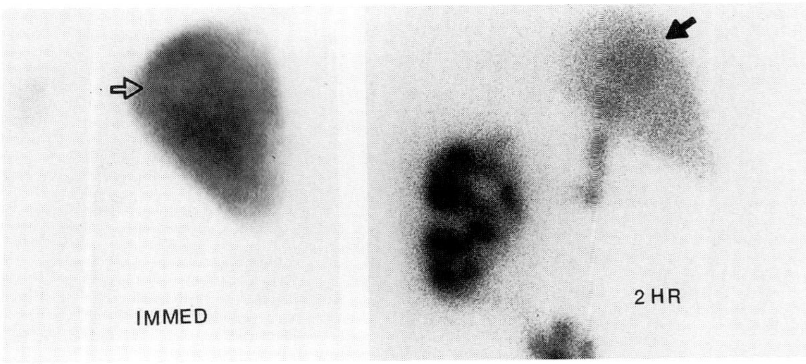

Figure 6. Technetium 99m IDA study diagnostic of hepatocellular carcinoma. The immediate image on the left shows a cold defect in the region of the known tumor. Delayed imaging 2 hr later shows increased uptake compared to adjacent liver.

gallium 67 is normally taken up diffusely in the normal liver, computer subtraction of the gallium 67 and Tc 99m SC studies can enhance visual detection of the hepatoma.

Hepatocellular carcinoma has a characteristic pattern on Tc 99m IDA cholescintigraphy that is different from that which has been described for FNH and hepatic adenoma, already discussed. Many hepatomas, particularly the larger ones, have increased blood flow that can be seen on the radionuclide flow phase. However, no tumor uptake is seen during the first 60 min of imaging. With delayed imaging at 2–4 hr, uptake in the malignant tumor can usually be seen (Fig. 6) (58, 59). The reason for this delayed pattern of uptake is that the malignant hepatocytes function poorly compared to normal liver, but they do function. This pattern is very specific and diagnostic.

Metastatic Liver Disease

Before the advent of CT, Tc 99m SC liver–spleen scans were used to diagnose tumor metastases to the liver and to follow patients' response to therapy. It is not commonly used for this today. Although today CT is the standard imaging modality for detection and follow-up of liver tumors, its sensitivity is surprisingly low, variously reported to be 38–93% (60). Most recent series report sensitivities of approximately 75% (61). Although it has been suggested that helical CT can improve on this, no large series have been reported with accuracy data.

Gallium 67 (Ga 67) citrate, a radiopharmaceutical used for tumor imaging since the 1970s, can detect malignant tumors within the liver in a manner similar to that described for hepatomas. A tumor that is cold on Tc 99m SC imaging will typically "fill in" with Ga 67. The mechanism of uptake in tumors is incompletely understood. Similar to iron, Ga 67 binds to transferrin in the blood, enters the tumor's extracellular fluid space via its leaky capillary endothelium, binds to tumor receptors, then is transported into the cell, where it binds to iron-binding proteins such as ferritin and lactoferrin, found in increased concentration in tumors. However, Ga 67 is not tumor specific nor can it differentiate tumor from infection. Its sensitivity for tumor detection varies, being quite high for lymphoma, melanoma, sarcoma, and lung cancer (>90%) (62), but lower for gastrointestinal and pelvic tumors.

In recent years the most common clinical indication for Ga 67 has been for tumor detection and localization in patients with Hodgkin's and non-Hodgkin's lymphoma. It has been used for presurgical tumor staging and as an indicator of the effectiveness of chemotherapy or radiation therapy. Continued uptake after therapy is consistent with residual tumor, whereas the lack of uptake suggests effective therapy (63). Gallium 67 can detect a variety of other malignant tumors with varying sensitivity.

Thallium chloride Tl 201 and Tc 99m sestamibi are two radiopharmaceuticals used routinely for radionuclide myocardial perfusion imaging to diagnose and evaluate coronary artery disease. However, these radiopharmaceuticals are also taken up by many benign and malignant tumors, for example, lymphoma, breast, and lung cancer. Both radiopharmaceuticals can detect tumors within the liver (64); however, data on their accuracy and clinical utility are limited (65). One report has shown that Tl 201 is taken up by low-grade lymphoma better than Ga 67 (66).

Indium In 111 Oncoscint is a radiolabeled monoclonal antibody approved by the FDA for clinical use for detection of colorectal and ovarian cancer. This B72.3 murine IgG antibody is directed against a high-molecular-weight glycoprotein, TAG-72, which is expressed in the majority of colorectal and ovarian carcinomas. For colorectal carcinoma, the two most common clinical indications are (1) a patient with a rising carcinoembryonic antigen titer but no tumor detected by the usual imaging methods, and (2) a patient with a single known metastasis, usually in the liver, that is potentially resectable. The Oncoscint study can confirm the presence of other metastases that would make the patient inoperable. The overall sensitivity of Oncoscint for tumor detection is 69%, specificity 76%, and positive predictive value 97% (67, 68). Although it is superior to CT for detecting tumors in the extrahepatic abdomen (66 versus 34%), it is less sensitive than CT for detecting tumors within the liver, 41 versus 84%. Large tumors within the liver usually image as photopenic (cold) defects, because normal uptake of the radiopharmaceutical by the liver is high. Smaller tumors may not be seen owing to the high liver background.

Indium In 111 Octreotide, a radiolabeled peptide and somatostatic receptor analogue, is used to image primary and metastatic neuroendocrine tumors derived from cells belonging to the amine precursor uptake and decarboxylation (APUDoma) system, for example, pancreatic islet cell tumors, carcinoid tumors, gastrinomas, medullary carcinoma of the thyroid, paragangliomas, neuroblastomas, and pheochromocytomas (69). Its overall accuracy is proved to be quite high in many tumors (86%) (Table 5). In a large multicenter series, In 111 octreotide was able to detect 82% of tumors within the liver (70).

Iodine I 131 MIBG (metaiodobenzylguanidine), a norepinephrine analogue, has been used for more than a decade to image and localize pheochromocytomas and neuroblastomas. Its sensitivity is approximately 90% and its specificity greater than 95% (71). It is generally considered to be superior to In 111 octreotide for this use, although they are both quite accurate. Pheochromocytomas are metastatic in about 10% of patients and distant metastases, including those in the liver, can be identified using this radiotracer (72). Iodine I 131 MIBG has also proved useful in localizing

Table 5. In 111 Octreotide scintigraphy sensitivity for tumor detection

Tumor Type	Sensitivity (%)
Gastrinoma	93
Insulinoma	46
Carcinoid	95
Small cell lung cancer	100
Non-small cell lung cancer	100
Non-Hodgkin's lymphoma	83
Hodgkin's disease	98
Breast cancer	68

neuroblastomas with a sensitivity of greater than 90% (73). The sensitivity for detecting carcinoid tumors is lower, about 50–60% (Fig. 7).

Intraarterial Chemotherapy of Hepatic Tumors

Technetium-labeled macroaggregated albumin (Tc 99m MAA) is the radiopharmaceutical used for lung perfusion imaging. However, it has also been used to evaluate the perfusion pattern of the liver in patients receiving intraarterial chemotherapy for treatment of primary and metastatic cancer of the liver (74). Successful application of

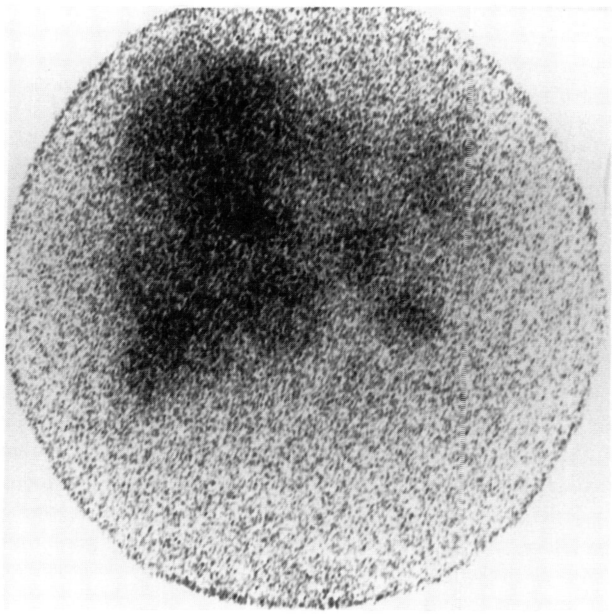

Figure 7. Metastatic carcinoid tumor diagnosed with I 131 MIBG. Multiple areas of inhomogeneously increased focal activity are noted throughout the liver.

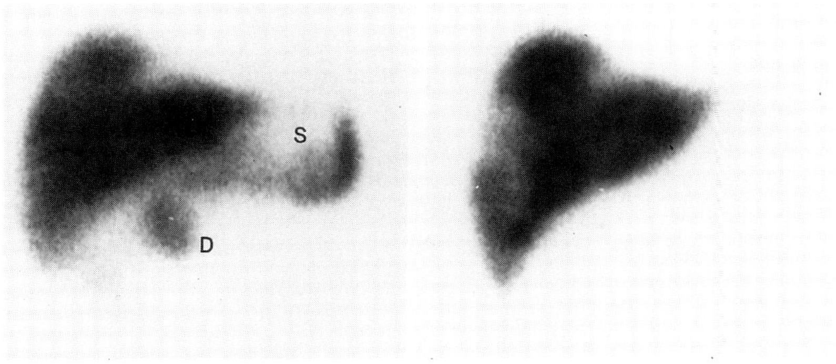

Figure 8. Technetium 99m MAA study in patient receiving intraarterial therapy for carcinoma of the colon metastatic to the liver. Left: In addition to liver perfusion, extrahepatic perfusion is seen in the stomach (S) and duodenum (D). Right: The percutaneously placed intraarterial catheter was repositioned. Now perfusion is limited to the liver.

this form of therapy requires that the drug be reliably and safely delivered to the tumor and liver. Although contrast angiography can document proper catheter placement, it is not a good indicator of blood flow at the capillary level. Improper positioning of the catheter results in inadequate perfusion of the tumor-involved liver and can result in extrahepatic perfusion to the stomach, pancreas, spleen, and bowel (74). This can lead to serious complications, including gastritis, ulceration, and hemorrhage. The Tc 99m MAA study can ensure that the chemotherapeutic agent will be directed to the tumor and liver and determine if there is any extrahepatic perfusion (Fig. 8). The Tc 99m MAA can be infused through a percutaneously placed or surgically placed infusion catheter. Intraarterial perfusion scintigraphy with Tc 99m MAA can be quite useful in differentiating patient symptoms suggestive of tumor progression from those caused by complications from extrahepatic perfusion of the chemotherapy.

REFERENCES

1. Meindok M, Langer B. Liver scan in Budd–Chiari syndrome. *J Nucl Med.* 1976; 17:365–369.
2. Feldman M. Hemangioma of the liver. *Am J Clin Pathol.* 1958;29:160–162.
3. Terriff BA, Gibney RG, Scudamore CH. Fatality from fine-needle aspiration biopsy of a hepatic hemangioma. *AJR.* 1990;154:203 (letter).
4. Kato M, Sugawara I, Okada A, et al. Hemangioma of the liver: diagnosis with combined use of laparoscopy and hepatic arteriography. *Am J Surg.* 1975;129:698–704.
5. Bree RL, Schwab RE, Glazer EM, Fink-Bennett D. The varied appearance of cavernous hemangioma with sonography, computed tomography, magnetic resonance imaging and scintigraphy. *Radiographics.* 1987;7:1153–1175.
6. Taboury J, Porcel A, Tubiana JM, Monnier JP. Cavernous hemangiomas of the liver studied by ultrasonography. *Radiology.* 1983;149:781–785.

7. Itah Y, Ohnishi S, Ohtomo K, et al. Hepatic cavernous hemangioma in patients at high risk for liver cancer. *Acta Radiol.* 1087;28:697–701.
8. Freeny PC, Marks WM. Hepatic hemangioma: dynamic bolus CT. *AJR.* 1986;147: 711–719.
9. Ferrucci JT. Liver tumor imaging. *Radiol Clin North Am.* 1994;32:39–54.
10. Stark DD, Felder RC, Wittenberg J, et al. Magnetic resonance imaging of cavernous hemangioma of the liver tissue-specific characterization. *AJR.* 1985;144:213–222.
11. Glazer GM, Aisen AM, Francis JR, et al. Hepatic cavernous hemangioma: magnetic resonance imaging. *Radiology.* 1985;155:417–420.
12. Ohtomo K, Itai Y, Yoshikawa K, et al. Hepatocellular carcinoma and cavernous hemangioma: differentiation with MR imaging. Efficacy of T2 values at 0.35 and 1.5 T. *Radiology.* 1988;168:621–623.
13. Birnbaum BA, Weignreb JC, Megibow AJ, et al. Definitive diagnosis of hepatic hemangiomas: MR imaging versus Tc-99m labeled red blood cell SPECT. *Radiology.* 1990;176:95–101.
14. Mitchell DG, Saini S, Weireb J, et al. Hepatic metastases and cavernous hemangiomas: distinction with standard- and triple-dose gadoteridol-enhanced MR imaging. *Radiology.* 1994;193:49–57.
15. Rabinowitz SA, McKusick KA, Strauss HW. 99mTc red blood cell scintigraphy in evaluating focal live lesions. *AJR.* 1984;143:63–68.
16. Moinuddin M, Allison JR, Montgomery JH, et al. Scintigraphic diagnosis of hepatic hemangioma: its role in the management of hepatic mass lesions. *AJR.* 1985;145:223–228.
17. Brodsky RI, Friedman AC, Maurer AH, et al. Hepatic cavernous hemangiomas: diagnosis with 99mTc-labeled red cells and single photon emission CT. *AJR.* 1987;148:125–129.
18. Itenzo C, Kim S, Madsen M, et al. Planar and SPECT Tc-99m red blood cell imaging in hepatic cavernous hemangiomas and other hepatic lesions. *Clin Nucl Med.* 1088;13:237–240.
19. Tumeh SS, Benson C, Nagel JS, et al. Cavernous hemangioma of the liver: detection with single-photon emission computed tomography. *Radiology.* 1987;164:353–356.
20. Kudo M, Ikekub K, Yamamoto K, et al. Distinction between hemangioma of the liver and hepatocellular carcinoma: value of labeled rbc-SPECT scanning. *AJR.* 1989;152:977–983.
21. Malik MH. Blood pool SPECT and planar imaging in hepatic hemangioma. *Clin Nucl Med.* 1987;12:543–545.
22. Brunetti JC, Van Heertum RL, Yudd AP, Cooperman AM. The value of SPECT imaging in the diagnosis of hepatic hemangioma. *Clin Nucl Med.* 1988;13:800–804.
23. Birnbaum BA, Weignreb JC, Megibow AJ, et al. Definitive diagnosis of hepatic hemangiomas: MR imaging versus Tc-99m labeled red blood cell SPECT. *Radiology.* 1990;176:95–101.
24. Ziessman HA, Silverman PM, Patterson J, et al. Improved detection of small cavernous hemangiomas of the liver with high-resolution three-headed SPECT. *J Nucl Med.* 1991;32:2086–2091.
25. Ginsberg F, Slavin JD, Spencer RP. Hepatic angiosarcoma: mimicking of angioma on three-phase technetium-99m red blood cell scintigraphy. *J Nucl Med.* 1986;27:1861–1863.
26. Edmondson HA. Tumors of the liver and intrahepatic bile ducts. In: Edmondson HA, Atlas of Tumor Pathology. Washington, DC: AFIP; 158:113–115.
27. Adson MA. Mass lesions of the liver. *Mayo Clin Proc.* 1986;61:362–366.
28. Kerlin P, Davis GL, McGill DB, et al. Hepatic adenoma and focal nodular hyperplasia: clinical, pathologic, and radiologic features. *Gastroenterology.* 1983;84:994–999.

29. Casarella WJ, Knowles DM, Wolff M, Johnson PM. Focal nodular hyperplasia and liver cell adenoma: radiologic and pathologic differentiation. *AJR.* 1978;131:393–402.
30. Welch TI, Sheedy PF, Johnson CM, et al. Focal nodular hyperplasia and hepatic adenoma: comparison of angiography, CT, US, and scintigraphy. *Radiology.* 1985;156:593–595.
31. Fishman EK, Farmlett E, Kadir S, Siegelman SS. Computed tomography of benign hepatic tumors. *J Comput Assist Tomogr.* 1982;6:642–645.
32. Rogers JV, Mack LA, Freeny, et al. Hepatic focal nodular hyperplasia: Angiography, CT, sonography and scintigraphy. *AJR.* 1981;137:983–989.
33. Foley WD, Berland LL, Lawson TL, Varma RR. Computed tomography of the liver. *Semin Liver Dis.* 1982;2:14–21.
34. Lee MJ, Saini S, Hamm B, et al. Focal nodular hyperplasia of the liver: MR findings in 35 proved cases. *AJR.* 1991;156:317–320.
35. Mathieu D, Rahmouni A, Anglade MC, et al. Focal nodular hyperplasia of the liver: assessment with contrast-enhanced turboFLASH MR imaging. *Radiology.* 1991;180:25–30.
36. Vilgrain V, Flejou JF, Arrive L, et al. Focal nodular hyperplasia of the liver: MR imaging and pathologic correlation in 37 patients. *Radiology.* 1992;184:699–703.
37. Arrive L, Flejou J-F, Vilgrain V, et al. Hepatic adenoma: MR findings in 51 pathologically proved lesions. *Radiology.* 1994;193:507–512.
38. Welch TJ, Sheedy HF, Johnson M, et al. Focal nodular hyperplasia and hepatic adenoma: comparison of angiography, CT, US, and scintigraphy. *Radiology.* 1985;156:593–595.
39. Lubbers PR, Ros PR, Goodman AD, Ishak KG. Accumulation of Technetium-99m sulfur colloid by hepatocellular adenoma. *AJR.* 1987;1438:1105–1108.
40. Tanasescu D, Brachman M, Rigby J, et al. Scintigraphic triad in focal nodular hyperplasia. *J Gastroenterol.* 1984;79:61–64.
41. Boulahdour H, Cherqui D, Charlotte F, et al. The hot spot hepatobiliary scan in focal nodular hyperplasia. *J Nucl Med.* 1993;34:2105–2110.
42. Gratz KF, Creutzig H, Brolsch C, et al. Choleszintigrapie zum nachweis der focal-nodularen hyperplasie der leber? *Chirurg.* 1984;55:448–451.
43. Kotzerke J, Schwarzrock R, Krischek, et al. Technetium-99m DISIDA hepatobiliary agent in diagnosis of hepatocellular carcinoma, adenoma and focal nodular hyperplasia. *J Nucl Med.* 1989;30:1278–1279.
44. Lisbona R, Rishkin S, Derbekyan V, et al. Role of scintigraphy in focally abnormal sonograms of fatty livers. *J Nucl Med.* 1988;29:1050–1056.
45. Schauwecker DS, Wass JL. Focal fatty infiltration of the liver: evaluation by planar and SPECT imagers. *Clin Nucl Med.* 1991;16:449–451.
46. Khedkar N, Pestikea B, Rosenblate H, et al. Large focal defect on liver/spleen scan caused by fatty liver and masquerading as neoplasm. *J Nucl Med.* 1992;33:258–259.
47. Marmolya GA, Miron SD, Eckhauser M, et al. Focal fatty infiltration of the liver appearing as a defect on a liver-spleen scintigram: case report. *Clin Nucl Med.* 1992;17:300–302.
48. Black RR, Winfield DF, Fernandez-Ulloa M. Solitary defect on liver sulfur colloid imaging secondary to focal fatty infiltration. *Clin Nucl Med.* 1989;14:603–605.
49. Patel S, Sandler CM, Rauschkoilb EN, McConnell BJ. Xenon-133 uptake in focal hepatic fat accumulation: CT correlation. *AJR.* 1982;138:541–544.
50. Baker MK, Scauwecker DS, Wenker JC, et al. Nuclear medicine evaluation of focal fatty infiltration of the liver. *Clin Nucl Med.* 1986;11:503–506.
51. Okuda K, Ryu M, Tobe T. Surgical management of hepatoma: The Japanese experience. In Wanebo HJ, ed. *Hepatic and Biliary Cancer.* New York: Marcel Dekker; 1987:219–238.

52. Henderson JM, Campbell JD, Olson R, et al. Role of computed tomography in screening for hepatocellular carcinomain patients with cirrhosis. *Gastrointest Radiol.* 1988;13: 129–134.

53. Lomas F, Dibos PE, Wagner HN. Increased specificity of liver screening with the use of 67-gallium citrate. *N Engl J Med.* 1972;286:1323–1329.

54. Suzuki T, Honjo I, Hamamoto K, et al. Positive scintiphotography of cancer of the liver wiht Ga-67 citrate. *AJR.* 1971;113:92–103.

55. James O, Wood EJ, Sherlock S. 67-Gallium scanning in the diagnosis of liver disease. *Gut.* 1974;15:404–410.

56. Nagasue N, Gallium scanning in the diagnosis of hepatocellular carcinoma: a clinicopathological study of 45 patients. *Clin Radiol.* 1983;34:139–142.

57. Lee VW, O'Brien MJ, Morris PM, et al. The specific diagnosis of hepatocellular carcinoma by scintigraphy; multiple radiotracer approach. *Cancer.* 1985;56:25–36.

58. Hasegawa Y, Nakano S, Ibuka K, et al. The importance of delayed imaging in the study of hepatoma with a hepatobiliary agent. *J Nucl Med.* 1984;25:1122–1126.

59. Lee VW, OBrien MJ, Devereau DF, et al. Hepatocellular carcinoma: uptake of 99m Tc-IDA in primary tumor and metastasis. *AJR.* 1984;143:57–61.

60. Ferruci JT, Stark DD. *Liver Imaging: Current Trends and New Techniques.* Boston: Andover Medical, 1990.

61. Bluemke DA, Soyer P, Fishman EK. Helical (spiral) CT of the liver. *Radiol Clin North Am.* 1995;33:863–886.

62. Neumann RD, Kemp JD, Weiner RE. Gallium-67 imaging for detection of malignant disease. In Sandler MP, Coleman RE, Wackers FJ, Patton JA, Gottschalk A, Hoffer PB, eds. Diagnostic Nuclear Medicine, 3rd ed. Baltimore: Williams and Wilkins; 1996:1243–1260.

63. Kaplan WD, Jochelson MWS, Herman TS, et al. Gallium-67 imaging: a predictor of residual tumor viability and clinical outcome in patients with diffuse large cell lymphoma. *J Clin Oncol.* 1990;8:1966–1970.

64. Nour R, Quinn RJ, Morris DL, Butler SP. Avid thallium-201 uptake in hepatic carcinoid metastases. *Eur J Nucl Med.* 1993;20:804–806.

65. Abdel-Dayem HM, Scott AM, Macapinlac HA, et al. Role of 201-Tl chloride and 99m Tc sestamibi in tumor imaging. In Freeman LM, ed. *Nuclear Medicine Annual 1994.* New York: Raven Press; 1994:181–234.

66. Waxman AD, Eller D, Ashook G, et al. Comparison of Ga-67 and thallium scintigraphy in peripheral and intrathoracic lymphoma. *J Nucl Med.* 1996;37:46–50.

67. Collier BD, Abdel-Nabi H, Doerr RJ, et al. Immunoscintigraphy performed with In-labeled CYT-103 in the management of colorectal carcinoma: comparison with CT. *Radiology.* 1992;185:179–186.

68. Doerr RJ, Abdel-Nabi H, Krag D, Mitchell E. Radiolabeled antibody imaging in the management of colorectal carcinoma. *Ann Surg.* 1991;214:118–124.

69. Krenning EP, Bakker WH, Kooij PM, et al. Somatostatin receptor scintigraphy with [111 In-DTPA-D-Phe1]- and [I-123-Tyr3]octreotide: the Rotterdam experience with more than 1000 patients. *Eur J Nucl Med.* 1993;20:716–731.

70. Krenning EP, Kewkkeboom DJ, Pauwels S, et al. Somatostatin receptor scintigraphy. In: Freeman LM, ed. *Nuclear Medicine Annual 1995.* New York: Raven Press, 1995.

71. McEwan AJ, Shapiro B, Sisson JC, et al. Radioiodobenzylguanidine for the scintigraphic location and therapy of adrenergic tumors. *Semin Nucl Med.* 1985;15:132–153.

72. Freitas JE. Adrenal cortical and medullary imaging. *Semin Nucl Med.* 1995;23:235–250.
73. Hoefnagel CA, Voute PA, de Kraker, et al. Radionuclide diagnosis and therapy of neural crest tumors using I-131 metaiodobenzylguanidine. *J Nucl Med.* 1987;28:308–314.
74. Ziessman HA, Thrall JH, Yang PJ, et al. Hepatic arterial perfusion scintigraphy with Tc-99m MAA. *Radiology.* 1984;152:167–172.

18

MAGNETIC RESONANCE IMAGING OF THE LIVER

Nikolaos L. Kelekis, M.D., and Richard C. Semelka, M.D.
University of North Carolina at Chapel Hill
Chapel Hill, North Carolina

Magnetic resonance imaging (MRI) is an excellent modality to detect and characterize focal liver masses and to evaluate diffuse liver disease. Among all focal liver lesions, MRI has the greatest advantage over computed tomography (CT) in the evaluation of hypervascular malignant lesions such as hepatocellular carcinoma or metastases from hypervascular primary tumors. Magnetic resonance imaging may be the most accurate nonoperative imaging modality to evaluate patients with suspected limited involvement of the liver with malignant disease who are considered candidates for partial hepatic resection. In many settings, however, MRI performs well as a problem-solving modality to characterize and determine the extent of focal liver lesions. Magnetic resonance imaging is accurate for the evaluation of diffuse liver disease and MR should be used to investigate patients with suspected iron deposition or fatty infiltration. Patients who are not candidates for contrast-enhanced CT examination (for example, patients with poor renal function of contrast allergy) should be studied with MRI.

TECHNIQUE

The minimum requirement for MRI of the liver is to perform T1-weighted and T2-weighted sequences, which highlight differences in relaxation of hepatic hydrogen protons when placed in a magnetic field. The normal liver on T1-weighted sequences has an intermediate signal intensity and is brighter than the normal spleen. With progressive T2-weighting the liver becomes darker than the spleen (Fig. 1). Contrast enhancement is important and the current standard approach is to administer a nonspecific extracellular contrast agent, gadolinium chelate, as a rapid bolus injection with serial imaging using a spoiled gradient echo (SGE) sequence.

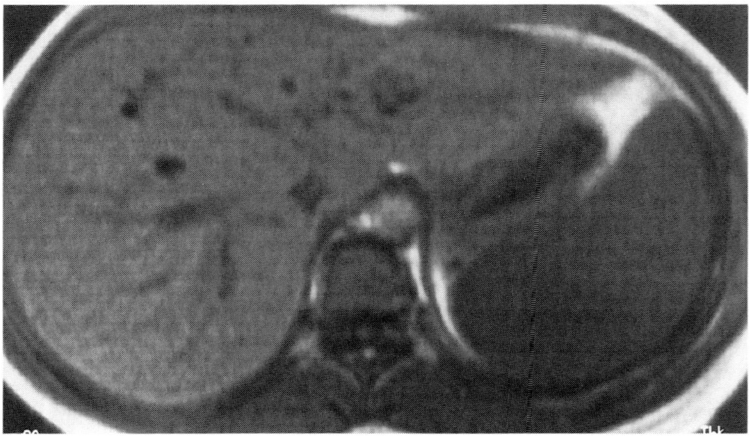

(A)

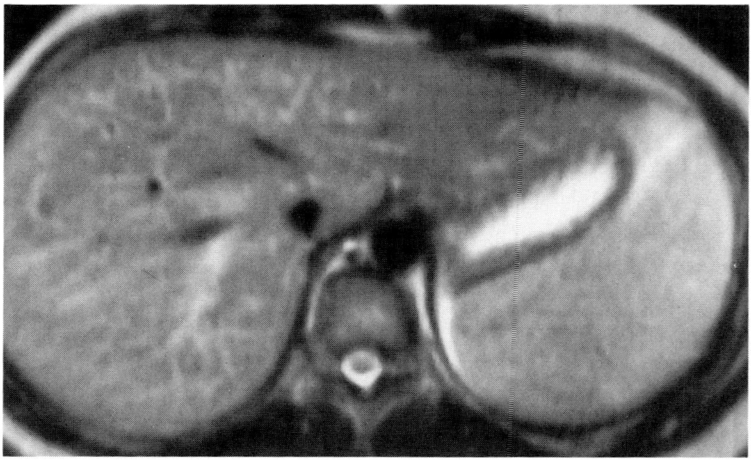

(B)

Figure 1. Normal liver and spleen on T1-weighted (A), T2-weighted (B), and immediate post-gadolinium (C, D, next page) images. In the absence of hepatic disease or iron overload, the normal liver is higher in signal intensity than the spleen on T1-weighted images (A) and slightly lower in signal intensity than the spleen on T2-weighted sequences (B). The liver parenchyma is minimally enhanced on the immediate post-gadolinium images, and contrast is identified in hepatic arteries and portal veins, but not in hepatic veins (arrows, C). Contrast present in the IVC is from the renal veins. The spleen (S) demonstrates normal arciform enhancement with dark and bright enhancing tissue.

Breathing artifact is the major problem with MR imaging of the abdomen, and various compensation techniques are useful to control this artifact. These include respiratory compensation, multiple averaging, fat suppression, anterior saturation, and most recently, navigator echoes. Breath-hold T1-weighted SGE sequence permits fast data acquisition, robust sequence performance, avoidance of breathing artifact, complete coverage of the liver in one breath hold, and good T1 weighting.

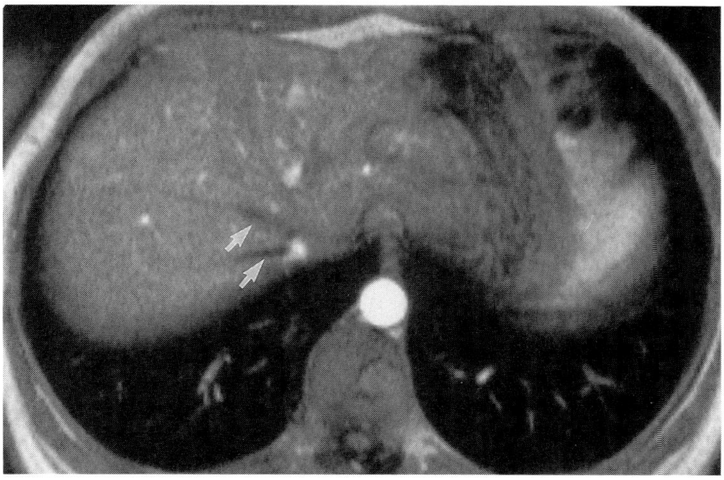

(C)

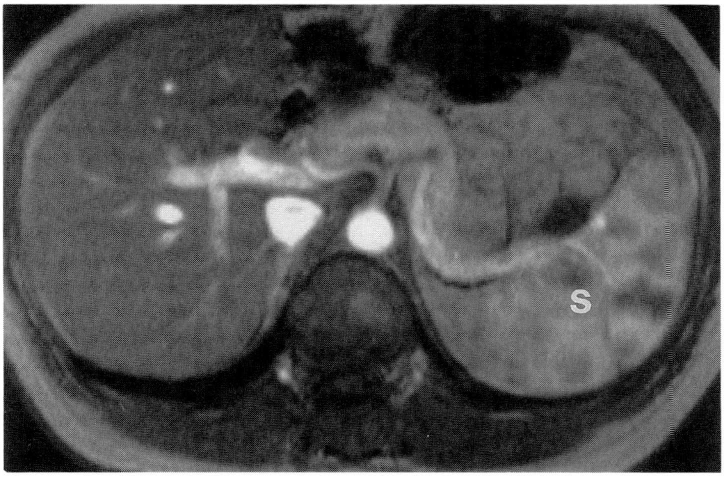

(D)

Figure 1. *(Continued)*

This sequence generates 14–22 sections in a 20-sec breath-hold period. The other important use of SGE is for dynamic gadolinium chelate imaging.

Out-of-phase T1-weighted imaging is generally useful for examining the liver for fatty infiltration. The presence of fatty infiltration results in diminution of signal intensity of the involved liver parenchyma or out-of-phase images.

T2-weighted imaging is most frequently performed as conventional spin-echo, or echo train spin-echo sequences (for example, fast spin-echo or turbo spin-echo sequences). A recently developed variation of turbo spin-echo termed half Fourier single shot turbo spin echo (HASTE) can acquire individual image sections in less than 1 sec per section. This sequence results in robust, reproducible image quality and is independent of breathing.

Contrast enhancement is performed by administering intravenously gadolinium–DTPA (0.1 mmol/kg), a nonspecific extracellular contrast agent, as a rapid bolus injection. SGE images are obtained immediately following contrast administration, and at approximately 1 and 5–10 min. On the immediate post-gadolinium images the liver is imaged in the capillary phase, where most of the contrast is provided by the hepatic arterial blood flow with minimal contribution from portal venous blood flow. This phase can be identified by the presence of contrast in hepatic arteries and portal veins but not in hepatic veins (Fig. 1), and is the most important phase of enhancement for detection and characterization of liver lesions. Malignant liver lesions derive their blood supply from hepatic arterial branches and their vascularized portions enhance more than liver parenchyma on these images. Images acquired 1 min post-contrast administration correspond to the portal phase of enhancement, in which the hepatic parenchyma enhances with contrast mainly derived from portal venous blood flow. This phase of enhancement provides additional information on the hemodynamic behavior of liver lesions, and because all vessels are enhanced, provides a reliable assessment of vessel patency. Bland thrombus on these images appears dark, near signal void, whereas tumor thrombus appears as intermediate to high signal intensity. The delayed, interstitial images acquired after 5–10 min post-gadolinium administration are helpful in showing the late enhancement features of lesions (for example, centripetal filling of hemangiomas, peripheral washout of metastases, late enhancement of fibrosis) and differentiating cysts from hypovascular metastases.

Magnetic resonance angiographic sequences may be occasionally useful in the examination of liver disease, especially in the setting of hepatic cirrhosis to examine for portal vein patency, direction of portal venous flow and presence of varices.

DIFFUSE LIVER PARENCHYMAL DISEASE

Fatty Liver

Magnetic resonance imaging is particularly effective in evaluating the liver of patients with fatty liver for the presence of focal lesions such as metastases. In this setting non-fat-suppressed T1-weighted images and fat suppressed T2-weighted images are useful to maximize contrast between liver and lesions.

Out-of-phase SGE is a highly accurate technique in the investigation of fatty liver, particularly in differentiating focal fatty infiltration from tumor (1, 2). When a lesion that is isointense or hyperintense to liver on in-phase SGE loses signal homogeneously on out-of-phase images the diagnosis of focal fat can be reliably established. Focal normal liver in the setting of diffuse fatty infiltration of the liver is shown by a focus of high signal in a background of diminished liver signal intensity on out-of-phase images (Fig. 2).

Portal Thrombosis

Tumor and bland thrombus may frequently be distinguished from each other by the observation that tumor thrombus is higher in signal intensity on T2-weighted

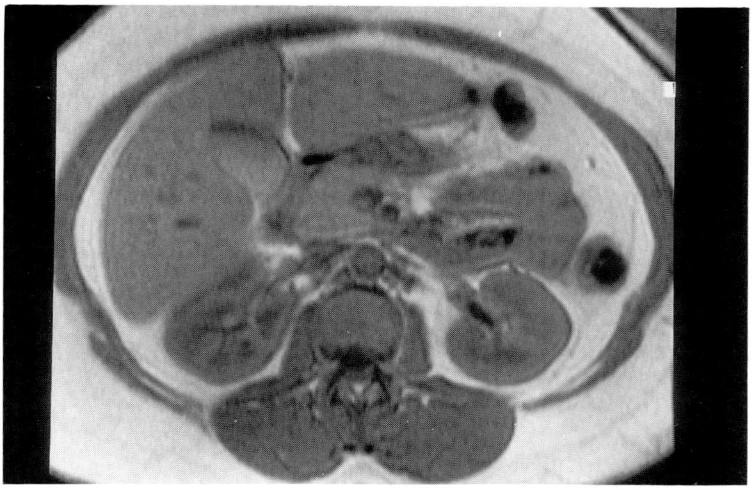

(A)

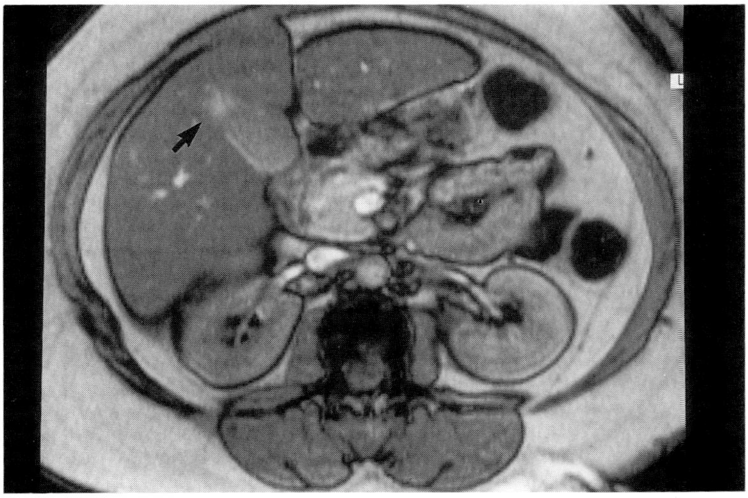

(B)

Figure 2. Fatty liver with focal sparing. In-phase (A), and out-of-phase (B) SGE images. The liver is homogeneous and has high signal intensity on the in-phase image (A). Signal intensity of the liver diminishes on the out-of-phase image (B) owing to the coexistence of water and fat protons in the same voxels. A focal spared area of normal liver immediately adjacent to the gallbladder retains signal intensity on the out-of-phase image (arrow, B).

images, and enhances with gadolinium. In comparison, bland thrombus is low in signal intensity on T2-weighted images, and does not enhance with gadolinium. Tumor thrombus is most frequently caused by hepatocellular carcinoma, although it may be also observed with metastases. Bland thrombus may be observed in the setting of cirrhosis and various inflammatory/infectious processes involving organs in the portal circulation, the most common cause being pancreatitis. Extrinsic compression of portal veins is most often caused by malignant tumors, but this may occur with benign tumors such as hemangiomas. Cholangiocarcinoma has a particular propensity to cause extrinsic compression and obstruction of portal veins. Lobar or segmental portal vein obstruction by tumor may cause discrete wedge-shaped regions of increased intensity on T2-weighted images and gadolinium-enhanced images (1, 3–7).

After administration of intravenous gadolinium, MR images may show transient increased enhancement of hepatic parenchyma in the areas with decreased portal perfusion during the capillary phase of enhancement, reflecting increased hepatic arterial supply due to an autoregulatory mechanism.

Cirrhosis

The most common underlying causes of cirrhosis in North America include alcoholism, viral hepatitis, and idiopathic hemochromatosis. Fibrosis and occasionally mild iron deposition occur in cirrhotic livers, which decrease hepatic signal intensity on T1- and T2-weighted images. Many cirrhotic livers may also possess regions of low signal on T1-weighted images and high signal on T2-weighted images secondary to hepatocellular damage and/or inflammation (8, 9).

Magnetic resonance images depict regenerative nodules with greater conspicuity than other imaging modalities. On T2-weighted images, regenerative nodules often are low in signal intensity relative to high-signal-intensity inflammatory fibrous septa or damaged liver (10). Approximately 25% of regenerative nodules accumulate iron more than the surrounding hepatic parenchyma, facilitating their identification as low signal on T2-weighted spin echo images and T2*-weighted gradient echo images (11). When regenerative nodules are not clearly visible, cirrhosis may be detected by noting irregular linear high-signal abnormalities on T2-weighted or late post gadolinium SGE images (12).

Budd–Chiari Syndrome

Absence of hepatic veins may be shown well by techniques in which flowing blood is signal void or by techniques in which flowing blood is high signal, such as time-of-flight techniques or portal phase gadolinium-enhanced SGE. Generally a combination of both approaches yields the highest diagnostic accuracy.

In acute onset Budd–Chiari syndrome the peripheral liver enhances less than central liver presumably owing to acute increased tissue pressure, which results in diminished blood flow of both hepatic arterial and portal venous systems. Increased enhancement of peripheral liver may be seen in chronic Budd–Chiari syndrome and may be due to a combination of decreased portal perfusion and dilatation of hepatic sinusoids.

INFECTIOUS DISEASES—PYOGENIC ABSCESS

Pyogenic abscesses are usually observed in the context of recent surgery, Crohn's disease, appendicitis, and diverticulitis (13). Characteristic gadolinium-enhanced

MR findings are low signal lesions with enhancing capsules (14). Abscesses typically have perilesional enhancement with indistinct outer margins on immediate post-gadolinium SGE images due to a hyperemic response in adjacent liver (Fig. 4).

HEPATIC TRANSPLANTATION

Although not extensively used at present, MRI provides substantial information for preoperative and postoperative evaluation of livers in transplant patients. MRI permits comprehensive preoperative evaluation of candidates for liver transplantation. Preoperatively, patency of the inferior vena cava (IVC), portal vein, hepatic artery, and common bile duct may be determined, and presence of malignant disease evaluated (15, 16). Extent of hepatic involvement, porta hepatis nodes, and distant disease may all be assessed in patients with malignant disease evaluated for possible transplantation.

The most common cause of early liver graft failure is rejection, and early diagnosis is essential to allow modification of immunosuppressive therapy (17). The differential diagnosis of rejection is extensive and includes biliary obstruction, cholangitis, ischemic injury, viral infection, and drug toxicity.

Periportal signal abnormalities are frequently apparent in transplanted livers. The most typical appearance is tissue that is low in signal on T1-weighted images and high in signal on T2-weighted images. Abnormal tissue is most prominent in the porta hepatis and extends along the branching portal tracts into the liver parenchyma (18). In many cases, this represents lymphocytic infiltration from rejection, but may also be caused by dilated lymphatics due to impaired drainage following surgery (19). When the tissue is particularly mass-like, post-transplant lymphoproliferative disease may be present. Inflammatory periportal tissue may also be observed in acute hepatitis, following biliary surgery, in various benign or malignant diseases, and in portal adenopathy (20).

Vascular complications, such as portal vein or IVC thrombosis or hepatic artery stenosis, are important causes of graft failure (21). Portal vein and IVC patency may be diagnosed reliably by MRI (22). Stenosis of veins is a not uncommon complication that does not necessarily lead to graft failure. Although hepatic artery patency may be documented by MRI in most cases, at present stenosis can not be reliably excluded by current techniques. Stenosis or obstruction of the biliary tree may also be demonstrated. Dilated bile ducts may be shown using techniques in which bile is low-signal, high-signal (MR cholangiography), or a combination of both.

Fluid collections are common after hepatic transplantation. Bile leaks may occur, sometimes associated with biliary strictures. Mucocele of the cystic duct remnant may develop and appears as a focal fluid collection adjacent to the hepatic duct (23). Magnetic resonance imaging is able to distinguish between hematomas and other fluid collections in hepatic allograft recipients, owing to the fact that extracellular methemoglobin, found in subacute hematomas, renders these fluid collections high in signal on T1-weighted images. As a result, hematomas are higher in signal than other fluid collections.

Magnetic resonance imaging is able to demonstrate a variety of morphological abnormalities in transplanted livers, and is able to identify various causes of graft

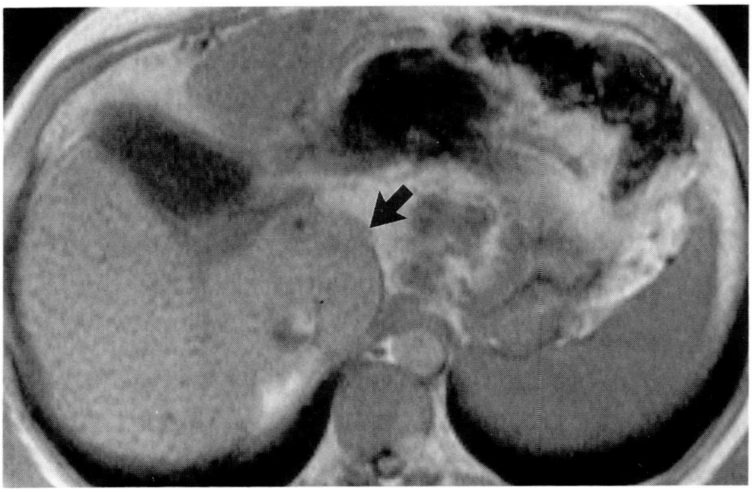

(A)

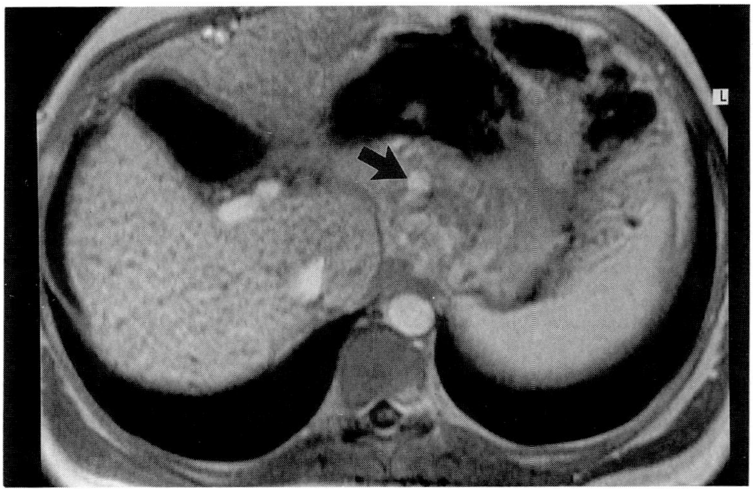

(B)

Figure 3. Regenerative nodules. SGE (A) and immediate post-gadolinium (B) SGE images. Multiple <1.0 cm nodules are scattered throughout the liver. Lesions are low in signal intensity of T1-weighted images (A), low in signal intensity of T2-weighted images (not shown), and low in signal intensity on post-gadolinium images (B). Additional findings of cirrhosis include hypertrophy of the caudate lobe (arrow, A), and varices along with the lesser curvature of the stomach (arrow, B). Immediate post-gadolinium SGE image in a second patient (C) demonstrates mulitiple low-signal <1 cm regenerative nodules throughout the liver (next page). Regenerative nodules are usually most conspicuous on immediate post-gadolinium images.

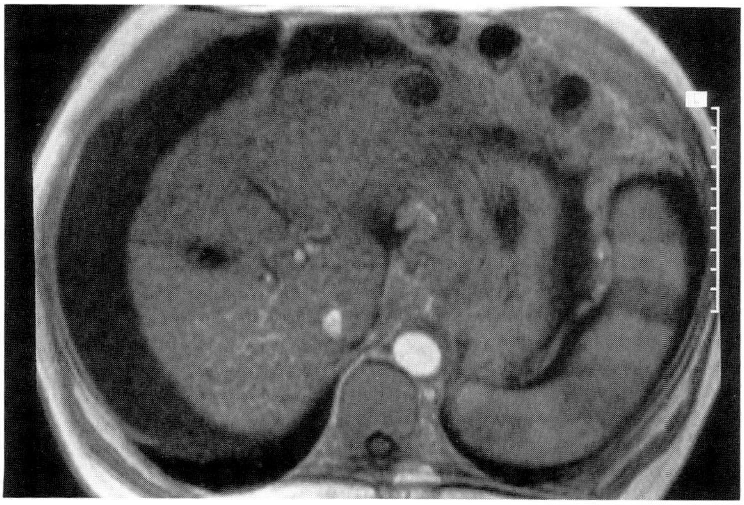

(C)

Figure 3. *(Continued)*

failure. At present, however, no specific MRI findings have been identified to establish or quantify transplant rejection. In the future, it is conceivable that hepatocyte specific agents may play a role in this determination.

BENIGN TUMORS

Hemangioma

Hemangiomas have long T1 and T2 values so they are low in signal intensity on T1-weighted images, high in signal on T2-weighted images, and maintain signal on longer TEs (for example, >120 msec) (24, 25). Hemangiomas have a well-defined lobular border with liver (24, 25). Hemangiomas typically enhance in a peripheral nodular fashion on dynamic serial gadolinium-enhanced MR images with slow progressive complete or nearly complete fill-in of the entire lesion at 10 min (Fig. 5) (26–28). Serial gadolinium-enhanced SGE images have been shown to be effective in distinguishing benign from malignant hepatic masses (29–30).

The most distinctive imaging feature of hemangiomas is the demonstration of a discontinuous ring of nodules immediately following gadolinium administration (29, 31, 32). Nodular enhancement is also frequently eccentric in location. Small hemangiomas with homogeneous enhancement may be indistinguishable from hypervascular malignant liver lesions such as hepatocellular carcinomas or leiomyosarcoma. The clinical history is important because patients with hypervascular malignant liver lesions usually have a known primary (33). Another variation in enhancement pattern seen in hemangiomas is that contrast enhancement may spread at a fairly rapid rate such that complete enhancement may occur at 1–2 min (31).

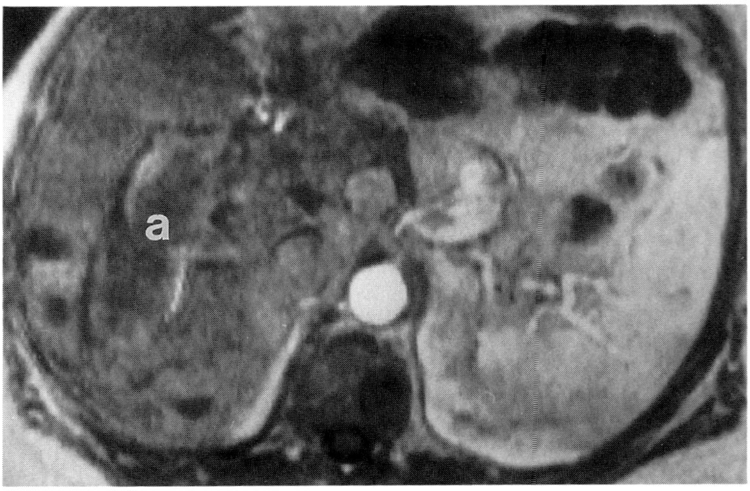

(A)

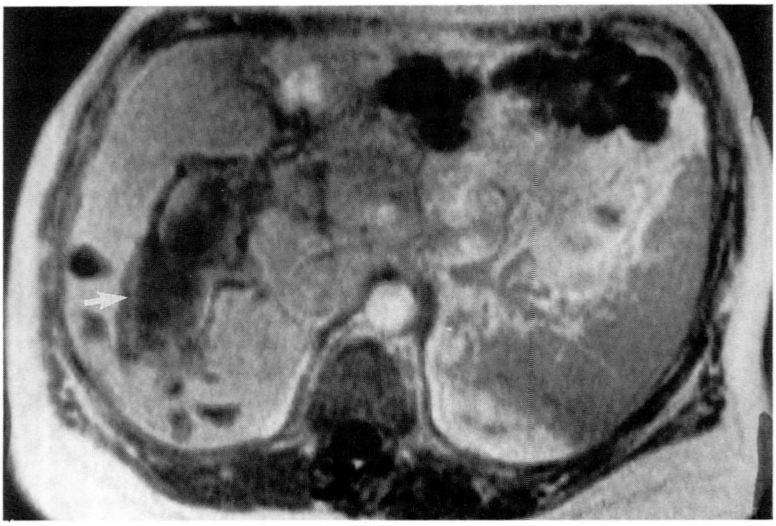

(B)

Figure 4. Bacterial liver abscesses. Immediate (A), and delayed (B) post-gadolinium SGE images. A low signal intensity, irregularly shaped lesion (a) with smaller peripheral hypointense lesions is noted on the immediate post-gadolinium image. Increased enhancement of the liver surrounding the lesions on the immediate post-gadolinium reflects hyperemic inflammatory parenchymal changes. The abscess capsule is identified on the delayed image (B) as a peripheral enhancing ring (arrow, B), reflecting late enhancement of fibrosis.

The MR appearances of small (<1.5 cm), medium (1.5–5.0 cm), and large (>5.0 cm) hemangiomas has been reported in a multi-institutional study (31). Among the 154 hemangiomas in 66 patients, 81 lesions were small, 56 medium, and 17 large. Hemangiomas were multiple in 68% of patients. All lesions were high in signal on T2-weighted images. Three types of enhancement patterns were observed: uniform high signal immediately following contrast (Type 1), peripheral nodular enhancement with centripetal progression to uniform high signal (Type 2), and peripheral nodular enhancement with centripetal progression with a persistent central scar (Type 3). Type 1 enhancement was observed only in small tumors. Types 2 and 3 enhancement were observed in all size categories. Type 3 enhancement was observed in 16/17 large tumors. This reflects the fact that giant hemangiomas most frequently have a central scar (Fig. 4) (31, 34), and the absence of a central scar should raise concern that the mass may represent another lesion. Large hemangiomas frequently have mildly complex signal intensity on T2-weighted images with frequent presence of low signal strands. In this multi-institutional study 68% of patients had multiple hemangiomas (31). A variation in the Type 2 enhancement pattern is that contrast enhancement may spread at a fairly rapid rate with complete enhancement at 1–2 min. Similar findings have also been described in an Asian patient population (35).

Cysts

Cysts are low signal on T1-weighted images and high signal on T2-weighted images and retain signal on longer TE (for example, >120 msec) T2-weighted images. Cysts do not enhance with gadolinium on MR images (Fig. 6). Delayed post-gadolinium images (up to 5 min) may be useful to ensure that lesions are cysts, not poorly vascularized metastases that show gradual enhancement (36).

Hepatic Adenomas

Approximately 90% of hepatic adenomas are found in young adult women (37, 38) and have a strong association with the use of birth control pills. Tumors may be multiple in 10–20% of the cases (39). Adenomas vary in signal intensity from mildly hypointense to moderately hyperintense (Fig. 7) on T1-weighted images, according to their fat content, and mildly hyperintense on T2-weighted images. They may be near isointense with liver on all imaging sequences, reflecting their similarity to liver parenchyma. Tumors may also have mixed high signal intensity on T1- and T2-weighted images owing to the presence of hemorrhage (40, 41). Characteristically tumors have a transient blush immediately following gadolinium chelate administration, which fades by 1 min.

Focal Nodular Hyperplasia

Focal nodular hyperplasia (FNH) is frequently found in adult females, however, 10–20% of cases occur in men (38). The tumors are not related to the use of birth control pills. Multiple lesions may be encountered as part of the multiple FNH syndrome, which consists of more than two FNH lesions and one or more of the

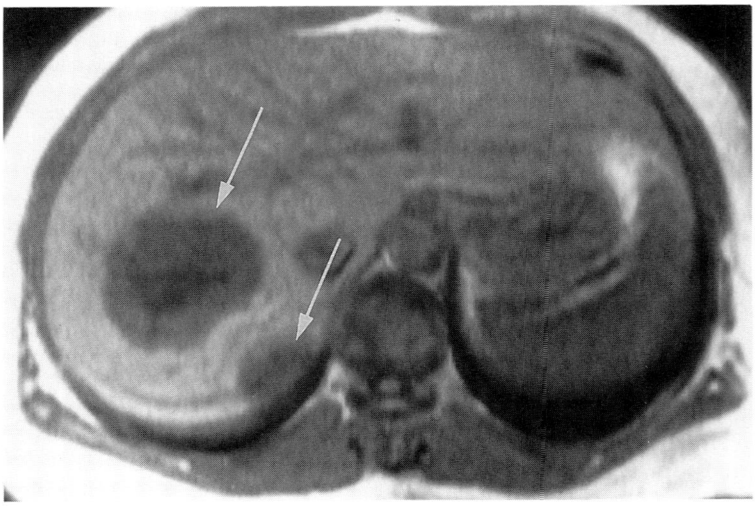

(A)

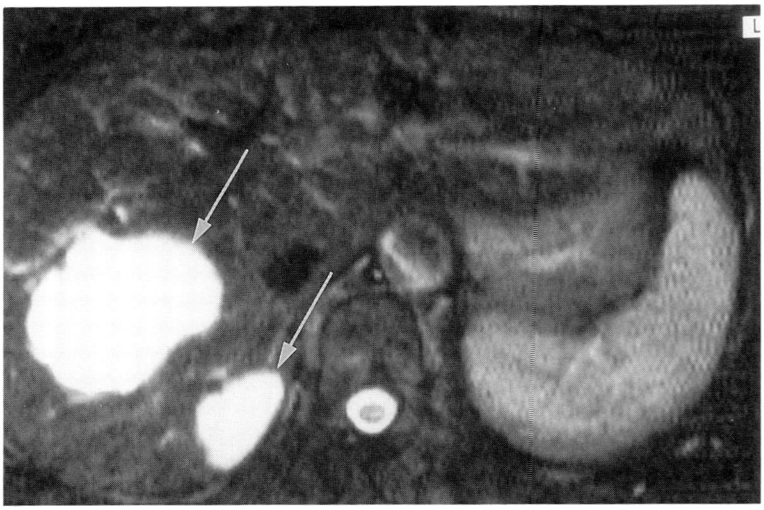

(B)

Figure 5. Hemangiomas of the liver. Precontrast SGE (A), T2FS (B), immediate post-gadolinium SGE (C, next page), and delayed post-gadolinium T1FS (D, next page) images. Two hemangiomas (arrows) are noted in the right lobe of the liver. They have rounded smooth borders, are low in signal intensity on precontrast SGE image and high in signal intensity on the T2FS image, and demonstrate a discontinuous ring of peripheral nodular enhancement on the immediate post-gadolinium image. On the delayed post-gadolinium image the smaller hemangioma enhances completely and is hyperintense compared to background liver, whereas lack of enhancement centrally in the larger hemangioma denotes the presence of a central scar. Note also that the central scar is of lower signal intensity compared to the periphery of the lesion on the precontrast SGE image (A).

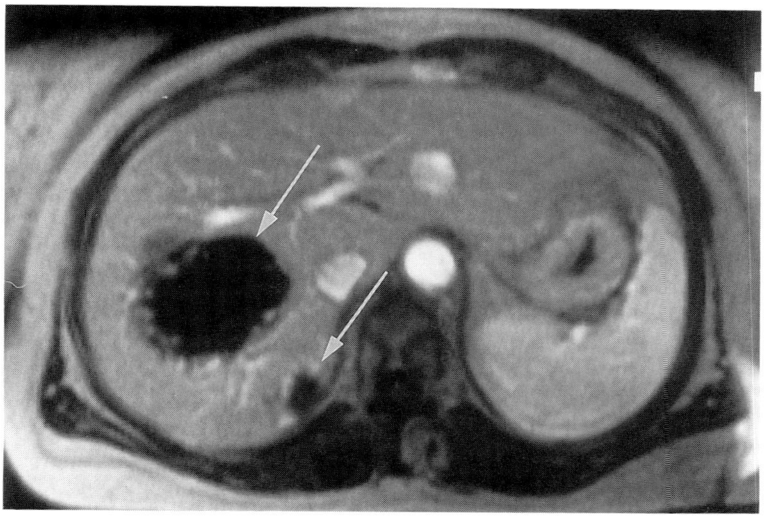

(C)

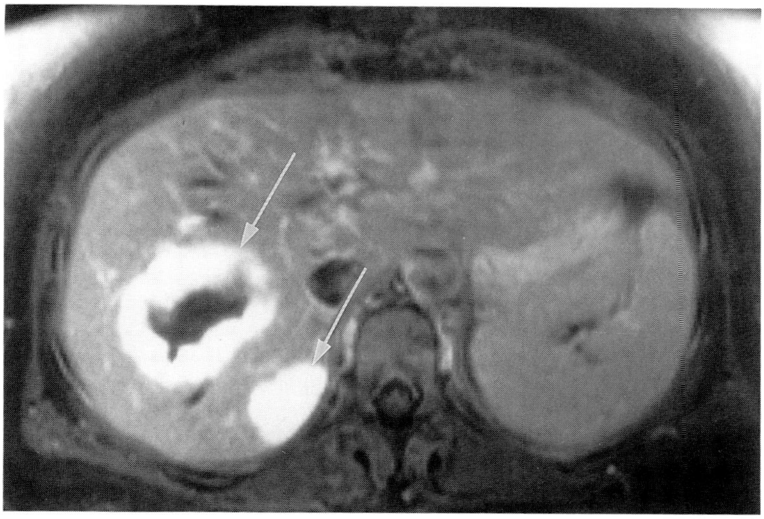

(D)

Figure 5. *(Continued)*

following lesions: hepatic hemangiomas, dysplastic systemic arteries, central nervous system vascular malformations, meningiomas, and astrocytomas (42).

The most frequent MR appearance on noncontrast images is slight hypointensity on T1-weighted images and slight hyperintensity on T2-weighted images, although tumors may be near isointense on these sequences. Unlike adenomas, FNH rarely has higher signal than liver on T1-weighted images. A high-signal central scar on T2-weighted images is a characteristic feature of FNH but is observed in only 10–49% of patients (43–46). The characteristic gadolinium enhancement feature of

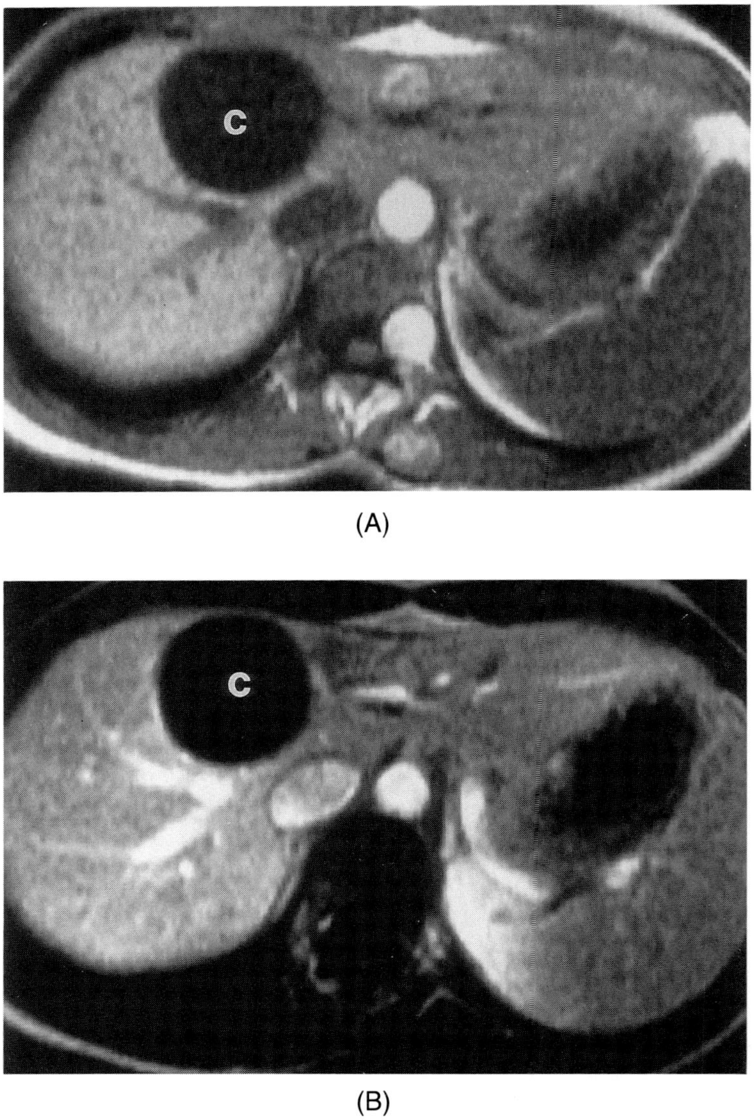

Figure 6. Simple liver cyst. Precontrast (A) and delayed post gadolinium (B) SGE images. The cyst is rounded and possesses smooth margins (c). Complete lack of enhancement is noted on the delayed post-gadolinium image (c), a finding characteristic of liver cysts.

these lesions is that they have an intense uniform blush on immediate post-gadolinium chelate images and fade rapidly to near isointensity (typically at 1 min post contrast) (Fig. 8) (47, 48).

Features that aid in the distinction between adenomas and FNH include the presence of a pseudocapsule, internal hemorrhage, or fat, which are features more typical for adenomas, and a central scar that shows delayed enhancement, which is more typical for FNH (40). Both lesions have an early transient tumor blush on gadolinium-enhanced images (26, 47, 48). These enhancement features must be viewed with caution because they represent features of well differentiated tumors

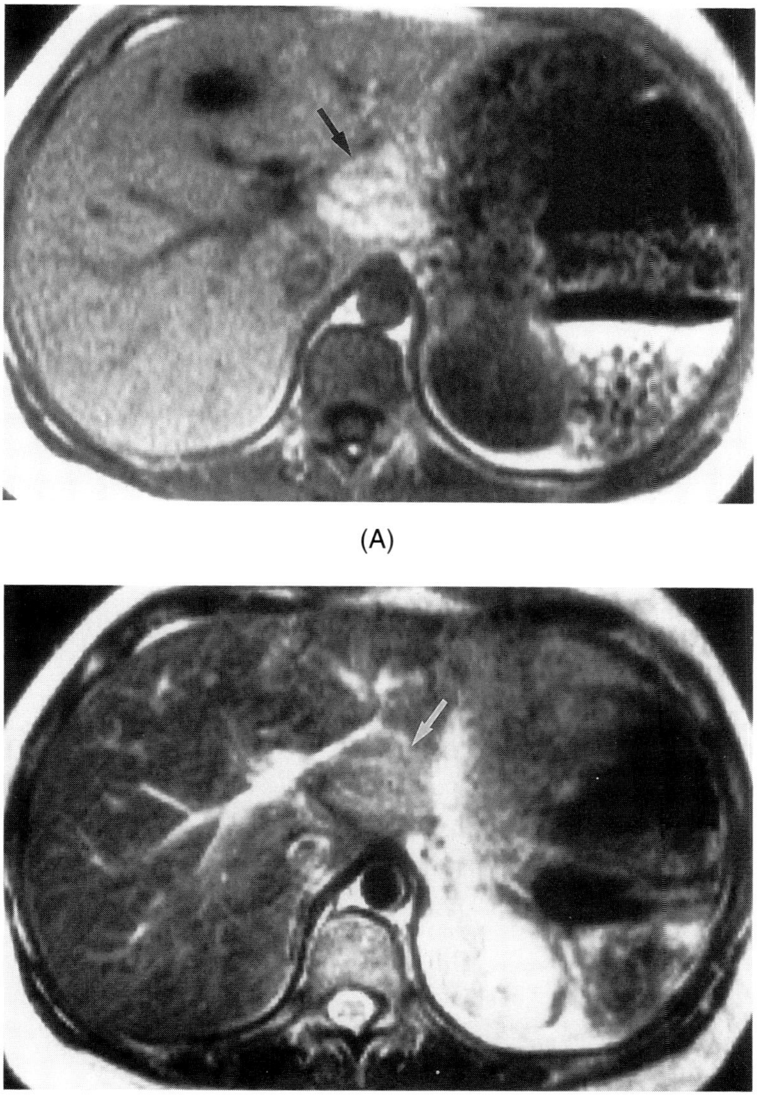

(A)

(B)

Figure 7. Fat containing hepatic adenoma. Precontrast SGE (A) and T2SE (B) images. The adenoma is moderately hyperintense on the SGE (arrow, A) and mildly hyperintense on the T2SE image owing to its fat content (arrow, B).

of hepatocellular origin, including well differentiated or early hepatocellular carcinoma.

MALIGNANT TUMORS

Liver Metastases

Liver metastases are the most common malignant tumors of the liver. Optimal imaging investigation involves both detection and characterization of liver lesions

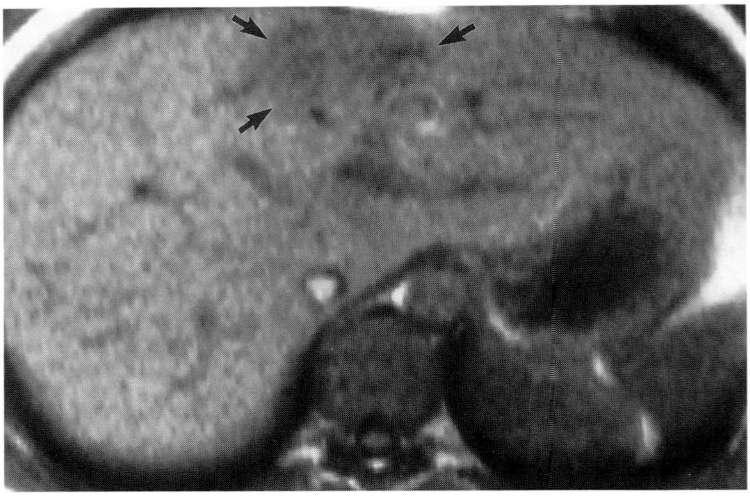

(A)

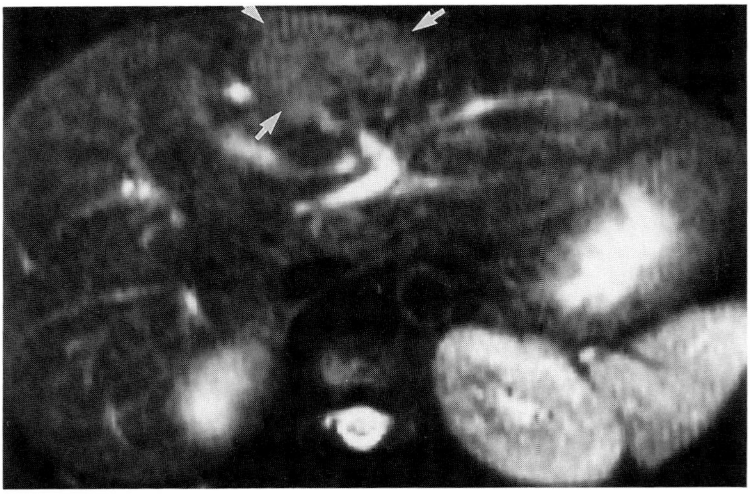

(B)

Figure 8. Focal nodular hyperplasia. Precontrast SGE (A), T2FS (B), immediate post-gadolinium SGE (C, next page), and 90-sec post-gadolinium SGE (D, next page) images. An FNH is present in the left lobe of the liver (arrows, A) which is minimally low in signal intensity on the precontrast SGE image and minimally hyperintense relative to liver parenchyma on the T2FS image (arrows, B). Intense transient homogeneous enhancement is evident on the immediate post-gadolinium image (arrows, C), which fades to isointensity on the more delayed post-gadolinium image (D). The top of a coexisitng hemangioma is partially imaged in the posterior segment of the right hepatic lobe.

(26, 49–51). Detection involves identification of the presence of lesions and the segmental extent of liver involvement (50). Demonstration that malignant disease has limited hepatic involvement may have a substantial impact on patient management. Survival of patients with colorectal metastases may be improved by partial hepatectomy if metastases are localized to three or fewer segments (52, 53).

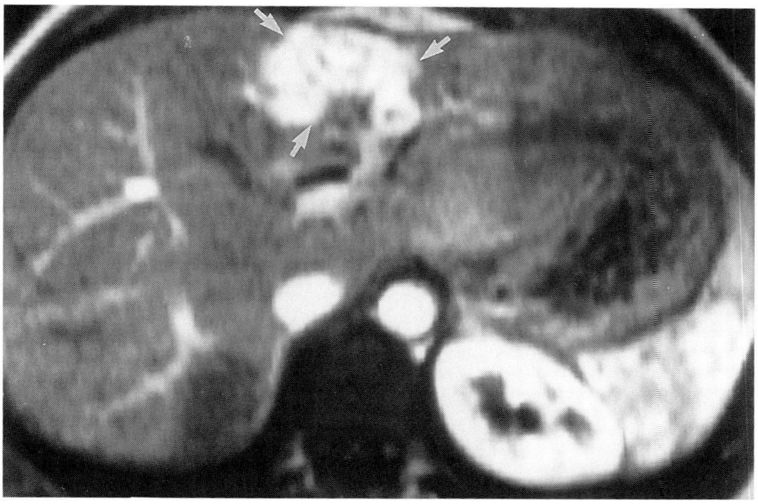

(C)

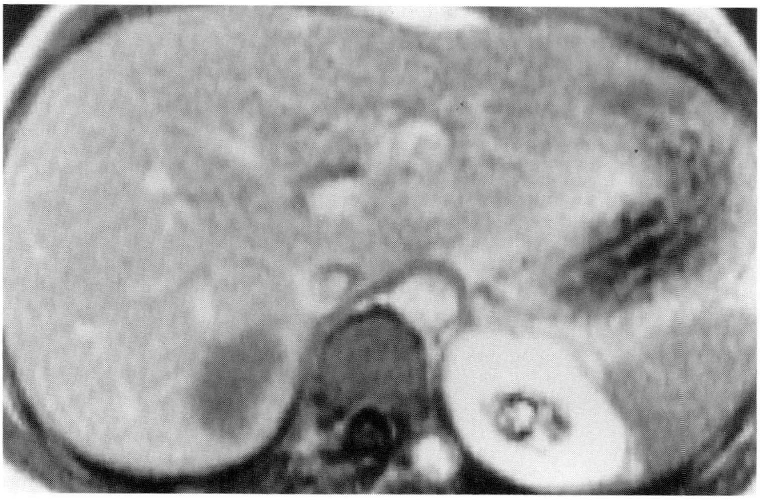

(D)

Figure 8. *(Continued)*

A previous study, which compared nonspiral dynamic contrast-enhanced CT and MRI employing T2-weighted fat suppressed (T2FS) spin echo, SGE, and dynamic serial post-gadolinium SGE images in 73 patients with clinically suspected liver disease, demonstrated greater lesion detection and characterization by MRI. Lesion detection was greatest with T2FS (272 lesions) and contrast-enhanced SGE (244 lesions), which was statistically greater than with CT (220 lesions) and SGE (219) ($p < .03$) (26). Lesion characterization was greatest with contrast-enhanced SGE (236 lesions) ($p < .01$), followed by CT (199 lesions), SGE (164 lesions), and T2FS (144 lesions).

A more recent comparison, between these MR sequences and dynamic nonspiral contrast-enhanced CT, in 20 patients with solitary hepatic metastases detected by CT, demonstrated that MRI detected more than 1 lesion in 6/20 (30%) of patients (54).

The importance of characterization of liver lesions is that patients with known primary malignancies may have small hepatic lesions that are not infrequently benign cysts or hemangiomas. Jones et al. reported on the detection of small (<15 mm) lesions in 254 of 1454 patients who underwent CT examination (55), and found that lesions in 51% of patients were benign despite the fact that 82% of patients had a primary malignancy. Patients may have a variety of lesions, which can be multiple and scattered throughout the liver; therefore the whole organ coverage per acquisition of SGE permits optimal evaluation of the entire liver with serial gadolinium enhancement.

In a recent study comparing spiral CT arterial portography (CTAP) and MRI employing the sequences described above, CTAP and MRI demonstrated 107 and 105 true positive, 11 and 0 false positive, 80 and 91 true negative, and 4 and 6 false negative segmental involvement, respectively. There was a significant difference ($p < .05$) in specificity of segmental involvement between MRI (1.0 ± 0) compared to CTAP (0.88 ± 0.05), and no other differences in sensitivity and specificity were observed. Total procedural cost was \$3,499 for CTAP and \$1,224 for MRI. Computed tomography arterial portography findings did not change patient management over MRI findings in any patient, but MRI findings resulted in a change in patient management over CTAP findings in seven patients (56).

Metastases vary substantially in appearance on T1- and T2-weighted images. Borders are usually irregular but may be sharp. Lesion shape is frequently irregular but may be round or oval. In general metastases are low in signal on T1-weighted images and modestly high in signal on T2-weighted images. Some metastases, particularly vascular metastases from islet cell tumors, pheochromocytoma and renal cell cancer or necrotic metastases may be high in signal on T2-weighted images, which may make distinction from hemangiomas difficult (24, 33, 57).

The typical enhancement feature of metastases is a peripheral ring of enhancement on immediate post-gadolinium chelate SGE images (33, 57). Enhancement not infrequently progresses centrally. Irregular or peripheral contrast washout is also observed (29, 33, 58).

Hypovascular Metastases

Metastases that are commonly hypovascular include metastases from colorectal cancer (Fig. 9), transitional cell cancer, and carcinoid tumors. Lymphoma and hepatocellular carcinomas are other malignant lesions that may also have this appearance. Malignant hypovascular metastases have diminished blood supply usually as a result of a fibrous/collagenous tumor matrix, coagulative necrosis, or monotonous dense cellularity. These lesions generally are low in signal on T1- and T2-weighted images, signal features comparable to muscle or fibrous tissue. These tumors are hypointense on T1-weighted images but may be isointense on T2-weighted images (59). Generally these tumors are most conspicuous on portal phase gadolinium-enhanced SGE images (59). Hypovascular metastases with liquefactive necrosis contain a large volume of extracellular fluid and may mimic cysts by appearing high in signal on T2-weighted images and near signal void immediately following gadolinium administration. Delayed post-gadolinium images demonstrate that the lesion borders become indistinct and lesions appear smaller owing to peripheral enhancement.

Hypervascular Metastases

Malignancies that frequently result in hypervascular liver metastases include renal, carcinoid, islet cell, leiomyosarcoma (Fig. 10), and melanoma (33). Malignancies that occasionally result in hypervascular liver metastases include bowel, breast, and lung cancer and rarely, other tumors such as ovarian carcinoma (Fig. 11). Magnetic resonance features of hypervascular metastases include high signal on T2-weighted images and intense peripheral ring of enhancement immediately following gadolinium administration (29, 33, 57). In many of these lesions, contrast progresses in a centripetal fashion (33). Dynamic serial gadolinium-enhanced MR images are especially important for lesion detection and characterization in patients with known vascular primary tumors. Vascular metastases from gastrinomas enhance with a uniform peripheral ring pattern on immediate post-gadolinium images. These metastases have a particular propensity to fade peripherally on more delayed images (57). Vascular metastases from renal cell cancer, bowel cancer, carcinoid, or nongastrinoma islet cell tumors tend to be irregular in size and shape and to enhance with a thick irregular rim that may gradually fill in. Characteristics of peripheral ring enhancement that suggest the diagnosis of a malignant lesion rather than a hemangioma include (1) early intense peripheral ring, (2) uniformity of the thickness of the ring, (3) jagged or serrated internal margin of the ring rather than a lobular margin, and (4) peripheral washout of the ring with presence of more central enhancement (29, 30, 33, 57, 58).

Small hypervascular metastases frequently enhance in a uniform fashion and fade to near isointensity by 1 min (33). Some small hemangiomas may enhance as rapidly; however, hemangiomas tend to retain contrast and remain high in signal for a more prolonged period. In patients with a known primary hypervascular malignancy, images should be acquired in more than one phase of gadolinium enhancement. The capillary phase of enhancement is the most important phase of image acquisition for both detection and characterization, and later phases assist with lesion characterization.

Hepatocellular Carcinoma

On MR images, hepatocellular carcinomas (HCCs) may have a variety of signal patterns on T1- and T2-weighted images. The most frequent appearance is minimally low signal on T1-weighted images and moderately high signal on T2-weighted images (60–68). HCCs may, however, range from hypo- to hyperintense on T1- and T2-weighted images. Early HCC is frequently high in signal on T1-weighted images and isointense on T2-weighted images (63–66). High signal on T1-weighted images on occasion is due to presence of fat, but many of these tumors do not contain fat; rather copper, copper-binding protein, or high protein content may be responsible for the high signal (64–66, 69). HCCs are frequently hypervascular and enhance in a diffuse heterogeneous fashion (33, 70, 71). The appearance on capillary-

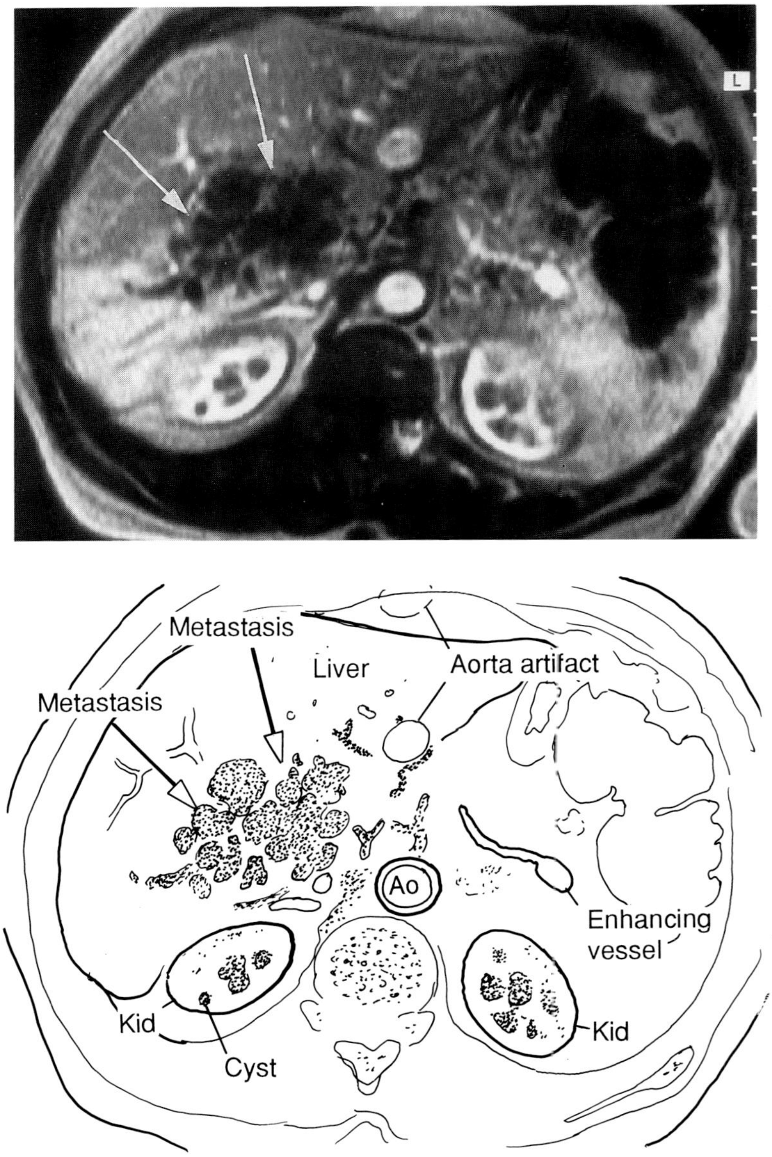

(A)

Figure 9. Hypovascular metastases from colon adenocarcinoma with portal vein thrombosis. Immediate (A) and 45 sec post-contrast (B, next page) images. A large metastasis is present in the right lobe of the liver which has the appearance of a cluster of grapes (arrows, A). Tumor thrombus is present in the posterior branch of the right portal vein (arrows, B). Associated intense transient enhancement is noted of the liver, subtended by the thrombosed portal vein on the immediate post-gadolinium image owing to compensatory increased hepatic arterial perfusion.

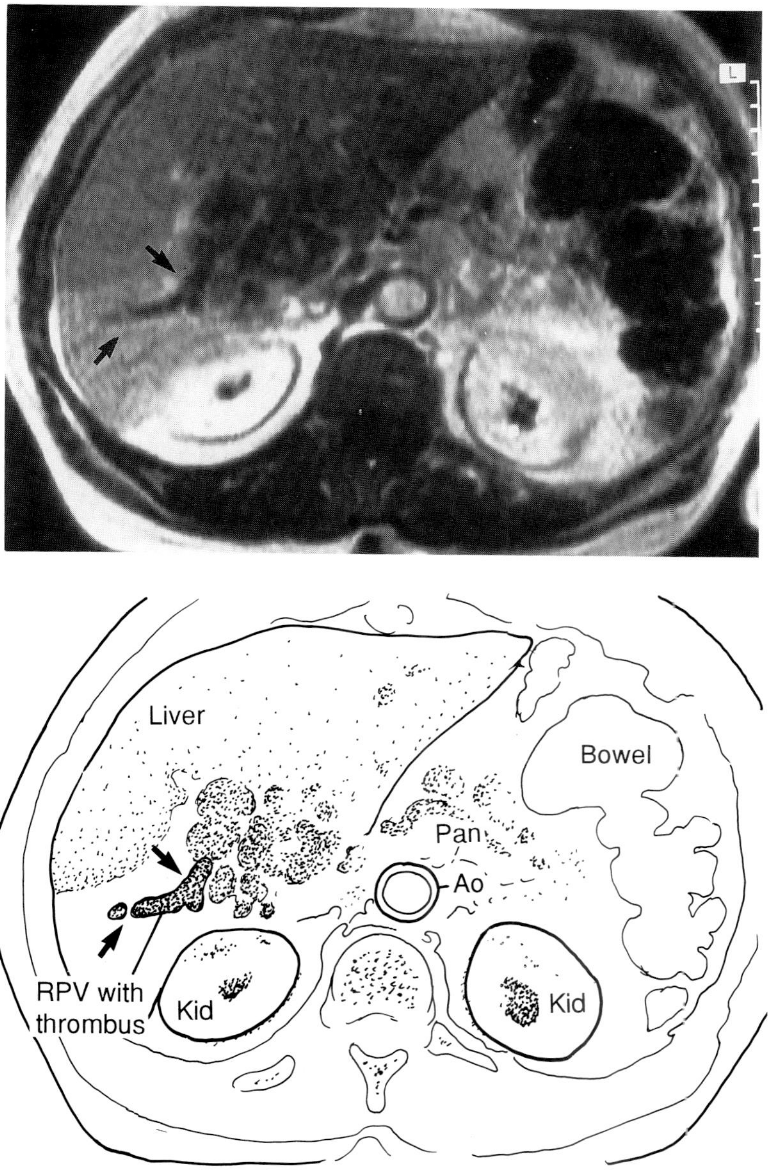

(B)

Figure 9. *(Continued)*

phase gadolinium-enhanced images often permits distinction of HCC from metastatic disease because HCCs typically demonstrate enhancing stroma throughout the entire tumor (Fig. 12), whereas metastases have peripheral enhancement (33). Small tumors may be apparent only on immediate post-gadolinium SGE images.

Tumor extension into portal or hepatic veins is observed in <50% of cases, but is common with large and advanced tumors. Pseudocapsules are often observed in

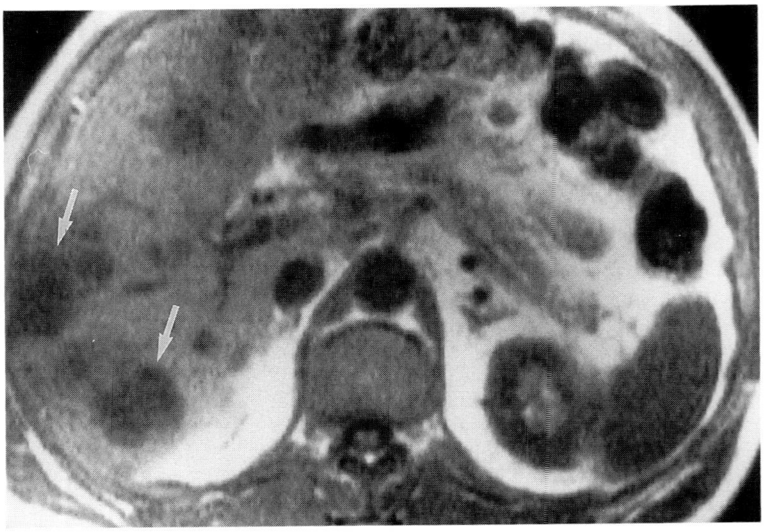

(A)

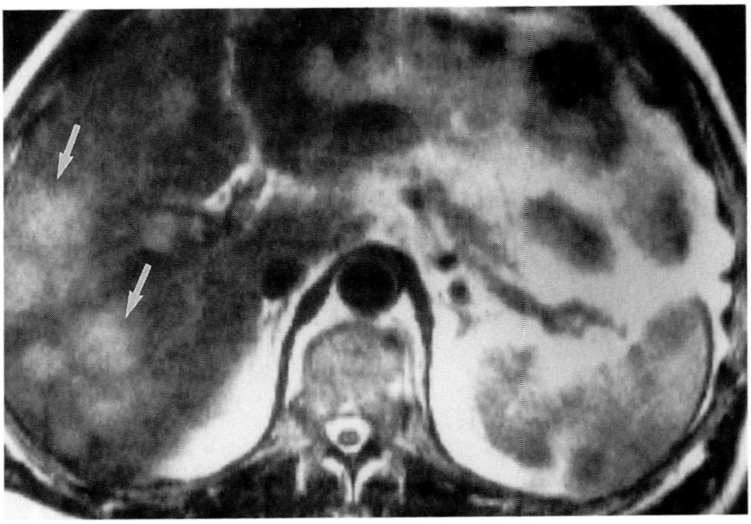

(B)

Figure 10. Hypervascular metastases from leiomyosarcoma. Precontrast SGE (A), T2 echo train spin echo (B), and immediate post-gadolinium SGE (C, next page) images. Multiple metastases (arrows) are scattered throughout the liver. The lesions have variable size, low signal intensity on the precontrast SGE image, and moderately high signal intensity on the T2-weighted image (B). Intense peripheral enhancement is demonstrated on the immediate post-gadolinium image (C).

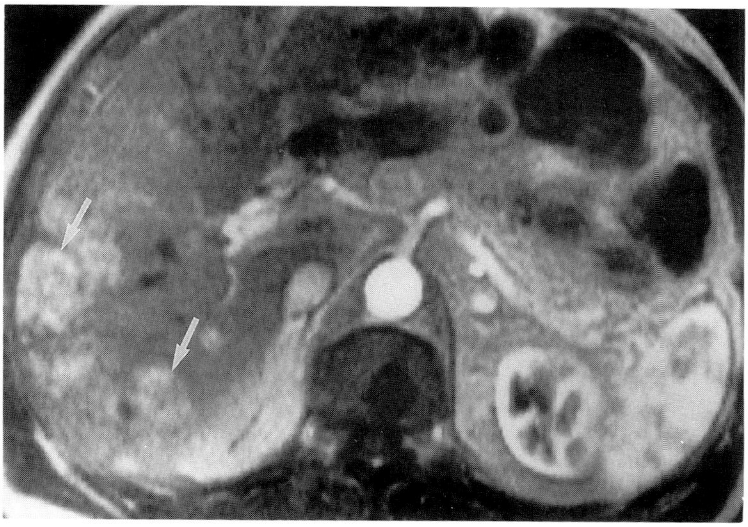

(C)

Figure 10. *(Continued)*

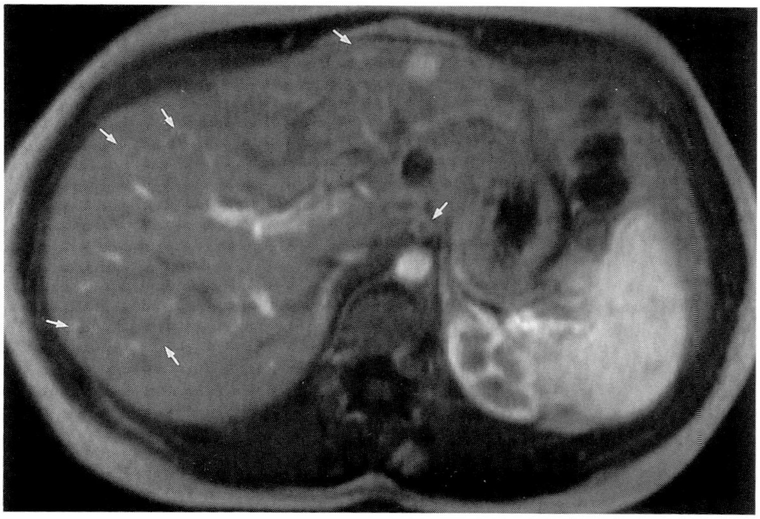

Figure 11. Hypervascular ovarian adenocarcinoma liver metastases. Immediate post-gadolinium SGE image. Multiple liver metastases are apparent throughout the liver on the immediate post-gadolinium SGE image. Distinct ring enhancement is apparent in lesions, many of which measure approximately 1 cm in diameter (arrows).

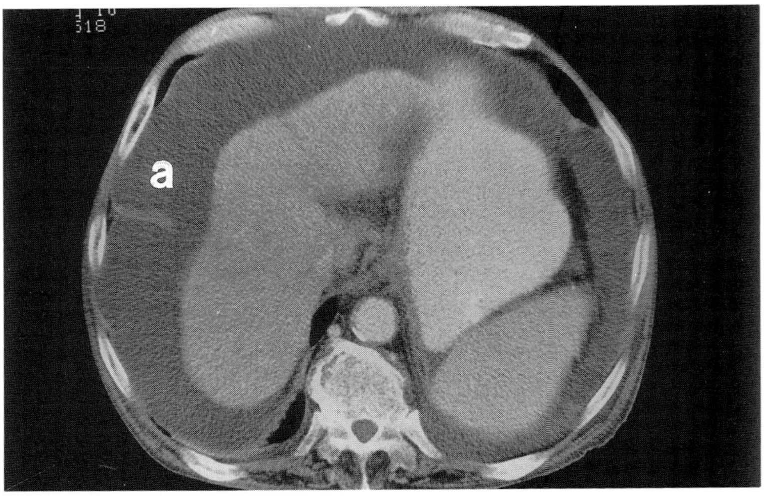

(A)

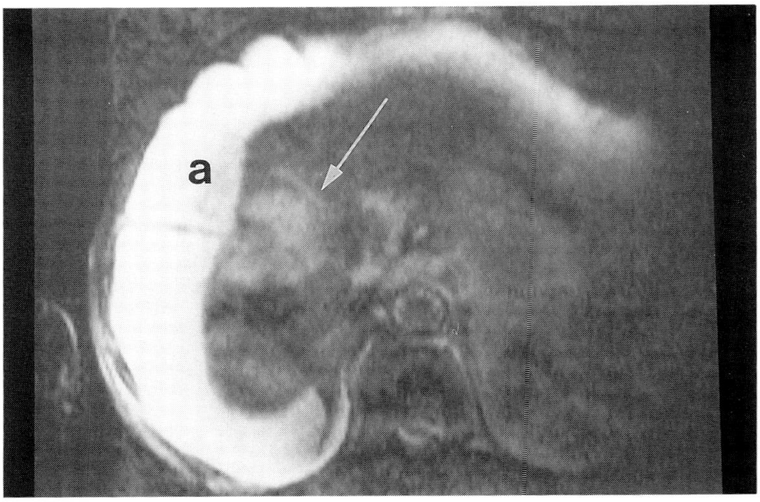

(B)

Figure 12. Hepatocellular carcinoma in a cirrhotic patient. Contrast-enhanced spiral CT (A), T2FS (B), and immediate post-gadolinium SGE (C, next page) images. Hepatic cirrhosis with decreased size of the liver, micronodular contour, and ascites (a) are identified on all images. The tumor is poorly visualized on the CT image. The hepatocellular carcinoma is identified on the MR images as an irregular mass that is heterogeneous and moderately high in signal intensity on the T2FS image (arrow, B) and possesses intense heterogeneous enhancement throughout its entirety on the immediate post-gadolinium SGE image (arrow, C).

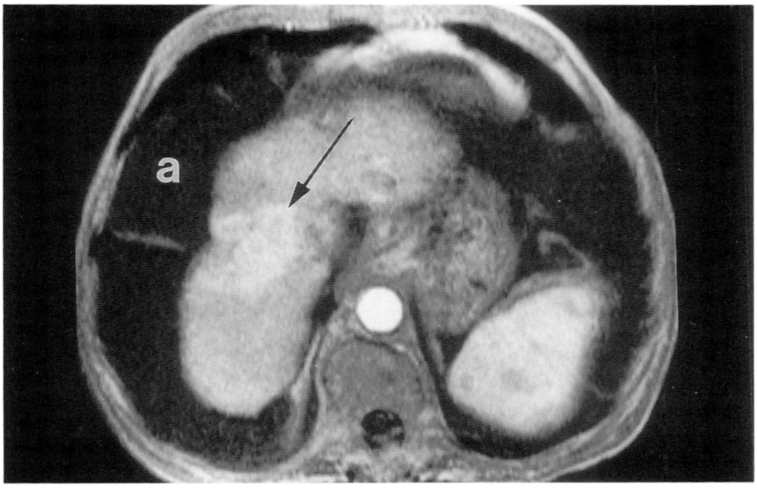

(C)

Figure 12. *(Continued)*

HCC, especially in early or well differentiated tumors. The typical signal intensity of a pseudocapsule is hypointensity on T1-weighted images, minimal hyperintensity on T2-weighted images, low signal on immediate post-gadolinium images, and increased enhancement on delayed images (71).

An uncommon type of HCC is the fibrolamellar HCC. This tumor is unusual in that it occurs in younger patients, frequently females, without underlying cirrhosis and has a better prognosis than HCC (72). Tumors are large, are usually low in signal intensity on T1-weighted images and heterogeneously high on T2-weighted images, and possess diffuse heterogeneous enhancement on immediate post-gadolinium images (73).

REFERENCES

1. Mitchell DG. Focal manifestations of diffuse liver disease at MR imaging. *Radiology*. 1992;185:1–11.
2. Mitchell DG, Kim I, Chang TS, et al. Fatty liver. Chemical shift phase-difference and suppression magnetic resonance imaging techniques in animals, phantoms, and humans. *Invest Radiol.* 1991;26:1041–1052.
3. Itai Y, Ohtomo K, Kokubo T, Okada Y, Yamauchi T, Yoshida H. Segmental intensity differences in the liver on MR images: a sign of intrahepatic portal flow stoppage. *Radiology*. 1988;167:17–19.
4. Lorigan JG, Charnsangavej C, Carrasco CH, Richli WR, Wallace S. Atrophy with compensatory hypertrophy of the liver in hepatic neoplasms: radiographic findings. *AJR*. 1988;150:1291–1295.
5. Carr DH, Hadjis NS, Banks LM, Hemingway AP, Blumgart LH. Computed tomography of hilar cholangiocarcinoma: a new sign. *AJR*. 1985;145:53–56.

6. Itai Y, Murata S, Jurosaki Y. Straight border sign of the liver: spectrum of CT appearances and causes. *Radiographics.* 1995;15:1089–1102.
7. Schlund JF, Semelka RC, Kettritz U, Eisenberg LB, Lee JKT. Transient increased segmental hepatic enhancement distal to portal vein obstruction on dynamic gadolinium-enhanced gradient echo MR images. *J Magn Reson Imaging* 1995;5:375–377.
8. Lehmann B, Fanucci E, Gigli F, Uhlenbrock D, Bartolozzi C. Signal suppression of normal liver tissue by phase corrected inversion recovery: a screening technique. *J Comput Assist Tomogr.* 1989;13:650–655.
9. Marti-Bonmati L, Talens A, del Olmo J, et al. Chronic hepatitis and cirrhosis: evaluation by means of MR imaging with histologic correlation. *Radiology.* 1993;188:37–43.
10. Ohtomo K, Itai Y, Ohtomo Y, Shiga J, Iio M. Regenerating nodules of liver cirrhosis: MR imaging with pathologic correlation. *AJR.* 1990;154:505–507.
11. Terada T, Nakanuma Y. Survey of iron-accumulative macroregenerative nodules in cirrhotic livers. *Hepatology.* 1989;10:851–854.
12. Mitchell DG, Lovett KE, Hann HW, Ehrlich S, Palazzo J, Rubin R. Cirrhosis: multiobserver analysis of hepatic MR imaging findings in a heterogeneous population. *J Magn Reson Imaging.* 1993;3:313–321.
13. Bertel CK, van Heerden JA, Sheedy PF. Treatment of pyogenic hepatic abscesses. Surgical vs percutaneous drainage. *Arch Surg.* 1986;121:554–558.
14. Mendez RJ, Schiebler ML, Outwater EK, Kressel HY. Hepatic abscesses: MR imaging findings. *Radiology.* 1994;190:431–436.
15. Finn JP, Edelman RR, Jenkins RL, et al. Liver transplantation: MR angiography with surgical validation. *Radiology.* 1991;179:265–269.
16. Nghiem HV, Winter TC, Mountford MC, et al. Evaluation of the portal venous system before liver transplantation: value of phase-contrast MR angiography. *AJR.* 1995;164: 871–878.
17. Demetris AJ, Lasky S, Van Thiel DH, Starzl TE, Dekker A. Pathology of hepatic transplantation: A review of 62 adult allograft recipients immunosuppressed with a cyclosporine/steroid regimen. *Am J Pathol.* 1985;118:151–161.
18. Lang P, Schnarkowski P, Grampp S, et al. Liver transplantation: significance of the periportal collar on MRI. *J Comput Assist Tomogr.* 1995;19:580–585.
19. Marincek B, Barbier PA, Becker CD, Mettler D, Ruchti C. CT appearance of impaired lymphatic drainage in liver transplants. *AJR.* 1986;147:519–523.
20. Matsui O, Kadoya M, Takashima T, Kameyama T, Yoshikawa J, Tamura S. Intrahepatic periportal abnormal intensity on MR images: an indication of various hepatobiliary diseases. *Radiology.* 1989;171:335–338.
21. Wozney P, Zajko AB, Bron KM, Point S, Starzl TE. Vascular complications after liver transplantation: a 5-year experience. *AJR.* 1986;147:657–663.
22. Dalen K, Day DL, Ascher NL, et al. Imaging of vascular complications after hepatic transplantation. *AJR.* 1988;150:1285–1290.
23. Zajko AB, Bennett MJ, Campbell VL, Koneru B. Mucocele of the cyctic duct remnant in eight liver transplant recipients: findings at cholangiography, CT, and US. *Radiology.* 1990;177:691–693.
24. Li KC, Glazer GM, Quint LE, et al. Distinction of hepatic cavernous hemangioma from hepatic metastases with MR imaging. *Radiology.* 1988;169:409–415.
25. Lombardo DM, Baker ME, Spritzer CE, Blinder R, Meyers W, Herfkens RJ. Hepatic hemangiomas vs metastases: MR differentiation at 1.5 T. *AJR.* 1990;155:55–59.
26. Semelka RC, Shoenut JP, Kroeker MA, et al. Focal liver disease: comparison of dynamic

contrast-enhanced CT and T-2 weighted fat-suppressed, FLASH, and dynamic gadolinium-enhanced MR imaging at 1.5 T. *Radiology.* 1992;184:687–694.

27. Schmiedl U, Kolbel G, Hess CF, Klose U, Kurtz B. Dynamic sequential MR imaging of focal liver lesions initial experience in 22 patients at 1.5 T. *J Comput Assist Tomogr.* 1990;14:600–607.
28. Quinn SF, Benjamin GG. Hepatic cavernous hemangiomas: simple diagnostic sign with dynamic bolus CT. *Radiology.* 1992;182:545–548.
29. Whitney WS, Herfkens RJ, Jeffrey RB, et al. Dynamic breath-hold multiplanar spoiled gradient-recalled MR imaging with gadolinium enhancement for differentiating hepatic hemangiomas from malignancies at 1.5 T. *Radiology.* 1993;189:863–870.
30. Hamm B, Thoeni RF, Gould RG, et al. Focal liver lesions: characterization with nonenhanced and dynamic contrast material-enhanced MR imaging. *Radiology.* 1994;190: 417–423.
31. Semelka RC, Brown ED, Ascher SM, et al. Hepatic hemangiomas: a multiinstitutional study of appearance on T2-weighted and serial gadolinium-enhanced gradient-echo MR images. *Radiology.* 1994;192:401–406.
32. Mitchell DG, Saini S, Weinreb J, et al. Hepatic metastases and cavernous hemangiomas: distinction with standard- and triple-dose gadoteridol-enhanced MR imaging. *Radiology.* 1994;193:49–57.
33. Larson RE, Semelka RC, Bagley AS, Molina PL, Brown ED, Lee JK. Hypervascular malignant liver lesions: comparison of various MR imaging pulse sequences and dynamic CT. *Radiology.* 1994;192:393–399.
34. Choi BI, Han MC, Park JH, Kim SH, Han MH, Kim CW. Giant cavernous hemangioma of the liver: CT and MR imaging in 10 cases. *AJR.* 1989;152:1221–1226.
35. Kim TK, Choi BI, Han JK, Jang H, Han MC. Optimal MR imaging protocol for hepatic hemangiomas: comparison of T2-weighted Fast and conventional SE and serial Gd-DPTA-enhanced GRE techniques. *Radiology.* 1995;197(P):175.
36. Semelka RC, Shoenut JP, Greenberg HM, Mickflickier AB. The liver. In: Semelka RC, Shoenut JP, eds. MRI of the Abdomen with CT Correlation. New York: Raven Press; 1993:13–41.
37. Kerlin P, David GL, McGill DB, Weiland LH, Adson MA, Sheedy PF. Hepatic adenoma and focal nodular hyperplasia: clinical, pathologic, and radiologic features. *Gastroenterology.* 1983;84:994–1002.
38. Shortell CK, Schwartz SI. Hepatic adenoma and focal nodular hyperplasia. *Surg Gynecol Obstet.* 1991;173:426–431.
39. Terminology of nodular hepatocellular lesions. International Working Party. *Hepatology.* 1995;22:983–993.
40. Paulson EK, McClellan JS, Washington K, Spritzer CE, Meyers WC, Baker ME. Hepatic adenoma: MR characteristics and correlation with pathologic findings. *AJR.* 1994;163:113–116.
41. Powers C, Ros PR, Stoupis C, Johnson WK, Segel KH. Primary liver neoplasms: MR imaging with pathologic correlation. *Radiographics.* 1994;14:459–482.
42. Wanless IR, Albrecht S, Bilbao J, et al. Multiple focal nodular hyperplasia of the liver associated with vascular malformations of various organs and neoplasia of the brain: a new syndrome. *Mod. Pathol.* 1989;2:456–462.
43. Lee MJ, Saini S, Hamm B, et al. Focal nodular hyperplasia of the liver: MR findings in 35 proved cases. *AJR.* 1991;156:317–320.
44. Vilgrain V, Flejou JF, Arrive L, et al. Focal nodular hyperplasia of the liver: MR imaging and pathologic correlation in 37 patients. *Radiology.* 1992;184:699–703.

45. Schiebler ML, Kressel HY, Saul SH, Yeager BA, Axel L, Gefter WB. MR imaging of focal nodular hyperplasia of the liver. *J Comput Assist Tomogr.* 1987;11:651–654.

46. Haggar AM, Bree RL. Hepatic focal nodular hyperplasia MR imaging at 1.0 and 1.5 T. *J Magn Reson Imaging.* 1992;2:85–88.

47. Mahfouz AE, Hamm B, Taupitz M, Wolf KJ. Hypervascular liver lesions: differentiation of focal nodular hyperplasia from malignant tumors with dynamic gadolinium-enhanced MR imaging. *Radiology.* 1993;186:133–138.

48. Mathieu D, Rahmouni A, Anglade MC, et al. Focal nodular hyperplasia of the liver: assessment with contrast-enhanced TurboFLASH MR imaging. *Radiology.* 1991;180: 25–30.

49. Rummeny EJ, Wernecke K, Saini S, et al. Comparison between high-field-strength MR imaging and CT for screening of hepatic metastases: a receiver operating characteristic analysis. *Radiology.* 1992;182:879–886.

50. Nelson RC, Chezmar JL, Sugarbaker PH, Murray DR, Bernardino ME. Preoperative localization of focal liver lesions to specific liver segments: utility of CT during arterial portography [see comments]. *Radiology.* 1990;176:89–94.

51. Mirowitz SA, Lee JK, Gutierrez E, Brown JJ, Heiken JP, Eilenberg SS. Dynamic gadolinium-enhanced rapid acquisition spin-echo MR imaging of the liver. *Radiology.* 1991;179:371–376.

52. Sugarbaker PH, Kemeny N. Management of metastatic cancer to the liver. *Adv Surg.* 1989;22:1–56.

53. Hughes KS, Rosenstein RB, Songhorabodi S, et al. Resection of the liver for colorectal carcinoma metastases. A multi-instutitional study of long-term survivors. *Dis Colon Rectum.* 1988;31:1–4.

54. Semelka RC, Shoenut JP, Ascher SM, et al. Solitary hepatic metastasis: comparison of dynamic contrast-enhanced CT and MR imaging with fat-suppressed T2-weighted, breath-hold T1-weighted FLASH, and dynamic gadolinium-enhanced FLASH sequences. *J Magn Reson Imaging.* 1994;4:319–323.

55. Jones EC, Chezmar JL, Nelson RC, Bernardino ME. The frequency and significance of small (less or equal to 15 mm) hepatic lesions detected by CT. *AJR.* 1992;158:535–539.

56. Semelka RC, Schlund JF, Molina PL, et al. Malignant liver lesions: comparison of spiral CT arterial portography and MR imaging for diagnostic accuracy, cost, and effect on patient management. *J Magn Reson Imaging.* 1996;1:39–43.

57. Semelka RC, Cumming MJ, Shoenut JP, et al. Islet cell tumors: comparison of dynamic contrast-enhanced CT and MR imaging with dynamic gadolinium enhancement and fat suppression. *Radiology.* 1993;186:799–802.

58. Mahfouz AE, Hamm B, Wolf KJ. Peripheral washout: a sign of malignancy on dynamic gadolinium-enhanced MR images of focal liver lesions. *Radiology.* 1994;190:49–52.

59. Semelka RC, Bagley AS, Brown ED, Kroeker MA. Malignant lesions of the liver identified on T1- but not T2-weighted MR images at 1.5 T. *J Magn Reson Imaging.* 1994;4:315–318.

60. Rummeny E, Weissleder R, Stark DD, et al. Primary liver tumors: diagnosis by MR imaging. *AJR.* 1989;152:63–72.

61. Matsui O, Kadoya M, Kameyama T, et al. Adenomatous hyperplastic nodules in the cirrhotic liver: differentiation from hepatocellular carcinoma with MR imaging. *Radiology.* 1989;173:123–126.

62. Rosenthal RE, Davis PL. MR imaging of hepatocellular carcinoma at 1.5 Tesla. *Gastrointest Radiol.* 1992;17:49–52.

63. Hirai K, Aoki Y, Majima Y, et al. Magnetic resonance imaging of small hepatocellular carcinoma. *Am J Gastroenterol.* 1991;86:205–209.
64. Kadoya M, Matsui O, Takashima T, Nonomura A. Hepatocellular carcinoma: correlation of MR imaging and histopathologic findings. *Radiology.* 1992;183:819–825.
65. Muramatsu Y, Nawano S, Takayasu K, et al. Early hepatocellular carcinoma: MR imaging. *Radiology.* 1991;181:209–213.
66. Ebara M, Watanabe S, Kita K, et al. MR imaging of small hepatocellular carcinoma effect of intratumoral copper content on signal intensity. *Radiology.* 1991;180:617–621.
67. Itoh K, Nishimura K, Togashi K, et al. Hepatocellular carcinoma: MR imaging. *Radiology.* 1987;164:21–25.
68. Yamashita Y, Fan ZM, Yamamoto H, et al. Spin-echo and dynamic gadolinium-enhanced FLASH MR imaging of hepatocellular carcinoma: correlation with histopathologic findings. *J Magn Reson Imaging.* 1994;4:83–90.
69. Kelekis NL, Semelka RC, Woosley JT. Malignant lesions of the liver with high signal intensity on T1-weighted MR images. *J Magn Reson Imaging.* 1996;6:291–294.
70. Yoshida H, Itai Y, Ohtomo K, Kokubo T, Minami M, Yashiro N. Small hepatocellular carcinoma and cavernous hemangioma: differentiation with dynamic FLASH MR imaging with Gd-DTPA. *Radiology.* 1989;171:339–342.
71. Mahfouz AE, Hamm B, Wolf KJ. Dynamic gadopentetate dimeglumine-enhanced MR imaging of Hepatocellular Carcinoma. *Eur Radiol.* 1993;3:453–458.
72. Craig JR, Peters RL, Edmondson HA, Omata M. Fibrolamellar carcinoma of the liver: a tumor of adolescents and young adults with distinctive clinco-pathologic features. *Cancer.* 1980;46:373–379.
73. Corrigan K, Semelka RC. Dynamic contrast-enhanced MR imaging of fibrolamellar hepatocellular carcinoma. *Abdom Imaging.* 1995;20:122–125.

19

HEPATIC ANGIOGRAPHY

Donald F. Denny, Jr., M.D.
The Medical Center at Princeton
Princeton, New Jersey

Safe, effective imaging of the hepatic vasculature became possible following the introduction of the catheter replacement system of Seldinger in 1953. The introduction of safer contrast agents, serial film changers, and automatic injectors all served to increase the safety and scope of hepatic angiography. Major advances in catheter and guide-wire technology have further expanded the range of vessels that can be selectively catheterized (1). Torqueable 4- and 5-French catheters are now the usual catheters used. Guide-wire advances include improved torqueability and low friction. Coaxial catheter systems have been developed for superselective vessel catheterization.

More recently, the rapid expansion of noninvasive imaging techniques has made hepatic angiography less important as a primary diagnostic modality. Sonography, computed tomography (CT), nuclear scintigraphy, and magnetic resonance imaging (MRI) are the principal modalities in current practice. Angiography continues to play an important role in the diagnosis and evaluation of a variety of conditions when noninvasive imaging is unable to provide sufficient information for diagnosis or treatment planning (2). Some examples include liver trauma, liver transplantation, primary neoplasms such as hepatocellular carcinoma and hemangioendothelioma, metastatic neoplasms such as endocrine tumors, focal nodular hyperplasia, and hepatic adenoma. Because celiac artery anatomy is highly variable, one of the most important roles of diagnostic hepatic angiography is to provide a road map prior to surgery. This is most often the case for patients undergoing liver transplantation or resection of hepatic neoplasms.

Perhaps more importantly, angiography has developed as an important therapeutic tool. Superselective catheterization has become considerably easier, allowing the interventional radiologist to deliver therapeutic agents via the catheter system while protecting noninvolved vascular beds. These uses include chemotherapy and embolization for neoplasms, and embolotherapy for traumatic injuries such as pseudoaneurysms and arteriovenous fistulas.

In the 1980s, there was an important shift in angiographic imaging technology from film-screen systems to digital subtraction angiography (DSA). With DSA, the image is recorded directly to a computer from the image intensifier; the images are immediately ready for review using television monitors. Because smaller amounts and concentrations of contrast are needed, the examination can be performed more safely and comfortably for the patient. Radiation dose per image is less. A larger number of angiographic runs can be performed in a shorter period of time, giving the radiologist and surgeon more data on which to form a judgment. However, DSA has less fine detail than the traditional film technique. This tradeoff has been shown to be acceptable, and hepatic angiography is now "conventionally" performed using DSA with a selective arterial catheter (3).

Two noninvasive imaging modalities are now challenging angiography by presenting angiography-like images. The first of these is MRI. Using MRI, no catheter or iodinated contrast is needed. Magnetic resonance angiography (MRA) uses the different signal characteristics of flowing blood versus static tissues to produce a series of cross-sectional images, most often in the axial plane. These images can then be reconstructed to show the angiographic perspective from a series of viewing angles. Using a computer work station, three-dimensional images can be created. The surrounding anatomic structures are not visible using the conventional sequences for MRA, and image resolution is limited. Artifacts from turbulent blood flow, vascular motion, breathing, and bowel movement all complicate image interpretation. Magnetic resonance angiography is a developing technique. Substantial progress has been made in recent years in improving the usefulness of MRA. Imaging the vessels of the head and neck, aorta, pelvis, extremities, and heart is very successful. Visceral MRA remains more limited. Computed tomographic angiography (CTA) is a very promising method for displaying the vascular anatomy without the use of a catheter (4). This requires a current-generation helical scanner with specialized software. Computed tomographic angiography uses a bolus of intravenous contrast delivered through an automatic injector; typical rates are 2–4 ml/sec for a volume of 50 to 125 ml, depending on the area being studied. Computed tomographic angiography can display two-dimensional data in any plane, and can show three-dimensional images from multiple perspectives. The image resolution is better than that of MRA, but inferior to DSA. A major advantage of CTA is that the surrounding anatomic structures are also visible, establishing the relationship of the vascular system to its environment. Unlike DSA or MRA, CTA does not allow arteries and veins to be separately studied; other than the rate and volume of contrast, the only other parameter affecting which vessels will be seen is the delay between injection and imaging. For providing a road map of the celiac, mesenteric, and portal systems, CTA may now be the modality of choice.

ANGIOGRAPHIC ANATOMY

The liver, unlike any other viscus, is supplied by two distinct circulations. The portal vein provides 75–80% of blood flow to the liver, with the hepatic artery providing the remaining 20–25%. The proportions are dynamic, for a decrease in either will result in an increase in the other. The portal vein, hepatic artery, and common hepatic duct enter the liver together in the porta hepatis (5). Within the liver, the three branch and travel together, forming the portal triad. The basic unit of the liver substance is the lobule. Surrounding the lobules are the branches of the hepatic artery and portal vein. These penetrate the lobule to empty into the sinusoids, which lie between the hepatocytes. The lobule drains via a central vein that travels to the base of the lobule, eventually joining an hepatic vein.

The hepatic artery most often is a primary branch of the celiac artery, which originates from the anterior border of the aorta at the T12–L1 level. In the standard anatomic description, the celiac artery branches into the splenic artery, left gastric artery, and common hepatic artery (Fig. 1). The common hepatic artery branches into the gastroduodenal artery and the proper hepatic artery. The proper hepatic artery then bifurcates within the porta hepatis into left and right hepatic arteries, which then further subdivide. The anatomy of the celiac artery and its branches is highly variable. This was studied and classified by Michels (6). The two most commonly seen variations are origin of the left hepatic artery from the left gastric artery (gastrohepatic trunk) in 10–12% (Fig. 2), and origin of the right hepatic artery from the superior mesenteric artery in 14% (Fig. 3). This anatomic variability poses a challenge to the angiographer in performing selective studies, to the surgeon in planning operative intervention, and to both in providing arterial chemotherapy. The superior mesenteric artery, which originates from the anterior aorta just below the celiac artery, is an important collateral pathway for the liver. In cases of celiac or common hepatic artery occlusion, flow to the liver is via the inferior to the superior pancreaticoduodenal arteries, to the gastroduodenal artery, to the proper hepatic artery.

Complications of hepatic arterial catheterization are spasm and dissection. The hepatic arteries are prone to vasospasm in response to passage of a guide wire or catheter. This is aggravated by the forces involved in passing guide wire and catheter through the often tortuous anatomy. In some cases, localized hepatic infarction occurs secondarily to arterial injury during catheterization (7). Small vessel coaxial systems are the best method of achieving superselective catheter placement.

Portal vein anatomy is quite constant. The portal vein forms from the junction of the superior mesenteric and splenic veins (Fig. 4). Angiographic study of the portal vein can be performed by several routes. Arterial portography is performed by intraarterial injection of a vasodilator such as tolazoline (25–50 mg) followed by a long contrast bolus into the celiac or superior mesenteric artery with delayed filming. This is the least invasive and most common route. It provides excellent visualization of the portal, splenic, and superior mesenteric veins, and varices in the case of portal hypertension. Arterial portography has replaced direct injection of the spleen for portography (splenic portography). Transhepatic portography is more invasive, improves vein opacification, and permits selective venography and venous sampling of portal, splenic, and mesenteric branches (Fig. 4). It is used most often for selective pancreatic vein sampling for localization of small pancreatic endocrine tumors. Complications of the transhepatic approach include bleeding at the hepatic puncture site, hemobilia, septicemia, and bile peritonitis. The patient should have normal or near-normal coagulation indices and be pretreated with intravenous antibiotics. A pledget of Gelfoam is frequently injected into the transhepatic track at the time the catheter is removed to assist in hemostasis.

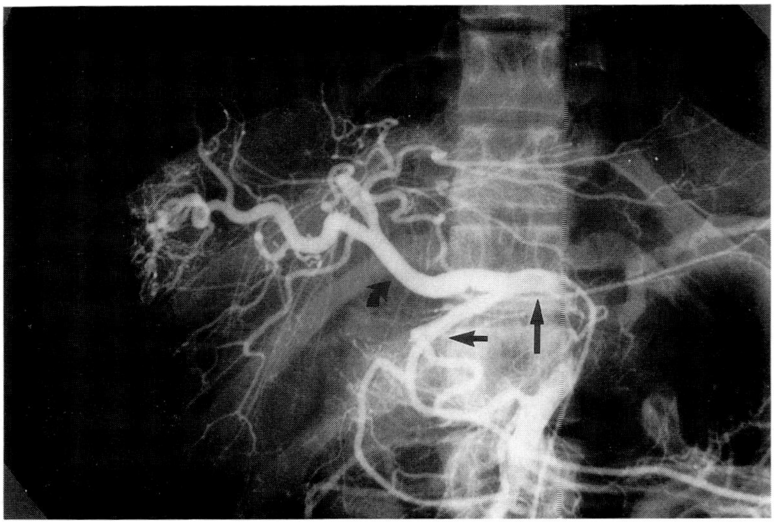

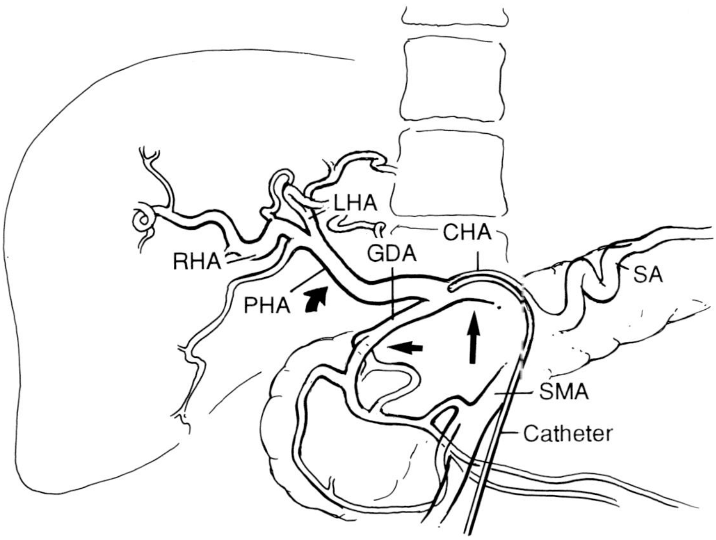

Figure 1. "Normal" hepatic artery anatomy shows the common hepatic artery (long arrow), gastroduodenal artery (short arrow), and proper hepatic artery (curved arrow). The proper hepatic artery bifurcates into left and right hepatic arteries.

Hepatic vein catheterization can be performed from a cranial or caudal approach. There are three principal hepatic veins: right, middle, and left. These join the inferior vena cava in the groove behind the liver, near the diaphragm: the veins course obliquely and caudally. Hepatic vein catheterization is performed for venography and pressure measurements in patients with cirrhosis (Fig. 5). The hepatic vein route is also used for liver biopsy in patients in whom standard percutaneous biopsy is contraindicated owing to coagulopathy or ascites (8).

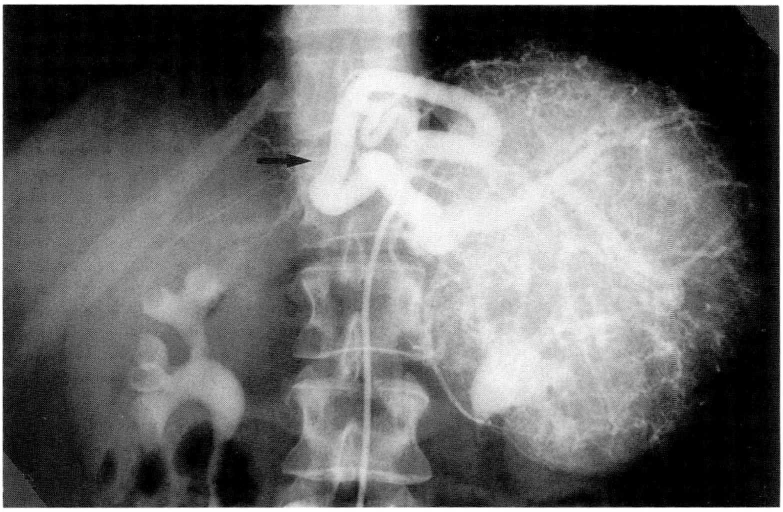

Figure 2. Left gastrohepatic artery. Large hypervascular hepatic mass in the left lobe with disordered tumor vascularity supplied by a hypertrophied left hepatic artery (arrow) originating from the left gastric artery. This mass was pathologically focal nodular hyperplasia.

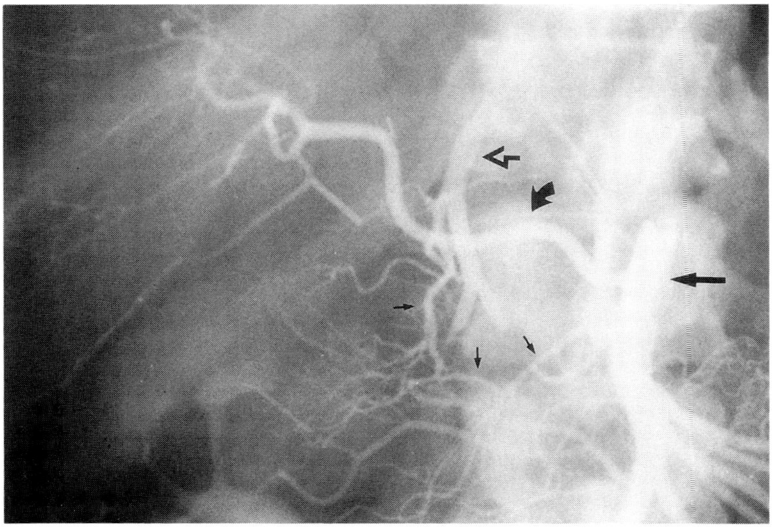

Figure 3. Replaced right hepatic artery. The right hepatic artery (curved arrow) originates from the superior mesenteric artery (straight arrow). Also seen is the gastroduodenal artery (open arrow) filling retrograde from the pancreaticoduodenal arcades (small arrows).

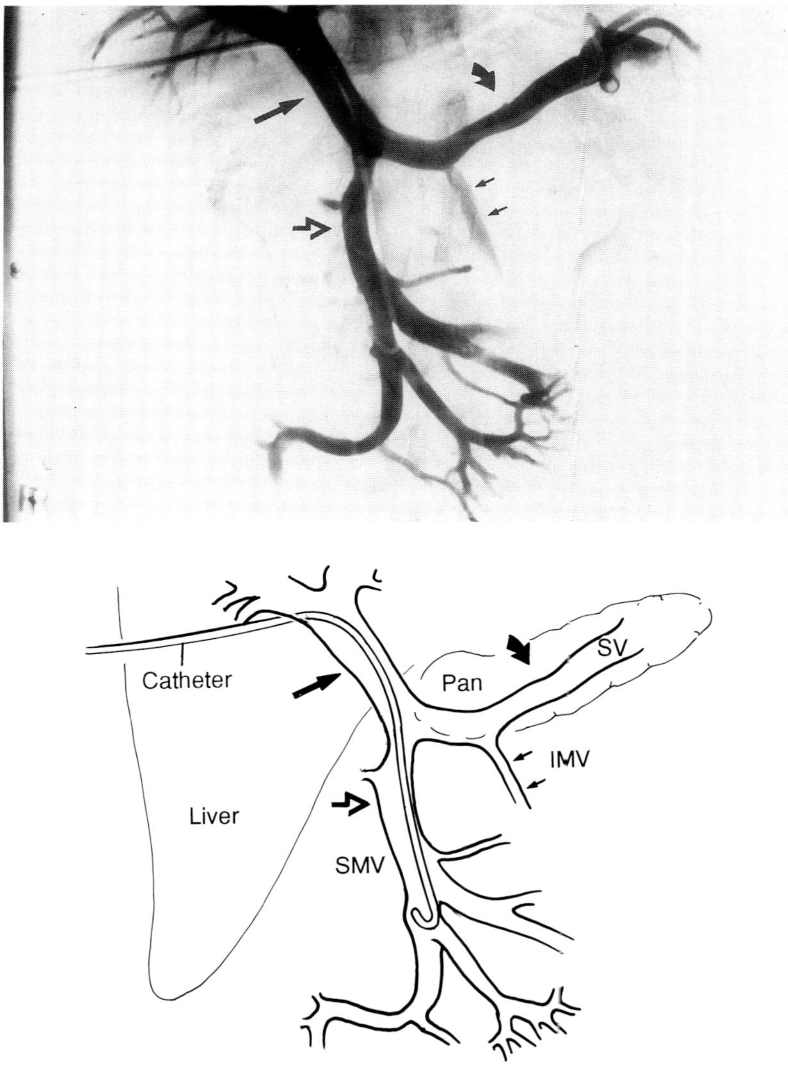

Figure 4. Portal venous system. A composite subtraction portal venogram performed by transhepatic portal vein catheterization shows the main portal vein (arrow), superior mesenteric vein (open arrow), splenic vein (curved arrow), and inferior mesenteric vein (small arrows).

NEOPLASMS

Primary and metastatic neoplasms of the liver are supplied primarily by the hepatic artery. Angiography plays a greater or lesser role in diagnosis depending on the specificity of noninvasive imaging studies and the vascularity of the neoplasm. Neovascularity has several angiographic characteristics that are present depending on the tumor type (Fig. 6). Tumor vessels are disorganized or chaotic within the tumor. Their size varies in an irregular fashion rather than in the normal pattern

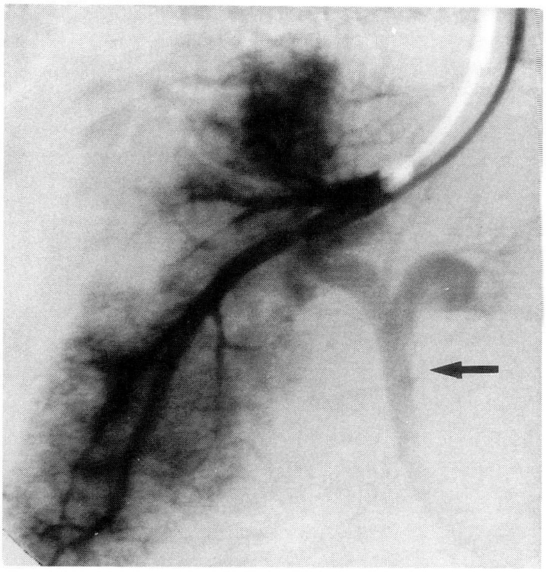

Figure 5. Hepatic venogram. Injection of the right hepatic vein using a balloon occlusion catheter shows parenchymal blush. This wedged injection also shows the right, left, and main (arrow) portal veins.

of larger to smaller vessels. This irregular size results from abnormal vessel growth or encasement by the neoplasm. Hypervascular tumors show an increased number and size of vessels within the mass. In addition, the artery supplying the neoplasm may be enlarged to compensate for the increased flow. Arteriovenous fistulas are seen with some neoplasms, particularly hepatocellular carcinoma. Vessels within a neoplasm often occlude abruptly. Normal vessels or tumor vessels on the periphery of the mass are displaced by it, resulting in a curved path not typical of normal arteries. The angiographic detection of hypovascular tumors is more difficult, because many of the findings of neovascularity are subtle or absent. In hypervascular tumors, the parenchymal phase of the arteriogram shows a "blush" corresponding to the neoplasm. Conversely, in hypovascular tumors such as colon carcinoma there is a hypoperfused area that fails to enhance to the same degree as normal tissue.

Intraarterial infusion of chemotherapy has been used in many clinical trials as a method of selectively increasing the concentration of agent within the hepatic mass, while maintaining a lower systemic concentration. More recently, chemoembolization has been used for hypervascular primary liver tumors such as hepatocellular carcinoma (HCC), and for hypervascular metastases such as endocrine tumors (for example, carcinoid) and ocular melanoma (9, 10). In chemoembolization, the combination of chemotherapeutic agent plus arterial embolization agent such as oily contrast (Lipiodol) and particles (for example, gelatin sponge, microfibrillar collagen) act to prolong the high tumor concentration of the drug while minimizing systemic concentration, and to make the tumor ischemic by direct arterial blockade.

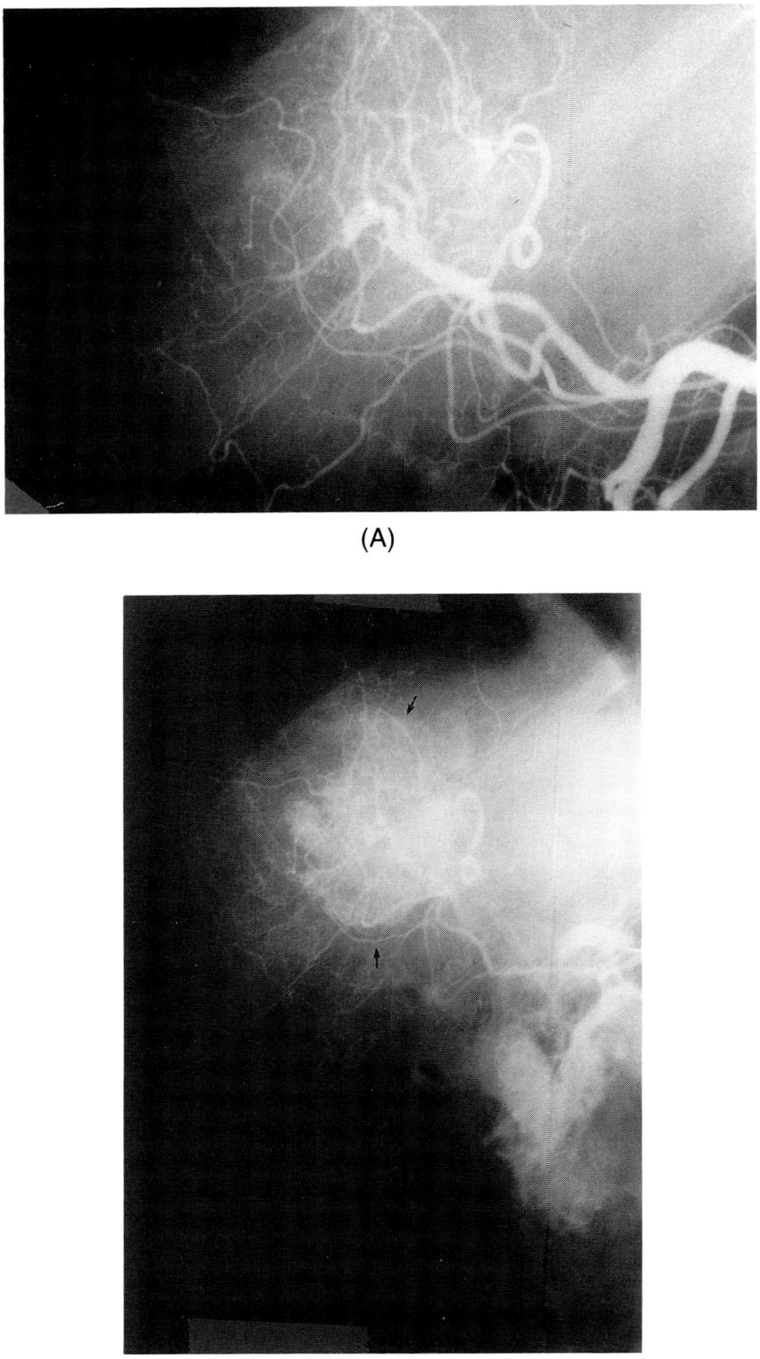

(A)

(B)

Figure 6. Hepatocellular carcinoma. (A) Irregular tumor vessels in a disorganized distribution within the mass in the right hepatic lobe. Note irregular vessel margins at multiple sites within the tumor. (B) Parenchymal phase shows tumor blush. Vessels on the periphery of the tumor are stretched and displaced around it (small arrows).

At one time, percutaneous temporary placement of an hepatic artery catheter was frequently performed for local infusion of chemotherapy. This is now more often performed surgically, using a subcutaneous infusion pump.

Hepatocellular Carcinoma

Hepatocellular carcinoma (HCC) is relatively uncommon in the United States, but is the most common cancer found in some parts of the world. It affects 1.25 million people worldwide, annually. In the United States, HCC is associated with cirrhosis in 50–80% of patients, most often alcoholic cirrhosis. Of cirrhotic patients in the United States, 5% eventually develop HCC. Worldwide, hepatitis appears to be the most common cause of HCC. Hepatocellular carcinoma is an intensely hypervascular tumor that shows disordered, chaotic tumor arteries with irregular borders (Fig. 6). Hepatic artery to portal venous shunting is common, as is tumor invasion into the portal venous system. Portal vein thrombosis may result. The hepatic arteries are displaced by the tumor mass, which is irregular and may be multifocal. The capillary phase of the angiogram shows a marked tumor blush. There may be small vascular lakes seen during the parenchymal phase.

Hepatocellular carcinoma derives its blood flow principally from the hepatic artery rather than the portal vein. The hepatic artery may be hypertrophied as a result. Portal vein studies may show only displacement of veins unless tumor invasion has occurred, in which case tumor thrombi will be seen. When angiography was the primary diagnostic modality for these tumors, intraarterial injection of a vasoconstrictor such as epinephrine (5–10 μg) was often used in difficult cases; the vasoconstrictor acts selectively on normal arterial branches, allowing easier visualization of tumor vessels. In current practice, HCC will already be suspected based on ultrasound and CT. Angiography may be done to provide additional support for the diagnosis and to provide a surgical road map for patients considered candidates for resection or transplant. More recently, angiography for HCC is being done for therapy. In the past 5 years, chemoembolization has become an important part of management for these patients (11, 12). A variety of chemotherapeutic agents are being used in combination with oily contrast (Lipiodol) and a particulate agent such as gelatin sponge (Gelfoam).

Colon Cancer

Colorectal carcinoma affects 155,000 new patients annually in the United States. Hepatic metastasis occurs in 50%, and the median survival after hepatic metastasis is only 6 months. The liver metastases are usually hypovascular by angiography. Angiography shows irregular, displaced vessels and peripheral enhancement (Fig. 7). Arteriovenous shunting is not seen. The tumors are easily seen by CT or sonography before becoming evident on angiography.

Chemoembolization protocols are in use for colorectal hepatic metastasis, but the efficacy of this technique is yet to be determined (9). This is reserved for patients who fail systemic chemotherapy and whose hepatic disease is considered unresectable. Hepatic metastases respond to systemic chemotherapy in 10–21% of patients. Regional chemotherapy using a surgically placed hepatic artery catheter and infusion pump increases the response of the tumor to chemotherapy in prospec-

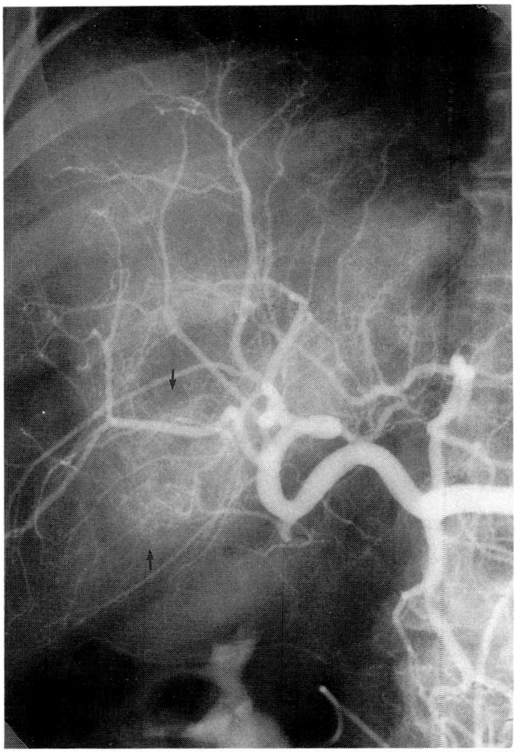

(A)

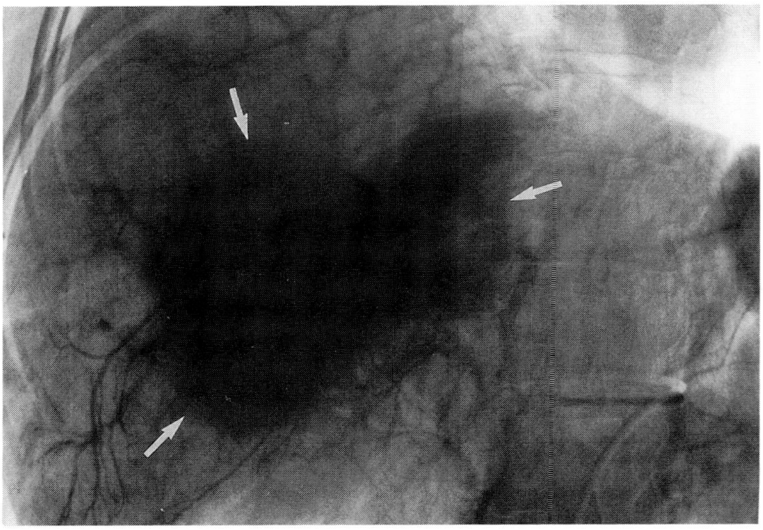

(B)

Figure 7. Colon carcinoma metastases. (A) Common hepatic arteriogram shows a minimally hypervascular mass (small arrows). (B) Parenchymal phase shows more extensive tumor blush than could be recognized on earlier phase.

tive randomized trials to 42–68%. However, these studies show no significant difference in survival rate between systemic and regional therapy. This lack of benefit is probably due to the high complication rate of regional therapy, including local toxicity (ulcer, biliary sclerosis), catheter-related complications, and biliary toxicity. To date, only limited series of patients treated with chemoembolization have been reported, none randomized. Lorenz reported responses in four of 11 patients treated using degradable starch microspheres and mitomycin-C (13). Civalleri reported five complete, five partial responses, and six patients with stable disease in 23 patients who received three or more cycles of treatment using mitomycin-C and starch microspheres via hepatic artery and portal vein (14). Sixteen of 39 patients were unable to receive therapy or had early interruption due to catheter-related problems. The median time to progression was 6 months, and the median length of survival was 16 months. Kameyama et al. compared the vascularity of the colorectal metastasis to the response to treatment using Lipiodol and cis-platinum (15). Treatment was effective in eight of 16 tumors judged hypervascular by Xenon 133 washout, but in only one of six judged hypovascular ($p < .05$). A large number of institutions are actively performing chemoembolization protocols for colorectal carcinoma.

Neuroendocrine Tumors

Like the primary tumor, metastatic neuroendocrine tumors are usually hypervascular, which assists in angiographic diagnosis and intervention. Although angiography occasionally identifies a small tumor deposit, diagnosis is most often made by noninvasive imaging methods. Angiographic characteristics are not specific. Displaced, irregular, enlarged feeding arteries are present. On parenchymal phase, there is a distinct nodular tumor blush. Arteriovenous shunting is not seen. Chemoembolization protocols may play a role.

TRAUMA

Although in the early 1970s hepatic angiography played a primary role in the evaluation of patients with suspected hepatic trauma, sonography and CT have supplanted angiography in current practice. Standard trauma protocols call for CT in the immediate evaluation of patients with abdominal trauma, either blunt or penetrating. Acute angiography is reserved for patients with diagnosed injury and hemodynamic instability despite resuscitation, owing to continuing hemorrhage from the hepatic injury. In this setting, angiography should be both diagnostic and therapeutic. Most patients with hepatic lacerations and blunt trauma do well without surgical or radiological intervention. Delayed angiography is indicated in patients with evidence of continuing signs and symptoms of vascular injury such as hemobilia or expanding subcapsular hematoma.

The principal vascular injuries seen at angiography are pseudoaneurysm (Fig. 8), arteriovenous fistula, and arteriobiliary fistula (16). Angiographic findings of liver contusion are elongation and straightening of arterial branches, delay in flow, and occasionally focal accumulation of contrast in affected segments. In liver laceration, findings include abrupt occlusion of arterial branches, contrast extravasation and pseudoaneurysm formation, arteriovenous fistula, and arteriobiliary fistula. In

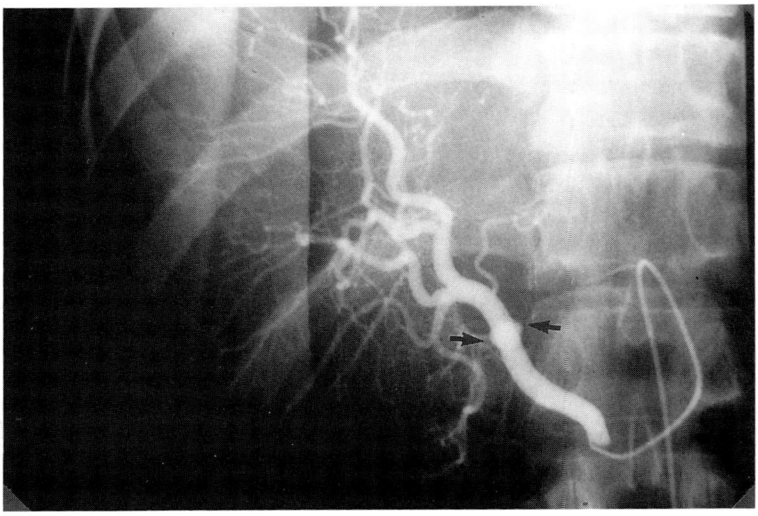

(A)

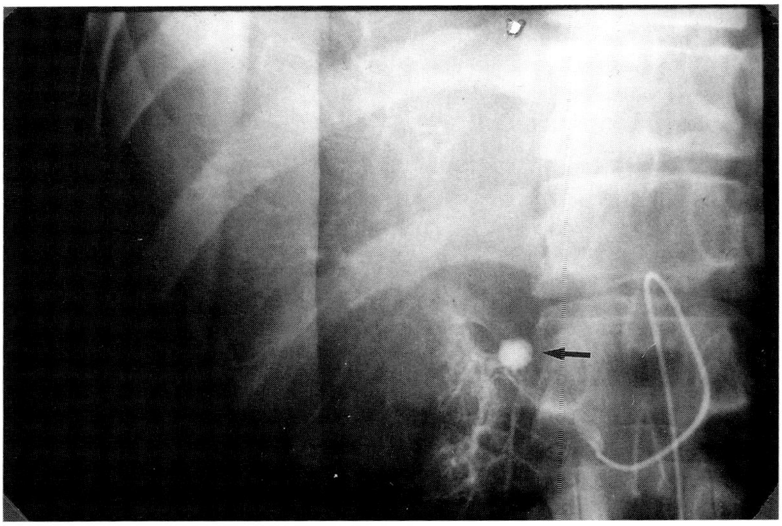

(B)

Figure 8. Pseudoaneurysm of a replaced right hepatic artery. (A) Pseudoaneurysm (arrows) is superimposed over the right hepatic artery. (B) After arterial washout, the pseudoaneurysm is more apparent (arrow). (C) Superior mesenteric arteriogram shows successful occlusion following embolization using two detachable balloons (arrows) bridging the pseudoaneurysm (next page).

subcapsular and intrahepatic hematoma, vessels are stretched around the avascular hematoma, whereas there may be focal areas of contrast extravasation at the interface between liver and hematoma. Subcapsular hematoma is readily recognized on arteriograms, but the precise vessel(s) responsible cannot usually be determined.

Vascular hepatic injury is frequently accompanied by biliary injury, with resultant

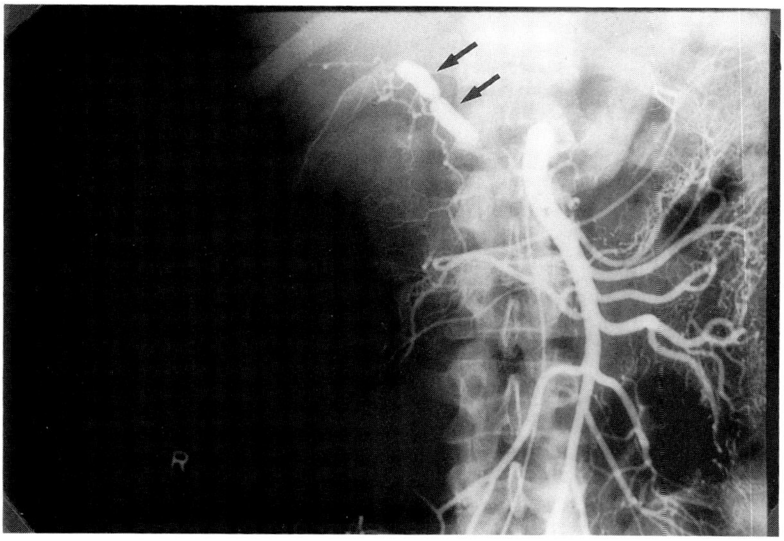

(C)

Figure 8. *(Continued)*

biloma. This presents as an avascular mass that on angiography may mimic a hematoma. Hepatobiliary radionuclide scanning demonstrates extravasation in cases of biloma.

Embolization of arterial injuries such as pseudoaneurysm, arteriovenous fistula, and arteriobiliary fistula is very successful and should be the initial intervention if conservative management is unsuccessful (17–19) (Fig. 8). Superselective catheterization is performed to provide specific intervention at the site of injury. Particulate agents such as gelatin sponge (Gelfoam), polyvinyl alcohol (Ivalon), and stainless steel embolization coils (Gianturco coils) are the ones most commonly used for embolotherapy of trauma. In this age of aggressive medical intervention, penetrating trauma sometimes occurs with iatrogenic procedures such as routine liver biopsy. This is treated expectantly, but may require angiographic intervention and management in the cases of persistent signs and symptoms (20).

FOCAL NODULAR HYPERPLASIA

Focal nodular hyperplasia (FNH) is a benign tumor of the liver of uncertain pathogenesis. 86% of patients are women, with a mean age of 35–39 years, but FNH has been reported in both pediatric and elderly patients. Patients often present with vague abdominal complaints. Typically solitary, the tumor is classically a white, hard, well-circumscribed mass composed of a central scar with radiating fibrous bands; between the bands normal-appearing hepatic tissue is interspersed. Kupffer cells are usually present. The radiographic appearance has been described by Rogers et al. (21) and Welch et al. (22). The mass is initially found at ultrasound or CT.

Technetium sulfur colloid scan can often provide a specific diagnosis, because more than 50% of FNH will show normal activity, unlike other liver tumors which normally show no activity. If scintigraphy and other noninvasive methods are equivocal, angiography should be performed. Classic angiographic findings are a hypervascular tumor with a dense parenchymal blush (16). The feeding artery penetrates to the center of the mass, then sends branches to the periphery in a spoke-like arrangement (Fig. 9). The artery supplying the mass is often enlarged. Arteriovenous shunting is not seen. Rogers et al. (21) reported characteristic angiographic findings in nine (82%) of 11 patients. Welch et al. (22) reported angiography in 18 patients with biopsy-proved FNH. Sixteen (89%) were hypervascular; hypertrophy of the feeding artery was seen in 11 (61%) (Fig. 2); capillary staining was intense in 16 (89%) and faintly increased in two (11%). Blood supply was central in four (22%), peripheral in eight (44%), and indeterminate in six (33%).

FNH is a benign condition that requires no treatment. However, in the absence of specific imaging findings, it may be difficult to distinguish from other conditions that require intervention, such as hepatic adenoma.

HEPATIC ADENOMA

Like FNH, hepatic adenoma occurs predominantly in women, with a mean age in the mid-thirties. Adenomas are associated with oral birth control pills in the majority of cases and are usually solitary. The tumor is composed of hepatocytes without Kupffer cells. As a result, it fails to take up technetium sulfur colloid, in contrast to FNH. Although this is a benign tumor, adenomas frequently contain areas of necrosis and hemorrhage. Computed tomography showed areas of acute hemorrhage within the tumor on noncontrast scans in five of 50 patients reported by Mathieu et al. (23). Patients commonly present with abdominal pain, although more vague symptoms of upper abdominal distress are also common. Intraabdominal hemorrhage can occur and the tumor has malignant potential. For these reasons, adenomas are commonly resected.

Angiographic findings vary. Most tumors are hypervascular with irregular areas of hypovascularity. Arteriovenous shunting is not seen. In the series of 13 cases reported by Welch et al. (22), nine were studied by angiography. The feeding artery was enlarged in four (44%). Three lesions (33%) had intense capillary staining but six (66%) did not. Blood supply was peripheral in six (66%) and indeterminate in three (33%).

The noninvasive differentiation of hepatic adenoma and FNH continues to challenge the physician. Progression of adenomas after discontinuing oral contraceptives was reported by Marks et al. in three cases (24); each of these cases had concurrent FNH and uterine leiomyomas. Although this would appear to be a rare event, another case of concurrent FNH and hepatic adenoma was reported by Friedman et al. (25).

VASCULAR LESIONS

A variety of primary vascular lesions affect the liver, the most common being hepatic cavernous hemangioma. These are composed of dilated, endothelial-lined

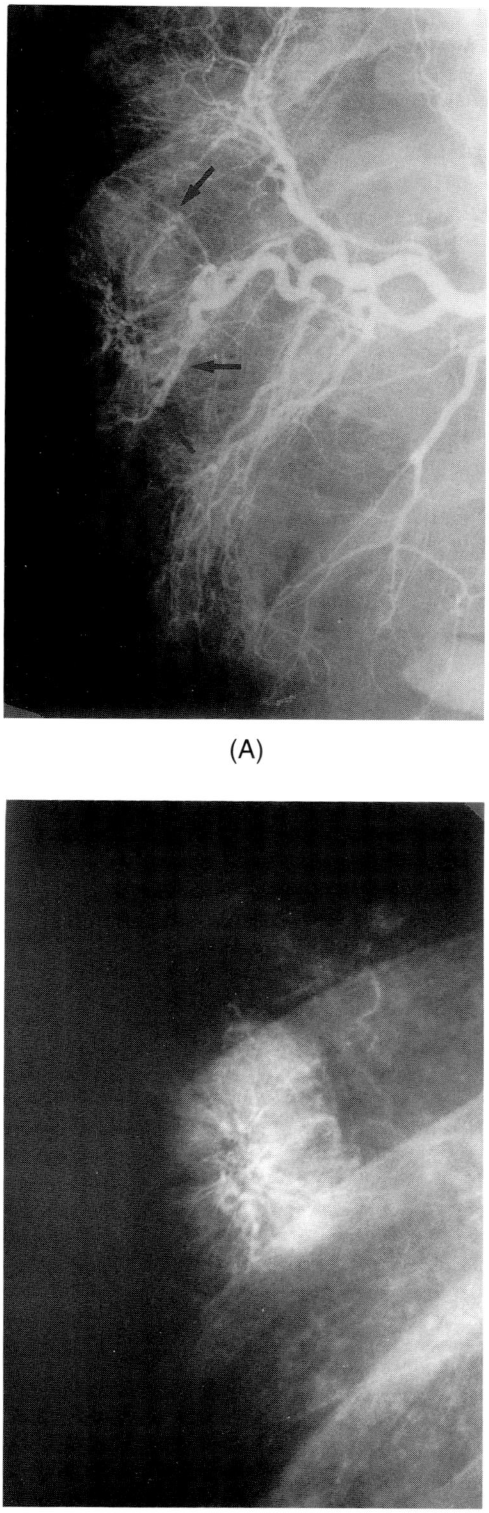

(A)

(B)

Figure 9. Focal nodular hyperplasia. (A) Arterial phase shows a mass displacing peripheral vessels (small arrows) with centrally radiating arteries. (B) Parenchymal phase shows radiating arteries and tumor blush.

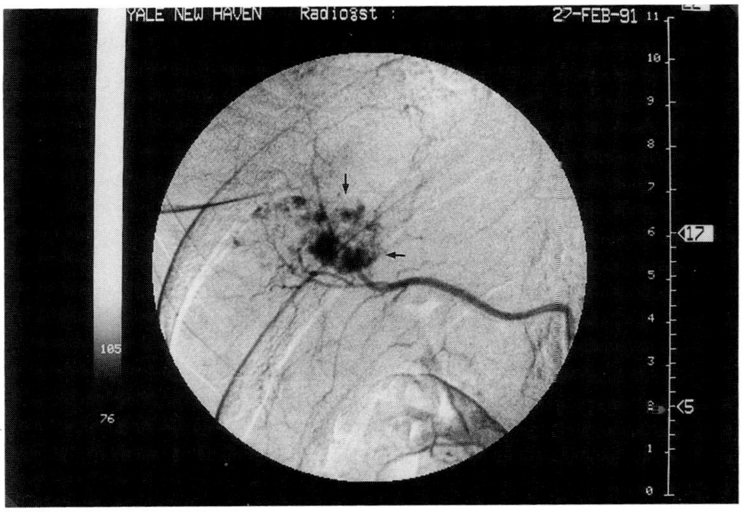

Figure 10. Hepatic hemangioma. Injection of an accessory right hepatic artery originating from the superior mesenteric artery shows the characteristic vascular puddling of a hemangioma (arrows).

spaces with very slow flow. They are single or multiple, and are usually less than 3 cm in size. Hemangioma is most often an incidental finding and does not cause clinical symptoms. The sonographic and CT appearances are both characteristic; if the results of these tests are equivocal, technetium-tagged red blood cell scan shows characteristic pooling. Incidental hemangiomas are frequently found at angiography (Fig. 10). The vascular spaces fill quite late, and persistence of contrast is seen well into the venous phase. Arteriovenous shunting is absent. Angiography plays little direct role, because the diagnosis is usually apparent on noninvasive tests (26).

Hereditary hemorrhagic telangiectasia (HHT) is an uncommon autosomal recessive disorder characterized by arteriovenous fistulas and telangiectasias of the brain, lungs, and gastrointestinal tract. Hepatic involvement was thought to be rare, but Bernard recently reported the findings in 11 such patients (27). Angiography showed hepatic artery enlargement in eight, disseminated intrahepatic telangiectasias in 10, and early hepatic vein opacification in seven. Hemodynamic studies performed in five patients showed a left-to-right intrahepatic shunt of 25 to 58% of cardiac output.

Hepatic artery aneurysms are infrequent and account for 19% of all splanchnic aneurysms (28). They are fusiform or saccular. 80% involve the extrahepatic artery, including 96% of those related to atherosclerosis. Because the lumen may be partially thrombosed, angiography can be falsely normal. Noninvasive tests such as ultrasound and CT may be more reliable in diagnosing this infrequent problem. Angiography, however, is needed to provide precise anatomic localization, and allows definitive therapy using embolization (29).

Budd–Chiari syndrome results from thrombosis of the hepatic veins or obstruction of the suprahepatic IVC. In most patients in the United States, thrombosis results from a hypercoagulable syndrome such as antiphospholipid antibody syndrome (30, 31). In its acute form, Budd–Chiari syndrome presents as fulminant

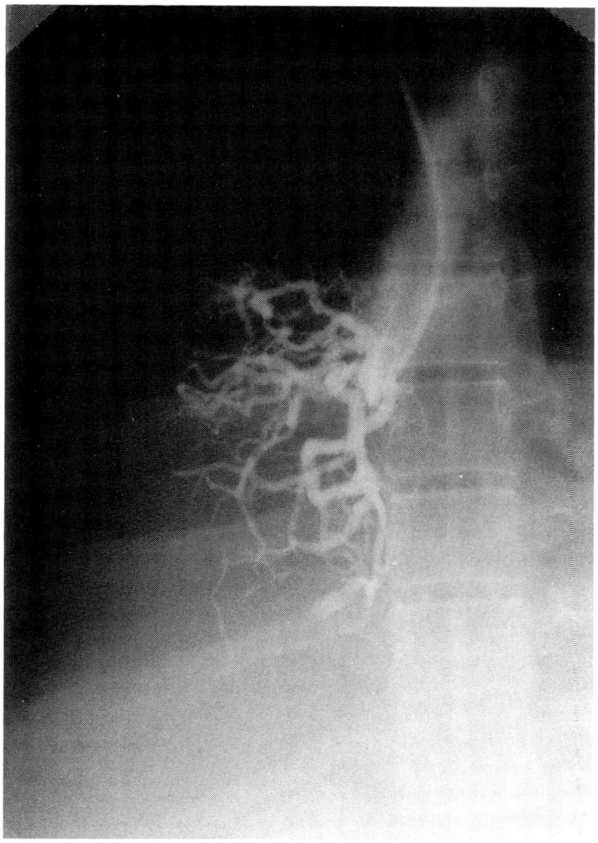

Figure 11. Budd–Chiari syndrome. Hepatic venography shows irregular, small hepatic veins. The main hepatic veins are occluded.

hepatic failure, portal hypertension, and ascites. In its less severe chronic form, the development of hepatic dysfunction is more insidious. Duplex sonography has become the initial tool for evaluating the status of the hepatic veins and inferior vena cava (IVC). Angiography continues to play a pivotal role in diagnosis and patient management. Webs of the suprahepatic IVC are associated with the chronic form of Budd–Chiari syndrome. Angioplasty and stent placement have been useful in these circumstances. Thrombolysis of the thrombosed veins has been reported, but because the process is usually subacute or chronic, this is of limited benefit. The usual treatment is surgical decompression by portal system to systemic vein bypass using porta-caval, meso-caval, or meso-atrial shunts. Hepatic venography in Budd–Chiari syndrome shows small, spiderlike, irregular veins, resulting from irregular recanalization of thrombosed veins (Fig. 11). At times, it will be impossible to catheterize the hepatic veins because of the thrombosis. Venography of the IVC may show webs. The intrahepatic segment of the IVC can be compressed by the caudate lobe, which is often enlarged in this condition.

HEPATIC TRANSPLANTATION

Hepatic angiography continues to play an important role in liver transplantation. As a preoperative test, angiography is able to map the celiac and mesenteric arteries, evaluate portal vein patency, flow direction, and size, and evaluate the inferior vena cava for patency and size (32–34). However, in recent years, duplex sonography has been very successful in performing many of these functions, and is sufficient in most patients. Taylor et al. reported successful ultrasound in 20 liver transplant candidates (35). Preoperative findings included tumors, portal vein occlusion, varices, biliary obstruction, and variant vascular anatomy. If there is any doubt after preoperative noninvasive evaluation, angiography should be done. Computed tomographic angiography is an effective alternative to angiography (36).

Angiography also plays an important role in the evaluation of the patient following hepatic transplant, but duplex sonography has replaced angiography as the primary method for post operative screening (37). Angiography is performed to evaluate portal vein and hepatic artery patency in cases of suspected thrombosis, and to diagnose aneurysms, pseudoaneurysms, and anastomotic strictures. Angiography is also performed for other suspected vascular abnormalities such as arteriovenous fistulas following liver biopsy, and can be therapeutic in such cases.

The arteriographic findings in transplant rejection include stretching, pruning, and narrowing of the hepatic artery branches and slow arterial flow (38) (Fig. 12). Although liver biopsy is the usual method for detecting rejection, it is important to recognize the arteriographic findings. White et al. retrospectively analyzed the arteriograms of 35 patients with rejection documented by biopsy (39). The hepatic arteriogram was abnormal in 30 (86%), including 11 with hepatic artery thrombosis. Intrahepatic branch vessel stenoses and occlusions were seen in four.

Splenic artery aneurysms occur in up to 10% of patients with cirrhosis and portal hypertension. Ayalon reported six splenic aneurysms in 71 patients receiving liver transplants (40). Five asymptomatic aneurysms were diagnosed by preoperative angiography, and one developed 3 months postoperatively. One patient experienced rupture 11 days post transplant. Splenic artery aneurysms in this group of patients usually occur in the distal third of the splenic artery or within the spleen and can be multiple. Their development appears to be related to the high splenic artery flow rate seen in patients with cirrhosis and portal hypertension. Larson reported two liver transplant patients with spontaneous development and regression of visceral aneurysms (41).

Visceral artery pseudoaneurysms following transplant occur at the sites of vascular anastomosis or at other sites. In 15 patients with pseudoaneurysms following organ transplant reported by Tobben et al., eight were at arterial anastomoses, and seven were nonanastomotic (42). Three of the eight anastomotic pseudoaneurysms were caused by infection. Of the seven nonanastomotic pseudoaneurysms, two were caused by infection and four by percutaneous biopsy. In this series, CT diagnosed pseudoaneurysm in 67% and sonography in 50%. Angiography visualized the abnormality in all cases, including three liver transplant patients with gastrointestinal bleeding in whom angiography was the only modality that detected the pseudoaneurysms.

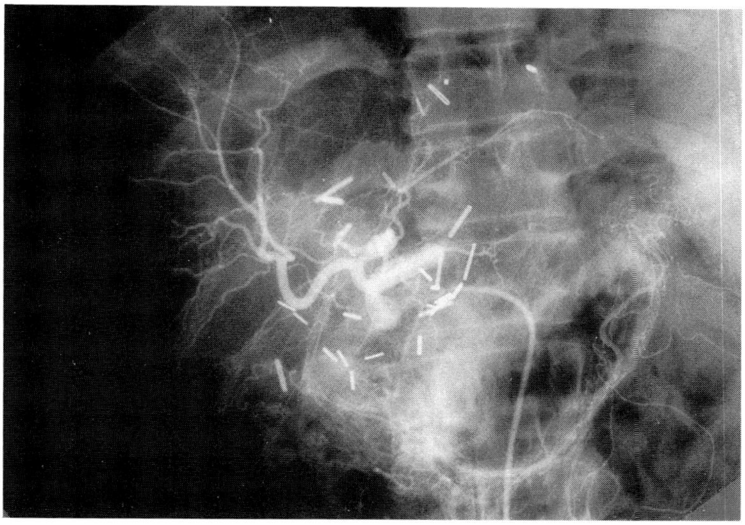

(A)

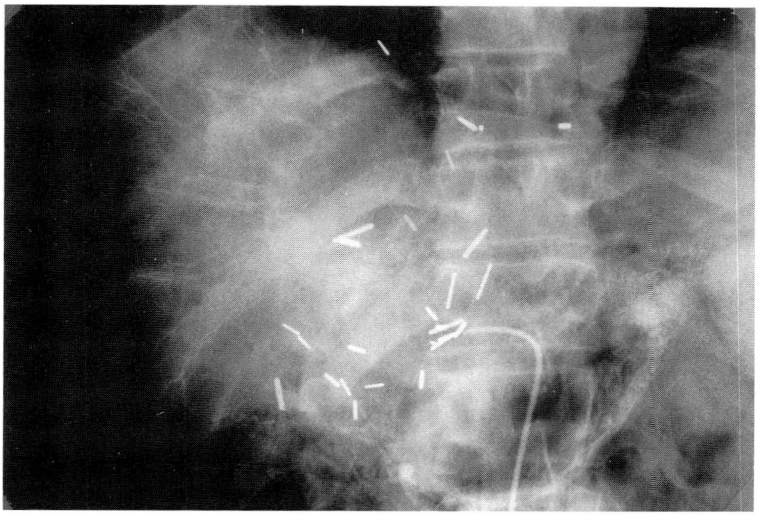

(B)

Figure 12. Transplant rejection. (A) Hepatic arteriogram shows severe pruning of the intrahepatic arteries. (B) Parenchymal phase shows late opacification of the hepatic arteries indicating slow flow.

PORTAL HYPERTENSION

Catheterization of the hepatic veins is performed in cirrhotic patients for venography and measurement of the free and wedged hepatic vein pressure (HVP) (43). A corrected wedged HVP (corrected sinusoidal pressure) is calculated by subtracting

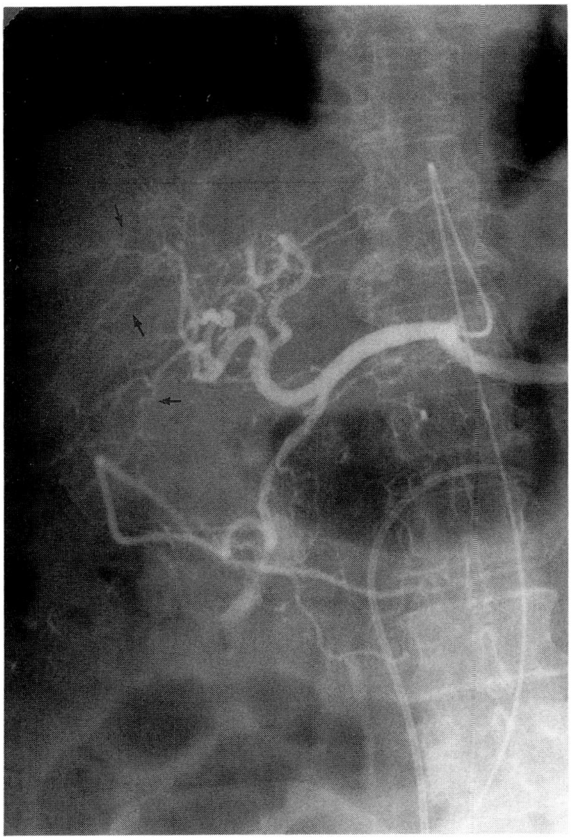

Figure 13. Cirrhosis. Hepatic arteriogram shows a small liver with tortuous "corkscrew" intrahepatic arteries (small arrows).

the IVC pressure at the level of the renal veins from the wedged HVP. The effect of beta blockers and other drugs in lowering wedged HVP has been measured in this way. The normal corrected HVP is less than 5 mm Hg.

Angiographic evaluation of patients is indicated prior to portal-systemic shunting (44). The evaluation includes celiac and mesenteric artery injections to diagnose anatomic variations, and arterial portography to assess the size of the portal vein and direction of flow within the mesenteric, splenic, and portal veins. If a distal spleno-renal shunt is contemplated, the left renal vein is studied. The free and wedged hepatic vein pressures are measured. In addition, the pressures in the low and high IVC and right atrium are measured to rule out a significant gradient that might affect shunt function. Hepatic arteriography in cirrhosis shows tortuous "corkscrew" intrahepatic arteries in a small liver (Fig. 13).

Following shunting, angiography is used to evaluate suspected shunt malfunction. Ultrasound is the primary screening method to evaluate the shunt, but depending on the anatomy, ultrasound may be unsuccessful in shunt visualization.

Splenic artery aneurysms occur in 10% of patients with portal hypertension and

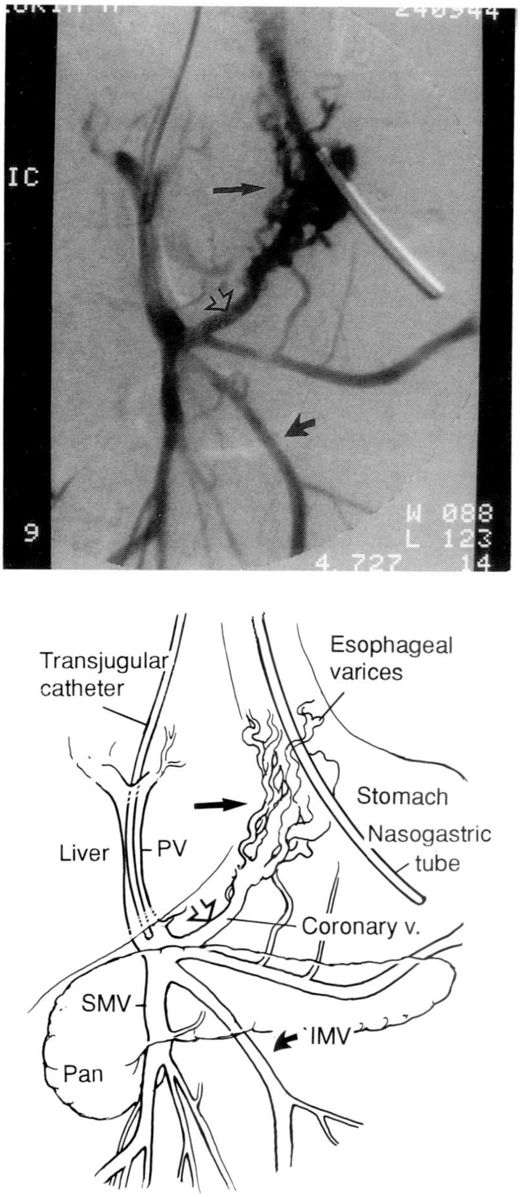

(A)

Figure 14. Transjugular intrahepatic portal systemic shunt. (A) Transjugular catheter entering the portal vein shows a dilated left coronary vein and esophageal varices (arrow). The inferior mesenteric vein fills, indicating hepatofugal flow (curved arrow). (B) A stent has been placed from the right hepatic vein to the right portal vein through the parenchymal track (next page). (C) Mesenteric venogram through the jugular catheter opacifies the mesenteric, portal, and hepatic veins. Because the portal system is decompressed, the esophageal varices no longer fill.

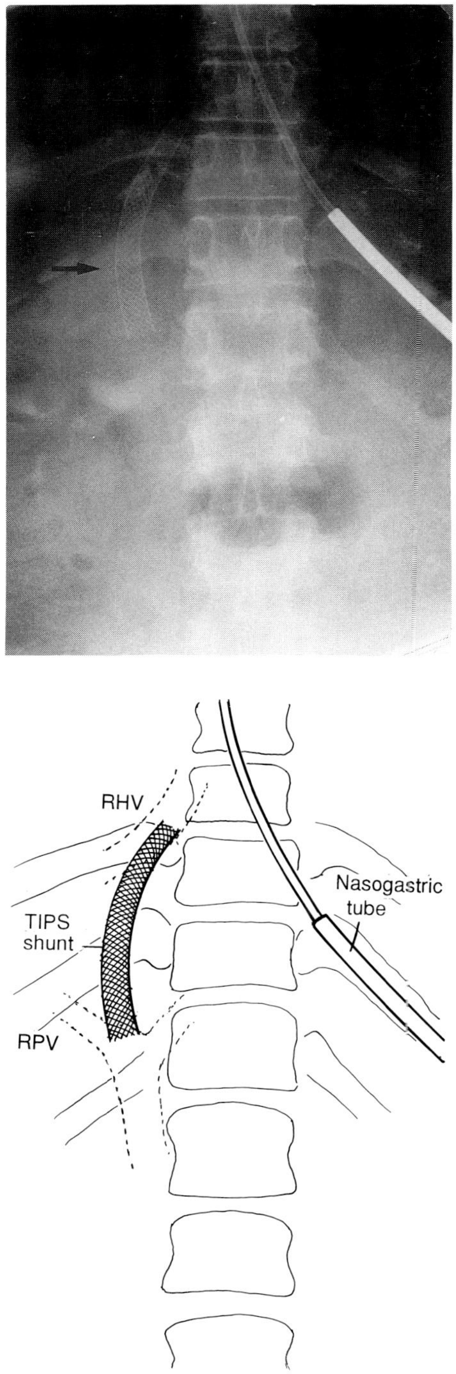

(B)

Figure 14. *(Continued)*

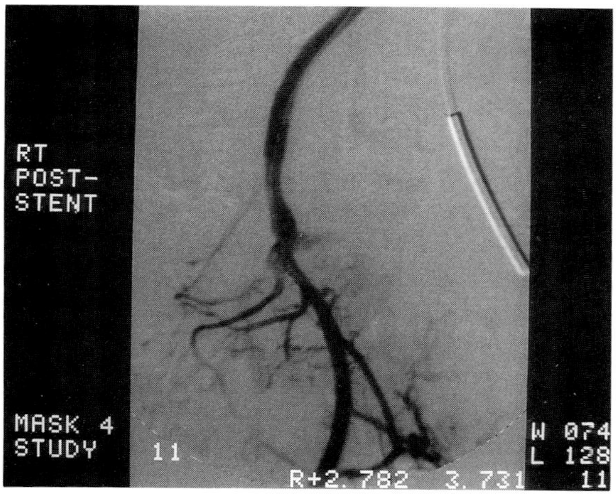

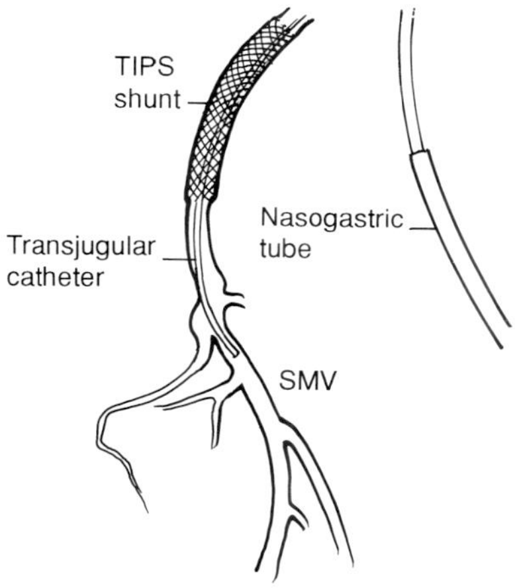

(C)

Figure 14. *(Continued)*

are thought to result from increased flow in the splenic artery (45). These are fusiform or saccular, single or multiple, and occur in the distal splenic artery or in intrasplenic branches.

Recently, transjugular intrahepatic portal vein catheterization has been used for percutaneous creation of a portal vein to hepatic vein shunt (TIPS) for the treatment of portal hypertension and variceal hemorrhage (46). In this approach, a curved needle and cannula are advanced from the jugular vein to the IVC, into a hepatic vein, through the liver parenchyma, and into the right or left portal vein. The liver parenchymal track is dilated and a metal stent is placed to maintain the track (Fig. 14). The current indications for TIPS are for the control of acute variceal hemorrhage in patients refractory to medical therapy, and as a bridge to hepatic transplant in patients with end-stage liver disease and variceal hemorrhage. The procedure is highly successful for control of hemorrhage. Similar to surgical shunts, new encephalopathy following the procedure is seen in 10–30% of patients but is usually well-controlled medically.

The principal procedural complications of TIPS are hemorrhagic. In the report of a prospective multi-center trial of 96 patients, Coldwell et al. reported inadvertent puncture of the liver capsule during passage of the cannula in 3%; although this should be self-limited if recognized early, one patient died (47). Catastrophic consequences follow accidental creation of a shunt between the hepatic vein and an extrahepatic part of the portal vein. Hemobilia can occur, but its incidence is impossible to determine because most of the patients are being treated for variceal hemorrhage and have guaiac-positive stools already. The principal delayed complication of TIPS is shunt closure. One-year primary patency rates are reported as 50–70%, with a primary assisted rate of 85% following correction by angioplasty and restenting. Because of this, the role of TIPS in long-term control of variceal hemorrhage is undetermined. Frequent screening using sonography at 3- to 6-month intervals is recommended for the first 2 years. Shunt closure occurs owing to intimal hyperplasia in the hepatic vein and neo-intimal hyperplasia in the stented track; shortening or repositioning of the stent can result in incomplete coverage of the track with delayed closure.

REFERENCES

1. Chuang VP, Soo CS, Carrasco CH, Wallace S. Superselective catheterization technique in hepatic angiography. *AJR.* 1983;141:803–811.
2. Dittman W. Hepatic angiography. *Semin Liver Dis.* 1982;2:414–418.
3. Flannigan BD, Gomes AS, Stambuk EC, Lois JF, Pais SO. Intra-arterial digital subtraction angiography: comparison with conventional hepatic arteriography. *Radiology.* 1983; 148:17–21.
4. Kuszyk BS, Heath DG, Ney DR, et al. CT angiography with volume rendering: imaging findings. *AJR.* 1995;165:445–448.
5. Pick TP, Howden R, eds. *Gray's Anatomy, American Edition.* New York: Bounty Books, 1977.
6. Michels NA. *Blood Supply and Anatomy of the Upper Abdominal Organs.* Philadelphia: Lippincott, 1955.
7. Porter B, Woodle ES, Ward RE. Hepatic perfusion abnormalities after liver transplantation. *Cardiovasc Intervent Radiol.* 1985;8:169–173.
8. Gamble P, Colapinto RF, Stronell RD, Colman JC, Blendis L. Transjugular liver biopsy: a review of 461 biopsies. *Radiology.* 1985;157:589–593.
9. Pentecost MJ. Transcatheter treatment of hepatic metastases. *AJR.* 1993;160:1171–1175.
10. Charnasangavej C. Chemoembolization of liver tumors. *Semin Intervent Radiol.* 1993; 10:150–160.
11. Matsui O, Kadoya M, Yoshikawa J, Gabata T, et al. Small hepatocellular carcinoma: treatment with subsegmental transcatheter arterial embolization. *Radiology.* 1993; 188:79–83.
12. Chung JW, Park JH, Han JK, Choi BI, Han MC. Hepatocellular carcinoma and portal vein invasion: results of treatment with transcatheter oily chemoembolization. *AJR.* 1995;165:315–321.
13. Lorenz M, Hermann G, Kirkowa-Rieman M, et al. Temporary chemoembolization of

colorectal liver metastases with degradable starch microspheres. *Eur J Surg Oncol.* 1989;15:453–462.

14. Civalleri D, Pector JC, Hakansson L, Arnaud JP, et al. Treatment of patients with irresectable liver metastases from colorectal cancer by chemo-occlusion with degradable starch microspheres. *Br J Surg.* 1994;81:1338–1341.
15. Kameyama M, Imaoka S, Fukuda I, Nakamori S, et al. Delayed washout of intratumor blood flow is associated with good response to intraarterial chemoembolization for liver metastasis of colorectal cancer. *Surgery.* 1993;114:97–101.
16. Baum S. Hepatic arteriography. In: Abrams HL, ed. *Abrams Angiography,* 3rd ed. Boston: Little Brown and Co; 1983:1500–1502.
17. Franklin RH, Bloom WF, Schoffstall RO. Angiographic embolization as the definitive treatment of post-traumatic hemobilia. *J Trauma* 1980;20:702–705.
18. Pais SO. Diagnostic and therapeutic angiography in the trauma patient. *Semin Roentgenol.* 1992;27:211–232.
19. Sclafani SJ, Shaftan GW, McAuley J, Nayaranaswamy T, et al. Interventional radiology in the management of hepatic trauma. *J Trauma.* 1984;24:256–262.
20. Vlahos L, Kalovidouris A, Gouliamos A, Kailidou E. Post-traumatic hemobilia. *Eur J Radiol.* 1991;13:199–202.
21. Rogers JV, Mack LA, Freeny PC, Johnson ML, Sones PJ. Hepatic focal nodular hyperplasia: angiography, CT, sonography, and scintigraphy. *AJR.* 1981;137:983–990.
22. Welch TJ, Sheedy PF 2d, Johnson CM, Stephens DH, et al. Focal nodular hyperplasia and hepatic adenoma: comparison of angiography, CT, US, and scintigraphy. *Radiology.* 1985;156:593–595.
23. Mathieu D, Bruneton JN, Drouillard J, Pointreau CC, Vasile N. Hepatic adenomas and focal nodular hyperplasia: dynamic CT study. *Radiology.* 1986;160:53–58.
24. Marks WH, Thompson N, Appleman H. Failure of hepatic adenomas to regress after discontinuance of oral contraceptives. An association with focal nodular hyperplasia (FNH) and uterine leiomyoma. *Ann Surg.* 1988;208:190–195.
25. Friedman LS, Gang DL, Hedberg SE, Isselbacher KJ. Simultaneous occurrence of hepatic adenoma and focal nodular hyperplasia: report of a case and review of the literature. *Hepatology.* 1984;4:536–540.
26. Clouse ME. Current diagnostic imaging modalities of the liver. *Surg Clin North Am.* 1989;69:193–234.
27. Bernard G, Mion F, Henry L, Plauchu H, Paliard P. Hepatic involvement in hereditary hemorrhagic telangiectasia: clinical, radiological, and hemodynamic studies of 11 cases. *Gastroenterology* 1993;105:482–487.
28. Paolella LP, Scola FH, Cronan JJ. Hepatic artery aneurysm: an ultrasound diagnosis. *J Clin Ultrasound.* 1985;13:360–362.
29. Jonsson K, Bjernstad A, Eriksson B. Treatment of hepatic artery aneurysm by coil occlusion of the hepatic artery. *AJR.* 1980;134:1245–1247.
30. Shill M, Henderson JM, Tavill AS. The Budd–Chiari syndrome revisited. *Gastroenterologist* 1994;2:27–38.
31. Dilawari JB, Bambery P, Chawla Y, Kaur U, et al. Hepatic outflow obstruction (Budd-Chiari syndrome). Experience with 177 patients and a review of the literature. *Medicine (Baltimore).* 1994;73:21–36.
32. Ledesma-Medina J, Dominguez R, Bowen A, Young LW, Bron KM. Pediatric liver transplantation. Part I. Standardization of preoperative diagnostic imaging. *Radiology.* 1985;157:335–338.

33. Cardella JF, Amplatz K. Preoperative angiographic evaluation of prospective liver recipients. *Radiol Clin North Am.* 1987;25:299–308.
34. Zajko AB, Bron KM, Starzl TE, Van Thiel DH, et al. Angiography of liver transplantation patients. *Radiology.* 1985;157:305–311.
35. Taylor KJ, Morse SS, Weltin GG, Riely CA, Flye MW. Liver transplant recipients: portable duplex US with correlative angiography. *Radiology.* 1986;159:357–363.
36. Winter TC 3rd, Freeny PC, Nghiem HV, et al. Hepatic arterial anatomy in transplantation candidates: evaluation with three-dimensional CT arteriography. *Radiology.* 1995; 195:363–370.
37. Segel MC, Zajko AB, Bowen A, Bron KM, et al. Hepatic artery thrombosis after liver transplantation: radiologic evaluation. *AJR.* 1986;146:137–141.
38. Dominguez R, Cuervas-Mons V, Van Thiel DH, Lecky JW, Starzl TE. Radiographic features of liver allograft rejection. *Gastrointest Radiol.* 1986;11:326–329.
39. White RM, Zajko AB, Demetris AJ, Bron KM, et al. Liver transplant rejection: angiographic findings in 35 patients. *AJR.* 1987;148:1095–1098.
40. Ayalon A, Wiesner RH, Perkins JD, Tominaga S, Hayes DH, Krom RAF. Splenic artery aneurysms in liver transplant patients. *Transplantation.* 1988;45:386–389.
41. Larson PA, Lipchik EO, Adams MB. Development and regression of visceral artery aneurysms following liver transplantation: case report. *Cardiovasc Intervent Radiol.* 1988;11:75–78.
42. Tobben PJ, Zajko AB, Sumkin JH, Bowen A, et al. Pseudoaneurysms complicating organ transplantation: roles of CT, duplex sonography, and angiography. *Radiology.* 1988;169:65–70.
43. Cavaluzzi JA, Sheff R, Harrington DP, et al. Hepatic venography and wedge hepatic vein pressure measurements in diffuse liver disease. *AJR.* 1977;129:441–446.
44. Henderson JM, Millikan WJ Jr, Galloway Jr. The Emory perspective of the distal splenorenal shunt in 1990. *Am J Surg.* 1990;160:54–59.
45. Puttini M, Aseni P, Brambilla G, Belli L. Splenic artery aneurysms in portal hypertension. *J Cardiovasc Surg.* 1982;23:490–493.
46. Kerlan RK, LaBerge JM, Gordon RL, Ring EJ. Transjugular intrahepatic portosystemic shunts: current status. *AJR.* 1995;164:1059–1066.
47. Coldwell DM, Ring EJ, Rees CR, et al. Multi center investigation of the role of transjugular intrahepatic portosystemic shunt in management of portal hypertension. *Radiology.* 1995;196:335–340.

20

SURGICAL SUMMARY: LIVER IMAGING

Russell J. Nauta, M.D.
*Georgetown University Medical Center
Washington, DC*

Choosing an imaging modality for an individual patient is compounded by the difficulty in determining whether a presumed advantage of one imaging modality over another is due to characteristics of the technology itself or to the sophistication of the interpreting radiologist. Although radiology units increasingly channel the interpretation of abdominal images to those proficient therein by custom or by training, one can readily envision, as with the surgical counterpart, a radiologist for whom no technological advance would improve interpretation—and conversely, one whose clinical acumen is such that sophisticated and accurate determinations could be made with very basic equipment. Moreover, and equally importantly for the clinician moved to research such matters, interpretation of sensitivity and specificity claims in the literature requires that the reader have a very clear sense of the technique and the machinery involved before endorsing or indicting a diagnostic modality for a given indication. For example, the number of clinically occult liver metastases found by surveillance computed tomography (CT) 10 years ago would be expected to be fewer than that found with bolus injection of contrast for a directed study performed on a more modern machine. False negative reports in the literature at that time should not be extrapolated to preclude the use of today's technology for surveillance CT.

The surgeon is in the best position to know the preoperative question he wishes the radiologist to answer, as well as what information will be available at laparotomy and therefore is unnecessary to acquire preoperatively (Fig. 1). Costly and redundant imaging can be avoided by clear communication of the clinical query from surgeon to radiologist and exclusion of the primary care doctor "trying to be helpful" from the selection of preoperative imaging studies.

Contemporary imaging modalities may thus be comparatively evaluated based on their ability to (1) identify clinically occult disease, (2) assist in accurately

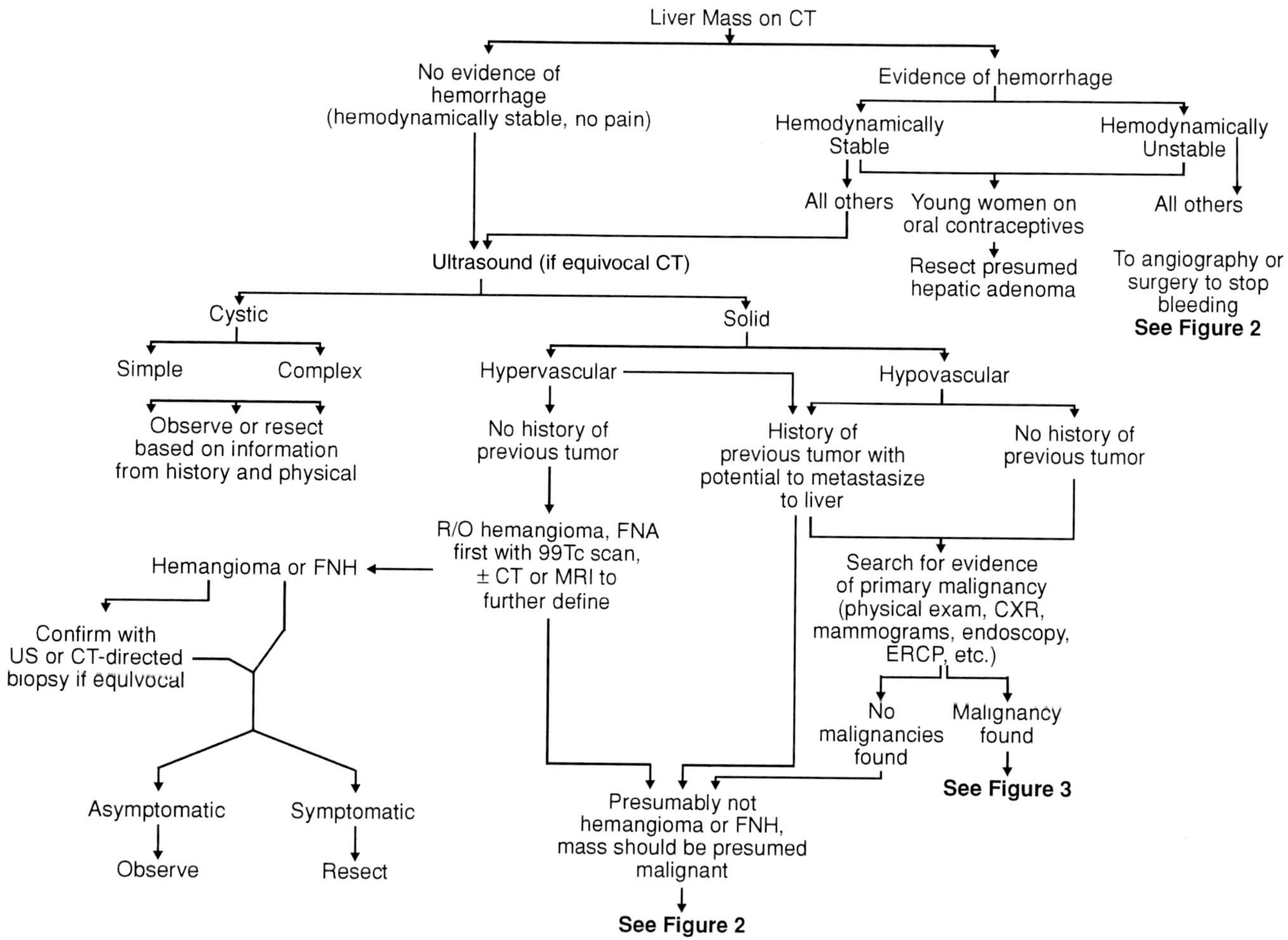

Figure 1. Although the solid liver mass on CT is treated with a high degree of suspicion, the enhancing patterns of hemangiomas and fibronodular hyperplasia should allow their distinction from tumor and permit nonoperative treatment. Most hepatic cysts are asymptomatic and require no surgical treatment, particularly in Western populations.

characterizing an identified lesion as benign or malignant, (3) help in the planning and conduct of an operative procedure, and (4) assess accurately margins of resection.

IDENTIFICATION OF CLINICALLY OCCULT DISEASE

The opportunity to identify clinically occult disease has traditionally existed in the three clinical surveillance settings of (1) routine cancer follow-up, (2) evaluation of the remainder of the liver when a large liver lesion is obvious, and (3) evaluation of masses found in scanning for other purposes ("incidentalomas"). A fourth opportunity to identify clinically occult disease has recently been utilized beyond the surveillance and perioperative setting with the more widespread use of intraoperative ultrasound (1, 2).

Acknowledging that benign disease may occur in patients with previous abdominal malignancy (false positives), the intent of liver imaging in patients with a previous history of resected malignancy is to identify and count "true positives" accurately, and thereby assess the potential for surgical cure. To accomplish this, one must both characterize the hepatic parenchymal disease and exclude extrahepatic disease; the latter may be difficult in abdomens wherein prior resections have altered standard radiological landmarks or where miliary metastatic patterns exceed imaging capabilities and preclude accurate radiological assessment.

Use of nuclear medicine studies has gradually given way to CT and magnetic resonance imaging (MRI) for follow-up cancer surveillance of previously resected abdominal malignancy (3). All three modalities seek to use vascularity as a means of distinguishing one growth from another. Although it is certainly true that primary hepatoma and metastatic deposits from islet cell tumors, melanomas, and renal cell carcinomas are more hypervascular than the more commonly occurring colorectal, gastric, pancreatic, and esophageal metastases (4), it is the clinical setting (that is, the histology of the previously resected primary) that will guide the clinician most. Because it is much more likely that a solid liver lesion discovered in a patient with a history of previous cancer is related to that cancer than to either hepatoma or a metastatic second primary, probabilities based on blood supply must yield to probabilities based on clinical history (5).

Clearly, if hepatic imaging is to be part of cancer surveillance follow-up, its utility should be maximized by adjusting the imaging modality for the clinical situation. The use of dynamic gadolinium enhancement imaging in MRI (6–8) and the accentuation of hepatic metastases on CT by bolus injection of the arteries supplying the portal venous system are examples of such tailoring (9, 10). The need for arterial catheterization in the latter procedure makes it somewhat less appealing than MRI if comparable detection rates are achieved; whether the two imaging modalities are equally sensitive remains a matter of debate in the literature (11–13).

As a practical matter, however, the question is best addressed by using CT (with its wider availability) and to a lesser extent MRI as the chief surveillance tool(s) (15). MR angiography can often answer questions previously asked of conventional angiography regarding proximity to major vessels, and can also create a "road map" for the operating surgeon.

The role of MRI is expanding because follow-up schemata for resected colorectal metastases are controversial with respect to their cost effectiveness (14), but this nihilism (in part, economically driven) must be balanced by the enthusiasm for the surgical cure of hepatic metastases that has evolved over the past three decades (16). The evaluation of extrahepatic disease when a known liver lesion is present, though crucial, is highly variable among the imaging modalities and no single study is uniformly superior. In fact, detailed physical examination of the abdomen, including careful pelvic and rectal examinations, may be superior to either of the two leading imaging modalities (CT and MRI) in detecting the presence of extrahepatic disease in the presence of known liver metastases (5, 17). For example, a Blumer's shelf in a patient with prior hysterectomy may be readily identified by physical examination, yet be occult radiologically because of postoperative changes in the pelvis.

The identification of small nodules within the liver when a larger nodule is obvious on imaging studies is critically important if a patient with advanced cancer is to be offered a potentially risky, yet potentially curative, operation. Although enhanced CT and MRI images may be useful preoperative imaging modalities in both this regard and in routine cancer follow-up surveillance, the more widespread use and availability of intraoperative ultrasound can lead to detection of as many as 11% more tumors than were suspected by preoperative imaging—most less than 2 cm in diameter. That some of these tumors would likely be discovered by careful examination and palpation of the mobilized liver or laparoscopic exploration, however, suggests that 11% is likely the upper limit of benefit attributable to the intraoperative ultrasound (18, 19). Human variability related to the experience of the ultrasonographer and the surgeon are likely to be stronger determinants in driving this occult detection figure up or down than further refinements in the technology.

CHARACTERIZATION OF A LESION AS BENIGN OR MALIGNANT

Sensitivity is clearly an important characteristic of an imaging modality. Once confirmed, however, the clinical question in lesion evaluation shifts from "Is it there?" to "What is it?" Whether in the evaluation of an "incidentaloma" discovered in imaging for other reasons, or in the evaluation of a directed surveillance study identifying a mass, imaging modalities are legitimately judged by how well they hone specificity—that is, how well they accurately characterize a discovered mass as benign or malignant.

In general, modalities that distinguish solid from cystic (of which diagnostic ultrasound is the cheapest and most reliable) and those that distinguish the hypervascular mass from the hypovascular mass are most useful in clinical practice. Despite very real differences in imaging, the major determinant of differentiation (for example, echinococcal cyst from congenital cyst) again derives from detailed knowledge of the patient's history and exposure, and the characteristics of the physical examination.

Were a laparotomy required for every biopsy, individual enhancement patterns might assume more importance; the availability of image-guided percutaneous and laparoscopic biopsies makes some—but not all—discussions about radiological differentiation moot. Hypervascular masses, including hepatomas, islet cell

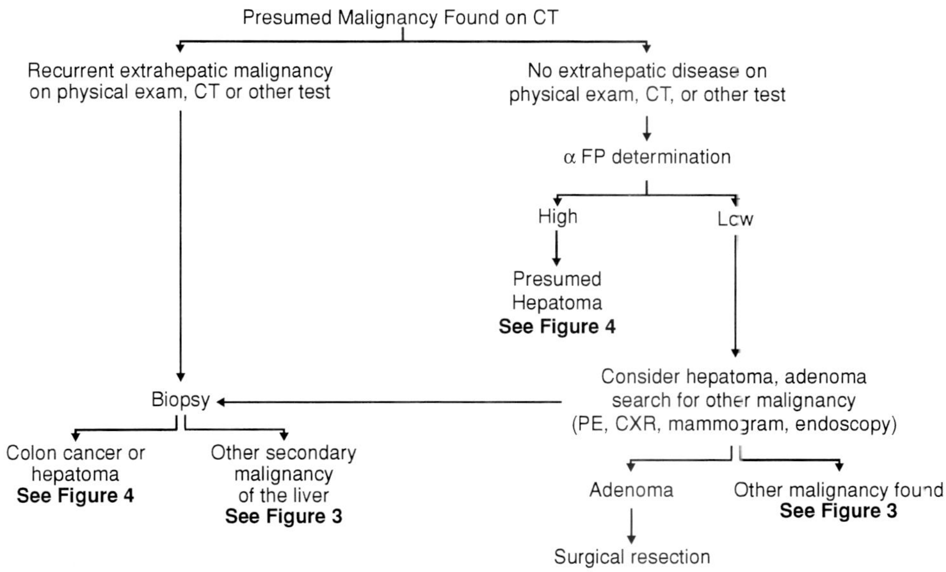

Figure 2. If the primary lesion is not amenable to biopsy, ultrasound or CT-guided biopsy of the hepatic lesion can expedite the work-up and avoid both superfluous discussions of enhancement patterns and diagnostic excesses.

tumors, fibronodular hyperplasia, hepatic adenoma, hereditary telangiectasias, melanoma, renal cell cancer, and hemangiomas, may often assume greater or lesser stature in the differential diagnosis of an imaged hepatic mass by the known or suspected concurrent or prior presence of a given primary tumor (Figs. 1–5). Although it is reasonable to believe that a hypervascular mass with a dense blush and a feeding artery penetrating to its center on MRI, CT, or angiography is fibronodular hyperplasia, this impression can be refined by an image-guided biopsy. Similarly, a young woman on birth control pills with a bleeding hepatic lesion likely has an hepatic adenoma, a patient with previous colon cancer developing hypovascular lesions in the liver should be considered to have colorectal metastases, and a patient with previous melanoma or hypernephroma with enhancing lesions in the liver should be considered to have metastases from these primaries. Although ultrasound-guided, CT-guided, or laparoscopic-guided biopsy can be correctly argued to be a more direct approach than the excessive analysis of subtle differences in imaging characteristics, the invasive route is not without bleeding risk in such lesions as hepatic adenoma, telangiectasias, and hemangiomas. Hemangiomas, in not lending themselves to percutaneous biopsy, and not often being "suspected" by a clinical syndrome, are a useful exception to the economy of imaging studies approach. They are well characterized by a number of complementary radiological studies including compression under ultrasound, bolus injection on CT or MRI, and enhancement studies in the nuclear medicine or digital subtraction angiography suite (20–22a). Inherent hazards in biopsy, though perhaps overestimated (23, 24), and confidence in the imaging modality for hormonally bland and characteristically

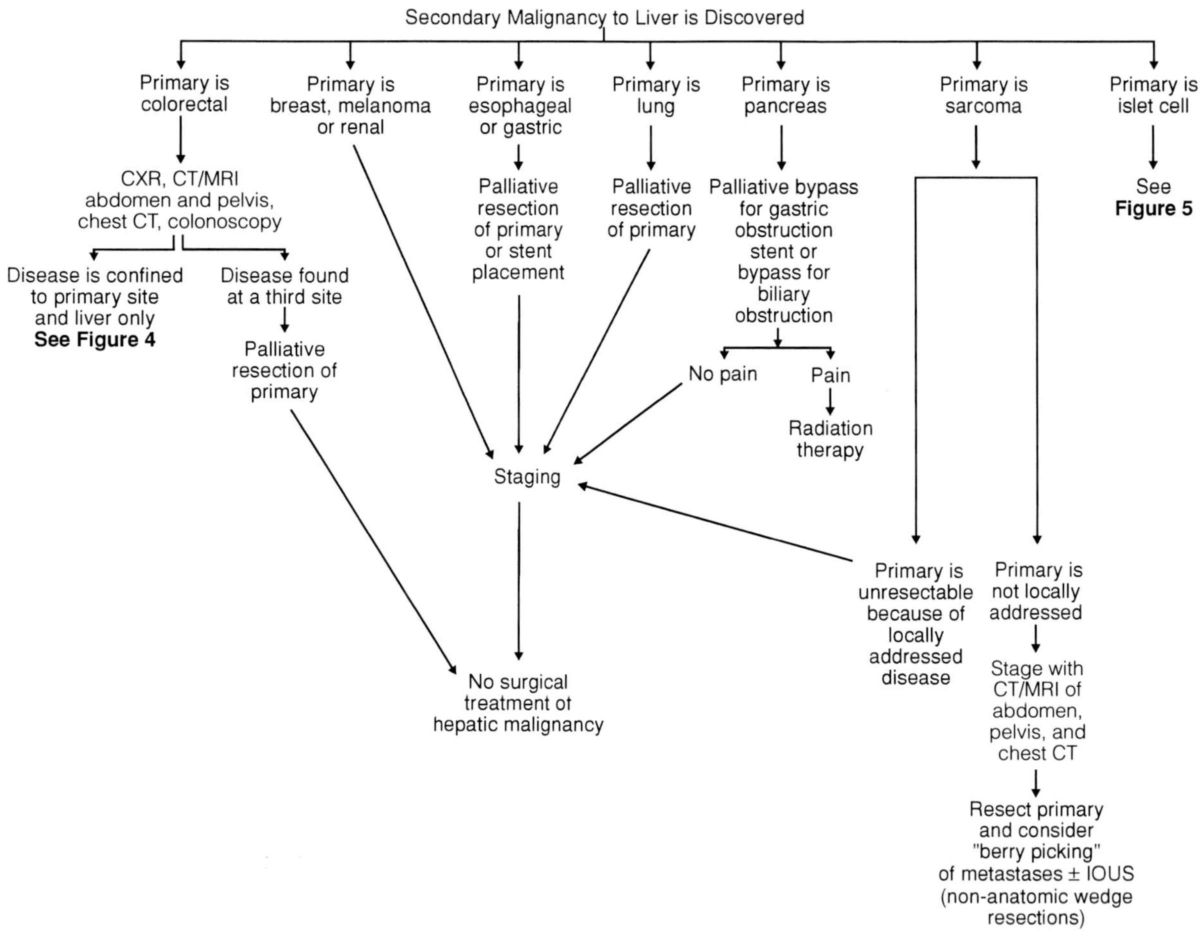

Figure 3. Hepatic metastasis represents an ominous course of disease progression in most human malignancy. Although longevity is demonstrable in colorectal metastasis resection, and symptoms may be improved in palliative resection of metastatic islet cell tumors, complete staging often demonstrates a systemic illness best addressed with systemic therapy.

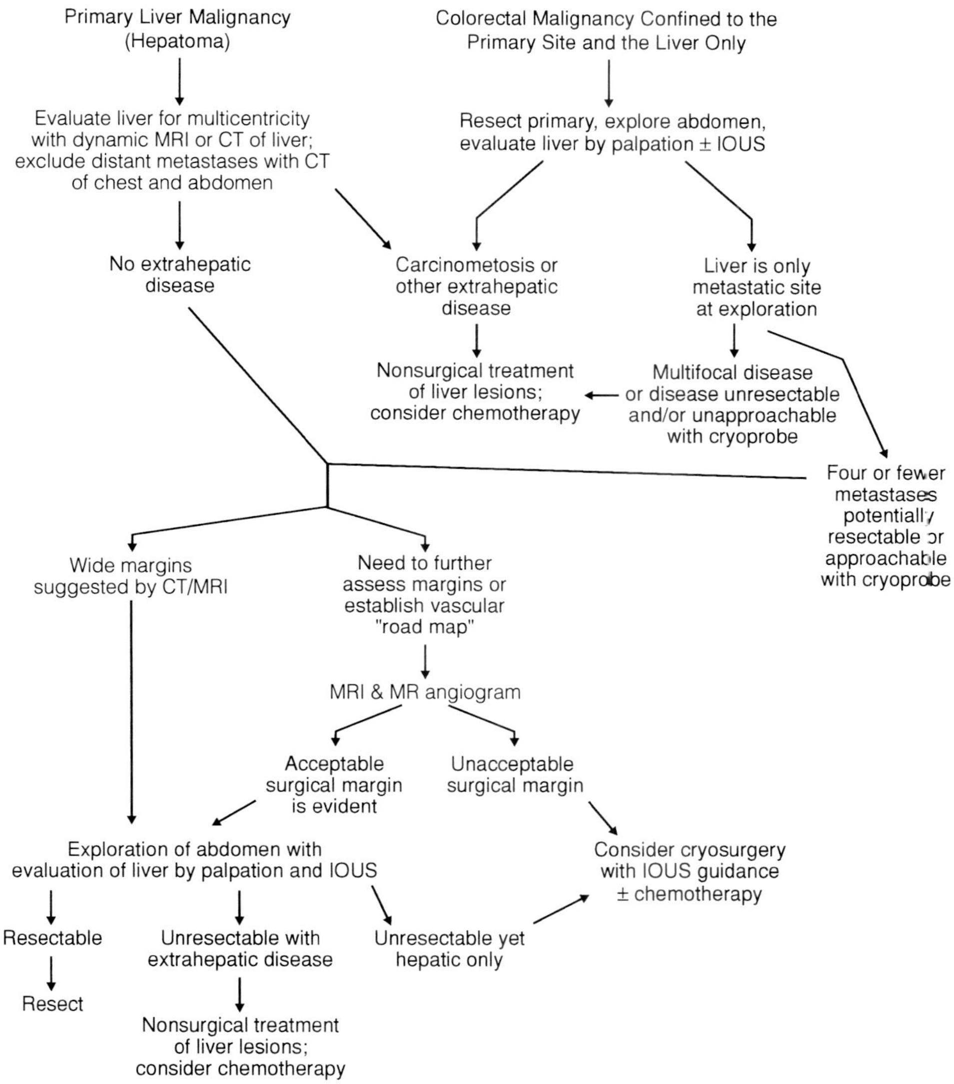

Figure 4. Diagnostic testing should identify the relationship of liver lesions to vital structures, but not delay operation. If staging proves to underestimate disease extent, local therapy should not be used to treat systemic illness.

enhancing masses should lead to a decision to observe the clearly characterized hemangioma (25, 26).

ASSESSMENT OF MARGINS OF RESECTION

Despite the relative lack of credible chemotherapeutic or radiotherapeutic alternatives in treatment of liver cancer, certain aspects of hepatic resection remain contro-

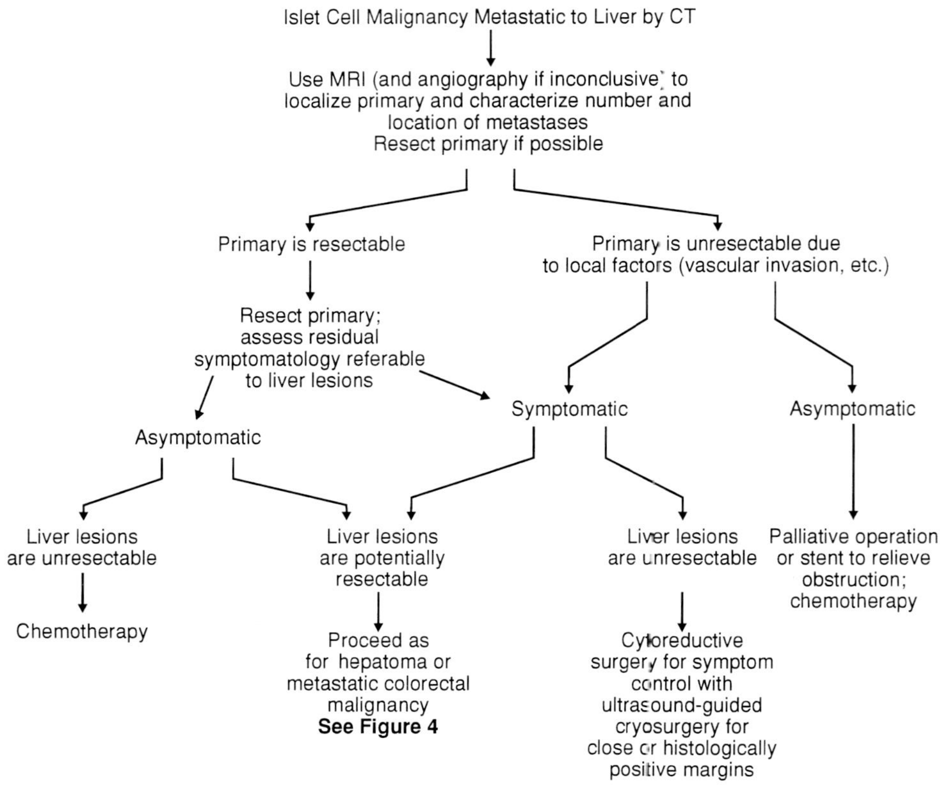

Figure 5. Management of symptoms attributable to islet cell tumors make noncurative resection acceptable in some instances.

versial. Early series of hepatic resection concentrated on the need to define variations in the arterial anatomy, and to conduct a resection that simply spared the contralateral lobe or remaining liver, often without regard for the size of the tumor-free margin (27, 28). Angiography initially played a prominent role, but as familiarity with the operation increased, angiography gave way to careful portal dissection as a means of establishing a "road map" for the operation (27). In circumstances where the need persists as a preoperative tool for liver surgery (for instance, hepatic transplantation, "re-do" ablative hepatic surgery), the accuracy and noninvasive characteristics of MRI are causing it to replace arteriography as the defining procedure of choice.

Steele et al. (29) have suggested that little to no survival advantage is conferred upon patients for whom the tumor-free resection margin at the transection point is less than 1.0 cm. This observation has led to the recruitment of imaging modalities to assess prospectively the anticipated surgical margin of resection and to utilize enhancement characteristics of those modalities (for example, the identification of hepatomas by MRI in cirrhotic livers) to predict resectability and clearance margins. Preoperatively, CT and MRI are more useful than arteriography, nuclear medicine, and ultrasound in margin assessment, but intraoperative ultrasound has recently been championed as an important tool for assessing the deeper margins of resection, particularly in the area of the inferior vena cava and hepatic veins (18, 19).

IMAGING MODALITIES AND CONTROVERSIAL SURGICAL PROCEDURES

Though hepatic surgery is generally acknowledged as increasing survival compared to historical controls, difficulties in patient accrual to no-treatment arms of clinical trials compromised its acceptance during its early years (30). Alternatives to ablative surgery, of which cryosurgery is the latest, also lack the imprimatur of a demonstrable advantage in a prospectively randomized, controlled clinical trial. Anecdotal experience with cryosurgery, however, has defined a role for intraoperative ultrasound in determining the development and margins of the "ice ball" as well as the relationship of the freeze zone to neighboring critical structures such as the porta hepatis and the inferior vena cava (31). Enthusiasm for regional infusion techniques favors arterial infusion of chemotherapeutic agents over portal venous infusion, but both have been unable to meet the standard of demonstrable survival advantage compared to systemic intravenous infusion. Regional infusion techniques are espoused for their theoretical appeal in delivering large doses of cytotoxic drugs by way of an artery that directly supplies the afflicted organ, which, in turn, clears them and maintains a nontoxic systemic level. The chemoembolization techniques currently enjoying a resurgence of support draw on the same desire to deliver treatment regionally while limiting systemic toxicity. All require accurate characterization of the hepatic inflow in order to plan catheter positioning accurately and to avoid complications of high-dose chemotherapy perfusion of adjacent organs. Depending on institutional capabilities, arteriography, digital subtraction angiography, and MRI angiography are used in combination to define the position of the metastases relative to the vessels for the percutaneous or implantable pump approach. The fewest number of imaging studies necessary to accomplish the task should be chosen. For example, if a standard angiographic approach is contemplated to place the catheter, there is little reason to precede it with MRI angiography.

Patency of the blood vessels for this purpose, as well as for assessment of vascular shunts, transjugular intrahepatic portosystemic shunts, and delineation of anatomy for hepatic transplantation remain potential roles for angiography, though Doppler ultrasound and the other modalities referenced represent the diminishing role for angiography with the wider availability of MRI.

SUMMARY

An imaging modality's primary use for the surgeon is in determining whether an operation can be performed in such a way as to meet its goals (32). The radiologist, therefore, is first charged with characterizing intrahepatic disease and excluding extrahepatic disease, and then with using an imaging modality suitable to answer the surgeon's questions regarding hepatic pathology. Clinically "blinded" radiologists function no better than clinically blind ones, and inquiry of the radiologist should not ask of the imaging modality information available from the history and physical examination; rather, imaging should refine a clinical impression using demonstrable characteristics between malignant and benign tissue's physical differences to garner relevant preoperative information. Importantly, the imaging modality should enhance, rather than duplicate, information from biopsy or from abdominal exploration. Approached in this way, the imaging modality will provide a cost effective (and therefore, defensible) prelude to the surgical conduct of effective therapy.

REFERENCES

1. Knol JA, Marn CS, Francis IR, et al. Comparisons of dynamic infusion and delayed computer tomography, intraoperative ultrasound, and palpation on the diagnosis of liver metastases. *Am J Surg.* 1993;165:81–88.
2. Boldrini G, deGaeteno AM, Giovannini I, et al. The systemic use of operative ultrasound for detection of liver metastases during colorectal surgery. *World J Surg* 1987;11:622–627.
3. Tempero M, Brand R, Holdeman K, Metzmoro A. New imaging techniques in colorectal cancer. *Semin Oncol* 1995;22:448–471.
4. Larson RE, Semelke RC, Bagley AS, Molin PL, Brown ED, Lee JK. Hypervascular malignant liver lesions: Comparison of various MR imaging pulse sequences and dynamic CT. *Radiology.* 1994;192:393–399.
5. Schwartz JH, Ellison EC. Focal liver lesions. Evaluation of solid neoplasms. *Postgrad Med.* 1994;95:157–160, 165–168, 171–174.
6. Semelke RC, Cumming MJ, Shoenut JP, et al. Islet cell tumors: comparison of dynamic contrast-enhanced CT and MR imaging with dynamic gadolinium enhancement and fat suppression. *Radiology.* 1993;186:759–802.
7. Whitney WS, Herfkens RJ, Jeffrey RB, et al. Dynamic breath-hold multiplasm spoiled gradient-recalled MR imaging with gadolinium enhancement for differentiating hepatic hemangiomas from malignancies at 1.5 T. *Radiology.* 1993;189:863–870.
8. Soyer P, Laissy JP, Silbert A, et al. Hepatic metastases: detection with multisection FLASH MR imaging during gadolinium chelate-enhanced arterial portography. *Radiology.* 1993;189:401–405.
9. Soyer P, Bluemke DA, Zeitonin G, et al. Detection of recurrent hepatic metastases affect partial hepatectomy: Value of CT combined with arterial portography. *AJR.* 1994;162:1327.
10. Soyer P, Roche A, Gad M, et al. Preoperative segmental localization of hepatic metastases: Utility of three-dimensional CT during arterial portography. *Radiology.* 1991;180:653–658.
11. Charnsangavez C. New imaging modalities for follow-up of colorectal carcinoma. *Cancer.* 1993;71(12 suppl):4236–4240.
12. Woodhouse CE, Ney DR, Sitzmann JV, Fishman EK. Spiral computed tomography with three-dimensional vohimetric rendering for oncologic surgery planning. A retrospective analysis. *Invest Radiol.* 1954;29:1031–1037.
13. Oi H, Murakami T, Kim T, Matsushita M, Kishimoto H, Nakamura H. Dynamic MR imaging and early-phase helical CT for detecting small intrahepatic metastases of hepatocellular carcinoma. *AJR.* 1996;166:369–374.
14. Steele G. Standard postoperative monitoring of patients after primary resection of colon and rectum cancer. *Cancer* 1993;71(12 suppl):4225–4235.
15. Ferrucci JT. Liver tumor imaging. *Cancer* 1991;67(suppl 4):1189–1195.
16. Hughes KS, Simon R, Songhoraboshi S, et al. Resection of the liver for colorectal

carcinoma metastases: a multi-institutional study of indications for resection. *Surgery.* 1988;103:278–288.

17. Schwartz JH, Ellison EC. Focal liver lesions, evaluation of solid neoplasms. *Postgrad Med.* 1994;95:157–160, 165–168, 171–174.
18. Machi J, Isomoto H, Yamashita Y, et al. Intraoperative ultrasonography in screening for liver metastases from colorectal cancer: Comparative accuracy with traditional procedures. *Surgery.* 1987;101;6:678–684.
19. Parker GA, Lawrence W, Horsley JS III, et al. Intraoperative ultrasound of the liver affects operative decision making. *Ann Surg.* 1989;209;5:569–577.
20. Middleton ML. Scintigraphic evaluation of hepatic mass lesions: emphasis on hemangioma detection. *Semin Nucl Med.* 1996;26:4–15.
21. Goldberg MA, Saini S, Hahn PF, Egglin TK, Mueller PR. Differentiation between hemangiomas and metastases of the liver with ultrafast MR imaging: preliminary results with T_2 calculations. *AJR.* 1991;157:727–780.
22. Leslie DF, Johnson CD, Johnson CM, Ilstrup DM, Harmsen WS. Distinction between cavernous hemangiomas of the liver and hepatic metastases on CT: values of contrast enhancement patterns. *AJR.* 1995;164:685–689.

22a. Semelka RC, Brown ED, Aschen SM, et al. Hepatic hemangiomas: a multi-institutional study of appearance on T2-weighted and serial gadolinium-enhanced gradient echo MR images. *Radiology.* 1994;192:401–406.

23. Baker ME. What is the most cost-effective imaging work-up for hepatic hemangiomas, and is it safe to obtain a biopsy of such a suspected hemangioma? *AJR.* 1994;163:1261.
24. Tung GA, Cronan JJ. Percutaneous needle biopsy of hepatic cavernous hemangioma. *J Clin Gastroenterol.* 1993;16:117–122.
25. Yamagata M, Karematsu T, Matsumoto T, Otsunomiya T, Ikeda Y, Sugimachi K. Management of hemangioma of the liver: comparison of results between surgery and observation. *Br J Surg.* 1991;78:1223–1225.
26. Gandolfi L, Leo P, Solmi L, Vitelli B, Verros G, Colecchia A. Natural history of hepatic hemangioma: clinical and ultrasound study. *Gut.* 1991;32:677–680.
27. Starzl TE, Bell RH, Beart RW, et al. Hepatic trisymentectomy and other liver resections. *Surg Gynecol Obstet.* 1975;141:429–437.
28. Fortner JG, Silva JS, Golberg RB, et al. Multivariant analysis of a performed series of 247 consecutive patients with liver metastases from colorectal cancer. 1. Treatment by hepatic resection. *Ann Surg.* 1984;199:306–316.
29. Steele G, Bledgy R, Mayer RJ, Linbland A, Petrelli N, and Wecvel D. A prospective evaluation of hepatic resection for colorectal carcinoma metastases to the liver: Gastrointestinal Tumor Study Group Protocol 6584. *J Clin Oncol.* 1991;9:1105–1112.
30. Silen W. Hepatic resection for metastases from colorectal carcinoma is of dubious value. *Arch Surg.* 1989;124:1021–1022.
31. Ravikumar TS, Steele G, Kane R, et al. Experimental and clinical observations on hepatic cryosurgery for colorectal metastases. *Cancer Res.* 1991;51:6323–6327.
32. Bennett WF, Bora JG. Review of hepatic imaging and a problem-oriented approach to liver masses. *Hepatology.* 1990;12(4, part 1):761–765.

IV

PANCREAS

21

TRANSABDOMINAL AND INTRAOPERATIVE ULTRASOUND OF THE PANCREAS

Jeffrey D. Neitlich, M.D., and Leslie M. Scoutt, M.D.
Yale University School of Medicine
New Haven, Connecticut

Pancreatic sonography plays an important role in the evaluation of acute and chronic pancreatitis, as well as pancreatic neoplasms. It also has utility as a guide for biopsy and therapeutic intervention. Although ultrasound (US) examination of the pancreas is less sensitive and specific than either computed tomography (CT) or endoscopic retrograde cholangiopancreatography (ERCP), it is often used as a first-line imaging technique as it is noninvasive, inexpensive, and portable. In some cases, such as for evaluation of cystic neoplasms of the pancreas, it is the most definitive imaging test available. Color and pulse Doppler capabilities have increased the usefulness of pancreatic US, particularly in the setting of pancreatitis where vascular complications such as splenic vein thrombosis occur. Intraoperative ultrasound of the pancreas is a relatively new field. Here the recent development of small, high-resolution transducers plays a critical role in lesion detection in certain clinical settings.

TECHNIQUE AND NORMAL ANATOMY

Ultrasound imaging of the pancreas is complementary to CT. Sonography is most effective when evaluating thin patients, whereas the pancreas is best imaged on CT when there is an abundance of perivisceral fat. Ultrasound is particularly useful in detecting subtle textural changes that may not be evident on either CT or magnetic resonance imaging (MRI). However, US is very operator dependent. Bowel gas and body fat are the two factors most likely to limit the US examination. Owing to the deep location of the pancreas, 2–3.5 MHz curved array transducers are generally required, although in thin patients or children higher-frequency transducers may be used. Distention of the stomach and duodenum with water or oral contrast agents (1) may be helpful, both by displacing gastric air and by providing an acoustic window. This is best accomplished by having the patient drink approximately 10 ounces of degassed water while in the upright position. Transverse and sagittal images of the body of the pancreas are best obtained through the distended gastric body. In the semi-upright right posterior oblique position, water fills the duodenum and antrum while air is displaced into the gastric fundus and evaluation of the pancreatic head is optimized. The tail of the pancreas may best be visualized through the splenic hilum.

The normal pancreas is oriented obliquely within the upper abdomen, with the head lying within the C-loop of the duodenum, the body anterior to the splenic vein, and the tail within the splenic hilum (Fig. 1). The normal pancreas has a variety of shapes and sizes. Usually the pancreas tapers from head toward tail, but some patients have a tail thicker than the body. The outer margin may be smooth or lobular. In adults, the normal pancreas is homogeneous in echotexture and is at least as echogenic as the liver at the same depth. As patients age, the pancreas becomes fatty and the echogenicity increases. This makes hypoechoic lesions easier to detect. The uncinate process of the pancreas is seen posterior to the superior mesenteric vein, and normally has a sharp, well-delineated medial margin that ends medial to the superior mesenteric artery.

The pancreatic duct may sometimes be visualized in normal patients as two parallel echogenic lines within the parenchyma (Fig. 1). The normal duct lumen should measure no more than 2 mm (2). In elderly patients, ductal ectasia may occur with no demonstrable source of obstruction. In this setting, it is necessary to exclude calculus, tumor, or chronic inflammation as the cause (3). Occasionally accessory pancreatic ducts are seen within the head and/or uncinate process. Whenever possible, it is useful to follow their course to the ampulla of Vater for confirmation.

PANCREATITIS

Acute pancreatitis is clinically defined as an acute inflammatory disease of the pancreas causing abdominal pain and associated with elevated serum or urinary pancreatic enzymes (4). This clinical picture is non-specific, however, and patients with acute cholecystitis, small bowel obstruction, bowel ischemia, and peptic ulcer disease may also present with abdominal pain as well as hyperamylasemia (5). Alcohol abuse and gallstones are the most common etiologies of pancreatitis, but other predisposing factors include drugs, hypercalcemia, hyperlipidemia, genetic predisposition, trauma, viral, ascariasis, postoperative (especially cardiac by-pass surgery), and prior endoscopic instrumentation (6). The clinical spectrum of acute pancreatitis ranges from a mild, self-limited illness to hemorrhagic/necrotizing pancreatitis which is a life-threatening condition. No definitive therapy exists, and survival is related to adequate supportive measures and prompt treatment of complications such as necrosis and/or infection.

The goals of imaging patients with clinically suspected acute pancreatitis are

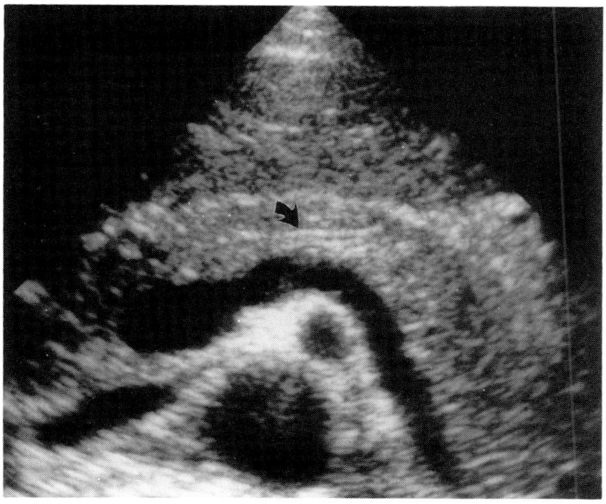

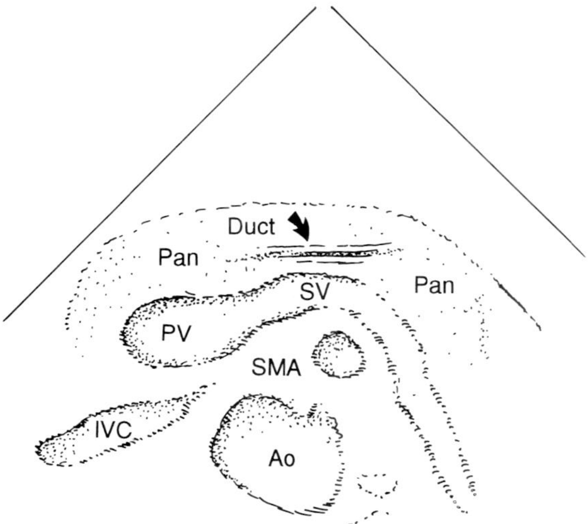

Figure 1. Normal pancreas: the normal pancreas is slightly more echogenic than the liver, and is well marginated. Here, the body and tail are seen anterior to the splenic vein. The normal pancreatic duct is less than 2 mm and is often identified by parallel, echogenic lines (arrow).

threefold. While imaging findings consistent with the diagnosis of acute pancreatitis can help secure the clinical diagnosis, other causes of abdominal pain should be excluded such as liver abscess, acute cholecystitis, bowel obstruction, or renal calculi. Second, potentially treatable causes of pancreatitis should be sought. For example, discovery of a common duct stone should triage the patient for surgical or endoscopic decompression unless the patient demonstrates significant clinical improvement within the first 24 to 48 hours. Finally, and perhaps most importantly, imaging has a significant role in the diagnosis and even treatment of complications of pancreatitis. The identification of ascites, pleural effusions, pseudocysts, hemorrhage, inflammation/necrosis/abscess, venous thrombosis, pseudoaneurysm, and gastrointestinal fistulae has important implications for patient management as well as prognosis. Pseudocysts and/or abscesses may be successfully treated by either CT- or US-guided percutaneous drainage. Although CT is the best overall survey technique, real-time as well as color Doppler US can be very useful for the evaluation of potential complications of acute pancreatitis.

Ultrasound examination of the pancreas may be difficult in the acute phase owing to abdominal pain and ileus. However, all patients, even patients who are likely to have pancreatitis on the basis of alcohol abuse, merit US examination immediately to rule out common duct stones. Both meticulous technique and persistence are required to achieve the diagnostic accuracy of 70–80% reported in the literature for evaluation of common duct stones (7–9).

Ultrasound findings in acute pancreatitis include decreased echogenicity and enlargement of the gland. However, because the maximal decrease in echogenicity occurs 2–5 days after the initial painful episode, the pancreas may appear normal immediately (first 24 hrs) following the onset of pain (10). Surrounding tissue planes may be indistinct and dilatation of the pancreatic duct (>2 mm) is frequently present and easily identified. Ultrasound examination should also include a search for fluid collections or phlegmon involving the lesser sac, anterior and posterior pararenal spaces, splenic hilum, and transverse mesocolon, particularly in patients with clinically severe disease. Of these, fluid collections in the lesser sac are the easiest to identify on US whereas the transverse mesocolon is the most difficult area to examine (11). The semi-erect right posterior oblique position is often extremely helpful, and the tail of the pancreas may be best visualized through the splenic hilum.

A fluid collection that persists for more than 6 weeks following a bout of pancreatitis develops a pseudocapsule of granulation and fibrous tissue and is called a pseudocyst (Fig. 2A). Sonographically, pseudocysts appear as well-marginated cystic collections with increased through transmission. Although typically anechoic, pseudocysts may contain septations or internal echoes due to debris, hemorrhage, or infection (see below). Many pseudocysts resolve spontaneously, but pseudocysts larger than 5 cm are prone to develop complications such as rupture, hemorrhage, or superinfection. Drainage is recommended for large or enlarging symptomatic pseudocysts, particularly with clinical evidence to suggest obstruction or infection (12, 13). Computed tomography is the most sensitive means of identifying extra pancreatic fluid collections. However, when visible on US, percutaneous diagnostic aspiration or drainage may easily and quickly be performed with US guidance. In addition, US is an efficient means of following fluid collections to ensure resolution. Percutaneous drainage of noninfected pancreatic pseudocysts has been reported to have a cure rate of 60–90% but requires an intact pseudocapsule as well as continuous drainage until the fistulous tract has closed (12–16).

Infected pancreatic pseudocysts, abscess, and infected pancreatic necrosis are the most serious complications of acute pancreatitis and require emergent percutaneous drainage or surgical debridement. Internal echoes, debris, air, mural irregularity, and infiltration of fat planes surrounding a mature pseudocyst suggest infection (Fig. 2B). Percutaneous drainage of infected pseudocysts has been reported to have a 90% success rate in the largest recently published series (14). Percutaneous drainage of a pancreatic abscess is controversial and more difficult. Multiple large-bore catheters are generally required with success rates reported ranging from 32

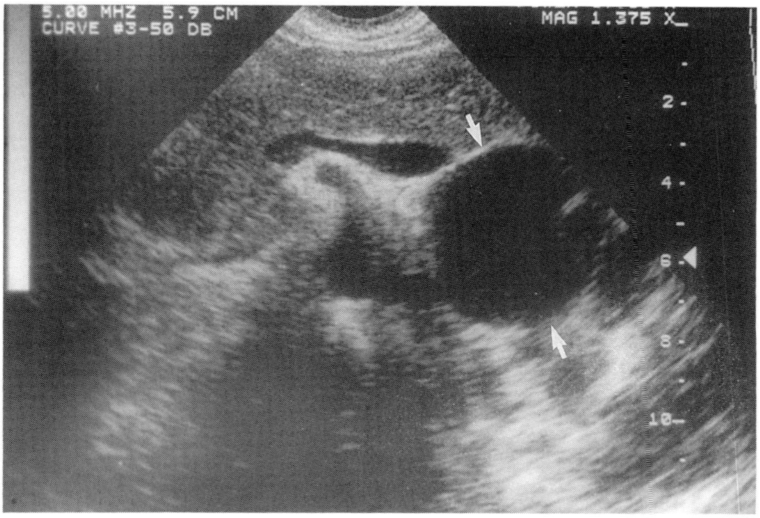

(A)

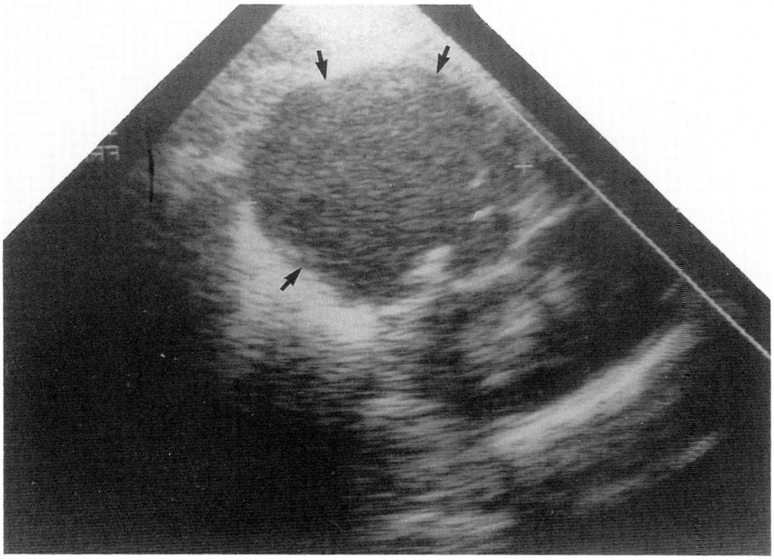

(B)

Figure 2. Pancreatic pseudocyst: (A) Well-circumscribed cystic mass (arrows) is seen in the pancreatic tail of a patient with pancreatitis. (B) cystic mass (arrows) containing echogenic debris. Note enhanced through transmission. This appearance can be seen with either infected or hemorrhagic pseudocysts.

to 79% (13, 17–19). A combined surgical and percutaneous approach may be necessary. On US, a pancreatic abscess may be recognized as a complex cystic area with a thick wall and often containing areas of increased echogenicity within the pancreatic bed. Air, ill-defined margins, and increased through transmission are common findings. Pancreatic necrosis is more easily diagnosed on CT than US

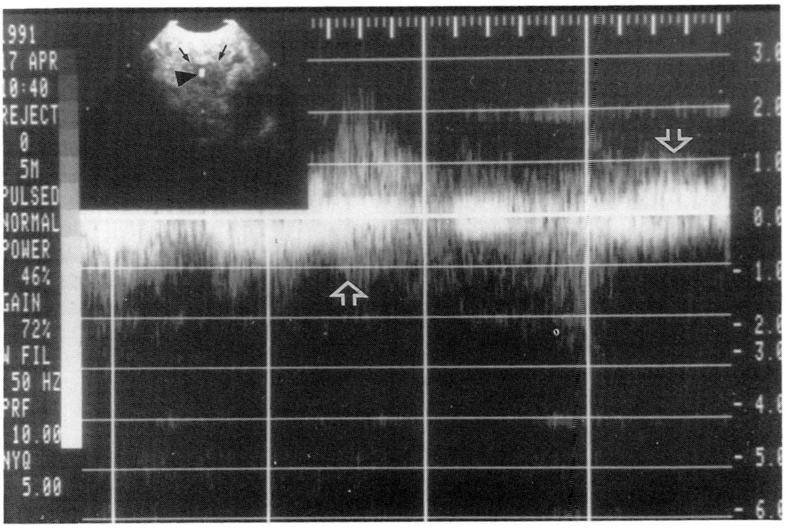

Figure 3. Pseudoaneurysm: pulsed Doppler ultrasound of a cystic mass (solid arrows) in a patient with chronic pancreatitis. The white rectangle (arrowhead) in the mass is the area being sampled. The tracing is consistent with actively flowing blood (open arrows). This mass was surgically proved to represent a splenic artery pseudoaneurysm. Courtesy of I. M. Ramos.

and appears as an area without contrast enhancement (20). However, fine needle aspiration (FNA) may be required to diagnose superinfection unless air bubbles are noted (21). Adequate treatment of infected pancreatic necrosis requires surgical debridement (22).

Hemorrhagic pancreatic tissue or fluid collections are typically very echogenic in the acute phase (23). Hemorrhagic pancreatitis carries a grave prognosis and US-guided aspiration or CT scanning can be helpful in confirming the diagnosis. Over time the US appearance of hemorrhage changes and becomes less specific. It may be difficult to determine if an ill-defined hypoechoic area represents old hemorrhage, necrosis, or infection. Similarly it may be impossible by imaging features alone to determine if debris or septations within a collection are due to hemorrhage or infection.

Real-time US with pulse and color Doppler may be very helpful in identifying vascular complications, such as pseudoaneurysms and venous thrombosis. On real-time examination pseudoaneurysms appear as complex cystic areas within or near the pancreas. Rapid change in size or echogenicity of a cystic mass should raise the suspicion of pseudoaneurysm formation or hemorrhage (24). Color or pulse Doppler demonstrates blood flow (25–28) (Fig. 3). The exact sensitivity of Doppler US in identifying pseudoaneurysms is unknown, but angiography is certainly required to diagnose those under 1 cm in diameter. Perivascular inflammation may lead to splenic vein thrombosis, which most commonly occurs in the portion of the splenic vein posterior to the pancreas. Findings on real-time US suggesting venous thrombosis are enlargement of the splenic vein with low-level internal echoes. Doppler US reveals no evidence of blood flow and collateral vessels or varices may be seen as well as infiltration of the surrounding fat planes.

Chronic pancreatitis is characterized by persistent or recurrent abdominal pain. Endocrine and/or exocrine functional abnormalities may develop as the disease progresses. Definitive diagnosis, particularly in mild cases, requires confirmatory correlative imaging with ERCP, CT, or US. On US the pancreas typically appears echogenic and inhomogeneous. The pancreatic duct is often dilated (29). However, the "double duct sign" may be noted in patients with pancreatic carcinoma as well (30). Focal areas of calcification representing stones within the pancreatic duct are the most specific US finding. Although CT is more sensitive than US for the detection of pancreatic calcification, the ability of ERCP to identify minimal ductal changes makes ERCP the most sensitive imaging tool for diagnosing chronic pancreatitis (29, 31).

Nearly 30% of patients with chronic pancreatitis have focal masses that must be differentiated from pancreatic carcinoma. If a pancreatic mass is echogenic or contains calcification, it is most often related to chronic pancreatitis (32). However, biopsy or ERCP is required to differentiate focal chronic pancreatitis from pancreatic carcinoma when a focal mass is hypoechoic.

PANCREATIC NEOPLASMS

Ductal Adenocarcinoma

Ductal adenocarcinoma of the pancreas accounts for 80–90% of all pancreatic neoplasms. In 1995, the American Cancer Society estimated that 24,000 new cases of pancreatic carcinoma would be diagnosed and that 27,000 related deaths would occur (33). The peak incidence occurs between the ages of 60 and 70 years. Presenting symptoms are nonspecific and include jaundice, back pain, weight loss, nausea, and fatigue. Pancreatic carcinomas occur most commonly in the head of the pancreas (60%); approximately 5% are diffuse, and the rest occur in the body and tail (34). Pancreatic carcinoma spreads locally in an aggressive fashion. Lesions that have infiltrated beyond the pancreas are not candidates for surgery and most patients are unresectable at presentation. Tumors in the head of the pancreas invade duodenum, common bile duct, and retroperitoneal tissue, where perineural, lymphatic, and ultimately vascular invasion will occur. Tumors in the body and tail of the pancreas invade stomach, spleen, peritoneum, colon, and left adrenal gland. Lymphangitic spread as well as hematogenous spread to liver and lung also frequently occur.

Pancreatic carcinoma is a lethal disease with a 5-year survival rate of less than 2% (35). Well-differentiated small tumors and tumors in the head of the pancreas have a slightly better prognosis. However, even patients who undergo surgical resection have a cure rate of less than 5–8% (36). Recently, Japanese authors have reported encouraging data that tumors <2 cm in diameter without peripancreatic infiltration or lymph node/liver metastases have a post-surgical 5-year survival rate of nearly 30% (37). The goals of diagnostic imaging include identification of a focal pancreatic mass, staging for determination of resectability, and FNA to confirm the diagnosis in a patient with unresectable tumor.

Ultrasound has been reported to have an 88–95% accuracy in determining the etiology and level of biliary obstruction in patients presenting with obstructive jaundice (38, 39). Ultrasound is most sensitive in detecting lesions in the head of

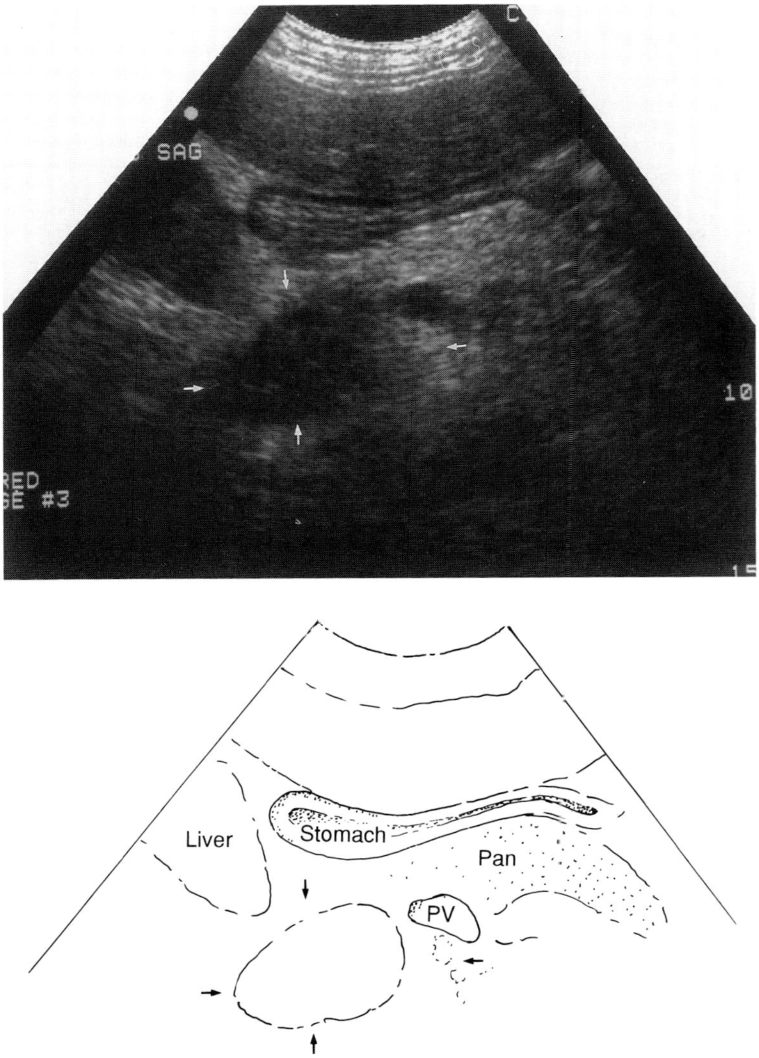

(A)

Figure 4. Adenocarcinoma of the pancreas: (A) A poorly marginated hypoechoic mass is seen in the pancreatic head (white arrows). (B, next page; C, page 436) Both the pancreatic duct (B) and common bile duct (arrow, C) are markedly dilated. (D) The splenic vein (arrowheads) is narrowed, suggesting tumor encasement of the vessel (page 436). (E) Multiple enlarged peripancreatic lymph nodes are seen (arrows) (page 436). Pathology: adenocarcinoma with portal and splenic vein invasion.

the pancreas because the body and tail may not be visualized in as many as 20–25% of patients (40). Sonographic findings of pancreatic carcinoma include a focal (rarely diffuse) hypoechoic, usually poorly marginated mass with associated dilatation of the pancreatic and/or common bile duct. However, these are nonspecific findings and may be seen with pancreatitis. Local and vascular invasion, hepatic and lymph

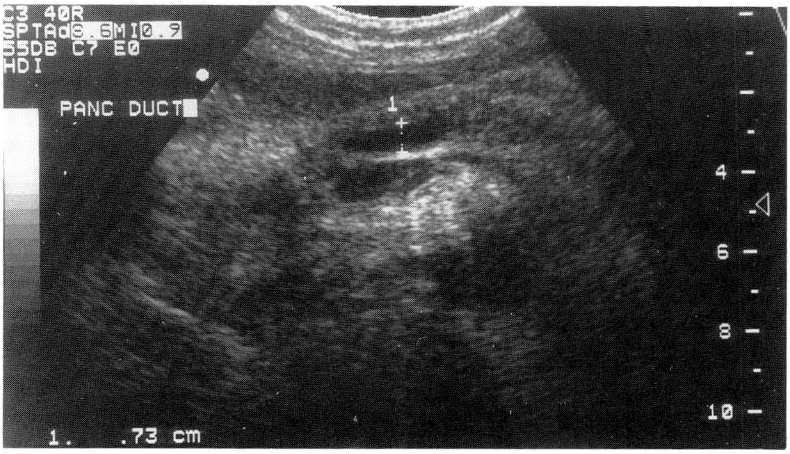

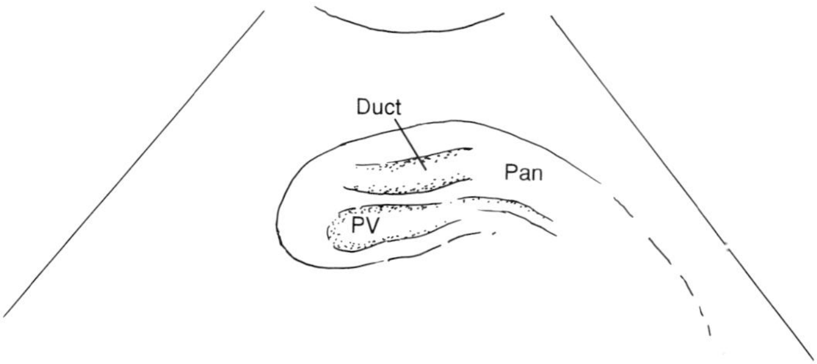

(B)

Figure 4. *(Continued)*

node metastases, and ascites are common ancillary findings and may also be documented on US examination (41) (Fig. 4).

Imaging findings that reliably predict unresectability include tumor larger than 2 cm, extracapsular extension, vascular invasion, lymphadenopathy, or metastatic disease. Computed tomography is clearly more sensitive than US in detecting spread of disease, and Freeny et al. (42) have reported that at least one of these findings was present in 92% of patients. Vascular involvement is most frequently seen (42). Whether detected by CT or US, these findings have a high positive predictive value for determining unresectability. However, the negative predictive value of these features is low. Many patients believed to be resectable on preoperative CT or US examination are found to have more extensive and unresectable tumor at surgery (42). When imaging findings suggest that the tumor is unresectable, percutaneous FNA is advocated to save the patient costly and debilitating surgery to confirm the diagnoses. Balen et al. (43) have shown that percutaneous biopsy does not adversely affect survival time for patients with inoperable pancreatic carcinoma. When a pancreatic mass is visualized on US, US-guided FNA has been reported to be more accurate than CT. Whether this is due to operator experience or real-time visualization during the procedure is not certain (44, 45).

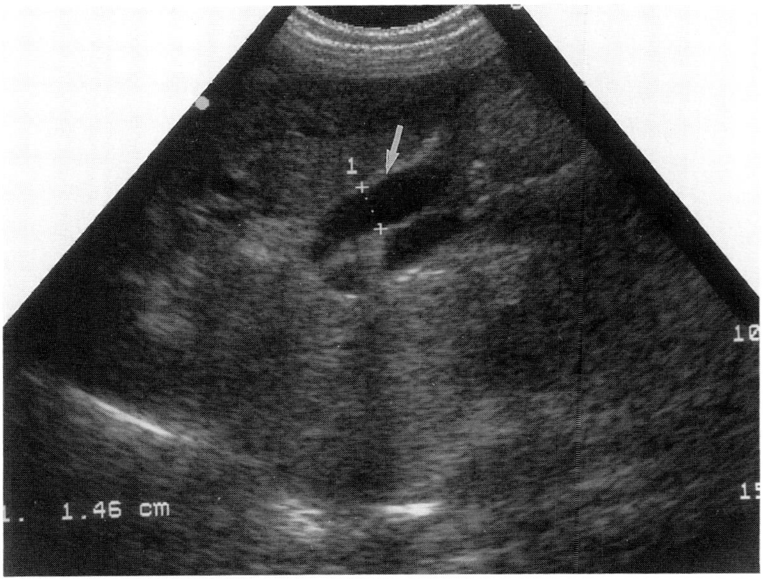

(C)

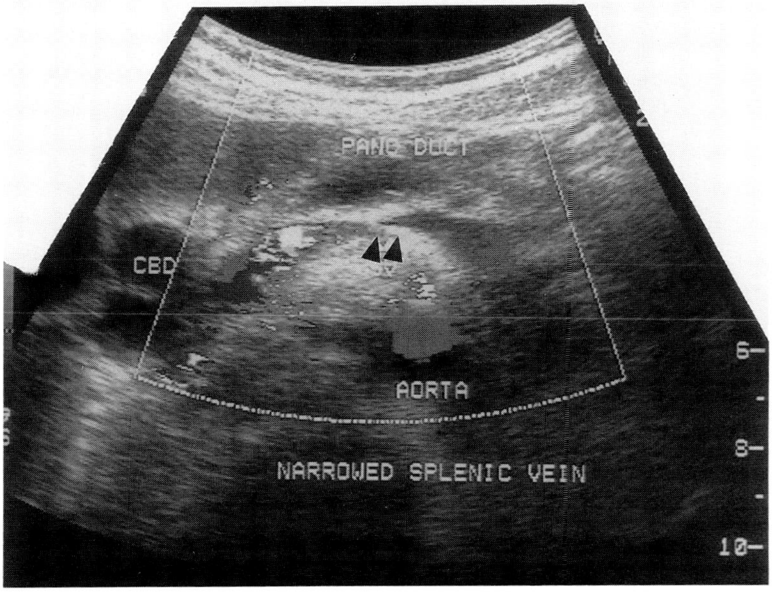

(D)

Figure 4. *(Continued)*

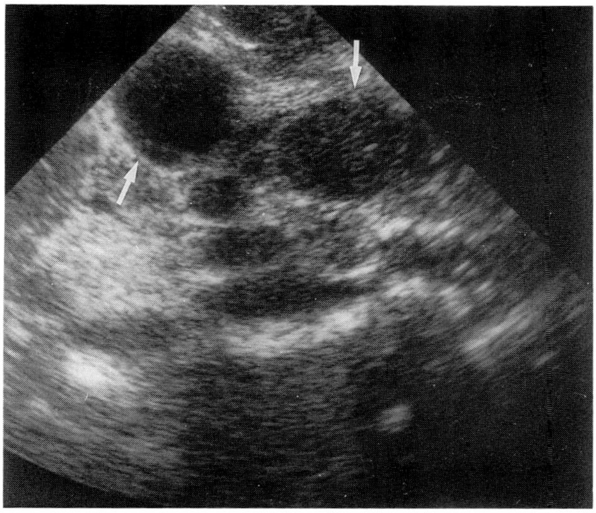

(E)

Figure 4. *(Continued)*

Endocrine Tumors of the Pancreas

Islet cell tumors of the pancreas derive from specialized cells within the pancreatic islets. These neoplasms may secrete hormones normally found in the adult pancreas (insulinoma, glucagonoma, somatostatinoma) or produce hormones found normally in fetal pancreas or other body parts (gastrinoma, VIPoma, carcinoid). Histology may be mixed and several peptides may be produced. Clinical presentation is related to the hormone produced. Patients with insulinomas present with hypoglycemia, gastrinomas with Zollinger–Ellison syndrome, glucagonomas with glucose intolerance and rash, and VIPomas with watery diarrhea/hypokalemic achlorhydria syndrome, for example. Islet cell tumors are small but very vascular tumors and are frequently multiple, particularly if associated with multiple endocrine neoplasia I syndrome. Insulinomas (60%) and gastrinomas (18%) are the most common islet cell tumors. Approximately 10% of insulinomas and 60% of gastrinomas are malignant. Other islet cell tumors are most often slow-growing malignant neoplasms, and metastases (most frequent to liver and lymph nodes) may be found at presentation (46, 47).

Radioimmunoassay and biochemistry establish the diagnosis. Imaging focuses on localizing the tumor because surgical excision may cure insulinomas and give patients with other islet cell tumors many years of symptom-free life (46, 47). Contrast-enhanced dynamic CT/MR angiography (because of increased tumor vascularity), portal venous sampling, as well as intraoperative US are more sensitive modalities than transabdominal ultrasound for the detection of these small lesions (48–52) (Table 1). In addition, because these lesions are often multiple, intraoperative US may be necessary to identify all lesions in order to guarantee surgical cure (53). On US examination these tumors appear as small, round or oval, well-

Table 1. Accuracy of techniques for localizing insulinomas

Authors	Year	Number of Patients	CT	Preoperative US	Angiography	Portal Venous Sampling	Palpation	IOUS
Gunther et al. (48)	1985	42	43	60	65	81	—	100
Grant et al. (49)	1988	36	27	59	55	—	—	90
Galiber et al. (50)	1988	52	30	61	54	—	91	84
Norton et al. (51)	1990	44	—	—	—	75	42	83
Bottger et al. (52)	1990	21	73	62	67	77	95	81

marginated, hypoechoic lesions. A hyperechoic capsule is sometimes seen. Malignant lesions may have an ill-defined border (46, 47). As many as 25–60% of insulinomas are detected preoperatively, whereas only 20% of gastrinomas are localized prior to surgery (48, 50, 54). Ultrasound examination may also be useful for identifying lymph node or liver metastases.

CYSTIC LESIONS OF THE PANCREAS

Congenital

Congenital cysts of the pancreas are rare and discovered most commonly in newborns. On ultrasound these appear as round anechoic structures with increased through transmission and no internal echoes. Ten percent of patients with adult polycystic kidney disease have multiple pancreatic cysts. Most often asymptomatic, these may be diffuse or localized and are rarely complicated by infection or hemorrhage. Patients with von Hippel–Lindau disease may also have numerous, although usually asymptomatic, pancreatic cysts (Fig. 5). Serous cystadenomas, islet cell tumors, and even adenocarcinomas have also been reported (55).

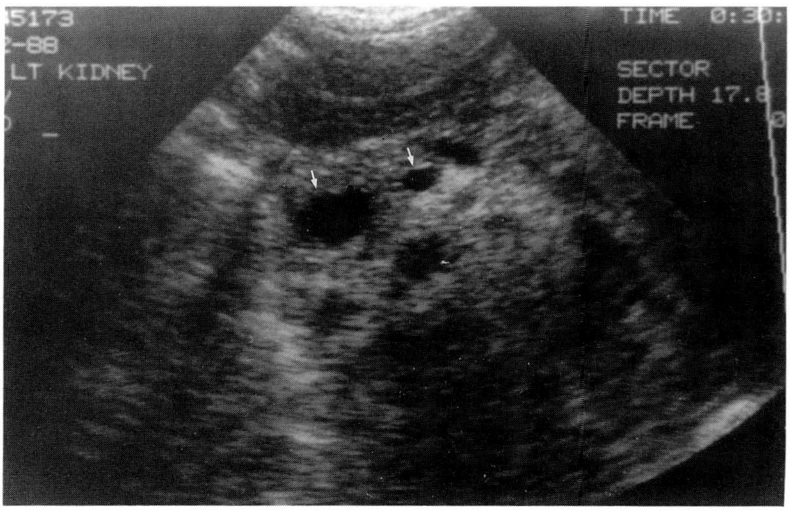

Figure 5. Multiple pancreatic cysts (arrows) in a patient with von Hippel–Lindau disease.

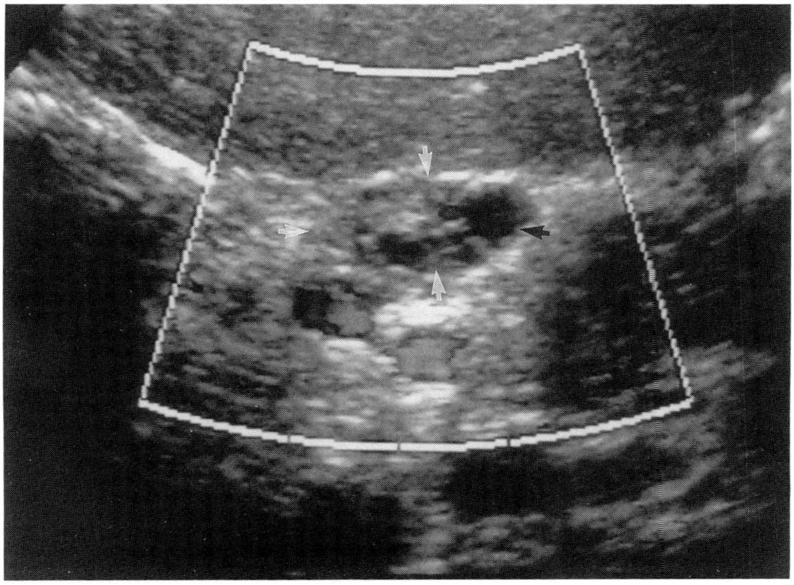

Figure 6. Cystic pancreatic neoplasm: a multilocular cystic mass is seen in the body of the pancreas which is well circumscribed and mildly echogenic (white arrows). The larger cysts (black arrow) are peripheral and measure less than 2 cm, typical for this lesion. Pathology: microcystic adenoma.

Cystic Neoplasm

Microcystic adenoma of the pancreas is a benign neoplasm occurring in older women. Patients present with nonspecific symptoms such as abdominal pressure or pain. These lesions are slow growing and may become quite large. Microcystic adenomas are composed of numerous small cysts (1 mm to 2 cm in size) filled with serous fluid, and 50% of patients have a characteristic central stellate scar that often calcifies (56–59). The size of the cysts determines the ultrasound appearance. When the cysts are smaller than 2 cm, a hyperechoic well-encapsulated mass with increased through transmission can be identified. A central calcified scar may rarely be seen. When the cysts are larger, discrete hypoechoic areas with increased through transmission are noted (56, 60) (Fig. 6).

Mucinous cystic neoplasms of the pancreas are considered potentially malignant if not frankly malignant at the time of diagnosis. These tumors occur in the middle-aged population, with a 10:1 female preponderance. They typically present with pain or abdominal mass and at pathology are irregular, lobulated masses with large cysts containing mucinous or hemorrhagic fluid and occasionally papillary projections. Mucinous cystic neoplasms occur most often in the tail or body of the pancreas (56, 58). On ultrasound examination a unilocular or multilocular cystic mass with good through transmission can be identified. Septations and mural nodularity are frequently observed and are seen better on US than on CT (56, 60). A mucinous ductectatic subtype has been described. This subtype is typically located in the uncinate process and mucoid plugs are seen in dilated branches of the pancreatic duct that communicate with the cyst. Endoscopic retrograde cholangio-

Table 2. Evaluation of cyst fluid indices in cystic pancreatic neoplasms[a]

Diagnosis	Viscosity	Glycogen	Amylase	CEA (ng/ml)	CA 15.3	CA 72-4	Cytology
Pseudocyst	Low	−	+	Low	Low	Low	−
Microcystic adenoma	Low	+	−	Low	Low	Low	50%+
Macrocystic adenoma	High	−	Often +	High	Low	Intermediate	Usually +
Cystadenocarcinoma	High	−	Often +	High	High	High	Usually +

[a] Modified with permission from Rosenfield, AT. Editorial: the evaluation of pancreatic cysts. *J Clin Gastroenterol.* 1995;20:94–95.

pancreatography may be required for definitive diagnosis (56). With careful and complete analysis, FNA of cystic pancreatic neoplasms has been reported to be extremely helpful in differentiation between pseudocysts and microcystic adenomas, which are benign lesions and may be followed, and between macrocystic adenomas, which are considered premalignant, and cystic pancreatic carcinomas, both of which require surgery (61) (Table 2).

INTRAOPERATIVE ULTRASOUND

Intraoperative US examination of the pancreas requires small scan-head configuration, high-frequency (7.5–10 MHz) linear array transducers with good near-field resolution. Occasionally saline baths may be necessary to visualize superficial lesions, and the uncinate process or pancreatic tail may have to be mobilized for complete evaluation. Intraoperative US (IOUS) is most efficacious in the localization of small, nonpalpable pancreatic neoplasms, particularly islet cell tumors, for resection or biopsy. A more limited role for IOUS has been described for evaluation of extrapancreatic spread of pancreatic adenocarcinoma and for surgical treatment of complications of acute pancreatitis.

Despite preoperative imaging techniques that include US, CT, MRI, and portal venous sampling, 10–20% of insulinomas are undetected even by experienced surgeons owing to their small size (53) (Table 1). Seventy percent of insulinomas measure 1.5 cm or less and 40% measure less than 1 cm (49). When lesions cannot be localized blind distal pancreatectomy is performed, but this is suboptimal owing to significant morbidity and the potential to miss lesions in the head of the pancreas (62). Several recent studies have reported that IOUS has an accuracy in detecting insulinomas ranging from 81 to 100% (48–52) (Table 1). On IOUS, islet cell tumors are typically small, round or oval, well-marginated hypoechoic lesions (Fig. 7). Malignancy is suggested if the tumor margin is irregular or indistinct. Intraoperative US is complementary to palpation, for IOUS has been reported to identify nonpalpable lesions and vice versa (50, 51). Galiber et al. (50) reported that IOUS and palpation had a combined sensitivity of 100%. In addition, Grant et al. (49) reported that IOUS provided information that influenced surgical management in 62% of patients. For example, accurate assessment of the proximity of a lesion to the pancreatic duct and blood vessels helps to avoid injury during dissection. In addition, identification of lymph node or liver metastases as well as size and extent of the lesion are important in determining if enucleation or more extensive pancreatic

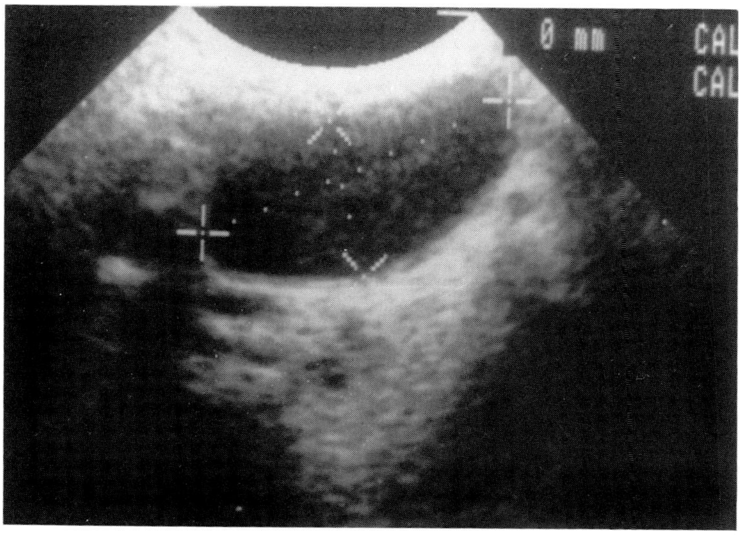

Figure 7. Islet cell tumor: Well-circumscribed hypoechoic mass in body of pancreas seen here on intraoperative ultrasound. Pathology: benign insulinoma.

resection is required (63). Intraoperative ultrasound is also extremely helpful in identifying or screening for multiple insulinomas. IOUS is less helpful in identifying extrapancreatic lesions, and less experience has been reported with other islet cell tumors. Preliminary studies have also shown IOUS effective in localizing gastrinomas, although the clinical significance of this information may be limited given that these tumors are more likely to be malignant (64).

In patients with ductal adenocarcinoma of the pancreas, IOUS may occasionally be helpful in identifying small nonpalpable lesions, evaluating extrapancreatic spread of disease to vascular structures, liver, and lymph nodes, and guiding intraoperative biopsy (65–67). Plainfosse et al. (67) reported a series of 22 patients with suspected pancreatic carcinoma in whom IOUS revealed two previously undetected carcinomas and was considered at least moderately helpful in evaluating extrapancreatic spread in 50% of patients, thereby helping to direct surgical management. Rifkin and Weiss (66) reported two patients with unexplained jaundice and dilated ducts without palpable masses in whom IOUS identified very small pancreatic carcinomas. Ultrasound features on IOUS of pancreatic carcinomas are similar to transabdominal imaging, with lesions appearing hypoechoic and poorly marginated.

In 1984 Siegel et al. (65) reported that IOUS was helpful in patients undergoing surgery for pancreatitis. In his hands, IOUS was judged to be useful in 69% of patients, primarily in identifying or excluding unsuspected pseudocysts and determining the relationship of fluid collections (pseudocysts/abscess) to the pancreatic duct or vascular structures.

REFERENCES

1. Lund PJ, Fritz TA, Unger EC, Hunt RK, Fuller E. Cellulose as a gastrointestinal US contrast agent. *Radiology.* 1992;185:783–788.

2. Parulekar S. Ultrasonic evaluation of pancreatic duct. *J Clin Roentgenol.* 1981;8:457.
3. Lawson T, Berland L, Foley W, et al. Ultrasonic visualization of pancreatic duct. *Radiology,* 1982;144:865.
4. Sarner M, Cotton PB. Classification of pancreatitis. *Gut.* 1984;25:756–759.
5. Moosa AR. Diagnostic tests and procedures in acute pancreatitis. *N Engl J Med.* 1984;311:639–643.
6. Ranson JHC. Etiological and prognostic factors in human acute pancreatitis: A review. *Am J Gastroenterol.* 1982;77:633–638.
7. Laing FC, Jeffrey RB, Wing VW. Improved visualization of choledocholithiasis by sonography. *AJR.* 1984;143:949–952.
8. Dong B, Chen M. Improved sonographic visualization of choledocholithiasis. *J Clin Ultrasound.* 1987;15:185–190.
9. Laing FC, Jeffrey RB, Wing VW. Biliary dilatation: defining the level and cause by real-time US. *Radiology.* 1986;160:39–42.
10. Freise J. Evaluation of sonography in the diagnosis of acute pancreatitis. In: Beger HG, Büchler M, eds. *Acute Pancreatitis.* Berlin: Springer-Verlag; 1987:118–131.
11. Jeffrey RB, Laing FC, Wing VW. Extrapancreatic spread of acute pancreatitis: new observations with real-time US. *Radiology.* 1983;147:185–188.
12. vanSonnenberg E, Casola G, Varney RR, Wittich GR. Imaging and interventional radiology for pancreatitis and its complications. *Radiol Clin North Am.* 1989;27:65–72.
13. Balthazar EJ, Freeny PC, vanSonnenberg E. Imaging and intervention in acute pancreatitis. *Radiology.* 1994;193:297–306.
14. vanSonnenberg E, Wittich GR, Casola G, et al. Percutaneous drainage of infected and noninfected pancreatic pseudocysts: experience in 101 cases. *Radiology.* 1989;170: 757–761.
15. Grosso M, Gandini G, Cassinis M, et al. Percutaneous treatment (including pseudocystogastrostomy) of 74 pancreatic pseudocysts. *Radiology.* 1989;173:493–497.
16. Matzinger F, Ho CS, Yee A, Gray R. Pancreatic pseudocysts drained through a percutaneous transgastric approach: further experience. *Radiology.* 1988;167:431–434.
17. Steiner E, Mueller PR, Hahn PF, et al. Complicated pancreatic abscesses: problems in interventional management. *Radiology.* 1988;167:443–446.
18. vanSonnenberg E, Wittich G, Casola G, et al. Complicated pancreatic inflammatory disease: diagnostic and therapeutic role of interventional radiology. *Radiology.* 1985;155:335–340.
19. Adams D, Harvey T, Anderson M. Percutaneous drainage of infected pancreatic and peripancreatic fluid collections. *Arch Surg.* 1990;125:1554–1557.
20. Beger H, Maier W, Block S, Büchler M. How do imaging methods influence the surgical strategy in acute pancreatitis? In: Malfertheiner P, Ditchuneit H, eds. *Diagnostic Procedures in Pancreatic Disease.* Berlin: Springer-Verlag; 1986:54–60.
21. Banks P. The role of needle-aspiration bacteriology in the management of necrotizing pancreatitis. In: Bradley E III, ed. *Acute Pancreatitis: Diagnosis and Therapy.* New York: Raven Press; 1994:99–103.
22. Büchler M, Uhl W, Beger H. Acute pancreatitis: when and how to operate. *Dig Dis Sci.* 1992;10:354–362.
23. Ates KB, Boyacioglu S, Tas I, et al. The ultrasonographic diagnosis of bleeding into a pancreatic pseudocyst. *Gastrointest Radiol.* 1991;16:178–180.
24. Vujic I. Vascular complications of pancreatitis. *Radiol Clin North Am.* 1989;27:81–91.

25. Kahn LA, Kamen C, McNamara MP Jr. Variable color Doppler appearance of pseudoaneurysm in pancreatitis. *AJR.* 1994;162:187–188.
26. Gooding GA. Ultrasound of a superior mesenteric aneurysm secondary to pancreatitis: a plea for real-time ultrasound of sonolucent masses in pancreatitis. *J Clin Ultrasound.* 1981;9:255–256.
27. Golzarian J, Braude P, Bank WO, et al. Case report: colour Doppler demonstration of pseudoaneurysms complicating pancreatic pseudocysts. *Br J Radiol.* 1994;67:91–93.
28. Falkoff GE, Taylor KJW, Morse S. Hepatic artery pseudoaneurysms: diagnosis with real-time and pulsed Doppler US. *Radiology.* 1986;158:55–56.
29. Bolondi L, LiBassi S, Gaiani S, Barbara L. Sonography of chronic pancreatitis. *Radiol Clin North Am.* 1989;27:815–833.
30. Ralls PW, Halls J, Renner I, Juttner H. Endoscopic retrograde cholangiopancreatography (ERCP) in pancreatic disease. *Radiology.* 1980;134:347–352.
31. Malfertheiner P, Büchler M. Correlation of imaging and function in chronic pancreatitis. *Radiol Clin North Am.* 1989;27:51–64.
32. DelMaschio A, Vanzulli A, Sironi S, et al. Pancreatic cancer versus chronic pancreatitis: diagnosis with CA 19-9 assessment, US, CT, and CT-guided fine-needle biopsy. *Radiology.* 1991;178:95–99.
33. Wingo PA, Tong T, Bolden S. Cancer statistics, 1995. *CA Cancer J Clin.* 1995;45:8–30.
34. Baert AL, Rigauts H, Marchal G. Ductal adenocarcinoma. In: Baert AL, ed. *Radiology of the Pancreas.* New York: Springer-Verlag; 1994:129–172.
35. Friedman AC, Krudy AG Jr, Shawker TH, et al. Pancreatic neoplasms. In: *Radiology of the Liver, Biliary Tract, Pancreas, and Spleen.* Baltimore: Williams and Wilkins; 1987:735–837.
36. Klöppel G, Maillet B. Classification and staging of pancreatic nonendocrine tumors. *Radiol Clin North Am.* 1989;27:105–119.
37. Tsuchiya R, Noda T, Harada N, et al. Collective review of small carcinomas of the pancreas. *Ann Surg.* 1986;203:77–81.
38. Gibson RN, Yeung E, Thompson JN, et al. Bile duct obstruction: radiologic evaluation of level, cause, and tumor resectability. *Radiology.* 1986;160:43–47.
39. Laing FC, Jeffrey RB Jr, Wing VW, et al. Biliary dilatation: defining the level and cause by real-time ultrasound. *Radiology.* 1986;160:39–42.
40. Freeny PC, Lawson TL. *Radiology of the Pancreas.* New York: Springer-Verlag; 1982:397–496.
41. Freeny PC. Radiologic diagnosis and staging of pancreatic ductal adenocarcinoma. *Radiol Clin North Am.* 1989;27:121–128.
42. Freeny PC, Marks WM, Ryan JA, et al. Pancreatic ductal adenocarcinoma: diagnosis and staging with dynamic CT. *Radiology.* 1988;166:125–133.
43. Balen FG, Little A, Smith AC, et al. Biopsy of inoperable pancreatic tumors does not adversely influence patient survival time. *Radiology.* 1994;193:753–755.
44. Brandt KR, Charboneau JW, Stephens DH, et al. CT and US-guided biopsy of the pancreas. *Radiology.* 1993;187:99–104.
45. DelMaschio A, Vanzulli A, Sironi S, et al. Pancreatic cancer versus chronic pancreatitis: diagnosis with CA 19-9 assessment, US, CT, and CT-guided fine-needle biopsy. *Radiology.* 1991;187:95–99.
46. King CMP, Reznek RH, Dacie JE, Wass JAH. Imaging islet cell tumors. *Clin Radiol.* 1994;49:295–303.
47. Rossi P, Allison DJ, Bezzi M, et al. Endocrine tumors of the pancreas. *Radiol Clin North Am.* 1989;27:129–161.

48. Gunther RW, Klose KJ, Ruckert K, et al. Localization of small islet-cell tumors with preoperative and intraoperative ultrasound, computed tomography, arteriography, digital subtraction angiography, and pancreatic venous sampling. *Gastrointest Radiol.* 1988; 10:145.
49. Grant CS, van Heerden J, Charboneau JW, et al. Insulinoma. *Arch Surg.* 1988;123:843.
50. Galiber AK, Reading CC, Charboneau JW, et al. Localization of pancreatic insulinoma: comparison of pre- and intraoperative US with CT and angiography. *Radiology.* 1988;166:405.
51. Norton JA, Cromack DT, Shawker TH, et al. Intraoperative ultrasonographic localization of islet cell tumors. A prospective comparison to palpation. *Ann Surg.* 1988;207:160–168.
52. Bottger TC, Weber W, Beyer J, Junginger T. Value of tumor localization in patients with insulinoma. *World J Surg.* 1990;14:107.
53. Dunnington GL. Intraoperative ultrasonography in abdominal surgery. *Surg Ann.* 1993;25:101–125.
54. Gorman B, Charboneau JW, James EM, et al. Benign pancreatic insulinoma: preoperative and intraoperative sonographic localization. *AJR.* 1986;147:929.
55. Choyke PL, Glenn GM, McClellan MW, Patronas NJ, et al. von Hippel-Lindau disease: genetic, clinical, and imaging features. *Radiology.* 1995;194:629–642.
56. Mathieu D, Guigui B, Valette PJ, et al. Pancreatic cystic neoplasms. *Radiol Clin North Am.* 1989;27:163–176.
57. Buck JL, Hayes WS. Microcystic adenoma of the pancreas. *Radiographics.* 1990; 10:313–322.
58. Ros PR, Hamrick-Turner JE, Chiechi MV, et al. Cystic masses of the pancreas. *Radiographics.* 1992;12:673–686.
59. Friedman AC, Lichtenstein JE, Dachman AH. Cystic neoplasms of the pancreas. *Radiology.* 1983;149:45–50.
60. Fugazzola C, Procacci C, Andreis IAB, et al. Cystic tumors of the pancreas: evaluation by ultrasonography and computed tomography. *Gastrointest Radiol.* 1991;16:53–61.
61. Rosenfield AT. Editorial: the evaluation of pancreatic cysts. *J Clin Gastroenterol.* 1995;20:94–95.
62. Mozell E, Stenzel P, Woltering EA, et al. Functional endocrine tumors of the pancreas: clinical presentation, diagnosis, and treatment. *Curr Probl Surg.* 1990;27:301–386.
63. Norton JA, Shawker TH, Doppman JL, et al. Localization and surgical treatment of occult insulinomas. *Ann Surg.* 1990;212:615–620.
64. Ruckert KF, Klotter HJ, Kummerle F. Intraoperative ultrasonic localization of endocrine tumors of the pancreas. *Surgery.* 1984;96:1045.
65. Siegel B, Machi J, Ramos JR, et al. The role of imaging ultrasound during pancreatic surgery. *Ann Surg.* 1984;200:486–493.
66. Rifkin MD, Weiss SM. Intraoperative sonographic identification of nonpalpable pancreatic masses. *J Ultrasound Med.* 1984;3:409.
67. Plainfosse MC, Bouillot JL, Rivaton F, et al. The use of operative sonography in carcinoma of the pancreas. *World J Surg.* 1987;11:654.

22

COMPUTED TOMOGRAPHY

Robert K. Zeman, M.D.
University of Vermont College of Medicine
Burlington, VT

Paul M. Silverman, M.D.
Georgetown University Medical Center
Washington, DC

Computed tomography (CT) has long been used to evaluate the pancreas for neoplastic and inflammatory conditions. Since 1992, helical (spiral) CT has been commercially available, and has proved to be a major technological breakthrough in the CT field (1, 2). This chapter reviews the CT approach to pancreatic disease, advantages and technical issues in helical CT, detection and characterization of pancreatic neoplasms, and assessment of pancreatitis and its complications (3).

DIAGNOSIS OF PANCREATIC DISEASE

Computed tomography is the dominant modality for screening evaluation of the pancreas for neoplasm and complications of pancreatitis. Although CT entails radiation exposure and the use of iodinated contrast material, it almost always results in a diagnostic study. Computed tomography allows visualization of the entire gland far more frequently than conventional transabdominal ultrasound. In the future, use of oral ultrasound contrast agents may allow transgastric acoustic transmission with better delineation of the relationship between the duodenum and pancreas. Visualization of the pancreatic tail, however, may continue to be hampered by the presence of gas within the jejunum and splenic flexure. Magnetic resonance imaging (MRI) is increasingly being used to evaluate the pancreas, but its role is generally limited to studying patients with contrast allergies or renal failure, or in whom the diagnosis is unclear using cross-sectional modalities or endoscopic retrograde cholangiopancreatography (ERCP).

ADVANTAGES OF HELICAL COMPUTED TOMOGRAPHY

Helical CT clearly has advantages over conventional scanning for evaluation of the pancreas (3). Despite the patient advancing through the gantry during the scan acquisition, high-quality images are possible because special reconstruction algorithms are used to correct for this motion (4) (Fig. 1). Because the scan acquisition requires no more than 30–40 sec, the entire scan may be completed while the circulating contrast level is at its peak. This maximizes the attenuation differences between normal pancreatic parenchyma and neoplasms. During helical scanning the patient is instructed to hold his or her breath during the entire acquisition of scan data. This serves to reduce misregistration artifacts. These artifacts occur frequently during conventional scanning owing to variation in the degree of patient inspiration as the breath is held for each individual slice. Misregistration makes it difficult to identify small pancreatic tumors when using conventional CT.

Because the helical acquisition is volumetric, the spacing or interval between reconstructed sections may be varied and may be selected by the radiologist even after the scan acquisition has been completed. Although the collimation is determined by the X-ray tube collimators at the time of acquisition, the spacing is independently selectable. Many scanners allow reconstruction spacing in increments as small as 0.5 cm. If the reconstruction spacing selected is less than the collimation, overlapping sections result. The ability to relocate scan sections offers great advantage for visualization of small pancreatic tumors, especially those that straddle two adjacent slices (Fig. 2). Similarly, short segments of vascular encasement may readily be evaluated using overlapping reconstruction. Overlapping reconstruction does not entail additional radiation exposure to the patient.

TECHNICAL ISSUES IN HELICAL COMPUTED TOMOGRAPHY

Many of the principles for the helical evaluation of the pancreas are based on years of experience using conventional scanning (5). Both oral and intravenous contrast agents are needed to produce an optimal examination of the pancreas. The gastrointestinal tract may be opacified either with dilute barium, water-soluble iodinated contrast or with a negative opacification agent such as water and an effervescent agent or a carbonated beverage. In patients in whom neoplasm is the primary concern, negative opacification of the duodenum may be helpful in recognizing tumor invasion of the duodenal wall. In the setting of pancreatitis we generally administer dilute barium so as not to confuse unopacified bowel loops with peripancreatic fluid collections. Precontrast, nonhelical sections are obtained to localize the pancreas prior to the helical acquisition.

A single helical "run" or "pass" is performed through the pancreas, using an exposure length of about 30 sec. Most patients can easily hold their breath for this interval. A collimation of 5 mm is used. Thicker sections may be used in the evaluation of patients with pancreatitis, but not for screening patients for neoplasm. Small tumors may not be evident on sections whose thickness approaches the size of the lesion. Most of the liver is included in the helical scan, but those portions that are not are scanned nonhelically immediately after the conclusion of the helical scan.

Intravenous contrast material should be administered at a minimum rate of 2

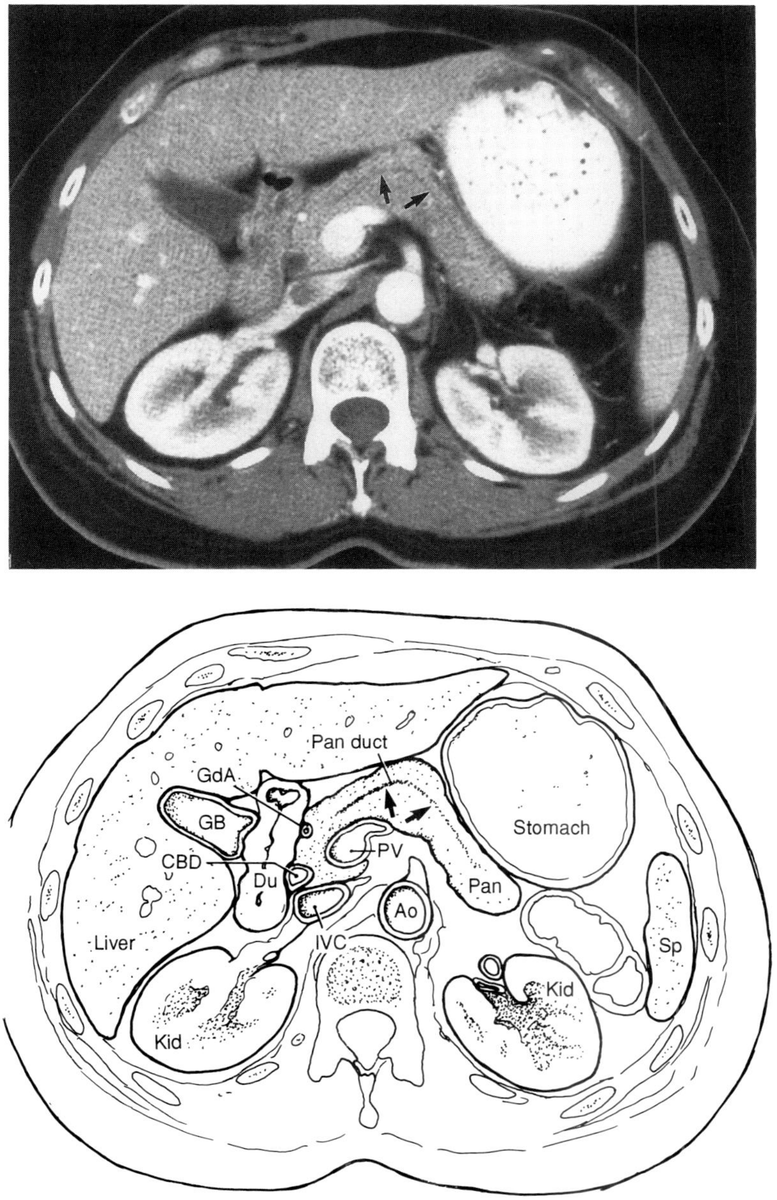

Figure 1. Excellent image quality obtained by helical scanning. This 5-mm section clearly shows the normal pancreatic duct (arrows). Despite the slightly broader section sensitivity profile of helical sections, excellent clinical image quality may be obtained. Courtesy of Robert K. Zeman, M.D. (3).

mL/sec and preferably at a rate of 3 mL/sec. The higher rate is used in patients in whom intravenous access can be obtained via a 20-gauge catheter. The lower injection rate is used in patients in whom only a 22-gauge needle or catheter may be placed. A minimum of 125 mL is needed to opacify the portal vein and enhance the liver adequately. The portal vein must be well opacified to recognize encasement

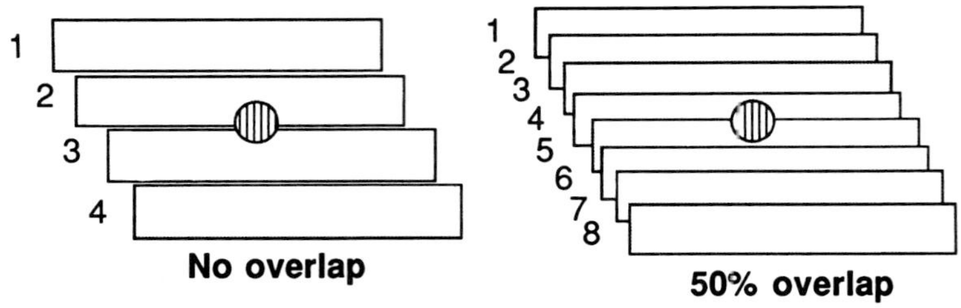

(A)

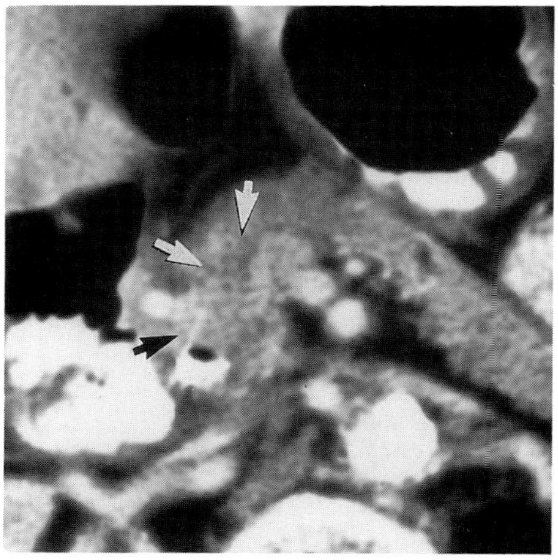

(B)

Figure 2. Use of overlapping sections. (A) Small lesions may not be well visualized, owing to partial volume averaging, when they straddle two adjacent sections (left). When overlapping scans are reconstructed, it is possible to visualize a small lesion better by centering it within the reconstructed slice (right). Reconstruction of overlapping slices increases the number of sections that the radiologist must interpret, so this technique is used selectively only when indicated. (B) Improved definition of cholangiocarcinoma by retrospectively shifting slice location of the helical CT scan. Helical CT scan obtained with 5-mm collimation reconstructed every 5 mm shows questionable fullness of the pancreatic head compared with caliber of rest of gland. The gland contour is irregular and of slightly lower attenuation (arrows). Biliary stent is present (C, next page). After retrospective overlapping reconstruction of the scans at 3-mm spacing, this slice was located 1 mm cephalad to that of Fig. 2B. Despite the slice location looking quite similar to that of 2B, note how the low attenuation of the mass (arrows) is accentuated and encasement of the pancreaticoduodenal vein branches draining into the gastrocolic trunk (arrowhead) is better defined. Slight changes in scan location can greatly affect appearance of small tumors. This patient had an unresectable cholangiocarcinoma of the distal bile duct infiltrating pancreatic head. Courtesy of *American Journal of Roentgenology* (2).

by tumor when present. Detection of hypovascular hepatic metastases from pancreatic carcinoma also requires optimal enhancement so as to identify small or infiltrative lesions. Some groups have reduced the volume of contrast even further (down to 90–100 mL) (6), but we would caution against this. The pancreas may show adequate enhancement with this volume of contrast, but the portal vein and liver do not. If the liver is not adequately enhanced, liver metastases may easily be overlooked (7, 8). Either 60% ionic contrast or 300 mgI/mL nonionic contrast material may be used.

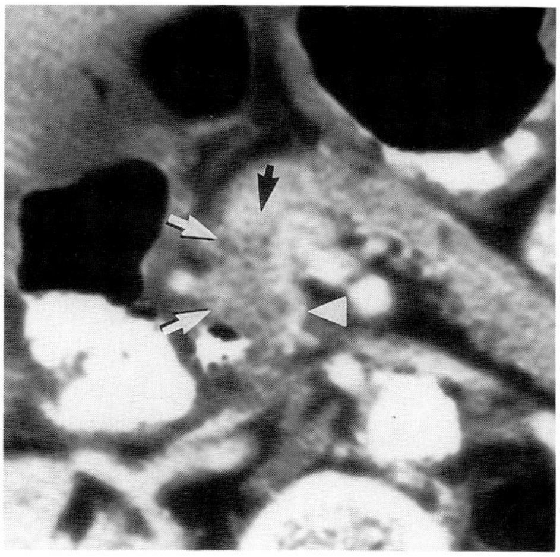

(C)

Figure 2. *(Continued)*

Some centers are injecting contrast material at rates up to 5.0 mL/sec. It has not been shown definitively that these high injection rates result in greater diagnostic accuracy than a 2–3 mL/sec contrast injection for the detection of pancreatic pathology. Biphasic scanning of the pancreas during both the arterial and portal venous phases may prove of value in the detection of small pancreatic lesions (11), but this too has not been conclusively shown to be superior to scans obtained only in the portal venous phase. In our practice we have seen some very small tumors exhibit progressive equilibration and "filling in" with contrast material between the arterial and venous phase, but this is quite rare. Most lesions enlarge the contour of the gland and are of lower attenuation than the normal pancreatic parenchyma in both the arterial and portal venous phase. Although scanning the pancreas during the arterial phase may prove to be a useful adjunct, portal venous phase scans will always be necessary for evaluation of the liver in patients with suspected pancreatic carcinoma (11).

DETECTION AND CHARACTERIZATION OF PANCREATIC NEOPLASMS

Pancreatic Adenocarcinoma

Pancreatic carcinoma is one of the most lethal neoplasms afflicting humankind; nearly 25,000 cases are reported each year in the United States with less than a 5% long-term survival. Even at presentation, the lack of a true capsule surrounding the tumor results in diffuse retroperitoneal infiltration and encasement of the splanchnic vessels in most patients. In order to be clinically useful, CT must play two important roles in the evaluation of pancreatic carcinoma. It must be capable of accurately detecting the presence of neoplasm, and the neoplasm must be accurately staged.

Although much progress has been made, detection of subtle vascular involvement and differentiation of T2 from T3 lesions remains problematic (12). Lesions with borderline vascular involvement generally require surgical exploration regardless of what the CT, endoscopic ultrasound (EUS), or MRI may show.

The hallmark of pancreatic carcinoma is focal enlargement with an asymmetric glandular contour. At times, tumor infiltrates the gland and produces diffuse enlargement. Secondary acute or chronic pancreatitis can also develop from pancreatic duct obstruction by neoplasm. In these cases, the gland may enlarge even further, and the presence of edema may cause the radiologist to overestimate the volume of tumor.

Most pancreatic cancers are of lower attenuation than normal-enhancing pancreatic parenchyma. Because helical scans are performed while the circulating contrast level is high, we are increasingly identifying small tumors that do not enlarge the contour of the gland, but represent an area of reduced attenuation (Fig. 2). This experience parallels that occurring using MRI with gadolinium enhancement. Although most carcinomas are of low attenuation, a small minority may actually be of increased attenuation and mimic hypervascular lesions such as islet cell carcinoma (see below). The radiologist must carefully scrutinize overlapping sections for subtle areas of decreased attenuation because this may be the only way to detect subtle tumors while they are still resectable.

Although areas of decreased attenuation within the pancreas often signify tumor, this is not always the case. In the setting of acute or chronic pancreatitis, areas of decreased or increased perfusion of the gland may occur, often in association with phlegmonous change. It is unusual for patients with carcinoma to present with pancreatitis, but this may occur. Whenever a low-attenuation mass in the inflamed pancreas persists, and is not clearly an evolving pseudocyst, percutaneous biopsy and/or ERCP is warranted. Focal fatty infiltration of the pancreas, as a manifestation of chronic atrophy, is also increasingly being recognized and should not be confused with tumor. This may especially occur in the dorsal anlage of the pancreas in patients with pancreas divisum (13).

Carcinoma often produces the so-called "double duct" sign. This refers to concomitant obstruction of the bile duct and the pancreatic duct (14) (Fig. 3). The diagnosis of malignant obstruction on CT is suggested when a focal tumor mass is present in association with high-grade, abrupt amputation of the bile duct and pancreatic duct. As on cholangiography, an abrupt transition zone at the level of a biliary or pancreatic duct stricture suggests malignancy (15). Whenever a pancreatic mass or "double duct" sign is identified, biopsy of the suspicious area is warranted.

There are three other types of lesions that may also produce the "double duct sign" (16, 17). Carcinoma of the ampulla can obstruct the intraduodenal segment of the bile duct as well as the pancreatic duct. At times cholangiocarcinoma may rarely extend outward from the distal bile duct to obstruct the pancreatic duct. Chronic pancreatitis may also result in a stricture of both the bile duct and the pancreatic duct. In our experience only 10% of patients with the "double duct sign" have chronic pancreatitis.

Resection of pancreatic carcinoma is precluded in patients with hepatic metastases, nodal involvement beyond the field of resection, or vascular encasement. Although the pancreaticoduodenal nodes are removed at the time of Whipple resec-

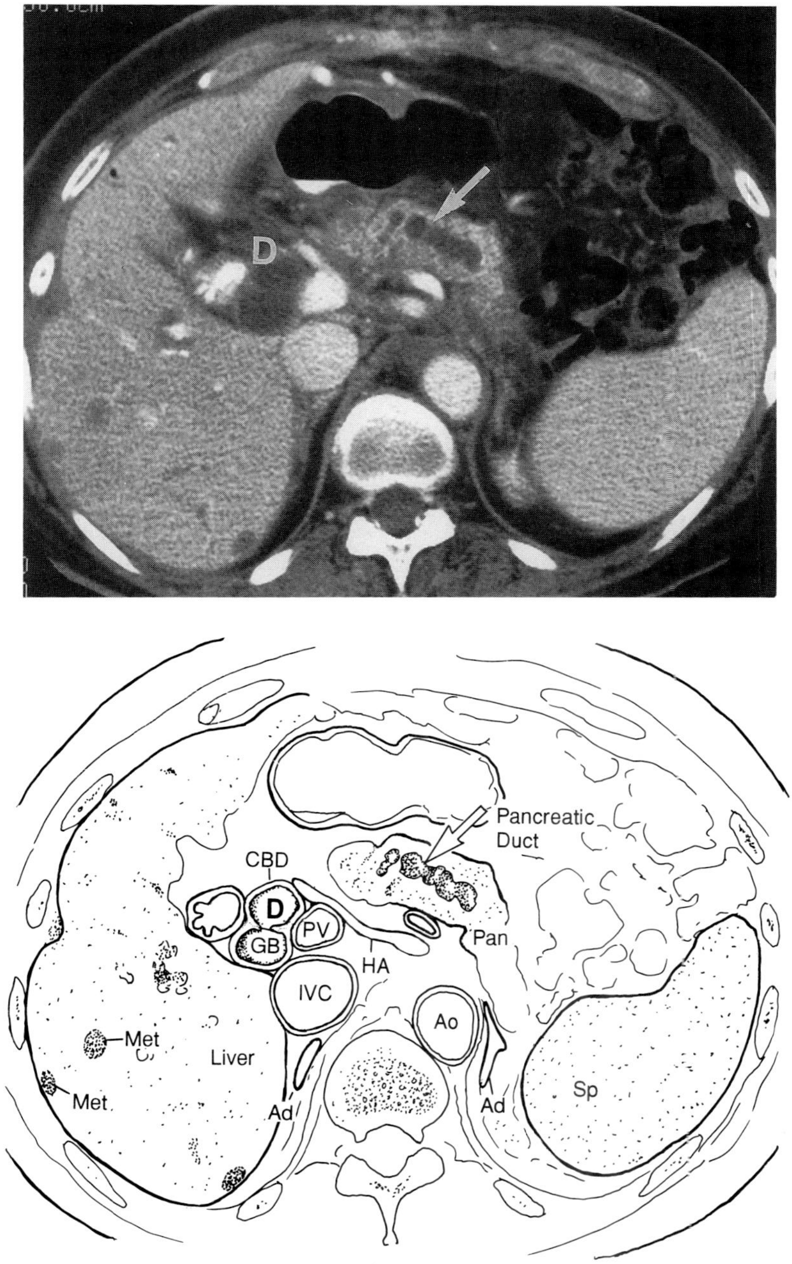

A

Figure 3. Obstruction of the pancreatic duct and bile duct by pancreatic carcinoma. (A) 5-mm collimation helical scan of the pancreas shows dilatation of the pancreatic duct (arrow) and bile duct (D). When both the pancreatic duct and bile duct are obstructed, the most likely etiology is pancreatic carcinoma. Chronic pancreatitis is much less likely to produce obstruction of both ducts. (B) On this section 1 cm below that of Fig. 3A a necrotic pancreatic carcinoma is present (M). There is flattening of the lateral edge of the superior mesenteric vein (arrow). The tumor was adherent to this surface of the vessel at surgery (next page). Courtesy of Robert K. Zeman et al. (1).

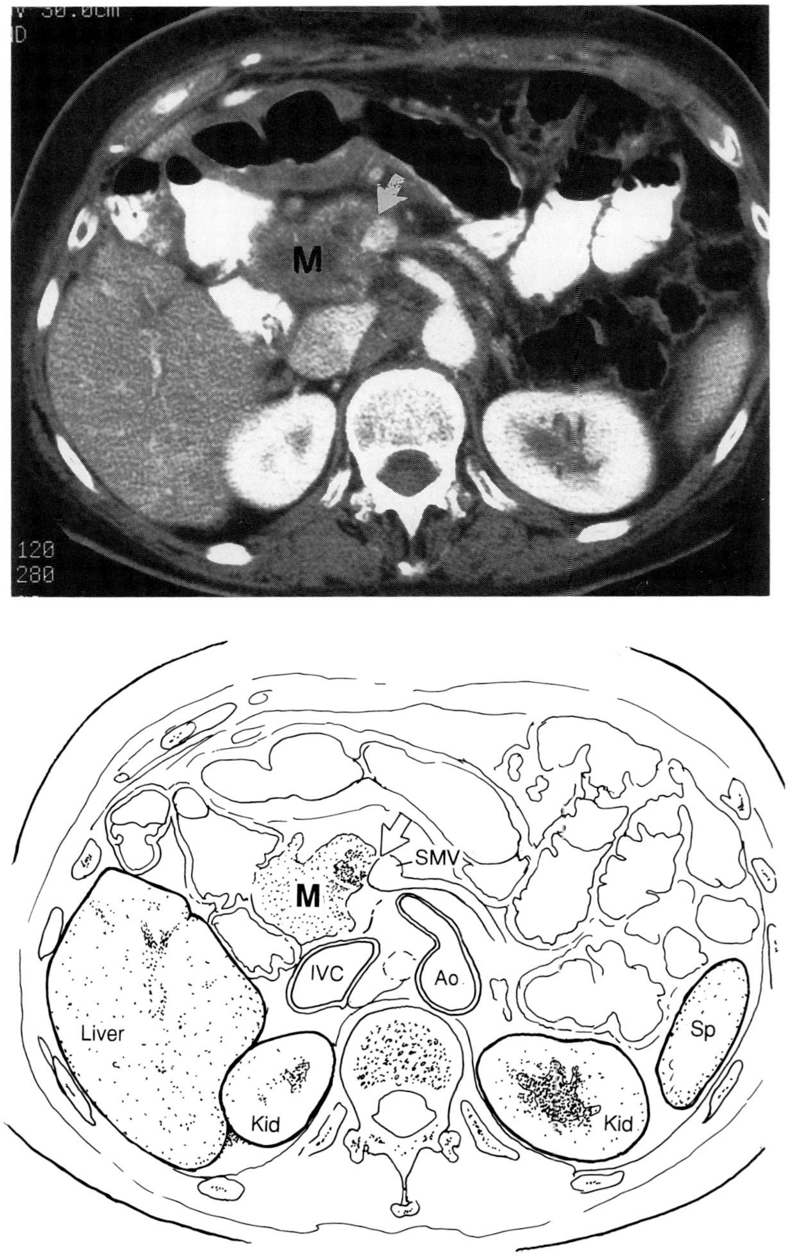

B

Figure 3. *(Continued)*

tion, the portal, celiac, and para-aortic nodes are not included in the resected specimen.

Both CT and EUS may characterize lesions using the TNM staging scheme suggested by the American Joint Committee on Cancer and the International Union Against Cancer (18). T1 lesions are confined to the pancreas (A < 2 cm, B > 2 cm); T2 lesions extend into the duodenum, bile duct, or peripancreatic tissues, and T3 lesions involve the major arteries or veins, stomach, spleen, or colon. Nodal disease is N0 (no regional nodes) or N1 (positive regional nodes). Distant disease is categorized as M0 (no distant disease) or M1 (positive for distant disease). Although this scheme does not address resectability per se, local disease that is T3 is generally not resectable.

Encasement of the major vessels implies nonresectability. The presence of overt caliber change of the superior mesenteric artery, celiac artery, portal vein, or superior mesenteric vein suggests vascular encasement (Fig. 4). Benign or well-encapsulated tumors may compress a vessel without encasing it; with pancreatic cancer, the tumor is almost always adherent to the vessel when a caliber change is identified. Even without a change in caliber, soft tissue obliteration of the fat planes surrounding the splanchnic vessels or subtle mass or "pad" effect on one surface of the vessels also implies tumor involvement, but with far less certainty than frank caliber change. In the presence of one of these less definitive signs of tumor spread, surgery is still warranted.

In most instances the axial sections adequately depict vascular encasement, but three-dimensional (3D) rendering of helical CT data may help clarify involvement of major vessels by tumor when uncertainty exists on the axially displayed sections. The 3D model also may be useful when the surgeon wants a preoperative vascular road map in lieu of a conventional arteriogram (19). Multiplanar reformatting provides much of the same information as 3D rendering (20), but the ability to view 3D models from any angle is somewhat more convenient than having to page through the various sections in a reformatted set of images.

Our scanning technique for evaluation of the splanchnic vessels is identical to our protocol for evaluation of the pancreas. Five-millimeter collimation sections are reconstructed at 2- or 3-mm intervals. These sections are then downloaded to a commercially available work station for volume rendering of the model. Generation of the model and post-processing, to enhance the vascular structures, take approximately 20–25 min. The physician participation and time required to process a model have been the two greatest limitations in the dissemination of this technology.

We believe that three-dimensional rendering may result in assessment of vascular encasement that may be superior to that obtainable by conventional arteriography. Both normal and abnormal vascular anatomy are clearly depicted on 3D views. Although conventional arteriography demonstrates the major arteries, opacification of the portal vein is indirect, via the mesenteric circulation. Subtle encasement of the portal vein by tumor can easily be overlooked, especially at the splenoportal confluence or if multiple overlying varices are present. Both arterial and venous anatomy may be mapped on a 3D model. Arterial anatomic variants are common. Replacement of the hepatic artery must be recognized so that aberrant arterial branches are not accidently sacrificed during surgery (Fig. 5). Ligation of a major hepatic arterial branch could jeopardize the blood supply of the common hepatic duct and result in subsequent failure of biliary–enteric anastomosis. Anomalies of

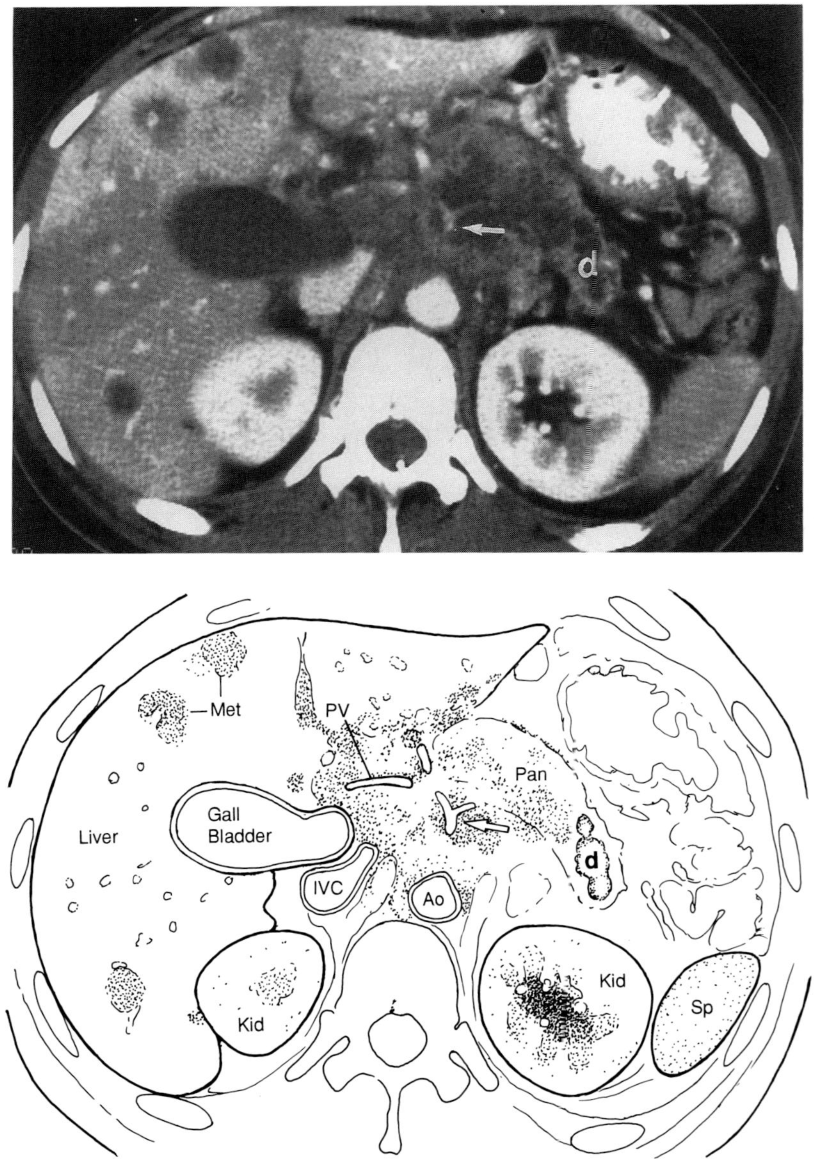

Figure 4. Extensive vascular encasement by pancreatic carcinoma. 5-mm collimation helical scan shows a large, infiltrative pancreatic carcinoma in the pancreatic body. There appears to be encasement of both the splenic and hepatic arteries distal to the celiac bifurcation (arrow). The pancreatic duct (d) is dilated and obstructed by the tumor mass. This type of vascular encasement signifies that the lesion will not be resectable. This patient also has hepatic metastases. Courtesy of Robert K. Zeman (3).

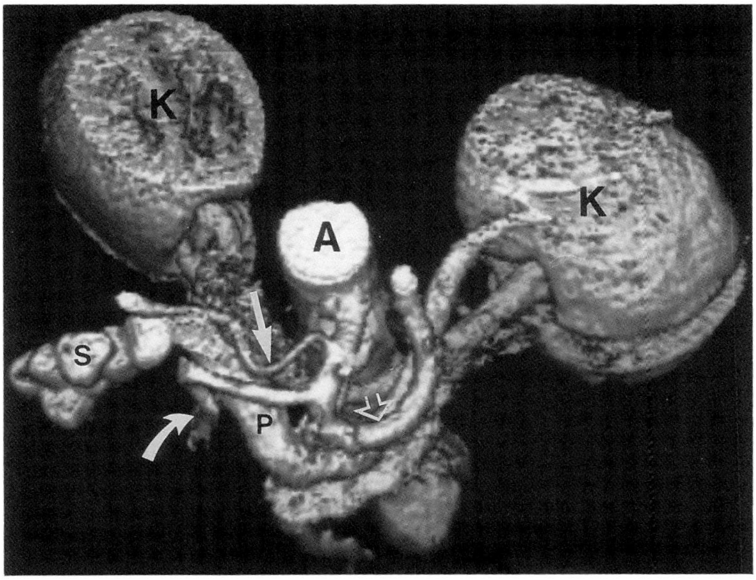

Figure 5. Aberrant origin of the hepatic artery. Surface model created from helical CT data, viewed from above, shows the hepatic artery (straight solid arrow) arising from the proximal part of the celiac axis and coursing behind the portal vein (P). This location is unusual: the artery normally passes anteriorly to portal vein. As the celiac axis bifurcates in this patient, it gives rise to the splenic artery (open arrow) and gastroduodenal artery (curved arrow). Ability to recognize anomalous branches of the hepatic artery is important for surgical planning, because these branches commonly supply arterial blood to the common hepatic duct. (K = kidneys, S = radiopaque gallstones of attenuation similar to that of enhanced vessels, A = aorta.) Courtesy of *American Journal of Roentgenology* (34).

the major veins also occur, but are less frequent than arterial anomalies. The most common venous anomaly is the inferior mesenteric vein joining the superior mesenteric vein (rather than the splenic vein) just below the splenoportal confluence.

Three-dimensional models readily demonstrate frank caliber changes of the arteries or veins (Fig. 6). The relative length of the encased vascular segment is also depicted. If portal vein encasement length is limited to 1–2 cm, grafting the vessel may be considered if no other disease is identified. This is technically difficult and is associated with significant morbidity. More often than not, other sites of nodal disease or peritoneal seeding are present that were not identified on CT. Most surgeons acknowledge that if frank vessel involvement is seen, it implies nonresectability. Subtle mass or "pad" effect on the surface of the vessel may signify tumor adherence in patients with pancreatic cancer (Fig. 7).

There has been much controversy over the relative merits of CT, MRI, and EUS in staging pancreatic carcinoma. In the absence of distant disease, encasement of the peripancreatic vessels is the single most common cause for pancreatic carcinoma being nonresectable. The ability of conventional CT to diagnose vascular involvement has varied greatly in reported series, and reflects variability in the technology that was used, scanning protocols, and the criteria of abnormality. Freeny and colleagues, in a study comparing dynamic CT and angiography, showed vascular

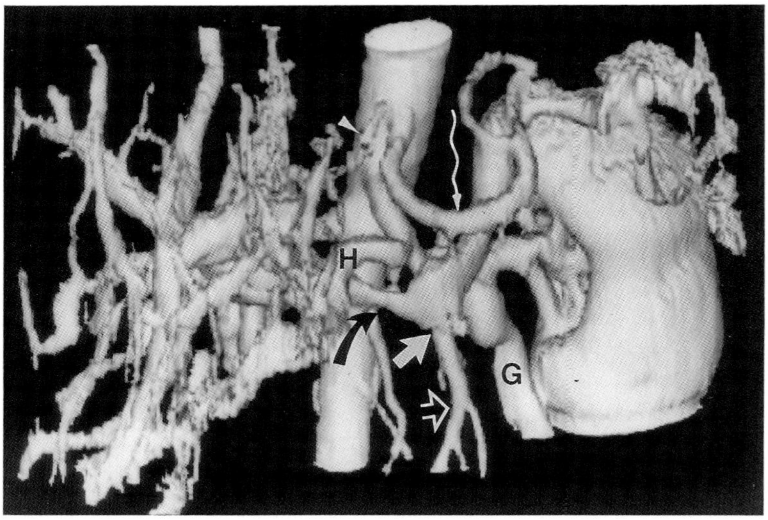

Figure 6. Involvement of the portal and superior mesenteric veins by pancreatic cancer. Surface model based on data from helical CT shows replacement of the hepatic artery (H), which shares a common trunk with the superior mesenteric artery (open arrow). The splenic artery (wavy arrow) arises from its own trunk, as does a small left hepatic artery (arrowhead). Tumor has caused amputation of the superior mesenteric vein (white arrow) just below the splenoportal confluence. The superior mesenteric artery can be seen coursing behind occluded mesenteric vein. The portal vein is also encased (curved black arrow) just above confluence. Although unusual, skip areas of vascular involvement may occur. The dilated gonadal vein (G) acts as a portosystemic collateral pathway. Courtesy of *American Journal of Roentgenology* (34).

involvement on CT in 15 of 16 patients in whom it was surgically confirmed (21). In a similar surgical series, Vellet et al. identified vascular invasion on CT in 31 of 39 patients, and portal venous invasion in 37 of 40 patients (22). In this same series MRI fared better, identifying 34 and 37 patients, respectively, in each of these categories. Warshaw and associates reported correct identification of vascular encasement on conventional CT in only 21 of 35 patients with pancreatic head neoplasms (23). These authors suggested that angiography played a complementary role in assessing vascular invasion. It correctly identified 25 of 35 patients with vascular involvement, many of whom did not have vascular invasion on CT. Muller found similar results with CT, missing small tumors and understaging T3 (vessel involvement) lesions (24).

Endoscopic ultrasound is far less available than helical CT, but is being utilized in some university centers to stage pancreatic neoplasms accurately. The pancreatic head is readily visualized by positioning the EUS probe in the gastric antrum or the second portion of the duodenum. Tio et al. have shown 93% accuracy in assessing vascular involvement and 92% accuracy for staging the local extent of disease (25). We believe that EUS compares favorably with conventional CT, but its accuracy has not been statistically shown in series comparing it with helical CT. In the future a prospective trial of these competing techniques correlated with surgical findings and survival data will have to be carried out before the true merits of these techniques can be proved.

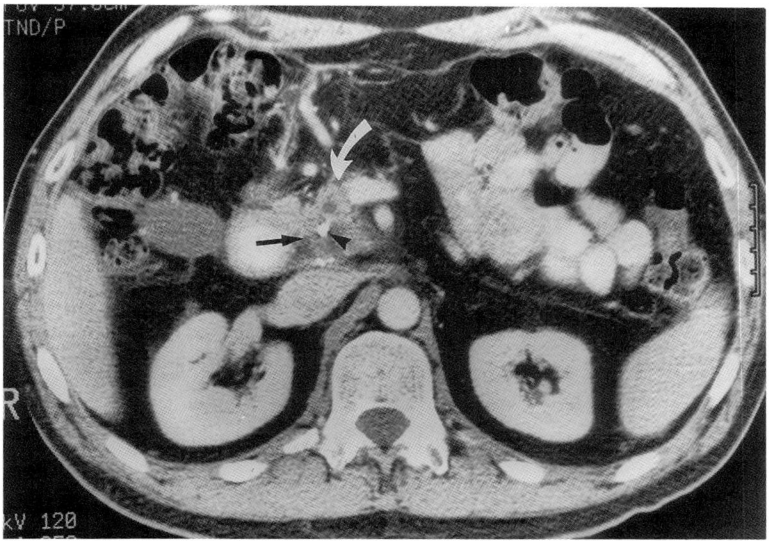

(A)

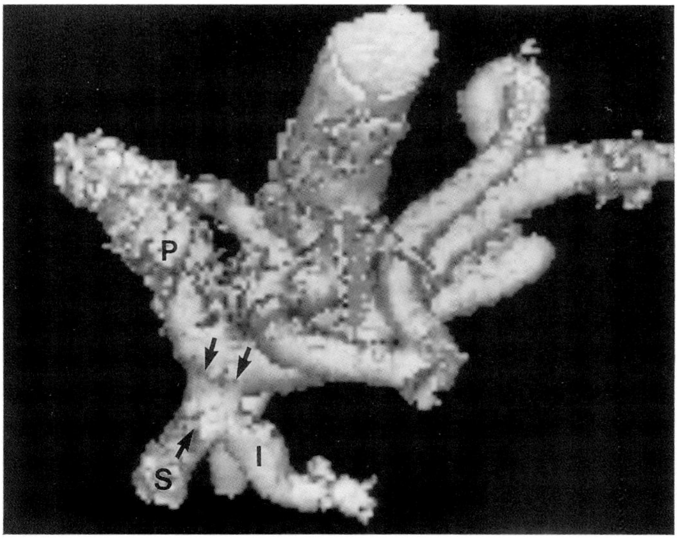

(B)

Figure 7. "Pad effect" on portal vein caused by tumor involvement. (A) Axial display of helical CT scan obtained through the pancreatic head shows a pancreatic mass (straight arrow). There is subtle "flattening" of the portal vein (curved arrow). Although a suggestion of a fat plane separating tumor from the vessel is present, it is difficult to say if the portal vein is encased (arrowhead = stent in bile duct). (B) Anterior oblique surface model of confluence region based on data from helical CT shows a "pad effect" (arrows), with impression on the splenoportal confluence. The finding is subtle, but surgical findings confirmed it represented vascular encasement (P = portal vein, S = superior mesenteric vein, I = inferior mesenteric vein). In pancreatic cancer, this type of pad effect signifies tumor adherence in our experience. Courtesy of *American Journal of Roentgenology* (34).

Regardless if 3D models or axially displayed sections are used to evaluate the peripancreatic vessels, the following approach has worked well in our attempt to distinguish surgical candidates from those with more advanced disease. If the patient has distant disease sites (hepatic metastases or regional nodes outside the field of possible resection), these along with the primary tumor are percutaneously biopsied. If distant disease is not present, our major focus in determining resectability is the splanchnic vessels. We deliberately err on the side of "undercalling" vascular involvement, in borderline cases, so as not to exclude patients from their one chance for cure. If the major vessels, however, are circumferentially surrounded by tumor or show a change in caliber, we do not recommend surgery, because resection is not possible even in the hands of the most skilled surgeon. All radiologists must clearly define their philosophical approaches to interpreting these kinds of cases in the context of developing a working relationship with their surgical colleagues.

Other Pancreatic Neoplasms

Islet Cell Tumors. The islet cells of the pancreas may give rise to a wide variety of functional and nonfunctional endocrine tumors (26). The functional tumors are generally small, and become symptomatic owing to their hormonal activity. The islet cell tumors include insulinoma, gastrinoma, glucagonoma, VIPoma, and somatostatinoma. The nonfunctional tumors typically present when they are larger in size, because they tend not to produce symptoms until they have compromised adjacent structures such as the bile duct or pancreatic duct. All islet cell tumors must be surgically removed, for between 10 and 80% (depending on the neuroendocrine cell line from which they are derived) are malignant.

The hallmark of islet cell tumors is their hypervascularity (27–29). Unfortunately, the tumor may be as little as 10 Hounsfield units greater than the surrounding pancreas on CT. This slight difference in attenuation may easily be overlooked if the images are not carefully reviewed. With conventional scanning techniques, visualization of tumor vascularity is highly variable owing to variation in the level of peak contrast enhancement. Because helical scanning results in higher levels of circulating contrast, hypervascular tumors are much more easily seen to be of higher attenuation than the surrounding gland (Fig. 8). By reconstructing overlapping sections from the helical scan data, our ability to see small tumors has also improved. Preliminary experience regarding the efficacy of helical CT in the evaluation of functional islet cell tumors is encouraging; future studies comparing helical CT with vascular sampling techniques (30), endoscopic ultrasound (31), and intraoperative ultrasound (32) should help clarify the relative merits of these techniques.

Cystic Neoplasms. There are two distinctly different types of cystic neoplasms of epithelial origin occurring in the pancreas, the microcystic adenoma and the mucinous cystic neoplasm (33–35). In the earlier literature the microcystic class of tumors was called serous cystadenoma, and the malignant form of mucinous neoplasms was called cystadenocarcinoma.

Microcystic adenomas tend to occur in elderly women. Tumors are equally distributed throughout the gland. The lesions tend to be large at the time of presentation. Multiple small cysts with a prominent radial distribution are identified. A central fibrotic scar with calcification may also be seen. The calcification may extend

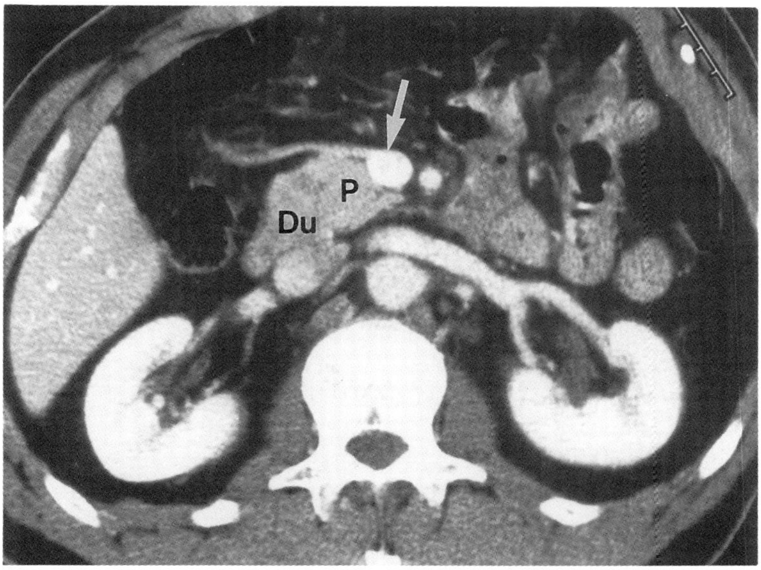

(A)

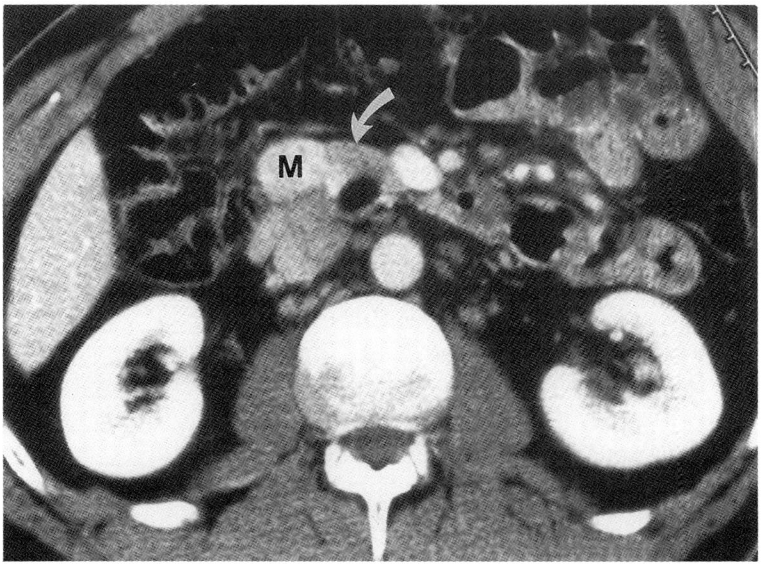

(B)

Figure 8. Malignant islet cell carcinoma. (A) This 5-mm collimation section shows a normal uncinate portion of the pancreas (P). The superior mesenteric vein (arrow) is identified in its usual position. (Du = duodenum). (B) This section 5 mm below that of Fig. 7A shows a small hypervascular mass (M) extending inferiorly from the uncinate. A small amount of normal pancreatic tissue (curved arrow) is seen interposed between the mass and the normal superior mesenteric vein. At surgery this proved to be a resectable malignant islet cell carcinoma. Courtesy of Robert K. Zeman et al. (1).

into the numerous cyst septations and fibrotic stroma surrounding the multiple cysts. This can create a calcified sunburst appearance on CT and plain films. When helical scans are performed with high levels of circulating contrast, the septations often show enhancement because of the vessels they contain. The multiple cysts can be expected to stand out as negative defects against the overall background of enhancing normal parenchyma (36). The major splanchnic vessels may be displaced or compressed by the neoplasm, but frank encasement or thrombosis is unusual.

Mucinous cystic neoplasms tend to occur in a slightly younger age group than the microcystic adenoma. This lesion is far more common in women than men (6:1). Most lesions are large at presentation and have a propensity for involvement of the pancreatic tail. Whenever a mucinous neoplasm is identified, it must be presumed malignant and excised unless distant metastases are present.

The CT diagnosis of mucinous cystic neoplasm can be difficult, but several key differences exist in the appearance of this lesion as compared to microcystic adenoma. The mucinous cystic neoplasm will usually have one or more dominant cysts up to several centimeters in diameter and may be associated with duct ectasia (37). Mural nodules, a prominent soft-tissue component, or a "shaggy" cyst wall may be present. The soft-tissue components may show dramatic enhancement associated with tumor vascularity. Although calcification is less common than in microcystic adenoma, we have seen several mucinous malignant lesions with scattered calcification.

Despite recent advances, it is unlikely that CT can uniformly distinguish benign from malignant cystic neoplasms. Although the appearance of some lesions clearly suggests microcystic adenoma, there is considerable overlap in the appearances of cystic lesions. We have seen patients with clusters of pancreatic pseudocysts that have closely mimicked the appearance of cystic neoplasms. The converse, a cystic neoplasm mimicking a pancreatic pseudocyst, is also all too common. Whenever a possible cystic neoplasm is identified, and there is no evidence of advanced disease on CT, an aggressive surgical approach is recommended.

ACUTE AND CHRONIC PANCREATITIS

There have not yet been large published series studying the use of helical scanning in acute or chronic pancreatitis. Because helical scanning allows the entire scan to be completed with high levels of circulating vascular contrast, it may be possible to recognize the vascular complications of pancreatitis with greater clarity than with conventional scanning. These complications include mesenteric vein thrombosis, portal vein thrombosis, and pseudoaneurysms of the celiac, gastroduodenal, splenic, or mesenteric arteries.

When high levels of circulating contrasts are present, the inherent vascularity of the pancreatic parenchyma may be assessed. In acute pancreatitis hyperemia of the gland is common. Areas devoid of decreased enhancement may indicate the presence of necrosis (38). Computed tomography is roughtly 80–90% accurate in detection of necrosis (39) (Fig. 9). There is increasing evidence supporting the relationship between pancreatic necrosis on CT and poor outcome in patients with acute pancreatitis. Balthazar and colleagues have suggested that the use of a CT severity index may help stratify patients at risk, and allow a more coherent approach to follow-

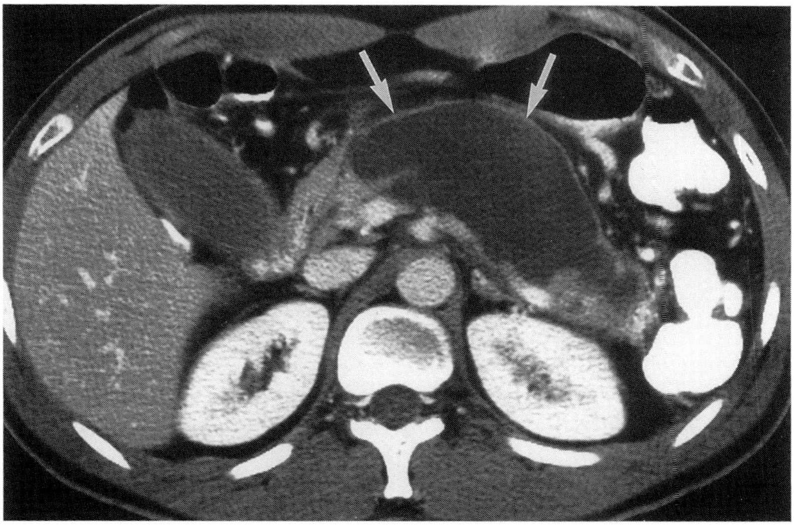

Figure 9. Sac necrosis of the pancreas following pancreatitis. Following a severe bout of pancreatitis, sac necrosis of the pancreas occurred (arrows). A well-defined fluid collection has replaced much of the pancreas. Only small amounts of enhancing parenchyma are still identified. The patient went on to develop pancreatic insufficiency. Courtesy of Robert K. Zeman (3).

up scanning (39, 40). In that series, patients with extensive necrosis had a 92% morbidity and 17% complication rate versus 0% mortality and 2% complications with minimal or no necrosis (39). Follow-up scanning (at 7- to 10-day intervals) is generally reserved for patients with significant pancreatic necrosis, fluid collections, or pancreatic gas. A well-defined enhancing rim surrounding intra- or extrapancreatic fluid suggests the presence of abscess. Aspiration and definitive drainage should be considered in the proper clinical setting. In the setting of trauma, areas devoid of vascularity within an otherwise well-enhanced gland may indicate hematoma or pancreatic fracture.

REFERENCES

1. Zeman RK, Brink J, Costello P, Davros WJ, Richmond B, Silverman PM, Vieco P. *Helical/Spiral CT: A Practical Approach.* New York: McGraw Hill Inc; 1994.
2. Zeman RK, Fox SH, Silverman PM, et al. Helical (spiral) CT of the abdomen. *AJR.* 1993;160:719–725.
3. Zeman RK, Silverman PM, Ascher SM, Patt RH, Cooper C, Al-Kawas F. Helical CT of the pancreas. *Radiol Clin North Am.* 1995;33:887–902.
4. Zeman RK, Zeiberg AS, Davros WJ, et al. Routine helical CT of the abdomen: image quality considerations. *Radiology.* 1993;189:395–400.
5. Megibow AJ. Pancreatic carcinoma: designing the examination to evaluate clinical questions. *Radiology.* 1992;183:297–303.

6. Dupuy DE, Costello P, Ecker CP. Spiral CT of the pancreas. *Radiology.* 1992;183: 815–818.
7. Heiken JP, Brink JA, McClennan BL, Sagel SS, Forman HP, DiCroce. Dynamic contrast-enhanced CT of the liver: comparison of contrast medium injection rates and uniphasic and biphasic injector protocols. *Radiology.* 1993;187:327–331.
8. Silverman PM, Cooper C, Zeman RK. Imaging of the liver: survey of prevailing techniques for conventional CT of the liver. *Abdom Imaging.* 1995;20:348–352.
9. Chambers TP, Baron RL, Lush RM, Dodd GD, Miller WJ. Hepatic CT enhancement: comparison of ionic and nonionic contrast agents in the same patients. *Radiology.* 1994;190:721–725.
10. Hollett MD, Jorgenson MJ, Jeffrey RB Jr. Quantitative evaluation of pancreatic enhancement during dual-phase helical CT. *Radiology.* 1995;195:359–361.
11. Silverman PM, O'Malley J, Tefft MC, Cooper C, Zeman RK. Conspicuity of hepatic metastases on helical CT: effect of different time delays between contrast administration and scanning. *AJR.* 1995;164:619–623.
12. Bluemke DA, Cameron JL, Hruban RH, et al. Potentially resectable pancreatic adenocarcinoma: spiral CT assessment with surgical and pathologic correlation. *Radiology.* 1995;197:381–385.
13. Zeman RK, McVay LV, Silverman PM et al. Pancreas divisum: thin-section CT. *Radiology.* 1988;169:395–398.
14. Zeman RK, Burrell MI. *Gallbladder and Bile Duct Imaging: A Clinical Radiologic Approach.* New York: Churchill Livingstone, Inc; 1987.
15. Pedrosa CS, Casanova R, Lezana AH, Fernandez MC. Computed tomography in obstructive jaundice. II. The cause of obstruction. *Radiology.* 1981;139:635–645.
16. Zeman RK, Silverman PM, Garra BS, Burrell MI, Buck JL. CT of the gallbladder and bile ducts. In: Silverman PS, Zeman RK, eds. *Contemporary Issues in Computed Tomography: CT and MRI of the Liver and Biliary System.* New York: Churchill Livingstone; 1990:183–221.
17. Ralls PW, Halls JM, Renner I, Juttner H. Endoscopic retrograde cholangiopancreatography (ERCP) in pancreatic disease. A reassessment of the specificity of ductal abnormalities in differentiating benign from malignant disease. *Radiology.* 1980;134:347–352.
18. American Joint Committee on Cancer. Exocrine pancreas. In: *Manual for Staging of Cancer.* Philadelphia: JB Lippincott Co; 1992:109–111.
19. Zeman RK, Davros WJ, Berman PM, et al. Three-dimensional models of the abdominal vasculature based on helical CT: usefulness in patients with pancreatic neoplasms. *AJR.* 1994;162:1425–1429.
20. Fishman EK, Wyatt SH, Ney DR, et al. Spiral CT of the pancreas with multiplanar display. *AJR.* 1992;159:1209–1215.
21. Freeny PC, Marks WM, Traverso LW. Pancreatic ductal adenocarcinoma: diagnosis and staging with dynamic CT. *Radiology.* 1988;166:125–133.
22. Vellet AD, Romano W, Bach DB, Passi RB, Taves DH, Munk PL. Adenocarcinoma of the pancreatic ducts: Comparative evaluation with CT and MR imaging at 1.5 T. *Radiology.* 1992;183:87–95.
23. Warshaw AL, Gu Z, Wittenberg J, Waltman AC. Preoperative staging and assessment of resectability of pancreatic cancer. *Arch Surg.* 1990;125:230–233.
24. Muller MF, Meyenberger C, Bertschinger P, Schaer R, Marincek B. Pancreatic tumors: evaluation with endoscopic US, CT, and MR imaging. *Radiology.* 1994;190:745–751.
25. Tio TL, Tytgat GNJ, Cikot RJLM, Houthoff HJ, Sars PR. Ampullopancreatic carcinoma: preoperative TNM classification with endosonography. *Radiology.* 1990;175:455–461.

26. Rossi P, Allison DJ, Bezzi M. Endocrine tumors of the pancreas. *Radiol Clin North Am.* 1989;27:129–161.
27. Gunther RW, Klose KJ, Ruckert K, Beyer J, Kuhn FP. Localization of small islet cell tumors. Preoperative and intraoperative ultrasound, computed tomography, arteriography, digital subtraction angiography, and pancreatic venous sampling. *Gastrointest Radiol.* 1985;10:145–151.
28. Krudy AG, Doppman JL, Jensen RJ et al. Localization of islet cell tumors by dynamic CT: comparison with plain CT. *AJR.* 1984;143:585–589.
29. Ros P, Baert A, Passariello R, et al. CT of functioning tumors of the pancreas. *AJR.* 1985;144:57–60.
30. Doppman JL, Shawker TH, Miller DL. Localization of islet cell tumors. *Gastroenterol Clin North Am.* 1989;18:793–804.
31. Rosch T, Lightdale CJ, Botet JF, et al. Localization of pancreatic endocrine tumors by endoscopic ultrasonography. *N Engl J Med.* 1992;326:1721–1726.
32. Norton JA, Cromack DT, Shawker TH, et al. Intraoperative ultrasonographic localization of islet cell tumors: a prospective comparison to palpation. *Ann Surg.* 1988;207:160–168.
33. Compagno J, Oertel JE. Microcystic adenomas of the pancreas (glycogen rich cystadenomas). A clinico-pathologic study of 34 cases. *Am J Clin Pathol.* 1978;69:289–298.
34. Compagno J, Oertel JE. Mucinous cystic neoplasms of the pancreas with overt and latent malignancy (cystadenocarcinoma and cystadenoma) *Am J Clin Pathol.* 1978;69:573–580.
35. Friedman AC, Lichtenstein JE, Dachman AH. Cystic neoplasms of the pancreas: radiological-pathological correlation. *Radiology.* 1983;149:45–50.
36. Buck JL, Hayes WS. Microcystic adenoma of the pancreas. *Radiographics.* 1990;10: 313–322.
37. Itai Y, Ohhashi K, Nagai H, et al. "Ductectatic" mucinous cystadenoma and cystadenocarcinoma of the pancreas. *Radiology.* 1986;161:697–700.
38. White EM, EM, Wittenberg J, Mueller PR, et al. Pancreatic necrosis: CT manifestations. *Radiology.* 1986;158:343–346.
39. Balthazar EJ, Robinson DL, Megibow AJ, et al. Acute pancreatitis: value of CT in establishing prognosis. *Radiology.* 1990;174:331–336.
40. Balthazar EJ, Freeny PC, vanSonnenberg E. Imaging and intervention in acute pancreatitis. *Radiology.* 1994;193:297–306.

23

MAGNETIC RESONANCE IMAGING OF THE PANCREAS

Nikolaos L. Kelekis, M.D., and Richard C. Semelka, M.D.
University of North Carolina at Chapel Hill
Chapel Hill, North Carolina

Magnetic resonance examination may be tailored to detect and characterize the complete range of pancreatic diseases. Breath-hold T1-weighted spoiled gradient echo, breathing-independent T2-weighted Half Fourier single shot turbo spin echo (HASTE), chemically selective fat suppression, and dynamic administration of gadolinium chelate have resulted in reproducible high image quality and generation of a broad variety of diagnostic information that has rendered magnetic resonance imaging (MRI) a comprehensive examination for pancreatic diseases (1–5). In this chapter we discuss the role of MRI in the investigation of common disorders of the pancreas.

TECHNIQUE

Our standard MRI protocol includes T1-weighted fat-suppressed imaging and spoiled gradient echo (SGE) (4, 6). The normal pancreas is hyperintense relative to liver on T1-weighted fat-suppressed images owing to the presence of aqueous protein in the glandular elements of the pancreas (4). In the past we reserved T2-weighted imaging of the pancreas for the investigation of associated liver metastases or for patients with islet cell tumors (1). With the introduction of breathing-independent T2-weighted HASTE imaging, we have incorporated this technique to demonstrate the pancreatic duct in assessing ductal obstruction or changes in duct caliber. This sequence is also useful to determine the complexity of pseudocyst fluid. Pseudocyst fluid that is mixed in signal intensity and lower in intensity than simple fluid suggests a high quantity of protein or necrotic material. The use of fat-suppressed T2-weighted spin echo (T2FS) improves the conspicuity of high-signal-intensity diseased tissue such as islet cell tumors. More recently, various bright bile MR

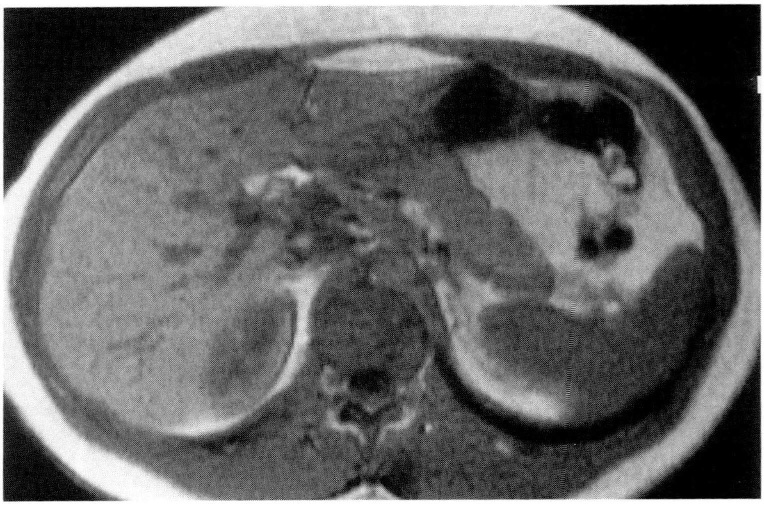

(A)

Figure 1. Normal pancreas. SGE (A), fat-suppressed T1-weighted spin echo (B, next page), immediate post-contrast SGE (C, page 468), and 45-sec post-gadolinium SGE (D, page 468) images. The pancreas is minimally higher in signal intensity than surrounding tissue on the precontrast SGE images (A). On the fat-suppressed T1-weighted spin echo image the normal pancreas has high signal intensity comparable to that of the normal renal cortex, which is considerably higher than liver and spleen (B). Immediate post-gadolinium SGE image (C) shows the uniform capillary blush of the pancreas, which is rendered higher in signal intensity than surrounding fat. On the 45-sec post-contrast image (D), signal intensity of the pancreas has decreased more than that of fat.

cholangiographic techniques have been introduced that generate three-dimensional data demonstrating the appearance of the biliary and pancreatic ducts (7).

Spoiled gradient echo (SGE) is acquired precontrast and immediately following rapid bolus injection of intravenous gadolinium-DTPA (gadolinium) while the patient is positioned in the bore of the magnet. The sequence is initiated immediately following a rapid normal saline flush. T1-weighted fat-suppressed SGE is repeated at 40 sec post-contrast, and SGE is repeated at 5 min. On immediate post-contrast images, the pancreas demonstrates a uniform capillary blush that renders it higher in signal intensity than liver and adjacent fat (4) (Fig. 1). On 5-min post-contrast SGE images, the pancreas has diminished signal intensity relative to fat.

DEVELOPMENTAL ANOMALIES

Pancreas divisum is the most clinically important and common major anatomic pancreatic variant. This results from the failure of embryologic fusion of the head and body of the pancreas. These portions of the pancreas have separate ductal systems; the head drained by the duct of Wirsung and the body by the duct of Santorini. The incidence of this anomaly varies between 1.3 and 6.7% of the population (8). The clinical importance of this anatomic variant lies in its occasional association with recurrent acute pancreatitis. Partial obstruction to the passage of

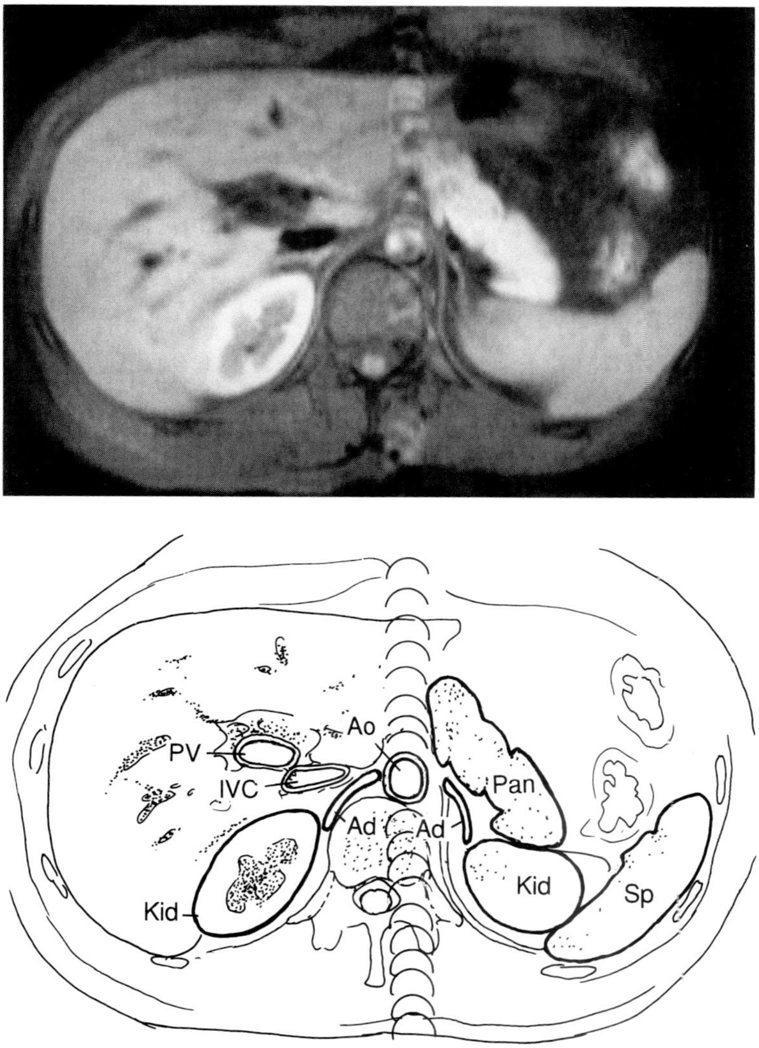

B

Figure 1. *(Continued)*

pancreatic exocrine secretions from the dorsal pancreas through the narrow orifice at the duodenum is considered to be the underlying cause. The partial obstruction may result in a leak of secretions into the pancreatic tissue causing pancreatitis. To date a definite diagnosis of pancreas divisum could be established only by endoscopic retrograde cholangiopancreatography (ERCP) with injection of both pancreatic ducts. Magnetic resonance cholangiopancreatography (MRCP) using a two-dimensional fast spin-echo sequence has been recently shown to have 100% diagnostic accuracy in 108 cases where correlation with ERCP was available (9). Magnetic resonance cholangiopancreatography (MRCP) is a noninvasive technique and re-

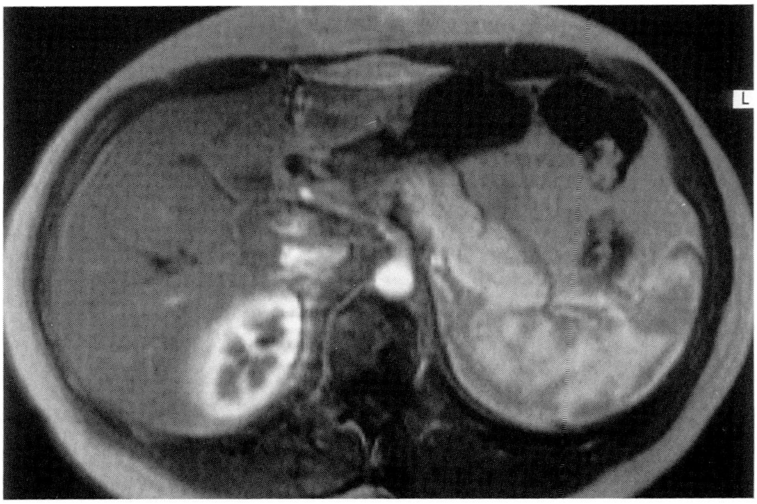

(C)

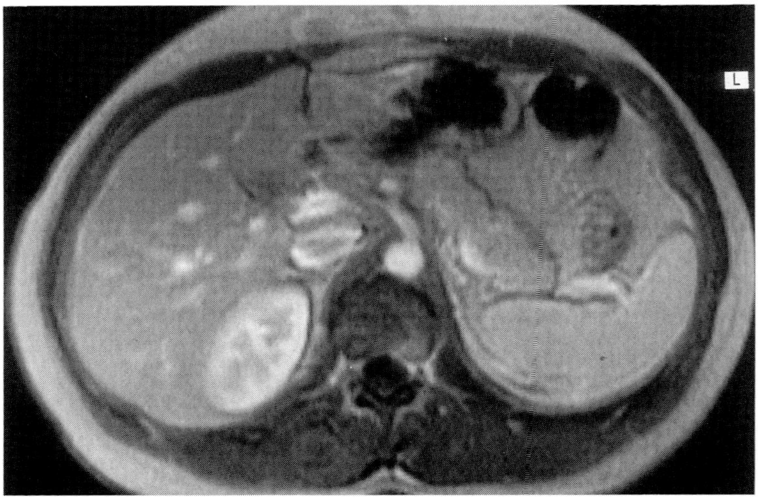

(D)

Figure 1. *(Continued)*

quires no contrast medium, and therefore may be an attractive method to evaluate for the presence of pancreas divisum.

MASS LESIONS

Adenocarcinoma

Detection of cancer is well performed by fat-suppressed T1-weighted images and immediate post-gadolinium SGE images (4). Normal pancreatic tissue is well deline-

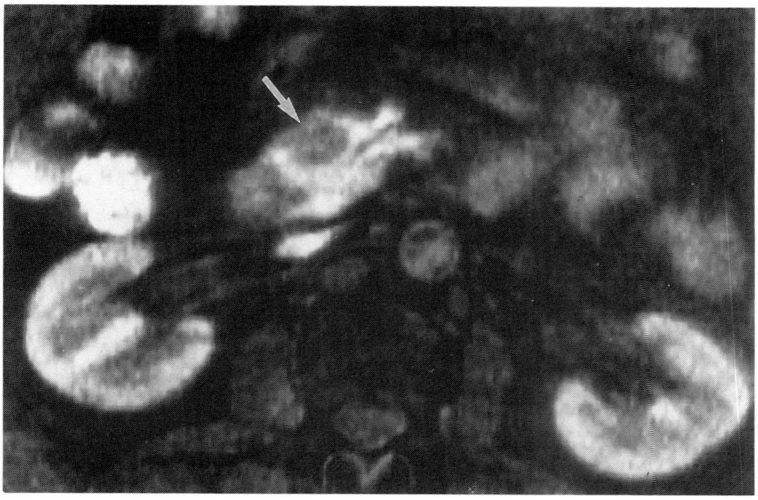

(A)

Figure 2. Small pancreatic adenocarcinoma. Precontrast fat-suppressed T1-weighted spin echo (A), immediate post-gadolinium SGE (B, next page), and post-contrast fat-suppressed T1-weighted spin echo (C, page 470) images. Fat-suppressed T1-weighted spin echo image shows a readily identified, well-defined hypointense mass that does not deform the contour of the organ (arrow, A). The mass enhances minimally (arrow, B) on the immediate post-gadolinium SGE image, reflecting the hypovascular, desmoplastic nature of the tumor. On the more delayed fat-suppressed T1-weighted spin echo image the tumor enhances slightly greater than background pancreas due to greater retention in the interstitial spaces (arrow, C). Reproduced with permission from Reference 1.

ated from tumors and tumor margins are well shown on MR images in the head, body, and tail regions. Fat-suppressed T1-weighted spin-echo or SGE images have inherently high contrast resolution for imaging of the pancreas and are well suited for the detection of small (1 cm) non-organ-deforming tumors. Pancreatic cancers enhance to a lesser extent than normal pancreatic tissue due to their desmoplastic, fibrotic composition (Fig. 2) (4). It is therefore critical in contrast-enhanced studies to exploit this difference in vascularity by imaging in the dynamic capillary phase of enhancement. Image section thinness is also helpful; however 8-mm sections may be sufficiently thin to detect even small (<1 cm) cancers owing to the high contrast resolution.

Pancreatic tissue distal to pancreatic cancers that obstruct the main pancreatic duct may be lower in signal intensity than normal pancreatic tissue owing to changes of chronic pancreatitis with decrease of proteinaceous fluid content (11). Chronically inflamed pancreas, however, enhances to a greater extent than pancreatic cancer on immediate post-gadolinium SGE images. Pancreatic cancer appears as a defined area of low signal intensity in a background of slightly higher-signal intensity chronically inflamed pancreatic tissue (Fig. 3). In addition, tumors frequently are large when they cause changes of chronic pancreatitis distally, and therefore diagnosis is not problematic.

Although pancreatic cancers are lower in signal intensity than pancreas on immediate post-gadolinium images, the appearance of cancers on >1 min post-gadolinium

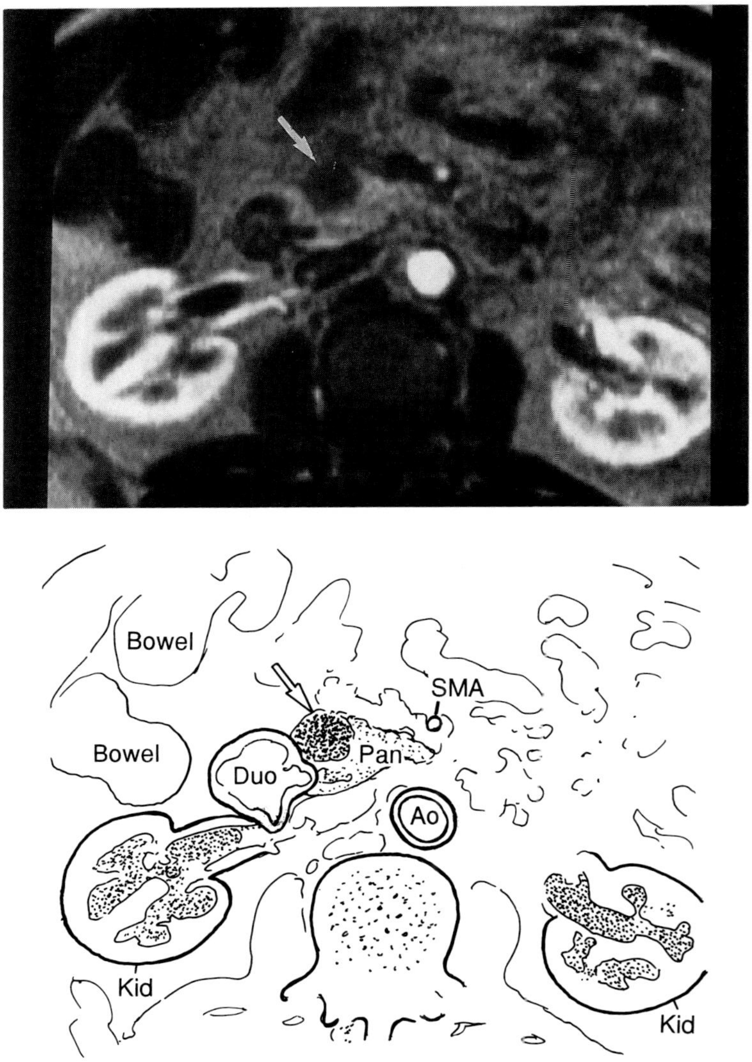

(B)

Figure 2. *(Continued)*

images is variable (Fig. 2). The enhancement of cancer relative to pancreas reflects the volume of extracellular space and venous drainage of cancers compared to pancreatic tissue.

A recent study compared single-phase spiral CT with MRI including noncontrast T1-weighted fat-suppressed spin echo and immediate post-gadolinium SGE for the detection or exclusion of pancreatic cancer in 16 patients with findings indeterminate for cancer on spiral CT (12). Immediate post-gadolinium SGE was found to be the most sensitive approach to detect pancreatic cancer, particularly in the head of the pancreas. Both immediate post-gadolinium SGE and T1-weighted fat-suppressed

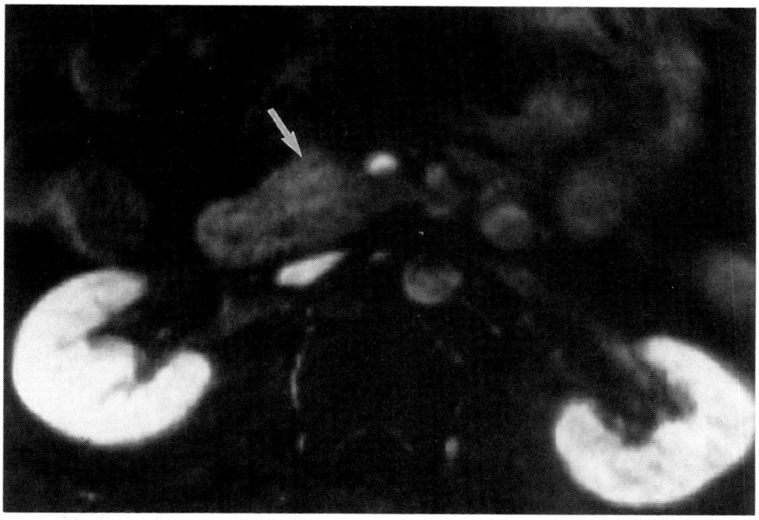

(C)

Figure 2. *(Continued)*

spin echo performed well at excluding cancer and both were significantly superior to spiral CT. These findings were similar to those reported by Gabata et al. (13), who compared these MR techniques to dynamic contrast-enhanced CT.

Noncontrast T1-weighted spin echo or SGE images are useful when staging pancreatic cancer for evaluation of peripancreatic tumor extension (14, 15). Tumor tissue is low in signal and contrasts well with high-signal peripancreatic fat. T1-weighted spin echo has been reported to be superior to dynamic contrast-enhanced CT for the determination of vascular encasement. Vascular patency may be evaluated by either a flow-sensitive gradient echo technique (16) or by dynamic gadolinium-enhanced SGE (Fig. 4). In general, detection of lymph nodes is well performed by MRI and CT. Magnetic resonance imaging may be superior for the detection of lymph nodes in thin or emaciated patients owing to the high intrinsic soft tissue resolution of T2FS and post-gadolinium fat-suppressed T1-weighted SGE images.

Assessment of liver metastases requires the addition of T2FS images. Liver metastases from pancreatic cancers generally have low signal intensity on conventional or fat-suppressed T1-weighted images, are minimally hyperintense on T2-weighted images, and demonstrate a faint irregular rim of enhancement on immediate post-gadolinium SGE images. The low signal intensity centers of metastatic lesions presumably reflect the desmoplastic nature of the primary tumor (2). The hypovascular nature of these metastases permits the distinction between these lesions and hemangiomas, even when lesions are 1 cm in diameter. The irregular rim enhancement distinguishes these lesions from cysts.

Patients with diminished renal function, iodine contrast allergy, or indeterminate or negative spiral CT findings with suspicion of small, non-organ-deforming cancers should be studied by MRI. Early detection of potentially curable tumors may

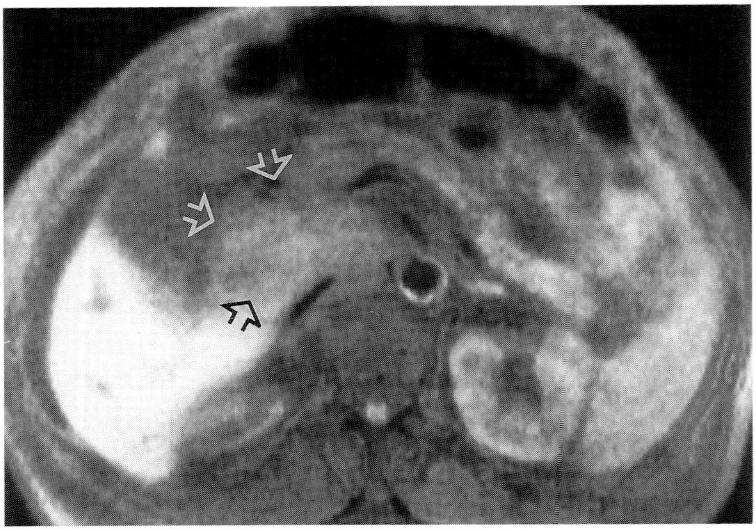

(A)

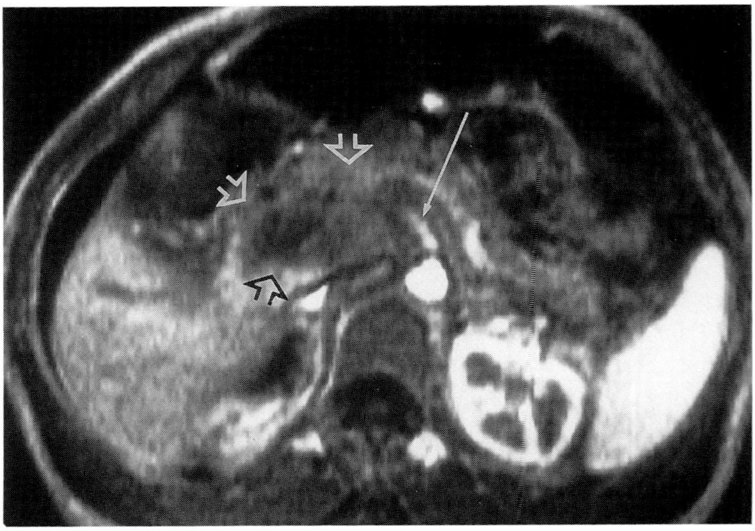

(B)

Figure 3. Pancreatic adenocarcinoma. Precontrast fat-suppressed T1-weighted spin echo (A), and immediate post-gadolinium SGE (B) images. A large irregular mass is seen in the head of the pancreas (open arrows, A, B). The mass is low in signal on the fat-suppressed T1-weighted spin echo image (A), and shows diminished contrast enhancement on the immediate post-gadolinium image (B). The tumor extends posteriorly into the aortocaval space, and encases the superior mesenteric artery (solid arrow, B). The dark periaortic tissue on the immediate post-gadolinium image corresponds to tumor extension.

result in improved patient survival, because surgery remains the main therapeutic treatment (17).

Islet Cell Tumors

Islet cell tumors are low in signal intensity on T1-weighted fat-suppressed images, demonstrate homogeneous or ring enhancement on immediate post-gadolinium SGE, and are high in signal intensity on T2FS images (1, 18, 19). They can be distinguished from ductal adenocarcinomas by their high signal intensity on T2FS images, greater enhancement on immediate post-gadolinium images, lack of vascular encasement, uncommon central necrosis in large tumors, lack of pancreatic duct obstruction, and presence of hypervascular liver metastases.

Insulinomas are frequently small at clinical presentation. They are most often hypervascular and their detection is facilitated by using techniques that evaluate dynamic contrast enhancement. Angiography with its superior spatial resolution has been shown to be superior to CT in the detection of these tumors (20). In a similar way MRI performs well in the detection of small insulinomas, owing to its superior soft tissue contrast resolution and greater sensitivity for the presence of intravenous contrast. Insulinomas are depicted on T1-weighted fat-suppressed images as low-signal intensity lesions in a background of high-signal-intensity normal pancreas. They have high signal intensity on T2FS images and possess intense homogeneous enhancement on immediate post-gadolinium images (Fig. 5) (19). Larger tumors exceeding 2 cm possess ring enhancement. Liver metastases from insulinomas typically have peripheral ring-like enhancement, although small metastases may enhance homogeneously.

Gastrinomas occur most commonly in the anatomic region termed "gastrinoma triangle," which is defined by the porta hepatis superiorly and the second and third parts of the duodenum inferiorly, and includes the head of the pancreas, duodenum, stomach, and lymph nodes (21).

Gastrinomas are not hypervascular as frequently as insulinomas. The better detection of gastrinomas compared with insulinomas on imaging studies is primarily due to the larger size of these tumors at presentation, which is approximately 4 cm compared with 2 cm for insulinomas. Conventional MRI has been limited in the detection of gastrinomas (22, 23).

Gastrinomas are low in signal intensity on fat-suppressed T1-weighted images and high in signal intensity on T2FS images and demonstrate peripheral ring-like enhancement on immediate post-gadolinium SGE images. This appearance is observed both in the primary lesion and in hepatic metastases, reflecting prominent peripheral vascularity and central hypovascularity (Fig. 6). These tumors are not hypervascular as frequently as insulinomas and on occasion may be cystic.

Islet cell tumor metastases to the liver in general are well shown on MR images. Gastrinoma metastases frequently are relatively uniform in size and shape and possess uniform ring enhancement on immediate post-gadolinium SGE images. Typically lesions are very high in signal intensity on T2FS images and have well-defined margins. Islet cell liver metastases are differentiated from hemangiomas by the relatively uniform ring-like enhancement pattern that fades with time (19). This appearance is better shown on MRI than CT images owing to the higher sensitivity of MRI to contrast enhancement, faster intravenous contrast injection,

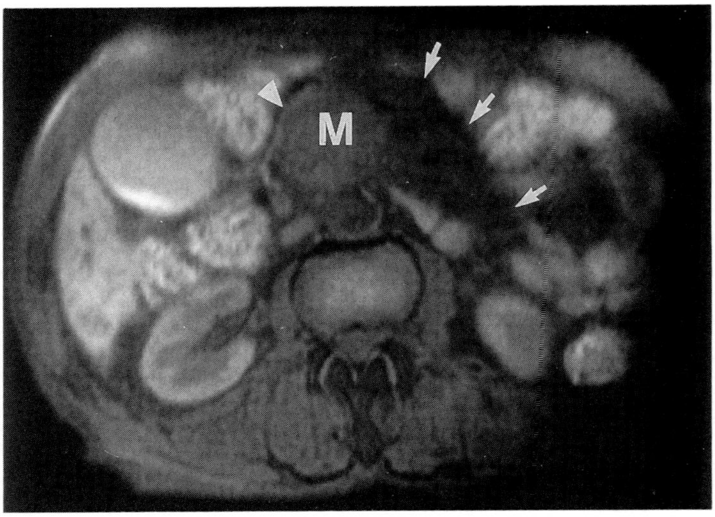

(A)

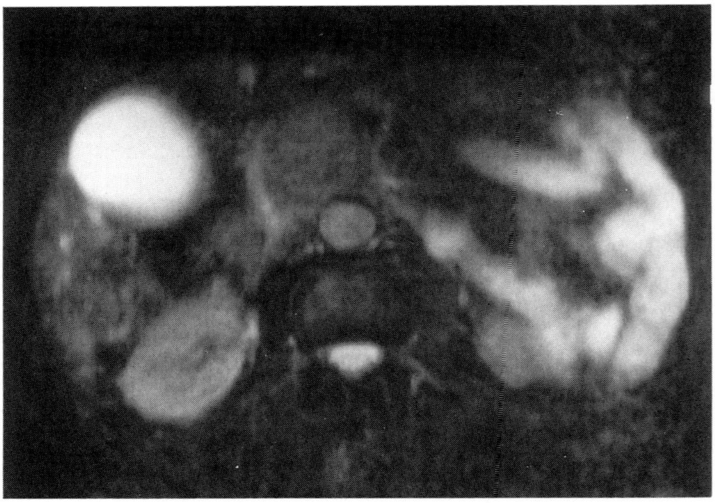

(B)

Figure 4. Pancreatic adenocarcinoma. Precontrast fat-suppressed T1-weighted spin echo (A), T2FS (B), and 45-sec post-gadolinium SGE (C, D, next page). A mass (M, A) enlarging the head of the pancreas is noted on the fat-suppressed T1-weighted spin echo image. The mass appears substantially hypointense on the fat-suppressed T1-weighted spin echo image compared to renal cortex. A thin zone of higher signal intensity remaining normal pancreatic parenchyma is noted in the anterolateral margin of the mass (arrowhead, A). The pancreatic head appears enlarged and low in signal intensity on the T2FS image; however, the signal intensity is nonspecific and there is no clear definition of the mass borders. On the 45-sec post-contrast SGE image the rounded mass shows diminished enhancement and is clearly defined. The mass abuts the superior mesenteric vein (arrow, C), which appears patent on the post-gadolinium SGE image. The main pancreatic duct is dilated and appears as a low-signal-intensity tubular structure (arrows, D) on the gadolinium-enhanced image at a higher tomographic level. Note that the parenchyma of the body and tail of the pancreas is low in signal intensity on the fat-suppressed T1-weighted spin echo image (arrows, A) compared to the renal cortex owing to chronic pancreatitis changes from the obstruction of the main pancreatic duct.

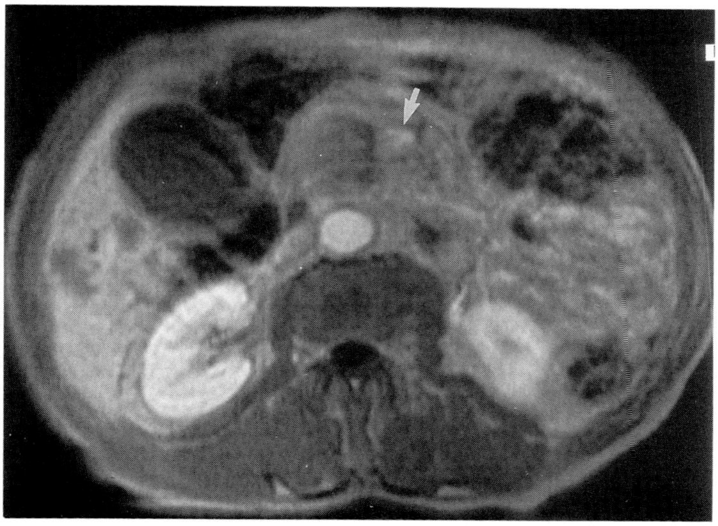

(C)

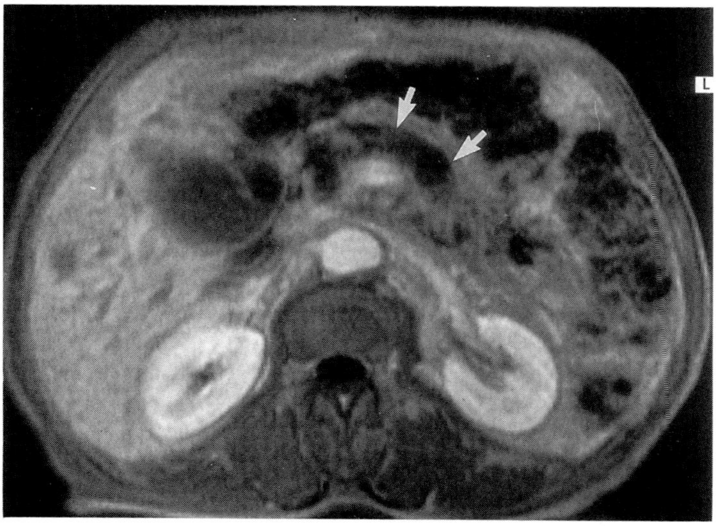

(D)

Figure 4. *(Continued)*

and greater imaging temporal resolution. The peripheral enhancing rim may be thin or thick, presumably due to differences in the degree of vascularity. Centripetal enhancement of metastases with associated peripheral washout may be observed on serial post-gadolinium images.

Glucagonomas, somatostatinomas, and adrenocorticotropin-secreting islet cell tumors are considerably rarer than insulinomas or gastrinomas. These tumors are frequently malignant, with liver metastases present at the time of diagnosis (21, 24). Tumors are large and heterogeneous on MR images: low in signal intensity on

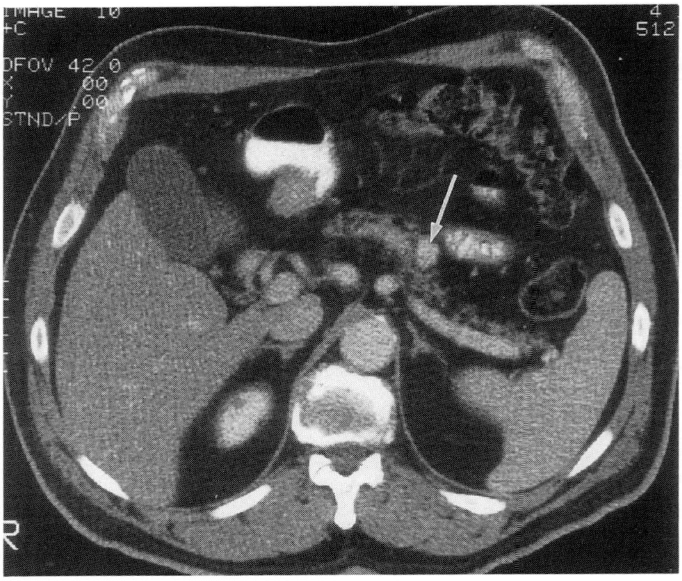

(A)

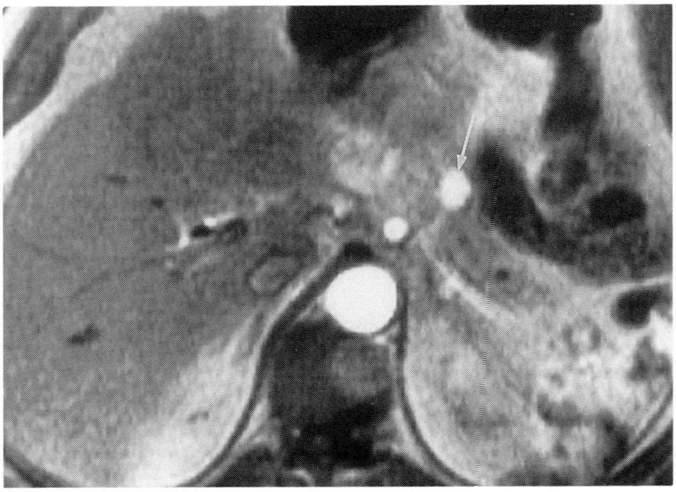

(B)

Figure 5. Insulinoma of the body of the pancreas. Contrast-enhanced dynamic CT (A) and immediate post-gadolinium SGE (B) images. Contrast-enhanced dynamic CT shows a 1.5-cm well defined rounded enhancing mass in the body of the pancreas (arrow, A). The mass is more conspicuous on the immediate post-gadolinium SGE image owing to intense enhancement, reflecting imaging at an earlier, capillary phase of enhancement and the superior sensitivity of MRI to the intravenous contrast agent (arrow, B). Reproduced with permission from reference 17.

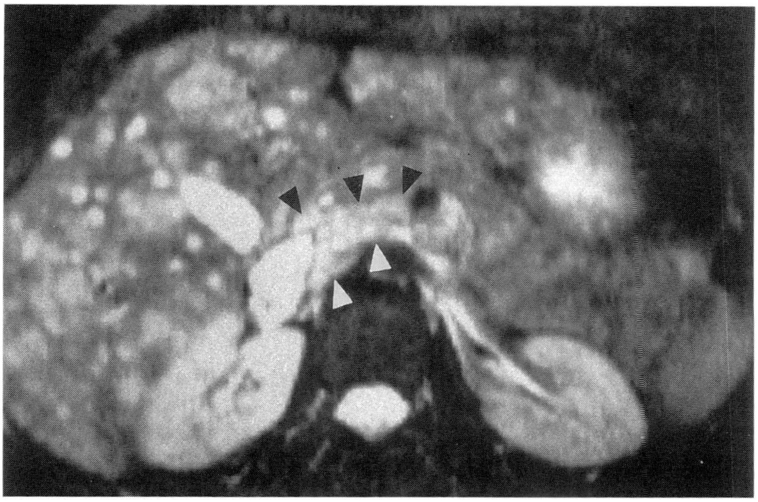

(A)

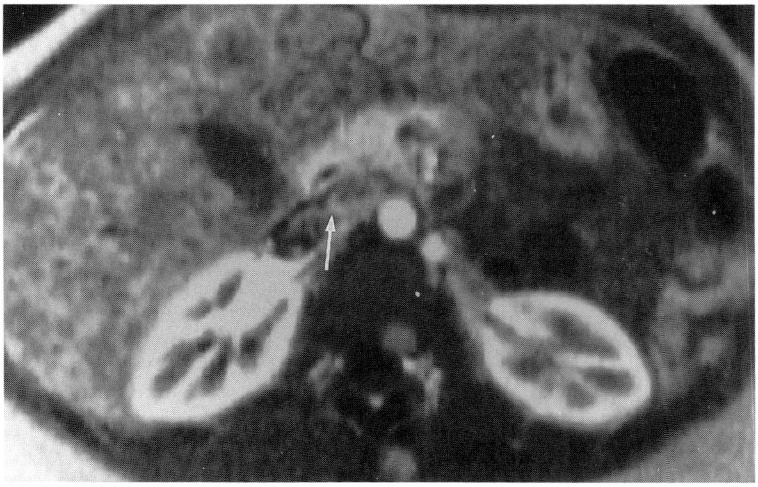

(B)

Figure 6. Gastrinoma with liver metastases. Fat-suppressed T2-weighted spin echo (A), and immediate post-gadolinium SGE (B) images. The tumor is located posterior to the head of the pancreas, has high-signal-intensity foci on the T2FS image (arrowheads, A) and ring enhancement (arrow, B) on the immediate post-gadolinium SGE image. Multiple hypervascular liver metastases are very high in signal intensity on T2FS and show intense ring enhancement on the immediate post-gadolinium SGE image. Note the similar appearance of the primary tumor to its liver metastases on all sequences. Reproduced with permission from Reference 17.

fat-suppressed T1-weighted and high in signal intensity on T2FS images (24). Tumors enhance heterogeneously with gadolinium. Liver metastases are heterogeneous in size and shape, unlike gastrinoma metastases, which are more uniform. Metastases possess irregular peripheral rims of enhancement on immediate post-gadolinium images.

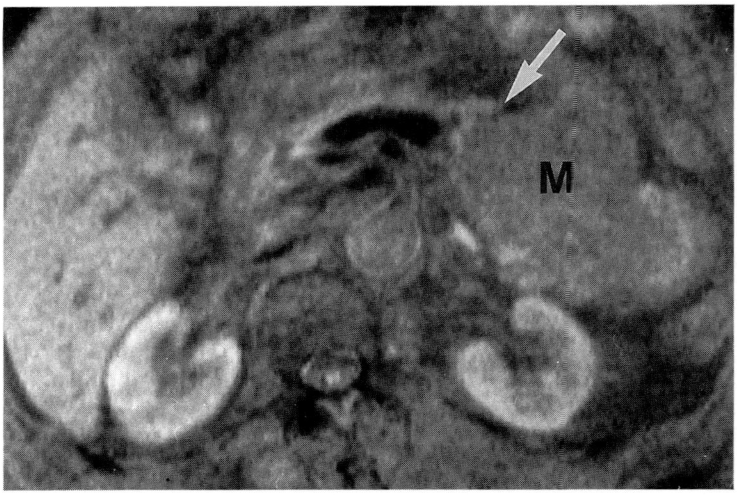

(A)

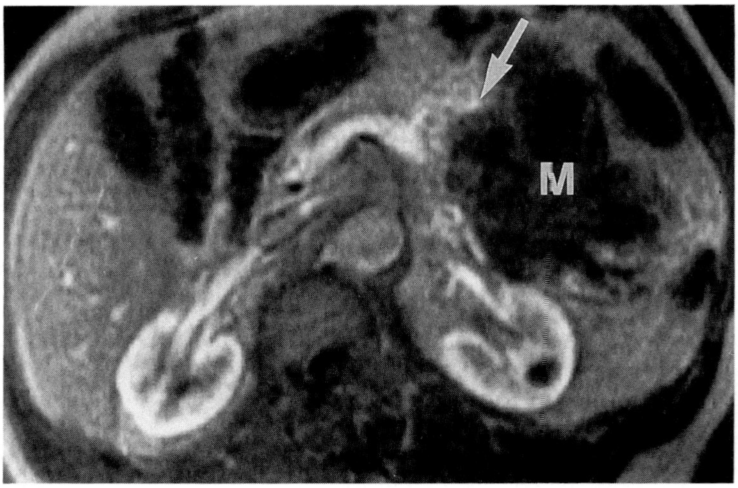

(B)

Figure 7. Microcystic cystadenoma. Fat suppressed T1-weighted spin echo (A) and immediate post-gadolinium SGE (B) images. Fat-suppressed T1-weighted spin echo image shows a 12-cm hypointense mass (M, A, B) arising from the tail of the pancreas. The mass shows minimal enhancement on the immediate post-gadolinium SGE image. The tumor is clearly shown to arise from the tail of the pancreas by the demonstration of a "beak sign" (arrow, A, B). Reproduced with permission from Reference 2.

Cystic Neoplasms

Two forms of cystic neoplasms are described: microcystic adenoma (formerly serous cystadenoma) and macrocystic adenoma (formerly mucinous cystadenoma).

Microcystic adenoma is a benign neoplasm characterized by multiple tiny cysts (25). This tumor frequently occurs in older patients and has an increased association with von Hippel–Lindau disease (25, 26). The tumor occasionally contains a central

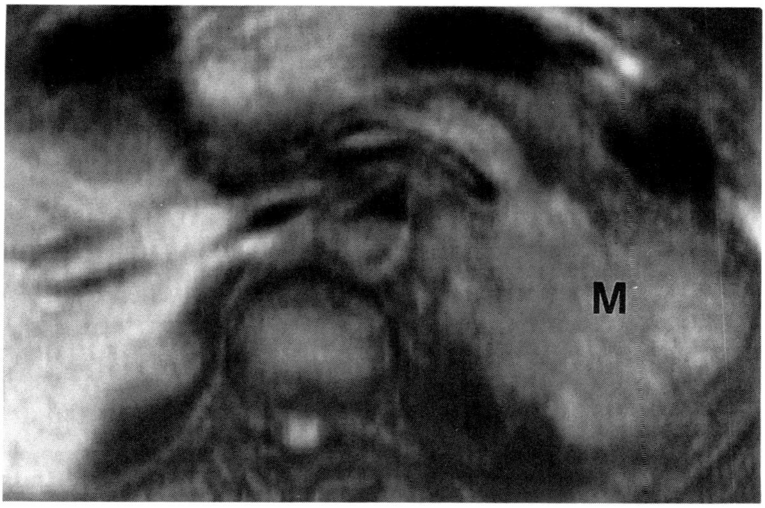

(A)

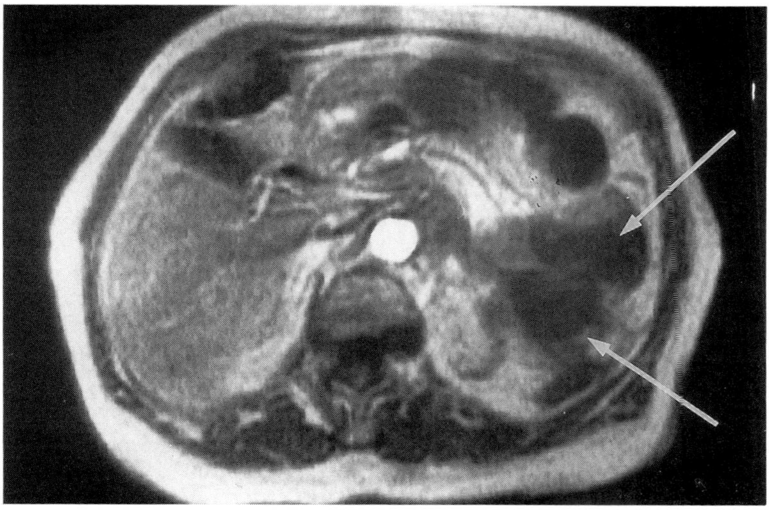

(B)

Figure 8. Macrocystic cystadenocarcinoma. Fat-suppressed T1-weighted spin echo (A), and immediate post-gadolinium SGE (B) images. Fat-suppressed T1-weighted spin echo image shows a large hypointense mass arising from the tail of the pancreas (M, A). Following gadolinium administration multiple large irregular signal-void defects (arrows, B) are noted in the mass consistent with cysts. Invasion of the spleen and multiple liver metastases are also present, confirming the malignant nature of this tumor. Reproduced with permission from Reference 2.

scar and ranges in size from 1 to 12 cm, with an average diameter at presentation of 5 cm. The lesion has either a smooth or nodular contour. On MR images the tumors are well defined and do not demonstrate invasion of fat or adjacent organs (Fig. 7) (27). On T2-weighted images multiple septations are apparent in the tumor, creating the appearance of a cluster of grapes. When the cysts measure less than

1cm in diameter then the diagnosis of microcystic adenoma can be made with confidence. Cysts that range in diameter between 1 and 2 cm may represent either micro- or macrocystic adenoma. Breath-hold or breathing-independent T2-weighted images possess the greatest clarity for defining the thin septations. Delayed enhancement of the central scar may occasionally be observed (2).

Macrocystic adenomas/adenocarcinomas are mucin-containing tumors that are malignant or have malignant potential (25, 27–29). They occur more frequently in females (6:1) and approximately one-half occur in patients between the ages of 40 and 60 years (29). These tumors usually are located in the body and tail of the pancreas; they are large (mean diameter 10 cm), multilocular, and encapsulated (27, 28). There is a great propensity for invasion of local organs and tissues. On T2-weighted images cysts typically are large, 2–5 cm in diameter, and irregular in shape. On gadolinium-enhanced fat-suppressed T1-weighted images, large, irregular cystic spaces separated by thick septa are demonstrated (Fig. 8). Macrocystic adenocarcinomas frequently show aggressive local invasion of adjacent organs such as stomach or spleen. The mucin produced by these tumors may result in high signal intensity on T1- and T2-weighted images of the primary tumor and metastases. The higher inherent soft tissue contrast of MRI compared to CT may result in better differentiation between microcystic and macrocystic cystadenomas because of clear definition of macrocysts in the latter tumor (27).

Metastases

Metastases may involve peripancreatic lymph nodes or may invade the pancreas. Primary malignancies include gastrointestinal, kidney, breast, lung, prostate, and melanoma. Renal cell carcinoma may metastasize many years following resection of the primary tumor. Magnetic resonance imaging in these patients reveals pancreatic masses that are high in signal intensity on T2-weighted images and show intense ring or, in small metastases, homogeneous enhancement on immediate post-gadolinium images (30). The metastatic deposits may be diffuse micronodular, multifocal, or solitary; clinical history plays an important role in establishing the diagnosis because these tumors may have an identical appearance with islet cell tumors (30). Melanoma metastases may be high in signal intensity on T1-weighted images owing to the paramagnetic properties of melanin (Fig. 9).

INFLAMMATORY DISEASE

Pancreatitis

Pancreatitis occurs secondarily to chronic alcoholism, gallstones, hypercalcemia, hyperlipoproteinemia, blunt abdominal trauma, penetrating peptic ulcer diseases, viral infections (most frequently Epstein–Barr), and certain drugs (31). Predisposition may also be inherited as an autosomal dominant trait (32).

Acute Pancreatitis

The MR findings in cases of uncomplicated acute pancreatitis are restricted to morphological changes (1). The pancreas may appear focally or diffusely enlarged,

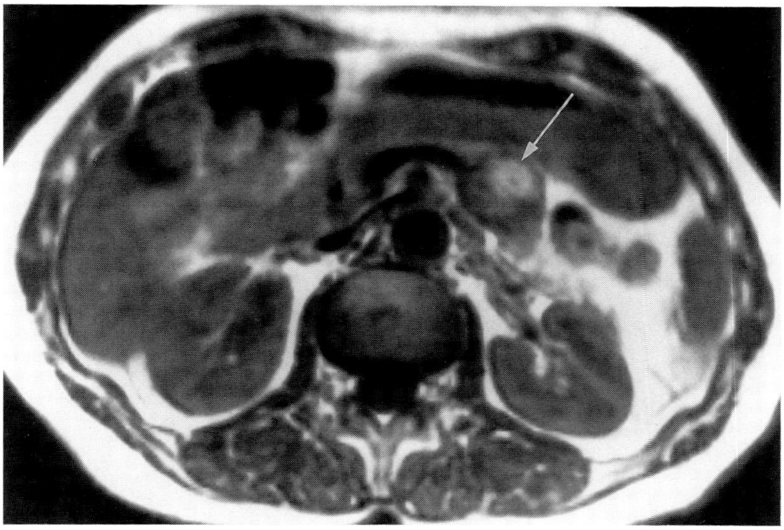

Figure 9. Melanoma metastasis. T1-weighted SE image shows a rounded mass in the tail of the pancreas (arrow). The mass is high in signal intensity owing to the paramagnetic properties of melanin. Reproduced with permission from Reference 1.

and this effect may be subtle. The presence of peripancreatic fluid is well shown on noncontrast SGE images as low-signal-intensity strands of fluid extravasation in a background of high-signal-intensity fat. Magnetic resonance imaging is sensitive for the detection of subtle changes of acute pancreatitis, particularly minor peripancreatic inflammatory changes (Fig. 10). The sensitivity of MRI may exceed that of CT, suggesting a role for MRI in the evaluation of patients with suspected acute pancreatitis and negative CT examination.

Percent pancreatic necrosis is an important prognostic indicator in patients with acute pancreatitis (33, 34). Dynamic gadolinium enhanced MRI may be useful for this determination. Complications of acute pancreatitis such as hemorrhage or pseudocyst formation are well depicted by MRI. Pseudocysts appear as low-signal-intensity or signal-void defects in a background of normal-signal-intensity pancreatic tissue on both SGE and fat-suppressed T1-weighted images; whereas hemorrhagic fluid collections are high in signal intensity on T1-weighted images. Pseudocysts complicated by infection or a large content of proteinaceous or necrotic material have moderate or mixed signal intensity on T2-weighted images compared to pseudocysts, which have a more simple fluid composition and are high in signal intensity. Signal intensity on T2-weighted images may provide information useful for therapeutic management.

Chronic Pancreatitis

Magnetic resonance imaging detects not only morphological findings but also the presence of fibrosis, reflected by a diminished signal intensity on T1-weighted fat-suppressed images and diminished enhancement on immediate post-gadolinium

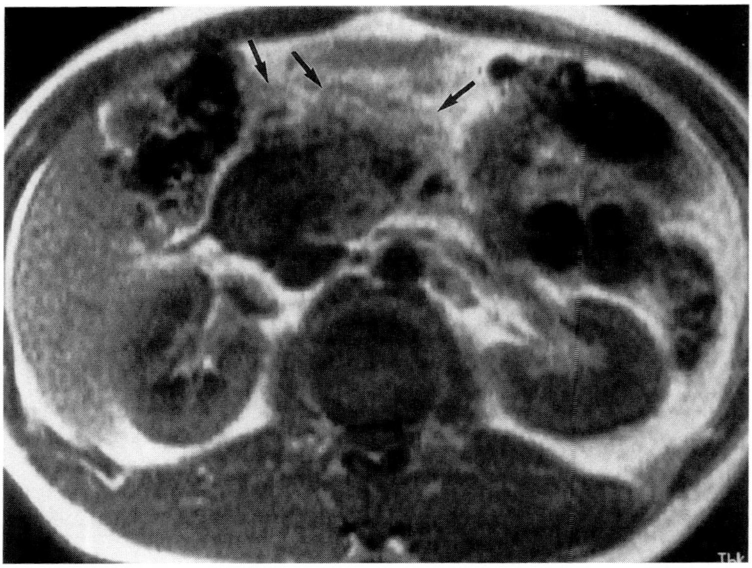

(A)

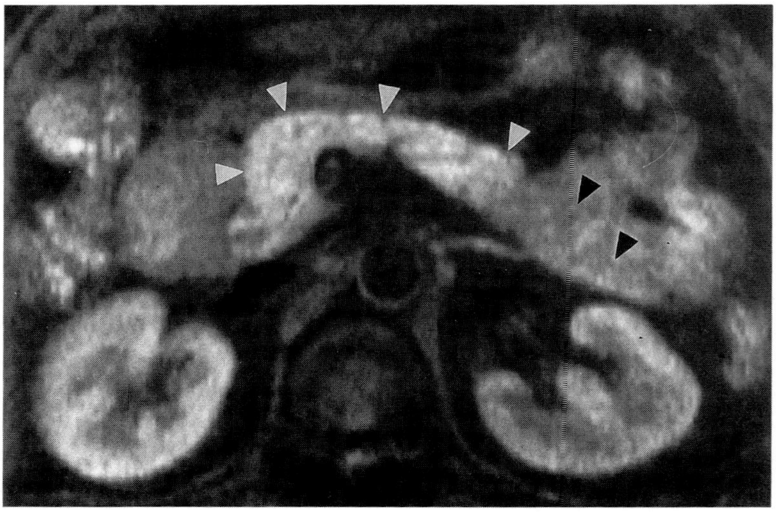

(B)

Figure 10. Acute pancreatitis. Precontrast SGE (A), fat-suppressed T1-weighted spin echo (B) and immediate post-gadolinium SGE (C, next page) images. Precontrast SGE image shows enlarged pancreatic head with subtle hypointense stranding in the peripancreatic fat (arrow, A). The immediate post-gadolinium SGE image shows an additional finding of free fluid (arrow, C) around the head of the pancreas (p, C) and duodenum (d, C) that is more conspicuous than on the precontrast SGE image. The precontrast fat-suppressed T1-weighted spin echo image from a higher level demonstrates normal high SI of the pancreas (arrowheads, B), suggesting that no fibrosis or devascularization is present. Reproduced with permission from Reference 4.

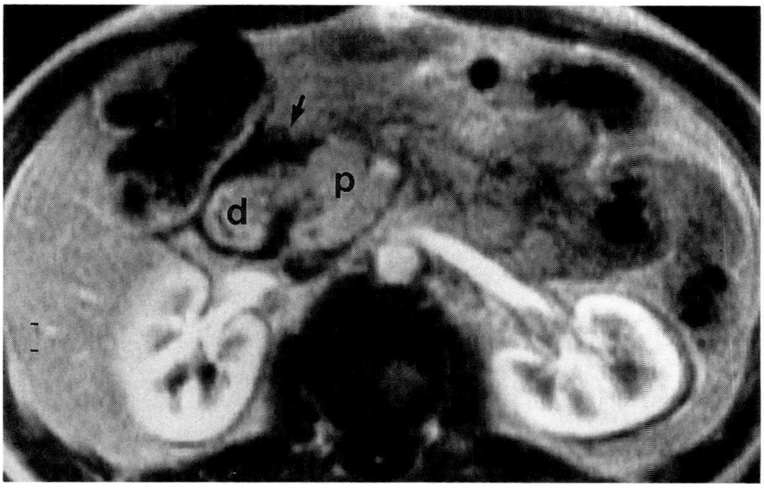

(C)

Figure 10. *(Continued)*

SGE images (Fig. 11) (35). In a report on 22 patients, including 13 with chronic calcifying pancreatitis and nine with presumed acute recurrent pancreatitis, differences between these groups were observed on T1-weighted fat-suppressed images and immediate post-gadolinium SGE images. All patients with pancreatic calcifications on CT examination had a diminished-signal-intensity pancreas on fat-suppressed T1-weighted images and abnormally low percent contrast enhancement on immediate post-gadolinium images. Patients with acute recurrent pancreatitis had signal-intensity features of the pancreas comparable to findings of normal pancreas. Because fibrosis is a precursor to the development of calcification, MRI may be able to detect chronic pancreatitis at an earlier stage than CT.

Chronic pancreatitis with associated focal enlargement of the gland may be difficult to distinguish from cancer on CT images. These two entities both demonstrate low signal intensity of the enlarged region of the pancreas on fat-suppressed T1-weighted images; however, on immediate post-gadolinium images, lack of a well-defined mass lesion and identification of signal-void cysts and calcifications usually permit the correct diagnosis of chronic pancreatitis to be made. Pseudocysts and cysts, sequelae of chronic pancreatitis, are well shown on gadolinium-enhanced fat-suppressed T1-weighted images (Fig. 12).

Pancreatic Transplants

Dynamic gadolinium-enhanced MRI has been advocated as a technique to assess rejection of pancreatic transplants. Percent enhancement in six normal grafts was 98 + 23% within the first minute, compared to 42 + 20% in six dysfunctional grafts (36).

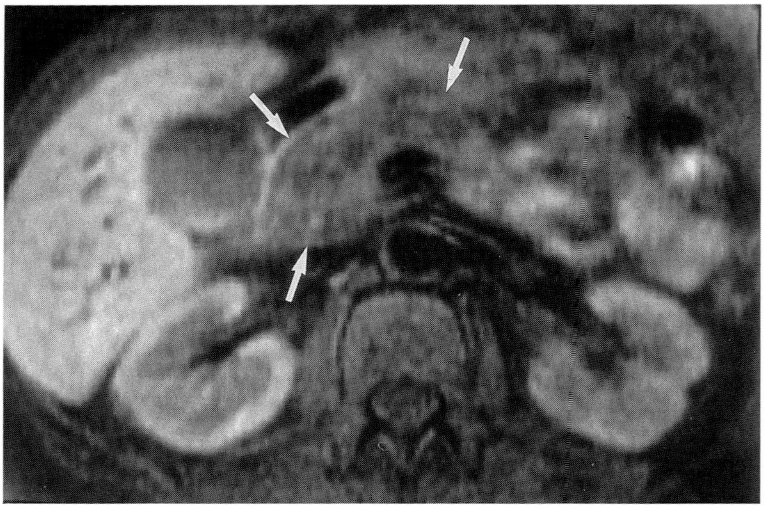

(A)

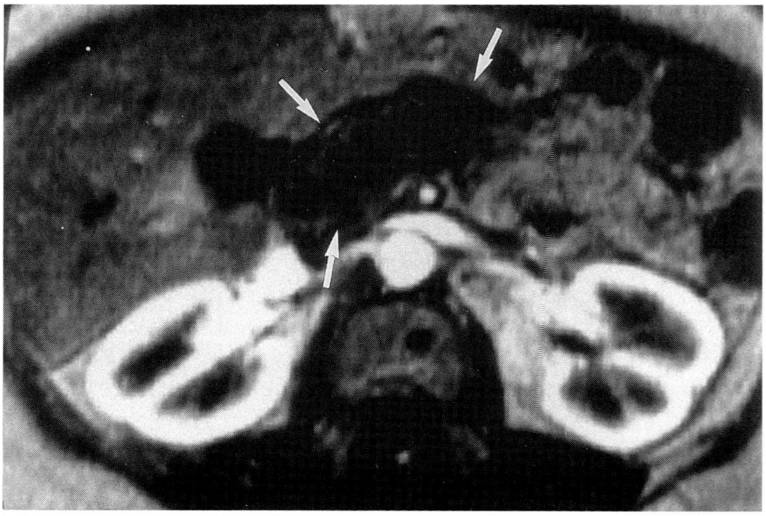

(B)

Figure 11. Chronic pancreatitis with calcifications and focal glandular enlargement. Fat-suppressed T1-weighted spin echo (A), immediate post-gadolinium SGE (B), and post-contrast fat-suppressed T1-weighted spin echo (C, next page) images. The head and neck of the pancreas are enlarged, have low signal intensity on the fat-suppressed T1-weighted spin echo image (arrows, A) and diminished contrast enhancement on the immediate post-gadolinium SGE image (arrows, B). Delayed enhancement consistent with fibrotic changes of chronic pancreatitis is noted on the post-contrast fat-suppressed T1-weighted spin echo image. Signal-void structures represent a combination of calcifications and dilated main pancreatic and common bile ducts (arrowheads, C). Reproduced with permission from Reference 2.

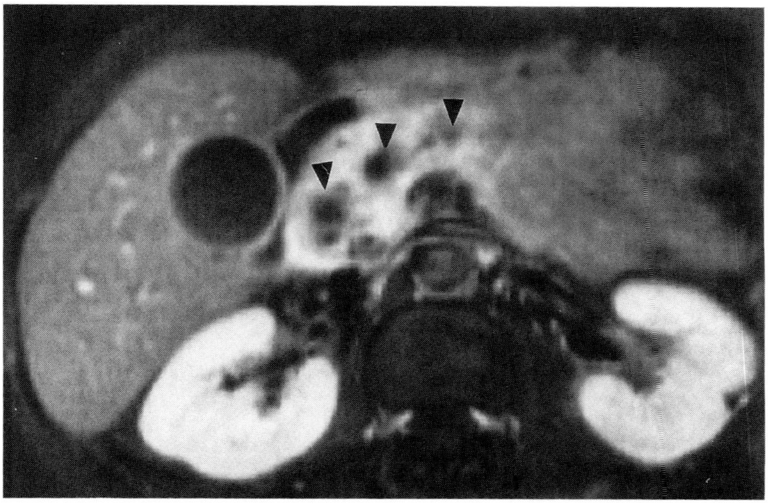

(C)

Figure 11. *(Continued)*

CLINICAL ROLE

Magnetic resonance imaging is able to provide a comprehensive evaluation of the pancreas, combining pancreatic parenchymal tomographic information with MR cholangiographic images. T1-weighted fat-suppressed images provide good contrast for the detection of small non-organ-deforming tumors and signal-intensity changes induced by chronic pancreatitis. T2FS images are helpful in the detection of islet cell tumors and in the evaluation of the liver for metastases. Fast echo train T2-weighted images, such as HASTE, define the pancreatic duct well, provide ERCP-like data, and are helpful in the determination of the level and cause of common bile duct obstruction in the region of the head of the pancreas. Immediate post-gadolinium SGE images depict pancreatic carcinomas owing to their hypovascular, desmoplastic nature, show diminished heterogeneous enhancement for chronic pancreatitis, and demonstrate the hypervascular blush or ring enhancement of islet cell tumors.

Patients should be considered for MR studies in the following settings: (*a*) elevated serum creatinine, allergy to iodine contrast, or other contraindications for iodine contrast administration; (*b*) focal enlargement of the pancreas with no definable mass on CT; (*c*) clinical history that is worrisome for malignancy and findings on CT that are equivocal or difficult to interpret; (*d*) failure to distinguish between chronic pancreatitis with focal enlargement and pancreatic carcinoma; (*e*) biochemical evidence of islet cell tumors but indeterminate findings on CT; and (*f*) a confusing clinical picture suggestive of pancreatitis and indeterminate findings on CT.

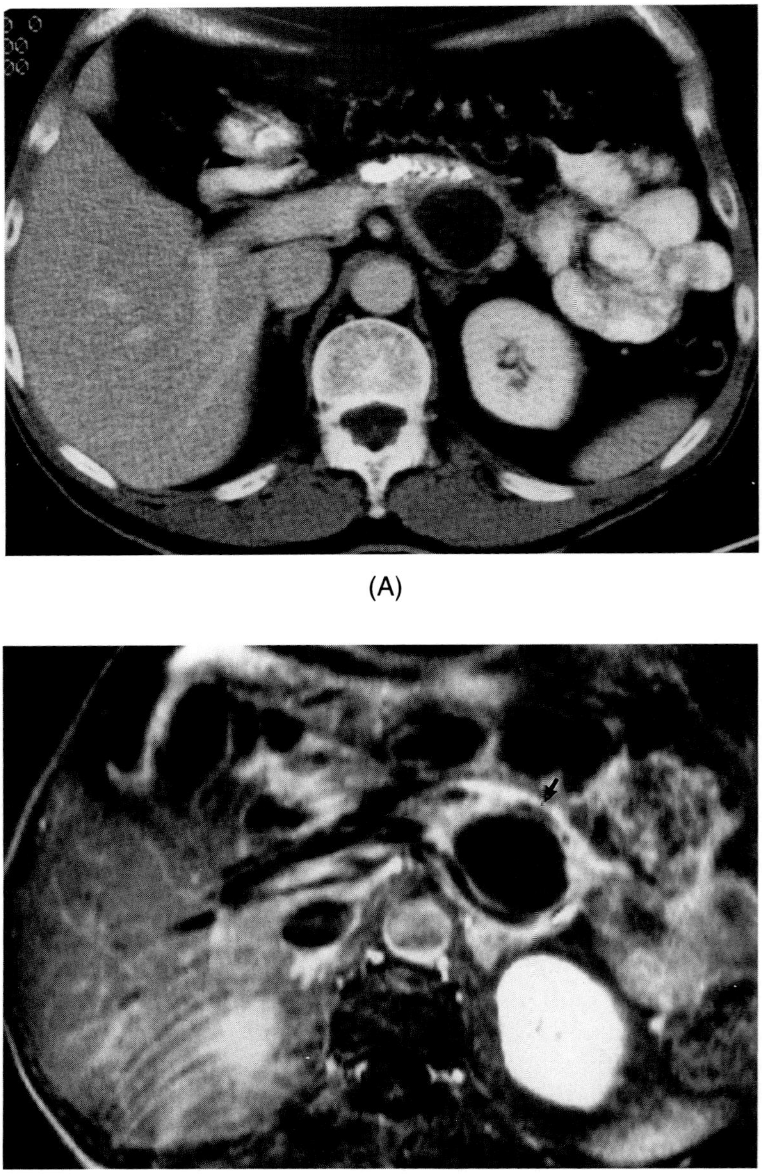

(A)

(B)

Figure 12. Chronic pancreatitis with pseudocyst. Contrast-enhanced 5-mm CT (A), and post-gadolinium fat-suppressed T1-weighted spin echo (B). The CT image shows extensive calcification along the wall of the pancreatic duct and the pseudocyst arising from the posterior aspect of the body of the pancreas. The MR image demonstrates that the pancreatic duct (arrow, B) is anterior in relation to the pseudocyst. Distinction between dilated duct and calcification could not be clearly made. Reproduced with permission from Reference 4.

REFERENCES

1. Semelka RC, Ascher SM. MRI of the pancreas—state of the art. *Radiology.* 1993;188:593–602.
2. Semelka RC, Shoenut JP, Kroeker MA, Micflikier AB. Pancreas. In: Semelka RC, Shoenut JP, eds. *Magnetic Resonance Imaging of the Abdomen with CT Correlation.* New York: Raven Press; 1993:84–98.
3. Mitchell DG, Vinitski S, Saponaro S, Tasciyan T, Burk DL Jr, Rifkin MD. Liver and pancreas: improved spin-echo T1 contrast by shorter echo time and fat suppression at 1.5T. *Radiology.* 1991;178:67–71.
4. Semelka RC, Kroeker MA, Shoenut JP, Kroeker R, Yaffe CS, Micflikier AB. Pancreatic disease: prospective comparison of CT, ERCP, and 1.5T MR imaging with dynamic gadolinium enhancement and fat suppression. *Radiology.* 1991;181:785–791.
5. Takehara Y, Ichijo K, Tooyama N, et al. Breath-hold MR cholangiopancreatography with a long-echo-time fast spin-echo sequence and a surface coil in chronic pancreatitis. *Radiology.* 1994;192:73–78.
6. Semelka RC, Simm FC, Recht M, Deimling M, Lenz G, Laub GA. MRI of the pancreas at high field strength—a comparison of six sequences. *J Comput Assist Tomogr.* 1991;15:966–971.
7. Reinhold C, Taourel P, Bret PM, Barkun AN, Atri M. MR cholangiography of choledocholithiasis by using a multicoil array and high resolution imaging parameters. *Radiology.* 1995;197:342.
8. Delhaye M, Engelholm L, Cremer M. Pancreas divisum: congenital anatomic variant or anomaly? Contribution of endoscopic retrograde dorsal pancreatography. *Gastroenterology.* 1985;89:951–958.
9. Bret PM, Reinhold C, Taourel P, Guibaud L, Atri M, Barkun AN. Pancreas divisum: evaluation with MR cholangiopancreatography. *Radiology.* 1996;199:99–103.
10. Siegelman ES, Mitchell DG, Outwater E, Munoz SJ, Rubin R. Idiopathic hemochromatosis: MR imaging findings in cirrhotic and precirrhotic patients. *Radiology.* 1993;188:637–641.
11. Sarles H, Sahel J. Pathology of chronic calcifying pancreatitis. *Am J Gastroenterol.* 1976;66:117–139.
12. Semelka RC, Kelekis NL, Molina PL, Scharp T, Calvo B. Pancreatic masses with indeterminate findings on spiral CR. Is there a role for MRI? *J Magn Reson Imaging.* 1996;6:585–588.
13. Gabata T, Matsui O, Kadoya M, et al. Small pancreatic adenocarcinomas: efficacy of MR imaging with fat suppression and gadolinium enhancement. *Radiology.* 1994;193:683–688.
14. Vellet AD, Romano W, Bach DB, Passi RB, Taves DH, Munk PL. Adenocarcinoma of the pancreatic ducts: Comparative evaluation with CT and MR imaging at 1.5T. *Radiology.* 1992;183:87–95.
15. Pavone P, Occhiato R, Michelini O, et al. Magnetic resonance imaging of pancratic carcinoma. *Eur Radiol.* 1991;1:124–130.
16. Patt R, Zeman RK, Nauta R, Ascher SM, Wooley P, Silverman P. Vascular encasement by pancreatobiliary neoplasms. Assessment with dynamic CT, spin-echo MR imaging and gradient echo MR imaging. *Radiology.* 1991;181(p):259.
17. Warshaw AL, Fernández-del Castillo C. Pancreatic carcinoma. *New Engl J Med.* 1992;326:455–465.
18. Mitchell DG, Cruvella M, Eschelman DJ, Miettinen MM, Vernick JJ. MRI of pancreatic gastrinomas. *J Comput Assist Tomogr.* 1992;16:583–585.

19. Semelka RC, Cummings M, Shoenut JP, Yaffe CS, Kroeker MA, Greenberg HM. Islet cell tumors: A comparison of detection by dynamic contrast-enhanced CT and MR imaging with dynamic gadolinium enhancement and fat suppression. *Radiology.* 1993;186:799–802.
20. Galiber AK, Reading CC, Charboneau JW, et al. Localization of pancreatic insulinoma: comparison of pre- and intraoperative US with CT and angiography. *Radiology.* 1988;166:405–408.
21. Mozell E, Stenzel P, Woltering EA, Rösch J, O'Dorisio TM. Functional endocrine tumors of the pancreas: clinical presentation, diagnosis, and treatment. *Curr Probl Surg.* 1990;27:304–385.
22. Frucht H, Doppman JL, Norten JA, et al. Gastrinomas comparison of MR imaging with CT, angiography, and US. *Radiology.* 1989;171:713–717.
23. Muller MF, Meyenberger C, Bertschinger P, Schaer R, Marincek B. Pancreatic tumors: evaluation with endoscopic US, CT and MR imaging. *Radiology.* 1994;190:745–751.
24. Kelekis NL, Semelka RC, Molina PL, Doerr ME. ACTH-secreting islet cell tumor: appearances on dynamic gadolinium-enhanced MRI. *Magn Reson Imaging.* 1995; 13:641–644.
25. Ros PR, Hamrick-Turner JE, Chiechi MV, Ross LH., Gallego P, Burton SS. Cystic masses of the pancreas. *Radiographics.* 1992;12:673–686.
26. Hough DM, Stephens DH, Johnson CD, Binkovitz LA. Pancreatic lesions in von Hippel–Lindau disease: prevalance, clinical significance, and CT findings. *AJR.* 1994;162:1091–1094.
27. Minami M, Itai Y, Ohtomo K, Yoshida H, Yoshikawa K, Iio M. Cystic neoplasms of the pancreas: comparison of MR imaging with CT. *Radiology.* 1989;171:53–56.
28. Friedman AC, Lichtenstein JE, Dachman AH. Cystic neoplasms of the pancreas: radiological-pathological correlation. *Radiology.* 1983;149:45–50.
29. Compagno J, Oertel JE. Mucinous cystic neoplasms of the pancreas with overt and latent malignancy (cystadenocarcinoma and cystadenoma): a clinicopathologic study of 41 cases. *Am J Clin Pathol.* 1978;69:573–580.
30. Kelekis NL, Semelka RC, Siegelman ES. MR imaging of pancreatic metastases from renal cancer. *J Comput Assist Tomogr.* 1996;20:249–253.
31. Steinberg W, Tenner S. Acute pancreatitis. *New Engl J Med.* 1994;1198–1210.
32. Kattwinkel J, Lapey A, DiSant'Agnese PA, Edwards WA, Jufty MP. Hereditary pancreatitis: three new kindreds and a critical review of the literature. *Pediatrics.* 1973;51:5–69.
33. Balthazar EJ, Robinson DL, Megibow AJ, Ranson JHC. Acute pancreatitis: value of CT in establishing prognosis. *Radiology.* 1990;174:331–336.
34. Johnson CD, Stephens DH, Sarr MG. CT of acute pancreatitis: correlation between lack of contrast enhancement and pancreatic necrosis. *AJR.* 1991;156:93.
35. Semelka RC, Shoenut JP, Kroeker MA, Micflikier AB. Chronic pancreatitis: MR imaging features before and after administration of gadopentetate dimeglumine. *JMRI.* 1993;3:79–82.
36. del Pilar Fernandez M, Bernardino ME, Neylan JF, Olson RA. Diagnosis of pancreatic transplant dysfunction: value of gadopentatate dimeglumine-enhanced MR imaging. *AJR.* 1991;156: 1171–1176.

24

PANCREATIC ANGIOGRAPHY

Donald F. Denny, Jr., M.D.
The Medical Center at Princeton
Princeton, New Jersey

As recently as the early 1980s, pancreatic angiography was described by Erik Boijsen (1) as ". . . the most reliable way to detect pancreatic disease." The development of sonography, computed tomography, endoscopic retrograde cholangiopancreatography, and magnetic resonance imaging has totally changed the playing field. Although angiography continues to play a role, it is much more limited. Angiography is indicated when the results of noninvasive imaging studies are inconclusive (2) and prior to pancreatic resection (3). Likewise, pancreatic venous sampling remains an important diagnostic tool, but its use is rare and largely confined to referral centers. This chapter describes the current role of these modalities in pancreatic cancer, islet cell tumors, pancreatitis, and other conditions.

ANGIOGRAPHIC ANATOMY

The pancreas is not supplied by any one distinct vessel. Rather, it receives arterial supply from several branches of the celiac and superior mesenteric arteries (SMA) that pass in the immediate vicinity of the organ. Anatomic variation is frequent (4). The celiac artery gives origin to the common hepatic and splenic arteries. The common hepatic artery passes superiorly to the head of the pancreas and gives rise to the gastroduodenal artery (GDA). The GDA passes laterally and inferiorly to the head and uncinate process of the pancreas and gives rise to two important pancreatic branches, the posterior and anterior superior pancreaticoduodenal arteries (Fig. 1). These anastomose with their respective counterparts, the inferior pancreaticoduodenal arteries, which originate from the SMA. Although the superior versions originate separately from the GDA, the inferior pancreaticoduodenal arteries arise as a common trunk from the posterior border of the SMA (Fig. 1) or from a proximal jejunal branch. The splenic artery runs along the superior surface of the body and tail of the pancreas. From it arise multiple small branches that penetrate

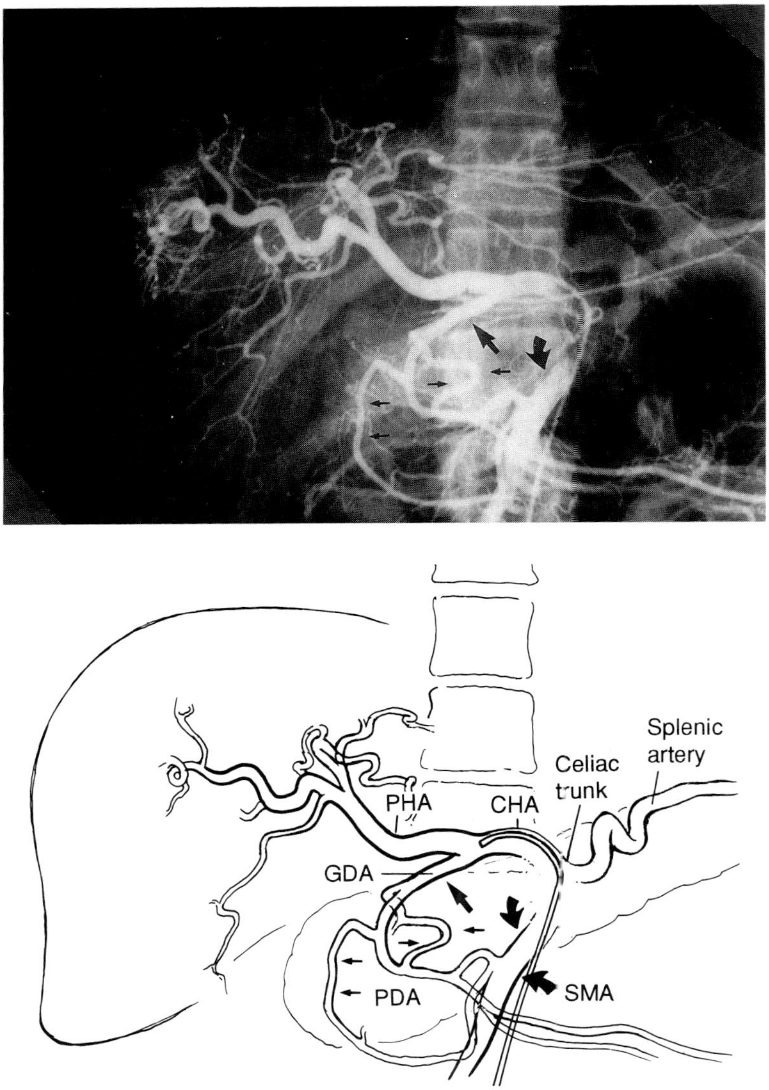

Figure 1. Pancreaticoduodenal arcades. Common hepatic artery injection shows filling of the gastroduodenal artery (large arrow) and pancreaticoduodenal arcades (small arrows). The superior mesenteric artery (curved arrows) is filling by flow from the superior to inferior pancreaticoduodenal arteries.

the pancreas in a vertical direction. The largest of these is termed the pancreatic magna. The dorsal pancreatic artery runs vertically from either the splenic or common hepatic artery to supply the midpancreas. It gives rise to the transverse pancreatic artery, which runs along the inferior aspect of the body and tail. There are commonly many interarterial anastomoses between branches within the organ.

Although venography of the pancreas is rarely done (5), venous sampling is more common. Knowledge of the venous anatomy is of primary importance for venous sampling in cases of suspected islet cell tumors. Venous drainage of the pancreas roughly parallels the arterial supply but is variable. There is considerable interconnection between draining veins. The main named veins are on the surface of the organ. The body and tail of the gland are drained superiorly through short veins that empty into the splenic vein. Inferiorly, the body and tail are drained by the transverse pancreatic vein, which joins the inferior or superior mesenteric vein, or the portal confluence. The head of the pancreas is drained dorsally by the posterior superior pancreaticoduodenal vein which empties into the main portal vein, and by the posterior inferior pancreaticoduodenal vein, which empties into the first jejunal vein or the superior mesenteric vein. The ventral head is drained by the anterior superior pancreaticoduodenal vein, which empties into the gastrocolic trunk, which in turn usually enters the SMV, and by the anterior inferior pancreaticoduodenal vein, which joins with its posterior counterpart to enter the first jejunal vein or SMV. Venous sampling is done by transhepatic catheterization of the portal vein.

Pancreatic angiography is performed using 4- or 5-French selective catheters. Injection of the aorta alone is insufficient for evaluation of the small arteries supplying the pancreas. A pancreatic arteriogram requires at the minimum injection of the celiac and superior mesenteric arteries. Selective injection of the GDA, splenic artery, dorsal pancreatic artery, and inferior pancreaticoduodenal trunk is often needed. If necessary, the operator may use a coaxial catheterization system with a 3-French catheter through a larger guiding catheter. The development of soft-tipped, steerable guide wires has been a significant aid to superselective catheterization. Complications of arteriography are infrequent. Spasm and dissection of a vessel are the primary concerns. Neither appears to be clinically important, perhaps owing to the rich interconnection of the vascular supply.

The introduction of digital subtraction angiography (DSA) into the practice of general diagnostic angiography has largely supplanted film-screen filming techniques (see Chapter 19). However, DSA is limited by inferior resolution when compared to film screen. In addition, motion of any body part may introduce artifacts that may obscure subtle tumors. This may be a particular problem for the pancreas because motion of gas in the stomach, small bowel, or colon may introduce artifacts mimicking a hypervascular lesion. Whether to use DSA or the traditional film-screen technique depends on various factors, including patient body habitus and cooperation, as well as operator preference. In a series reported by Hoevels, intra-arterial DSA and conventional film-screen angiography had equivalent results in 60% of patients with pancreatic or periampullary carcinomas; DSA was superior in 26% owing to improved visualization of the splanchnic veins, whereas it was inferior in 14% because of motion artifacts (6). Regardless of which system is employed, high-quality filming with magnification is necessary for satisfactory visualization.

Injection of a vasoconstrictor such as epinephrine (5–10 mcg) or vasopressin (0.5–1.0 international unit) into the celiac or SMA prior to angiography may enhance pancreas and tumor visualization by selectively constricting gastric, splenic, and mesenteric branches. Simultaneous injection of the celiac and SMA also has been suggested.

ADENOCARCINOMA

The primary angiographic findings of pancreatic adenocarcinoma are artery and vein encasement and displacement. Encasement is manifested by irregular stenosis and occlusion. Displacement may be difficult to detect given the large degrees of variation seen in the area. The primary tumor is usually hypovascular, so that tumor neovascularity may be absent. Tumor blush and arteriovenous shunt are absent. There is extensive literature describing the sensitivity and specificity of pancreatic angiography in the diagnosis of adenocarcinoma (5). Much of it is now moot, because noninvasive imaging using sonography, computed tomography, and magnetic resonance imaging provide direct visualization. Vessel encasement is also found in chronic pancreatitis, and it may be difficult to distinguish these two angiographically. Irregular vessel stenosis may also be caused by atherosclerosis and fibromuscular dysplasia, but involvement of other nonpancreatic vessels should help to distinguish this from primary pancreatic disease.

Angiography is performed prior to surgery to evaluate the arterial anatomy and to predict operability and prognosis (7); anatomic variation that may affect the surgical approach is frequent in this area. Preoperative arteriography may reduce the morbidity of pancreatic resection (8). If unsuspected celiac occlusive disease is present, pancreaticoduodenectomy may sacrifice critical visceral collaterals unless vascular bypass is performed (9). Evidence of encasement of the peripancreatic arteries or veins is an indicator of nonresectability. Because the main vessels are superficial to the pancreas, involvement indicates spread beyond the gland. In a prospective study of 88 patients studied using computed tomography (CT), magnetic resonance imaging (MRI), angiography, and laparoscopy, the combination of CT and angiography showed a pancreatic head tumor to be nonresectable in 87%. When all test results were negative, 78% of pancreatic head tumors were resectable, whereas only 5% were resectable if any test was positive (10).

Provocative work comparing endosonographic ultrasound with angiography and noninvasive imaging suggests that endosonography may be the most accurate in assessing resectability of pancreatic carcinoma (11).

ISLET CELL TUMORS

Islet cell tumors may be benign or malignant. The tumors may produce insulin, glucagon, gastrin, vasoactive intestinal peptide (VIP), or nothing. If the tumor secretes an active hormone, clinical signs develop while the primary tumor is still small. The primary tumor and metastases are hypervascular, and show a prolonged tumor blush (Fig. 2). High-quality magnification and subtraction films may be needed to show this, because the tumors are usually small. A blush in the tail of the pancreas must be distinguished from an accessory spleen.

Angiography continues to play an important role in the diagnosis of these infrequent tumors. In a prospective report comparing MRI, CT, sonography, and angiography, Pisegna et al. reported a 59% sensitivity for angiographic detection of primary gastrinoma, compared to sonography 19%, MRI 25%, and CT 28% (12). The combination of CT, sonography, and MRI had a sensitivity rate of only 38%.

Venous sampling complements angiography and noninvasive testing, and may localize an abnormality in the absence of a positive finding on arteriography. Gunther et al. reported a series of 31 insulinomas less than 2 cm in size (13). Sonography was successful in localization in 60%, CT in 43%, angiography in 65%, and pancreatic venous sampling in 81%. Intraoperative sonography correctly local-

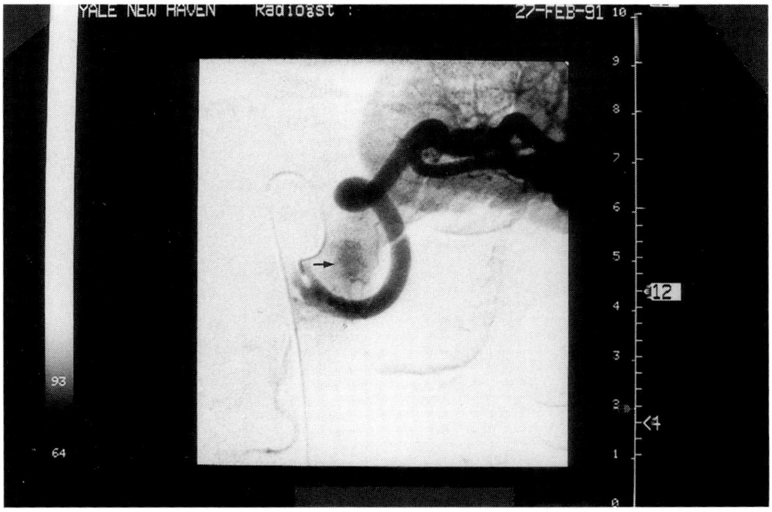

Figure 2. Insulinoma. Splenic artery injection shows a small hypervascular insulinoma of the pancreas (arrow).

ized nine of nine cases studied. Cho et al. reported successful localization of insulinomas using pancreatic venous sampling in 10 of 10 patients; angiography was successful in only two (14). In Cho's series, three of 10 adenomas could not be palpated intraoperatively. Daggett et al. reported 33 patients with insulinomas and took a more skeptical view. Angiography was successful in nine of 18 cases, but all insulinomas could be palpated at surgery; in their hands, venous sampling was successful in only two of eight patients studied (15). To summarize, pancreatic venous sampling is a complex, tedious procedure whose results vary depending on the technical performance of the procedure; it should be performed in patients with functional islet cell tumors with uncertain localization from noninvasive tests and angiography.

Moore et al. reported a case of angiographic embolization in a patient with recurrent insulinoma following primary resection (16). This approach may be useful when surgery is contraindicated.

PANCREATITIS

Angiography is used in the evaluation of vascular complications of pancreatitis (17, 18). The most common is pseudoaneurysm, which most often involves the splenic or gastroduodenal artery (Fig. 3). Hemorrhage without pseudoaneurysm may occur when the inflammation of pancreatitis causes erosion of an artery into the pancreatic duct (19) or into a pseudocyst (20). Compression or thrombosis of the splenic, portal, or mesenteric veins may occur secondarily to pancreatitis, and can be diagnosed angiographically. In addition to diagnosis, angiographic embolization may be used to aid in management of hemorrhage (21). In the initial evaluation of hemorrhage associated with pancreatitis, CT and sonography are indicated. Sonography with

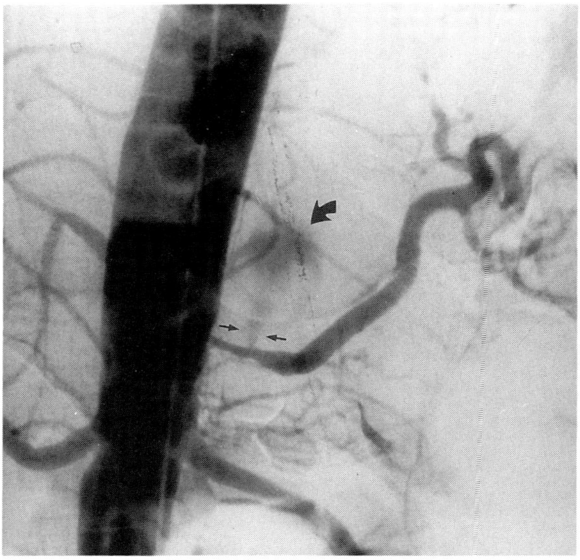

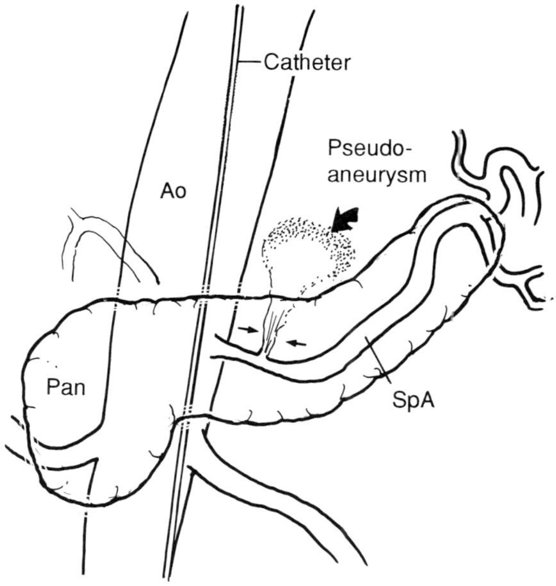

A

Figure 3. Pseudoaneurysm of the splenic artery from pancreatitis. (A) Aortogram shows irregular encasement of the proximal splenic artery and a jet of contrast (small arrows) filling a pseudoaneurysm (curved arrow). (B) CT shows the pseudoaneurysm (straight arrow) lying behind the stomach with central contrast (curved arrow) and peripheral thrombus (next page).

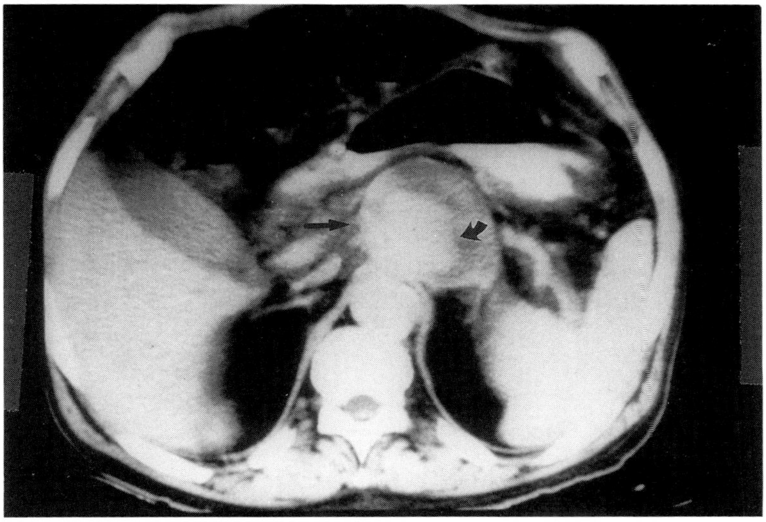

(B)

Figure 3. *(Continued)*

Doppler may reveal evidence of an aneurysm or pseudocyst. Computed tomography shows both of these; in addition, by evaluating the Hounsfield value of a fluid collection, CT may show evidence of acute hemorrhage.

The angiographic findings of pancreatitis are similar to those seen in pancreatic carcinoma. There is irregular arterial stenosis and occlusion. Displacement of vessels by the inflammatory mass may be present, but is difficult to diagnose with certainty owing to anatomic variability. Neovascularity is absent, as is usually true for carcinoma. Hypervascularity and arterioportal shunting have been reported (22). Occasionally, diagnostic angiography may be useful in evaluation of atypical masses in the region of the pancreas. Tongio et al. reported two cases of pseudocyst presenting in the region of the kidney; angiography was useful in determining that these were not of renal or other visceral origin (23).

Embolization of pseudoaneurysms related to pancreatitis has been reported by multiple authors. Jaschke et al. reported three such cases (24). Kolt and Wise reported a single case of successful embolization of a pseudoaneurysm of the gastroduodenal artery related to alcoholic pancreatitis with pseudocyst (25). Vujic et al. reported three patients with varying angiographic presentations in whom hemorrhage was successfully treated with embolization (26). Vujic observed that the angiographic findings may not show active extravasation at the time of study; observation of vascular abnormalities such as pseudoaneurysm and encasement helps in the choice of vessel to be embolized.

OTHER CONDITIONS

True aneurysms of the pancreatic arteries are infrequent. Chiang reported four cases of inferior pancreaticoduodenal aneurysms (27). The three patients who presented as acute hemorrhage were treated successfully by embolization. One asymptomatic aneurysm with anatomy unfavorable for embolization was treated surgically.

The indications for angiography in cases of cystic neoplasms such as cystadenoma and cystadenocarcinoma are similar to those for carcinoma. Mucinous cystic neoplasms are hypovascular; CT and sonography play the primary role in their characterization (28).

Iatrogenic hemorrhage through the pancreatic duct may be seen following gastric surgery. Vujic et al. reported a case of hemorrhage from the left gastric artery stump into a pseudocyst following subtotal gastrectomy; angiography showed pancreatic duct opacification and duodenal hemorrhage (29).

REFERENCES

1. Boijsen E. Pancreatic angiography. In: Abrams HL, ed. *Abrams Angiography,* 2nd ed. Boston: Little, Brown, 1983:1427.
2. Stanley RJ, Sagel SS, Evens RG. The impact of new imaging methods on pancreatic arteriography. *Radiology.* 1980;136:251–253.
3. Levin DC, Wilson R, Abrams HL. The changing role of pancreatic arteriography in the era of computed tomography. *Radiology.* 1980;136:245–249.
4. Toni R, Favero L, Mosca S, Ricci S, et al. Quantitative clinical anatomy of the pancreatic arteries studied by selective celiac angiography. *Surg Radiol Anat.* 1988;10:53–60.
5. Rosch J, Keller FS. Pancreatic arteriography, transhepatic pancreatic venography, and pancreatic venous sampling in diagnosis of pancreatic cancer. *Cancer.* 1981;47(6 suppl):1679–1684.
6. Hoevels J, Busch HP, Beyer-Enke S. Intra-arterial DSA versus conventional angiography in assessing the resectability of pancreatic and periampullary carcinomas. ROFO *Fortschr Geb Rontgenstr Nuklearmed.* 1987;146:291–294.
7. Karp W, Lunderquist A, Tylen U, Ishe I. Angiography and ultrasound examination in the evaluation of pancreatic lesions. *Acta Radiol [Diagn] (Stockh).* 1980;21(2A):169–176.
8. Thomford NR, Chandnani PC, Taha AM, Chablani VN, Busnardo AC. Anatomic characteristics of the pancreatic arteries. Radiologic observations and their clinical significance. *Am J Surg.* 1986;151:690–693.
9. Thompson NW, Eckhauser FE, Talpos G, Cho KJ. Pancreaticoduodenectomy and celiac occlusive disease. *Ann Surg.* 1981;193:399–406.
10. Warshaw AL, Gu ZY, Wittenberg J, Waltman AC. Preoperative staging and assessment of resectability of pancreatic cancer. *Arch Surg.* 1990;125:230–233.
11. Rosch T, Dittler HJ, Lorenz R, Braig C, et al. The endosonographic staging of pancreatic carcinoma. *Dtsch Med Wochenschr.* 1992;117:563–569.
12. Pisegna JR, Doppman JL, Norton JA, Metz DC, Jensen RT. Prospective comparative study of ability of MR imaging and other imaging modalities to localize tumors in patients with Zollinger–Ellison syndrome. *Dig Dis Sci.* 1993;38:1318–1328.
13. Gunther RW, Klose KJ, Ruckert K, Beyer J, et al. Localization of small islet-cell tumors. Preoperative and intraoperative ultrasound, computed tomography, arteriography, digital subtraction angiography, and pancreatic venous sampling. *Gastrointest Radiol.* 1985;10:145–152.
14. Cho KJ, Vinik AI, Thompson NW, Shields JJ, et al. Localization of the source of hyperinsulinism: percutaneous transhepatic portal and pancreatic vein catheterization with hormone assay. *AJR.* 1982;139:237–245.

15. Daggett PR, Goodburn EA, Kurtz AB, Le Quesne LP, et al. Is preoperative localisation of insulinomas necessary? *Lancet.* 1981;1(8218);483–486.

16. Moore TJ, Peterson LM, Harrington DP, Smith RJ. Successful arterial embolization of an insulinoma. *JAMA.* 1982;248:1353–1355.

17. Vujic I. Vascular complications of pancreatitis. *Radiol Clin North Am.* 1989;27:81–91.

18. Savastano S, Feltrin GP, Antonio T, Miotto D, et al. Arterial complications of pancreatitis: diagnostic and therapeutic role of radiology. *Pancreas.* 1993;8:687–692.

19. Ribbans WJ, Pounder RE, Lindsay I. Haemorrhage through the ampulla of Vater. *Postgrad Med J.* 1985;61:533–535.

20. Bender JS, Levison MA. Pseudoaneurysm of the gastroduodenal artery arising within a pancreatic pseudocyst. *Ann Vasc Surg.* 1992;6:171–172.

21. Vujic I, Anderson MC, Meredith HC, Cullom JW. Successful embolization of the dorsal pancreatic artery to control massive upper gastrointestinal hemorrhage. *Am Surg.* 1980;46:184–186.

22. Kitagawa K, Takashima T, Matsui O, Kadoya M, et al. Marked hypervascularity and early arteriovenous shunting with portal vein filling in chronic relapsing pancreatitis. *Gastrointest Radiol.* 1986;11:56–60.

23. Tongio J, Wenger JJ, Barth M, Warter P. Pseudocysts of the pancreas presenting in the kidney region. A report on two cases. *Semin Hop.* 1980;56:453–456.

24. Jaschke W, Hoevels J, Menges HW, Georgi M. Diagnosis and therapy of bleeding aneurysms of the parapancreatic arteries. *ROFO Fortschr Geb Rontgenstr Nuklearmed.* 1988;148:619–623.

25. Kolt S, Wise A. Embolisation in the management of parapancreatic pseudoaneurysm—a case report. *Australas Radiol.* 1992;36:65–67.

26. Vujic I, Andersen BL, Stanley JH, Gobien RP. Pancreatic and parapancreatic vessels: embolization for control of bleeding in pancreatitis. *Radiology.* 1984;150:51–55.

27. Chiang KS, Johnson CM, McKusick MA, Maus TP, Stanson AW. Management of inferior pancreaticoduodenal artery aneurysms: a 4 year, single center experience. *Cardiovasc Intervent Radiol.* 1994;17:217–221.

28. Friedman AC, Lichtenstein JE, Dachman AH. Cystic neoplasms of the pancreas. Radiological-pathological correlation. *Radiology.* 1983;149:45–50.

29. Vujic I, Jones WN 3d, Bradham GB, Meredith HC. Angiogram demonstration of gastrointestinal bleeding through the pancreatic duct. *Gastrointest Radiol.* 1980;5:43–45.

25

ERCP AND ENDOSCOPIC ULTRASOUND OF THE PANCREAS

Gregory G. Ginsberg, M.D.
University of Pennsylvania Health Systems
Philadelphia, PA

Cuong C. Nguyen, M.D.
Mayo Clinic Scottsdale
Scottsdale, Arizona

The past 20 years have witnessed tremendous advances in the endoscopic diagnosis and treatment of pancreatic diseases. The development of endoscopic retrograde cholangiopancreatography (ERCP) allowed, for the first time, radiographic imaging of the pancreatic duct without requiring laparotomy. Today, ERCP has become the "gold standard" for imaging the pancreatic duct as well as the biliary tree. An assortment of pancreatic tissue sampling techniques and the application of endoscopic therapies have become routine. Endoscopic ultrasonography (EUS) is a more recent advance that has been found particularly well suited for the evaluation of the pancreas. It allows high-resolution imaging of all portions of the pancreatic parenchyma and the main pancreatic ductal system, as well as surrounding lymph nodes and vascular structures. It is an effective tool in the diagnosis and staging of pancreatic cancer and has an emerging role in the evaluation and management of non-neoplastic pancreatic diseases.

INSTRUMENTATION

Endoscopic Retrograde Cholangiopancreatography

Endoscopic retrograde cholangiopancreatography is a technically demanding procedure performed by gastrointestinal endoscopists to evaluate diseases of the pancreatico-biliary tree. Although it is widely available, technical success and image quality are operator dependent and may vary considerably, based on the endoscopist's training and experience. In experienced hands, it is generally a safe and well tolerated, minimally invasive, outpatient procedure.

The fasting patient is placed in a modified prone position on a fixed fluoroscopic unit. Conscious sedation, typically with intravenous midazolam and meperidine, is administered. A side-viewing flexible duodenoscope is used. This endoscope is modified with an elevator lever that allows additional "up–down" directional movement of instruments passed through the working channel of the endoscope. This side-viewing endoscope allows an "en face" view of the major papilla. The standard diagnostic duodenoscope has a working channel of 2.8 mm and an outside diameter of 11.5 mm. Larger therapeutic duodenoscopes have a working channel of 4.2 mm and an outside diameter of 12.5 mm. State-of-the-art electronic video endoscopes allow image projection, storage, retrieval, and reproduction.

Ductal cannulation is usually achieved with a standard Teflon catheter of 5-French gauge (1.7 mm) with a slightly rounded radiopaque distal tip passed through the working channel of the endoscope. By maneuvering the tip of the endoscope and the elevator, the cannula is positioned for insertion into the major papilla. Radio-opaque contrast is then injected under fluoroscopic observation. Numerous catheter modifications and guide wires are available to facilitate selective duct cannulation. In expert hands, selective cannulation of the biliary and pancreatic ducts is feasible in 90% of cases. The risk of procedure-related pancreatitis is 1.3–7.4% (1, 2). Conditions that contribute to difficult or impossible ductal cannulation include duodenal stenosis, Bilroth II anastomosis, papillary stenosis, and an uncooperative patient.

Two immediate advantages of ERCP for the evaluation and management of pancreatic disease are its ability to (1) visualize the ampulla of Vater, and (2) apply therapeutic or tissue-sampling techniques adjunctively to a diagnostic study. In addition to pancreatography and cholangiography, the major and minor papillae are inspected for gross abnormalities (Fig. 1). A number of therapeutic and tissue sampling techniques have evolved such as stone removal, dilation and stenting of strictures, pseudocyst drainage, intraductal brush cytology, needle aspiration, and forceps biopsy sampling.

Endoscopic sphincterotomy utilizes an electrocautery wire to transect the sphincter choledochus or the sphincter pancreaticus. Indications for sphincterotomy include retained or recurrent common bile duct stones, papillary stenosis, biliary dyskinesia, ampullary tumors, choledochocele, strictures, and ductal leaks. Strictures can be dilated with rigid or pneumatic dilating devices. Finally, rigid plastic or expandable metallic stents may be placed in the pancreatic or biliary tree in the management of benign or malignant disease.

Endoscopic Ultrasound

Endoscopic ultrasound (EUS) was first conceived and developed as a technology to improve imaging of the pancreas; it combines the technologies of flexible endoscopy with that of high-frequency ultrasonography. Higher-frequency ultrasound maximizes spatial resolution, but at the cost of reduced tissue penetration. Attaching the ultrasound transducer to the tip of flexible endoscope (1) allows placement of

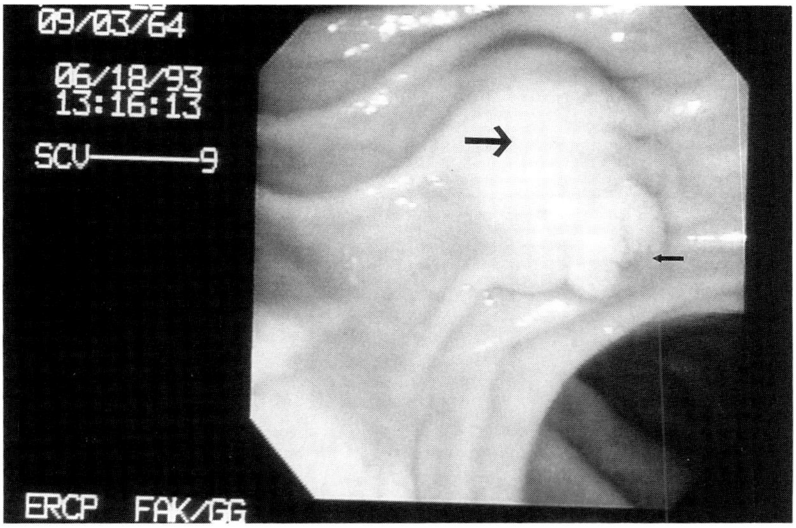

(A)

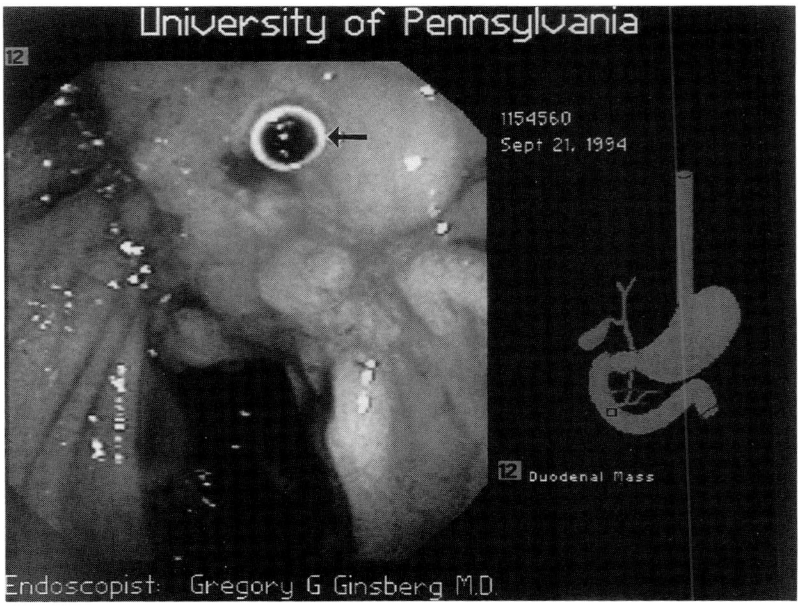

(B)

Figure 1. (A) Normal ampulla of Vater. The papillary orifice is designated by the small arrow. The intraduodenal segment of the common bile duct is designated by the large arrow. (B) Abnormal major papilla. This is an ampullary carcinoma arising from adenomatous dysplasia. A stent has been placed in the bile duct to relieve obstruction (arrow).

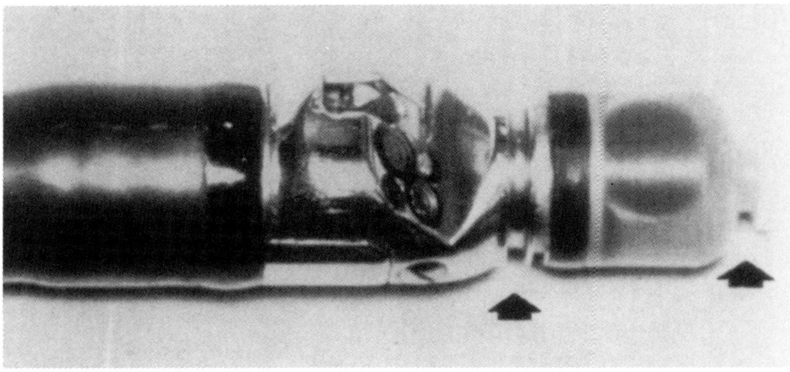

(A)

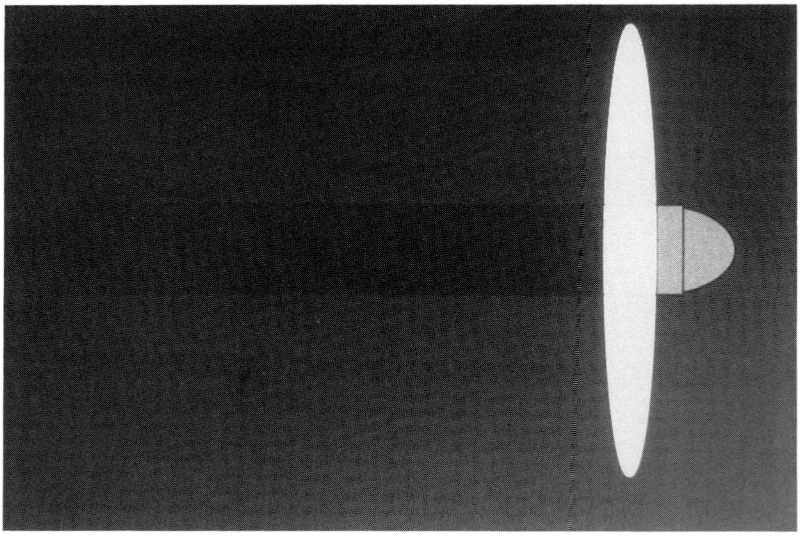

(B)

Figure 2. (A) Olympus GFUM20 echoendoscope. An ultrasound transducer is mounted to the tip of a modified fiber optic endoscope. The transducer is driven by a motor to spin on a 360° axis. A latex balloon is placed over the transducer (into slots designated by arrows) which is filled with water to enhance acoustic coupling. (B) 360° radial scanning allows cross-sectional imaging of the bowel wall and neighboring structures.

the transducer in close proximity to the tissue of interest in order to take advantage of high-frequency ultrasound, and (2) circumvents the traditional impediments of transabdominal ultrasonography such as interposing skin, bowel gas, and bone.

The most commonly used instrument for performing EUS is the Olympus GF-UM-20 (Olympus America, Inc., Lake Success, NY). This is a radial scanning echoendoscope (Fig. 2). A single-element transducer is attached to the tip of a fiber optic endoscope. The transducer is rotated mechnically 360° around the axis of the endoscope. Images are transmitted at two frequencies, 7.5 and 12 MHz, and are created in a plane perpendicular to the endoscope shaft. The endoscope is a modified standard fiber-optic endoscope with viewing optics at a 45° angle, rather than straight ahead. A disposable latex balloon is fitted over top of the ultrasound transducer. This can be filled with water to allow coupling between the organ of interest and the ultrasound transducer. The Olympus echoendoscope has an outside diameter of 13 mm with rigid tip of 2 cm in length. The ultrasound images are displayed on a dedicated monitor. A computer keypad allows images to be frozen for accurate measurements, labeling, and further documentation.

An alternative type of echoendoscope developed by the Pentax Corporation in conjunction with Hitachi incorporates a linear array transducer providing sector scanning along the axis of the endoscope. The transducer is made up of multiple piezoelectric elements aligned on a curved surface. The angle of scanning is 100° (Fig. 3). A disposable balloon condom is placed over the ultrasound head to allow coupling of the transducer and the gut wall. Unique to the Pentax echoendoscope is the construction of a 2-mm biopsy channel that allows an aspiration needle to course along the direction of imaging. This enables real-time ultrasound-guided fine needle aspiration for cytology. Also unique to the Pentax/Hitachi system are several features including pulse Doppler, color flow Doppler, and variation of the focal length.

The Olympus GFUM-20 is the most commonly used instrument for pancreatic cancer evaluation and staging. However, studies comparing the use of the linear array with the radial scanning echoendoscope have demonstrated parity. More often, the Pentax linear array scope is used to facilitate ultrasound-guided, real-time, fine needle aspiration of pancreatic masses and celiac or peripancreatic lymph nodes.

Through-the-scope ultrasound probes are small diameter (2-mm) flexible probes designed to pass through the working channel of an endoscope. This feature obviates the need for a specialized, dedicated scope and allows endoscopically directed localization of the ultrasound tip. These probes may be passed, independently or over a guide wire, into the biliary or pancreatic ducts (Fig. 4). Frequencies of 7.5, 12, 15, and 20 MHz have been used.

Endoscopic ultrasound is an outpatient procedure performed in the fasting patient with conscious sedation similarly to ERCP. With the patient in the left lateral decubitus position, and appropriate level of intravenous endoscopic conscious sedation achieved, the endoscope is passed blindly through the oropharynx and then under endoscopic visualization through the esophagus, stomach, and into the descending duodenum. Using a standard straightening technique, the endoscope is advanced into the second portion of the duodenum where the ampulla of Vater is visualized endoscopically. Thereafter, the echoendoscope is advanced so that positioning of the transducer is distal to the papilla, at which time endosonographic imaging begins.

Localization of the surrounding structures provides anatomic orientation. In this location the aorta is seen in cross-section at the 5 o'clock position and the inferior vena cava at the 7 o'clock position (Fig. 5A). On withdrawal of the echoendoscope, the head of the pancreas is examined from the horizontal, descending, and bulbar duodenum. The body and the tail of the pancreas are imaged from the inferoposterior gastric wall in the antrum and body of the stomach. Inflation of the water-filled balloon or filling the duodenal or gastric lumen with water may be necessary to achieve acoustic coupling.

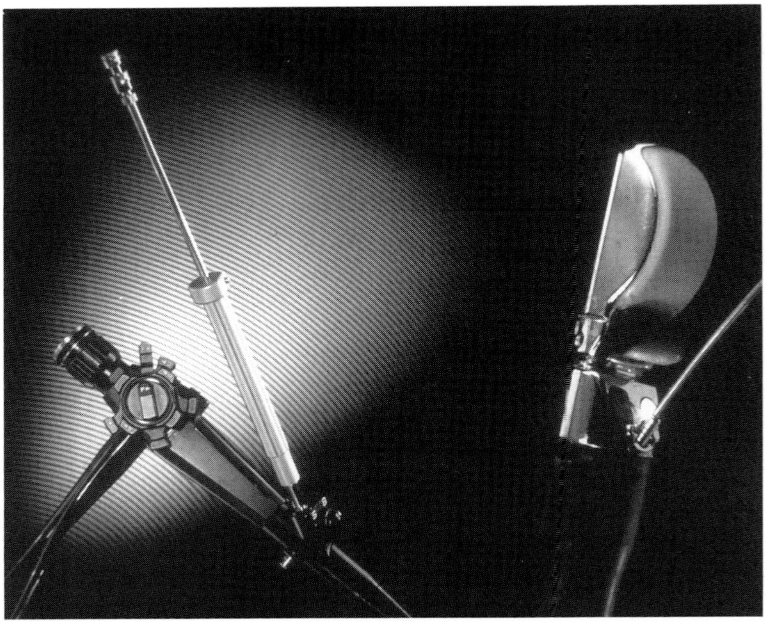

(A)

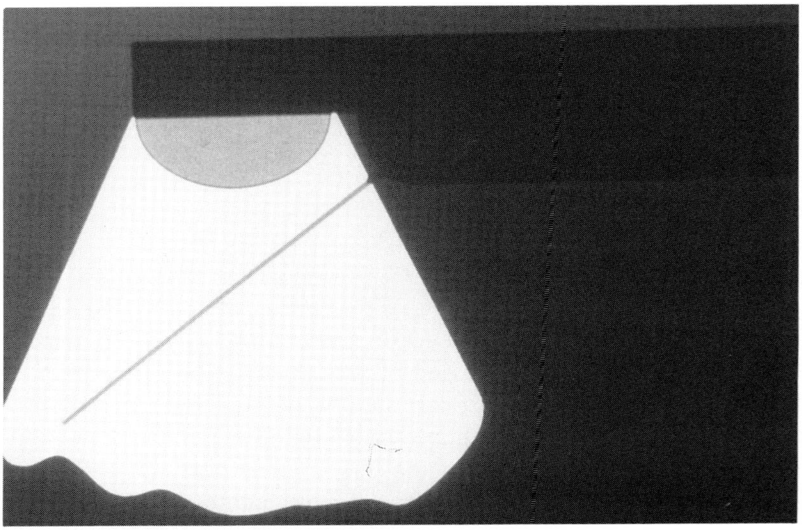

(B)

Figure 3. (A) Pentax FG-32PUA (Pentax Precision Instrument Corp., Orangeburg, NY) endoscope shown here with 22-gauge GIP aspiration needle (GIP Medizin ¯echnik, Grassau, Germany). (B) The linear array echoendoscope provides a 100° angle of imaging. The aspiration needle is directed into the field of image allowing real-time, ultrasound-guided tissue sampling.

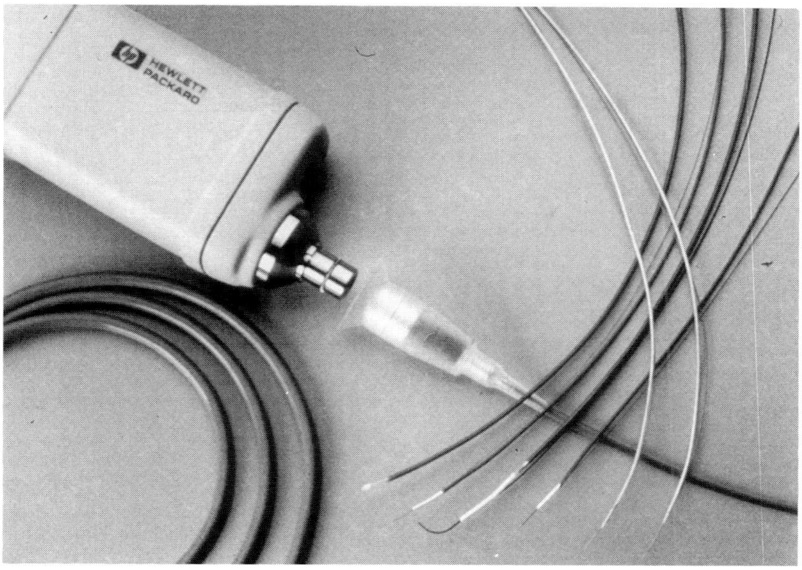

Figure 4. Through-the-scope ultrasound probes (Microvasive Inc, Boston Scientific Corp., Natick, Massachusetts) can be passed directly or over a guide wire into the biliary or pancreatic ducts under endoscopic guidance.

The ventral pancreas is seen with the main pancreatic duct (Wirsung's duct) coursing through it. The portal vein, splenic vein, and splenoportal confluence should be identified. The trifurcation created by the splenic and superior mesenteric veins joining to form the portal vein is often visualized (Fig. 5B). However, the superior mesenteric vein may not always be assessed because of its distance from the transducer. On pulling back into the duodenal bulb, the common bile duct can be readily identified ventral to the portal vein. The hepatic artery may be seen from this location. The remainder of the head and the genu of the pancreas are visualized from the duodenal bulb position. Pulling back into the antrum, the proximal pancreatic body is seen and the remaining body and tail region is observed by traversing the posterior gastric wall (Fig. 5C). The splenic vein is nearly universally seen as the transducer is withdrawn along the posterior gastric wall. This can be traced to its origin in the splenic hilum. The splenic artery runs a tortuous course ventral to the splenic vein and is smaller in diameter. The dorsal pancreatic duct is found approximately 1 cm ventral to the splenic vein. When the transducer is withdrawn more proximally in the stomach, the celiac axis can be imaged arising from the aorta. The bifurcation of the celiac axis into the splenic artery and hepatic artery has a classic "whale's tail" or "seagull" appearance (Fig. 5D). Successful identification of the celiac axis is achieved in 97% of cases (3). The inability to identify the celiac axis when accessing patients with pancreatic carcinoma should raise a suspicion of celiac axis invasion.

Pancreatic imaging by endosonography is difficult and proficiency requires intensive training and experience. A stepwise disciplined examination is necessary to obtain satisfactory images from all portions of the pancreas, and to evaluate the large vessels of the region. Individual anatomic variations increase the challenge.

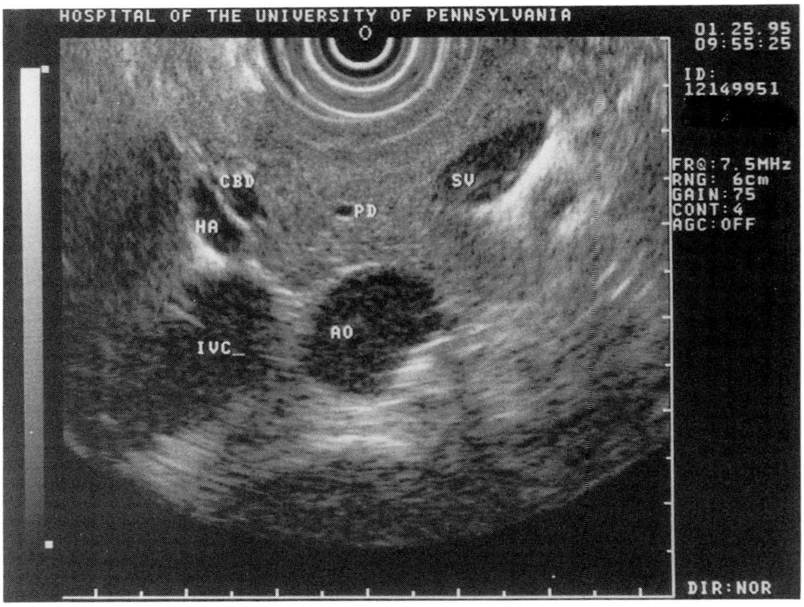

(A)

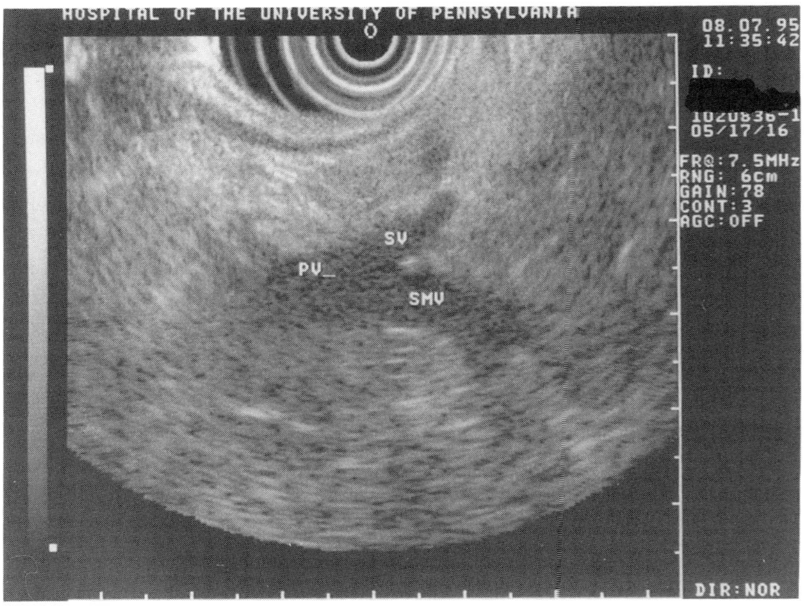

(B)

Figure 5. (A) The pancreatic head is first imaged from the duocenum. Orientation is provided by identifying the great vessels (AO = aorta, IVC = inferior vena cava, CBD = common bile duct, HA = hepatic artery, PD = pancreatic duct, SV = splenic vein, SA = splenic artery). (B) The confluence of the splenic vein (SV) and the superior mesenteric artery (SMV) can be seen below the pancreatic head where they meet to form the portal vein (PV). (C) Imaging of the genu, body, and tail regions of the pancreas are obtained from transantral positioning (next page). (D) The celiac axis is seen posterior or superior to the pancreas through the posterior gastric body (next page).

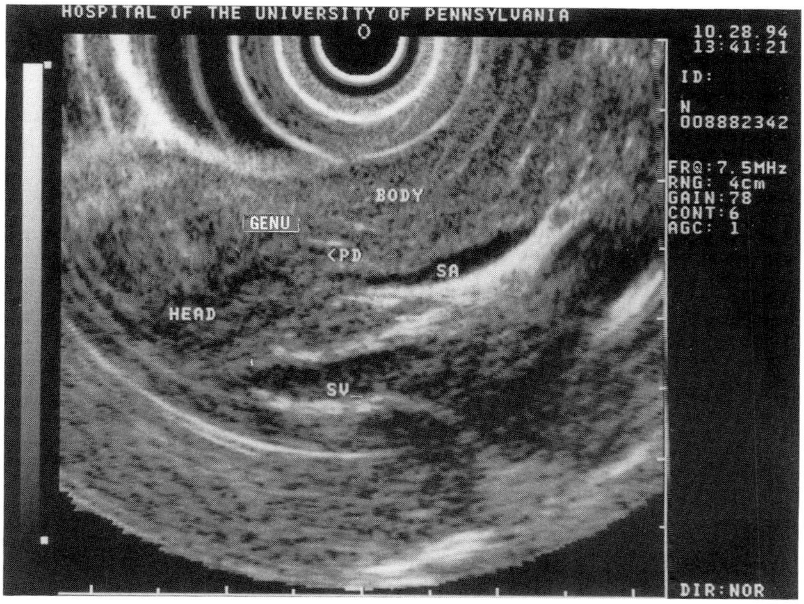

(C)

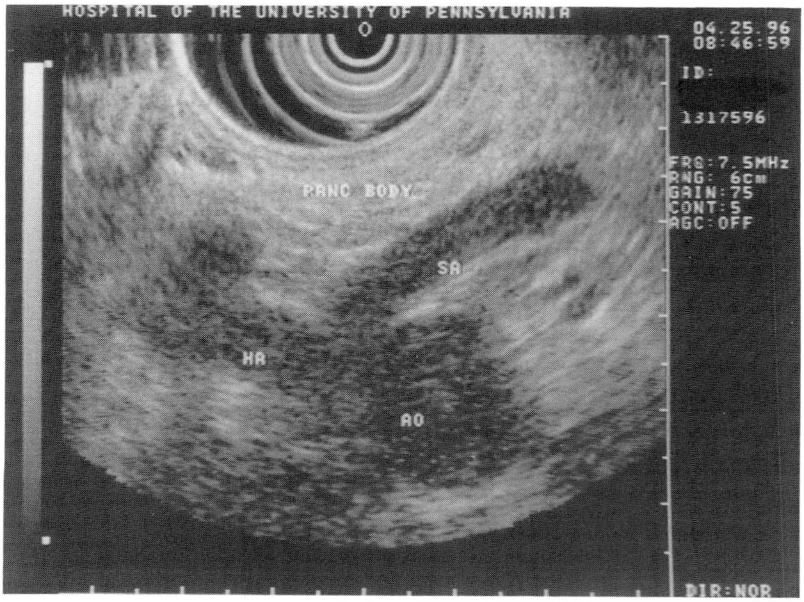

(D)

Figure 5. (*Continued*).

Limitations of EUS evaluation of pancreas include (1) luminal stenosis, (2) uncooperative patient, and (3) prior abdominal surgeries, such as Bilroth II or Whipple procedures. Endoscopic ultrasound, like other ultrasound technology, assesses the tissue echo character and is not a substitute for histopathology.

PANCREATIC CANCER

Adenocarcinoma of the pancreas occurs with an incidence of 0.01%; however, it is the fourth leading cause of cancer death in American men and women. The 5-year survival rate for the disease is only 2–5%. This poor survival rate is the result of the apparent widespread dissemination of malignant cells during the preclinical phase such that, by the time most patients present with symptoms, they already have advanced incurable disease. In spite of the dismal outlook, new strategies for staging and treatment of pancreatic cancer offer some encouragement. In particular, EUS allows improved diagnosis and localization of small (<2–3 cm) lesions and more accurately detailed staging information. The early identification of small pancreatic cancers not seen by other conventional imaging studies is important because this group of patients may achieve a 5-year survival rate of 30% with attempted curative resection. The result of improved staging is earlier, and more precise selection of treatment based on true tumor stage.

Endoscopic Retrograde Cholangiopancreatography

More than 80% of pancreatic carcinomas originate from the pancreatic duct epithelium. Endoscopic retrograde pancreatography, which enables examination of the main pancreatic duct, as well as the secondary and tertiary side branches, is a sensitive and specific means for evaluating pancreatic carcinoma. The normal pancreatic duct measures 2–4 mm in the head and body of the pancreas, tapering to 1–2 mm in the tail (Fig. 6). Pancreatographic features suggestive of cancer include (1) obstruction or abrupt cutoff of the duct (50%), (2) stenosis with proximal dilatation (35%), (3) tapering or gradual narrowing of the duct (8%), and (4) cavitation of the pancreatic duct from tumor necrosis (7%) (4). Another feature is the disappearance of secondary ducts adjacent to the stenosis.

When cannulation is successful, the diagnostic accuracy for pancreatic cancer is reported to be between 85 and 95% (5–7). Niederau and Grendell reported a sensitivity and specificity of ERCP for detecting malignant lesions as 92 and 95%, respectively (8). Because pancreatography images only the ductal system, small tumors arising in the parenchyma are likely to be missed. Patients with pancreatic cancer may have a normal pancreatogram in 2–12% of cases (9). Distinguishing ductal changes attributed to pancreatic carcinoma versus chronic pancreatitis may be difficult, resulting in an inaccurate diagnosis in up to 8% of cases (7).

The majority of pancreatic cancers involve the head (75%). Body and tail lesions make up 20 and 5% of cases, respectively. The cholangiogram is apt to be abnormal in up to 95% of pancreatic carcinomas involving the head, and up to 75% of carcinomas of the body (10). Pancreatic carcinoma may cause common bile duct distortion by direct invasion or by extrinsic compression. Concomitant stenosis or obstruction of the bile duct and the pancreatic duct, the radiological "double duct

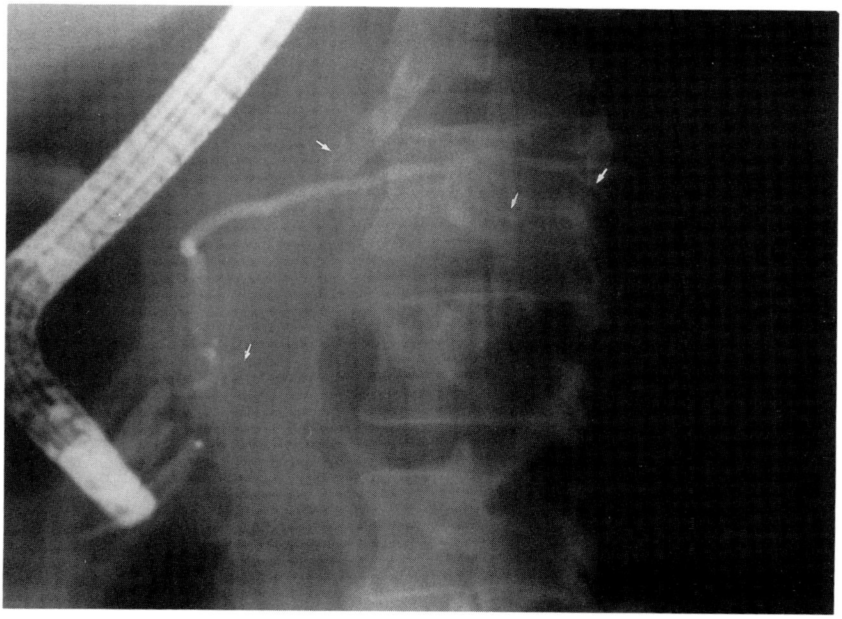

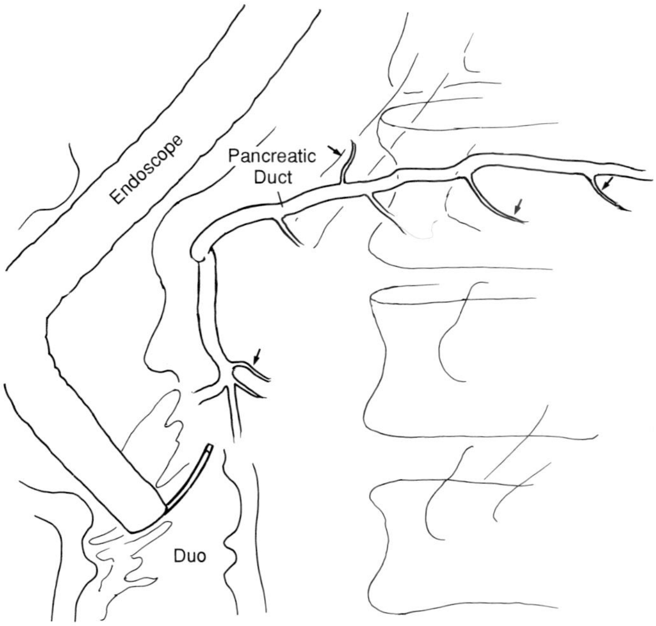

Figure 6. Normal pancreatogram. The ventral and dorsal ducts are smooth without stricture, dilatation, or filling defects. The side branches are smooth and taper into secondary and tertiary radicals (arrows).

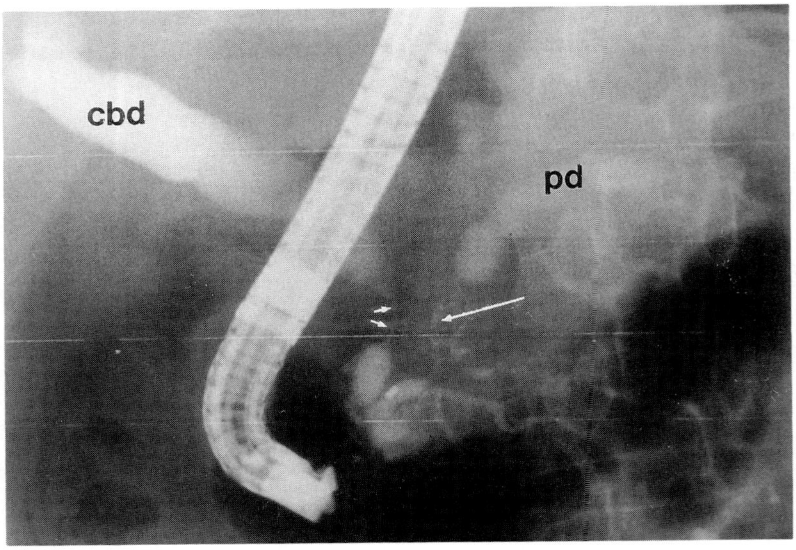

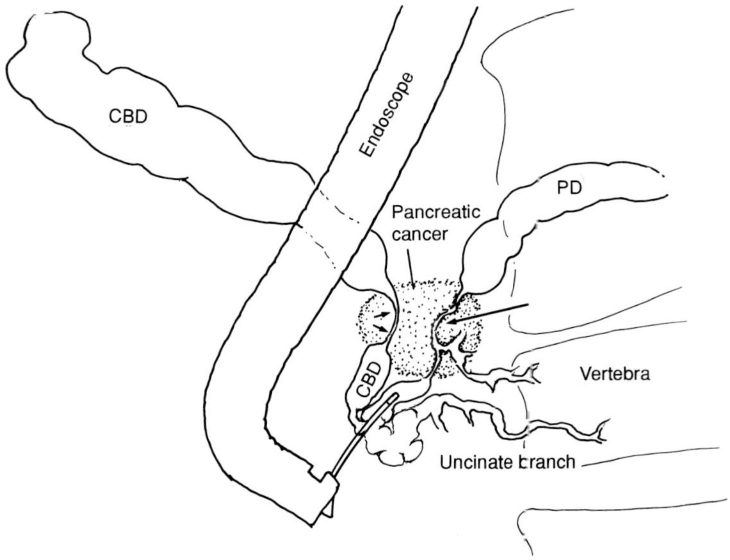

Figure 7. Double duct sign. There is concomitant stricture of the common bile duct (short arrows) and main pancreatic duct (long arrow) with prestenotic dilatation. This finding is associated with pancreatic head carcinoma.

sign," is seen in approximately 80% of cases (Fig. 7). The double duct sign was initially proposed as a specific indicator of pancreatic cancer; however, it may be seen in benign disease as well (11). In patients who present with painless jaundice 85% of tumors are of pancreatic origin, 6% of distal common bile duct carcinoma, and 4.5% each of duodenal and ampullary carcinomas (12).

Distinguishing a benign biliary stricture (papillary stenosis, inflammatory, primary sclerosing cholangitis, chronic pancreatitis) from a neoplastic stricture may be difficult. Frick et al. reported that abrupt obstruction or cutoff of the duct, shorter stricture length (<15 mm), and irregular contour of the stenosis are features associated with malignancy (13). Conversely, long stenotic segments (approximately 30 mm) and smooth gradual tapering of the stenosis are characteristic of benignity. Other features suggestive of pancreatitis rather than pancreatic cancer include (1) multiple stenoses of the main pancreatic duct, (2) intraductal calculi, (3) irregularities and ectasia of the secondary branches, and (4) the presence of a pseudocyst.

There is an increased incidence of pancreatic cancer in patients with chronic pancreatitis. Differentiating pancreatic carcinoma in the presence of concurrent chronic pancreatitis is particularly challenging. Shemesh et al. reported their results assessing pancreatograms in 45 subjects with chronic pancreatitis and 10 with chronic pancreatitis and coexisting pancreatic carcinoma (14). All patients with chronic pancreatitis and coexisting cancer had pancreatic duct strictures greater than 10 mm long, whereas those patients with chronic pancreatitis alone had pancreatic duct strictures measuring less than 5 mm. Pancreatic calcifications were present in 50% of patients with coexisting carcinoma and only 26% of patients with chronic pancreatitis alone, surprisingly. New onset of abdominal pain and weight loss within the preceding 2–3 months were clinical features predictive of the presence of carcinoma. These findings contradict those of Frick et al. above and highlight the limitations of pancreatography in distinguishing benign versus malignant strictures (13, 14).

Although some features of the pancreatogram are highly suggestive of malignancy versus chronic pancreatitis, there are no pathognomonic characteristics to distinguish the two processes. Therefore, in most cases, adjunctive studies to access abnormalities of the pancreatic parenchyma or to obtain tissue must be performed to achieve a definitive diagnosis. When a stricture is identified at the time of ERCP, efforts should be made to obtain diagnostic tissue.

Endoscopic retrograde cholangiopancreatographic-facilitated cytological analysis from ductal washings, brushings, needle aspirate, and biopsies achieve an accurate tissue diagnosis in only up to 60% of cases in most series (15–19). When direct brushing is performed in pancreatic duct strictures, pancreatic neoplasms can be detected with a frequency as high as 85% (18).

There is growing interest in the use of genetic and molecular markers in the diagnosis of pancreatic cancer. A high incidence of point mutations of the K-*ras* codon has been identified by gene analysis. Although the number of patients studied are small, initial results show promise. In a report by Berthelemy, this group found K-*ras* mutations in pure pancreatic juice collected during ERCP in none of 24 patients with no pancreatic disease, none of 29 patients with nontumoral pancreatic disease, that is pancreatitis, and 17 of 22 patients with pancreatic cancer (77%) (20).

Tumor-associated antigens have also been studied to access their value in diagnosing pancreatic cancer, particularly distinguishing malignant from benign pancreatic disease. Gentiloni et al. described the diagnostic value of a newly discovered antigen 90K. In 19 patients with pancreatic cancer, 20 patients with chronic pancreatitis, and seven controls with cholelithiasis, pancreatic juice 90K protein when used in combination with serum CA 19-9 correctly identified 84.2% of pancreatic cancers and 90% of chronic pancreatitis cases (21).

Unfortunately, ERP facilitates the diagnosis of the majority of pancreatic tumors only at a stage when they are clinically apparent. Although it is useful in the diagnosis of small tumors in the ampullary region at early stages when other imaging studies are negative, it is otherwise not useful for the early diagnosis of other small pancreatic tumors. Pancreatography offers no staging information because it is an inaccurate means of assessing tumor size or extent, nor does it provide information regarding resectability, nodal involvement, or distant metastases. These shortcomings and the emergence of endoscopic ultrasonography have diminished the role of endoscopic retrograde pancreatography in the diagnosis and staging of suspected pancreatic cancer.

Endoscopic Palliation of Pancreatic Carcinoma

Given the overall poor prognosis of patients with pancreatic carcinoma and the absence of therapeutic regimens that reliably prolong and enhance the quality of life, palliation is the goal in most patients. Endoscopic transpapillary biliary stent insertion is now a widely available means of achieving palliation of biliary obstruction secondary to pancreatic carcinoma. Successful biliary drainage by this method can be achieved in 80–90% of cases with low procedure-related morbidity and mortality (Fig. 8).

Several comparisons have demonstrated the superiority of endoscopic biliary stent placement over the percutaneous route. Speer et al. in a randomized, prospective trial compared percutaneous versus endoscopic methods for stent insertion in 75 patients (22). The endoscopic method had a higher success rate for relief of jaundice with fewer complications. Several randomized trials have compared surgical bypass with endoscopic stenting in patients with unresectable lesions (23–25). These three prospective, comparative trials demonstrated similar success rates for decompression of biliary obstruction and overall survival. Additionally, they consistently reported lower morbidity and 30-day mortality rates in patients treated with endoscopic drainage compared to surgical bypass.

Recurrent jaundice due to stent clogging occurs more frequently in the endoscopically treated patients. However, this can be routinely managed with a stent exchange. The average patency of the 10-French plastic stent most commonly used is 6 months. Thus patency is usually maintained for the life-span of the majority of patients. Most studies have demonstrated that the patency rate affects approximately one-fifth of patients with malignant jaundice. Finally, in a small percentage of patients treated endoscopically, surgery may ultimately be required to palliate gastric outlet obstruction owing to duodenal compression from infiltrating carcinoma. These data support the philosophy that surgical bypass should be reserved for those patients in whom preoperative staging suggests the potential for curative resection but are found to be unresectable at the time of laparotomy, or in those patients with duodenal obstruction at the time of presentation. Others have suggested that patients in whom a longer survival was predicted, based on younger age, absence of comorbid disease, and earlier-stage tumors, are more likely to benefit from operative therapy versus those patients with shorter life expectancies who are better served by endoscopic therapy (26). Lastly, a retrospective review by Brandabur et al. reported that patients who underwent operative versus nonoperative treatment for

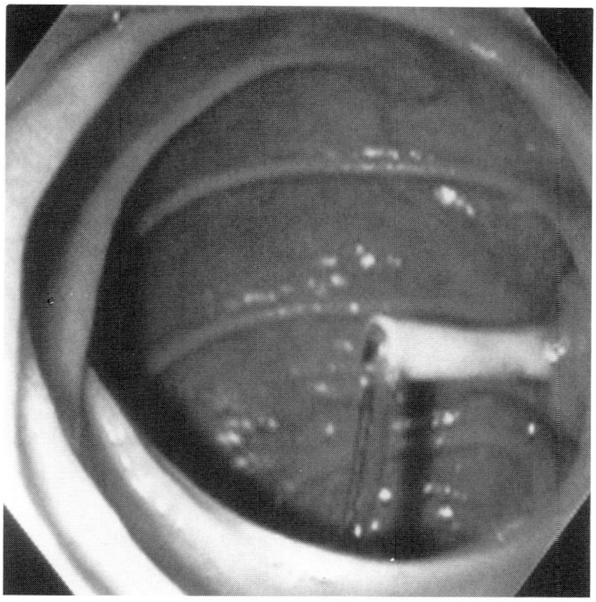

(A)

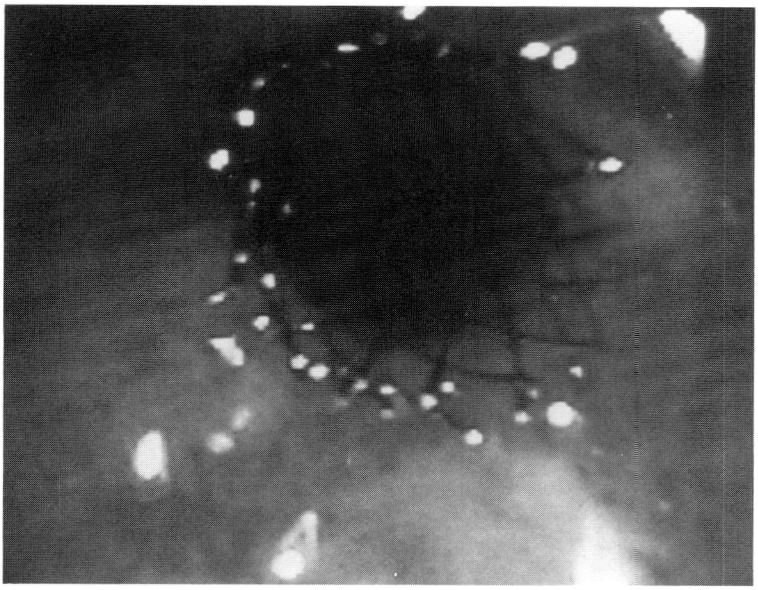

(B)

Figure 8. (A) A freshly placed plastic endobiliary stent has free flow of bile from a common bile duct previously obstructed by pancreatic carcinoma. (B) Expandable metal endoprosthesis may be delivered endoscopically and expand up to 10 mm diameter.

Table 1. Sensitivity of EUS in the diagnosis of pancreatic cancer with comparisons to transabdominal ultrasound, CT, ERCP, and MRI[a]

Authors	No. Patients	Sensitivity (%)				
		EUS	TAUS[b]	CT	ERCP	MRI
Muller et al. (84)	22	94	—	89	—	83
Forsmarch et al. (85)	26	77	44	68	86	—
Giovanini and Seitz (86)	30	100	48	69	—	—
Kallimanis et al. (87)	32	92	66	74	88	—
Akahoshi[c] et al. (88)	43	93	72	70	84	—
Palazzo et al. (31)	49	96	65	69	—	—
Nakaizu et al. (89)	49	94	78	65	—	—
Yasuda et al. (90)	50	100	78	86	94	—
Rösch et al. (28)	76	99	87	77	90	—
Total	377	95	67	76	86	83
<2–3 cm	86	97	57	51	80	67

[a]Modified from Reference 28 with permission of Thomas Rösch.
[b]TAUS = transabdominal ultrasound.
[c]Stratified for tumors <2–3 cm.

biliary obstruction generated significantly higher mean cost between the time of diagnosis and death (27).

Endoscopic Ultrasound

Endoscopic ultrasound is an effective tool for the evaluation of a suspected pancreatic lesion. It is currently one of the most sensitive imaging modalities for the diagnosis of pancreatic cancer (Table 1). Endoscopic ultrasound is indicated when a pancreatic lesion is suspected based on clinical history and other imaging modalities; it is not intended to be a screening test for pancreatic cancer. Its clinical usefulness is as an adjunct to cross-sectional imaging when pancreatic cancer is suspected. In the patient who presents with painless jaundice, ERCP should first be performed to relieve biliary obstruction as well as to provide the diagnostic cholangiographic and pancreatographic studies. Cross-sectional imaging should be performed to assess the presence and extent of a pancreatic lesion, as well as to assess for the presence of abdominal adenopathy and distant metastasis. Endoscopic ultrasound should be employed when ERCP or cross-sectional imaging studies are equivocal or when staging information is deemed inadequate. Furthermore, in patients deemed unresectable by preoperative staging techniques, EUS-guided fine needle aspiration (FNA) provides histological diagnosis, which, at most institutions, is the prerequisite for the commencement of chemotherapy or radiation therapy.

Pancreatic carcinoma typically appears as a hypoechoic mass with an inhomogeneous internal echo architecture and irregular borders (Fig. 9). However, in very large and very small tumors the echo pattern may be mixed and somewhat variable. Carcinomas tend to have irregular margins, sometimes with extending pseudopodia,

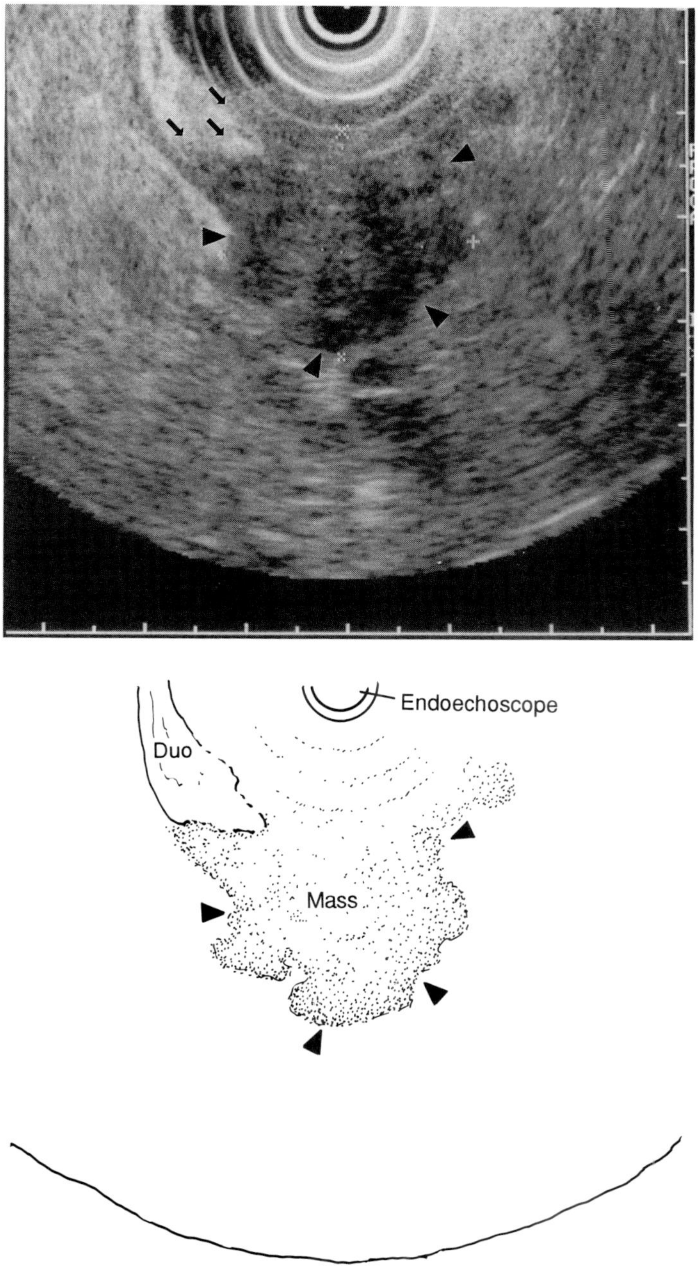

Figure 9. EUS image of pancreatic carcinoma. Typically hypoechoic, the lesion (arrowheads) has an irregular margin and is seen here to invade the duodenal wall (arrows).

Table 2. TNM staging for pancreatic cancer

	Primary Tumor (T)
TX	Primary tumor not assessable
T0	No evidence of tumor
T1	Tumor limited to pancreas
T1a	Tumor less than 2 cm
T1b	Tumor greater than 2 cm
T2	Tumor extending into duodenum, bile duct, or pancreatic tissue
T3	Tumor extending into stomach, spleen, colon, or adjacent large vessels
	Regional Lymph Nodes (N)
NX	Regional lymph nodes not assessable
N0	No regional lymph node metastasis
N1	Regional lymph node metastasis
	Distant Metastasis (M)
MX	Distant metastasis not assessable
M0	No distant metastasis
M1	Distant metastasis

but smaller lesions may have smooth margins. With a high negative predictive value, EUS is a very helpful imaging modality for excluding pancreatic malignancy (28).

Although EUS has high sensitivity and specificity in the diagnosis of pancreatic tumors, it is much less reliable in distinguishing malignancy versus benignity of the lesion. Focal inflammatory processes may have a similar hypoechoic pattern and irregular margins of demarcation (29, 30). Whereas earlier reports with smaller number of patients were more promising, more recent, larger series demonstrate EUS to be no more accurate than CT or ERCP in the differentiation between pancreatic cancer and focal chronic pancreatitis (28, 31–33). Analysis of echo patterns did not reveal any significant differences to help distinguish malignancy versus focal chronic pancreatitis. Fortunately, advances in the EUS technology have now enabled the endoscopist to obtain cytology at the same setting and provide histological information for the diagnosis.

Endoscopic Ultrasound Staging for Pancreatic Cancer. Endoscopic ultrasound is an accurate means to assess the size and extent of a pancreatic mass. The American Joint Committee on Cancer (AJCC) has promoted the TNM staging system to achieve consistency in assessing prognosis and response to therapies. Endoscopic ultrasound is particularly accurate for assessing the T stage or extent of the primary tumor. In this system, T1 tumors are limited to the pancreas, with T1a tumors being less than 2 cm in diameter, and T1b tumors greater than or equal to 2 cm in diameter; T2 tumors demonstrate infiltration of the duodenal wall, common bile duct, and peripancreatic tissue; T3 tumors infiltrate the gastric wall, spleen, colon, or mesenteric or portal vessels (Table 2) (Fig. 10).

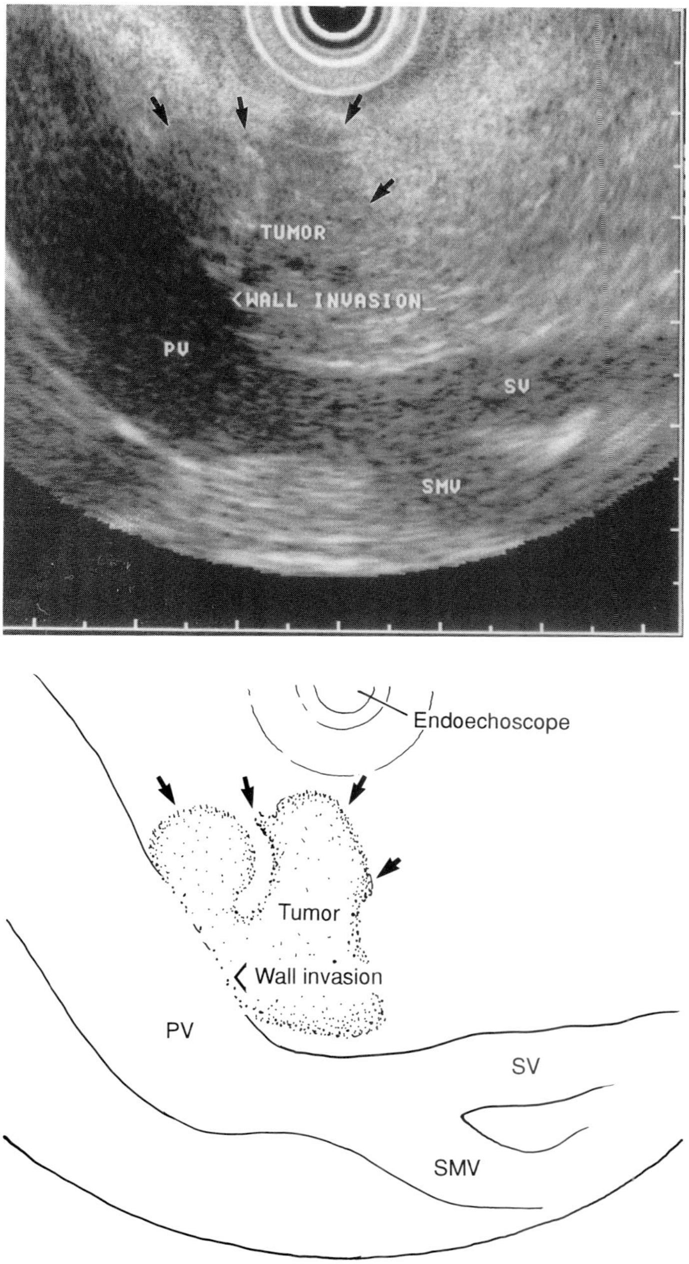

Figure 10. T3 pancreatic head carcinoma. The lesion (arrows) is observed to invade the portal vein (PV) directly just beyond the confluence of the splenic vein (SV) and the superior mesenteric vein (SMV). This finding generally confers unresectability.

Table 3. T and N stage accuracy of EUS for pancreatic cancer with surgical/histopathological confirmation[a]

Authors	No. Patients	Accuracy (%) T Stage	Accuracy (%) N Stage
Grimm et al. (91)	26	85	72
Tio et al. (92)	36	92	72
Kallimanis et al. (93)	32	78	66
Rösch et al. (94)	35	94	80
Wiersema et al. (95)	39	76	82
Muller et al. (84)	22	82	64
Akahoshi et al. (88)	25	64	48
Gress et al. (86)	59	87	80
Kadish et al. (34)	30	84	76[b]
Rösch et al. (96)	35	69	60[c]
Total[d]	339	81	70[d]

[a]Modified from reference 96 with permission of Thomas Rösch.
[b]N stage available in only 29.
[c]N stage available in only 20.
[d]N stage available in only 325.

Regional and celiac adenopathy (N stage) can be identified with high sensitivity. The specificity for lymph node involvement is lower, however, for the distinction between metastatic and reactive adenopathy remains problematic. Lymph nodes may be seen arising in the peripancreatic tissue, along the surrounding vasculature and the celiac axis. Endosonographic appearances that correlate with malignancy include round shape, hypoechogenicity, well-demarcated borders, and size greater than 1 cm. Because it is unusual to see lymph nodes around the normal pancreas, the identification of any lymph node should raise suspicions. Distant metastasis (M stage) cannot reliably be assessed by EUS.

Endoscopic ultrasound is a sensitive and highly accurate means of staging pancreatic tumors. Comparative studies have demonstrated superiority in T and N staging of pancreatic cancer compared to other imaging modalities. Table 3 details the T and N staging accuracy of pancreatic cancer with surgical confirmation from the larger series. T and N staging accuracy by EUS compares favorably to that of CT scan and MRI (Table 4). The accuracy of EUS for various T and N stages is displayed

Table 4. Accuracy of EUS versus CT and MRI for T and N stage assessment of pancreatic cancer from combined series[a]

Stage	No. Patients	Accuracy (%) EUS	Accuracy (%) CT	Accuracy (%) MRI[b]
Tumor	173	86	43	67
Nodal	223	71	53	56

[a]Data from References 31, 84, 88, 94, 97, and 98.
[b]Data for only 35 patients for T stage and 29 patients for N stage.

Table 5. Staging accuracy of EUS in pancreatic cancer by T and N stage[a]

Stage	No. Patients	Accuracy of EUS (%)
T1	27	82
T2	78	81
T3	91	85
N0	94	80
N1	156	78

[a]Data from References 31, 84, 86, 91–94, and 99.

in Table 5. Staging errors most frequently occur between stages T2 (overstaging) and T3 (understaging); however, therapeutic consequences are much more dependent on this differentiation.

Assessment of vascular invasion is probably the most important parameter of determining resectability in pancreatic cancer. Most surgeons believe that invasion of a portal vein determines lesion unresectability. Endoscopic ultrasound has been demonstrated to be superior to CT scanning, MRI, and even angiography (Table 6). We recently reported our blinded assessment of vascular invasion by EUS, helical CT scanning, MRI with gadolinium, and digital angiography. In our series angiography was superior to CT or MRI for accessing vascular invasion, and EUS was superior to all modalities with a positive predictive value of 85% and a negative predictive value of 92%, compared to 50% respectively, for angiography (34). Assessing vascular invasion becomes more difficult in larger pancreatic tumors because of the echo reduction experienced in large tumors.

Impact of Endosonographic Staging of Pancreatic Cancer. Endoscopic ultrasound plays a significant role in the management of pancreatic cancer by improving tumor detection, differentiating malignant from benign disease, and assessing resection status. Gress et al. confirmed the hypothesis that EUS staging of pancreatic cancer correlates with survival (35). Their findings demonstrated that patients with T1 lesions benefited from surgical management. Patients with T2 lesions demonstrated a trend toward improvement with operative management. No benefit was

Table 6. Accuracy of EUS in detecting vascular invasion confirmed operatively and compared to angiography

Authors	No. Patients	EUS (%)	Angiography (%)
Yasuda et al. (97)	29	79	72
Kadish et al. (99)	25	88	50
Snady et al. (100)	30	97	80
Rösch et al. (101)	40	95	85
Akahoshi et al. (88)	25	79	81
Total	149	88	74

observed with surgical management versus medical management in patients with T3 lesions. There was improved survival in surgically treated patients with T1-N0.

Endoscopic ultrasound, when used in the appropriate clinical setting, significantly changes the management in about one-third of patients either by making the diagnosis or by changing an incorrect diagnosis of tumor stage (36). If EUS is used following initial cross-sectional imaging studies to evaluate resectability, a significant number of angiographies and their attendant costs and morbidity will be avoided. EUS has been demonstrated to have an accuracy rate of up to 88% in determining resectability (37), whereas Warshaw and Fernandez-Del Castillo reported that by using CT, laparoscopy, and angiography, they correctly predicted resectability in only 78% of cancers in the head of the pancreas upon laparotomy (38). Finally, EUS was more sensitive than CT scanning for assessing response to combined chemo-radiation therapy (39).

Endosonographically Guided Fine Needle Aspiration. A definitive tissue diagnosis of pancreatic cancer is important for patient management. Traditionally, tissue can be obtained via the percutaneous route, during ERCP, or by operative means. Unfortunately, all these approaches are imperfect. Specifically, percutaneous FNA of the pancreas using ultrasound or CT for guidance has a sensitivity of only 50–80% (40). Complications such as pancreatitis, bleeding, cholangitis, and sepsis can occur (0–7%) (41, 42). Furthermore, there has been concern that intraperitoneal spread of tumor may be provoked by percutaneous needle aspirate attempts, although this has not been substantiated by others (43, 44). Similarly, tissue sampling via ERCP techniques also has a rather low sensitivity of 60% as described above. When these techniques fail, the physician is often left to recommend operative assessment. Laparoscopy identifies patients with peritoneal and liver metastasis below the resolution of imaging studies. However, open laparotomy is typically required to obtain tissue from a discrete pancreatic lesion. Endoscopic ultrasound-guided, real-time, fine needle aspiration is a welcome addition to the armamentarium for obtaining a histological diagnosis from a pancreatic lesion.

Endoscopic ultrasound-guided FNA is performed using a linear array echoendoscope. Pancreatic head and genu lesions are best sampled from transduodenal approach with the tip of the echoendoscope in the duodenal bulb or the second portion of the duodenum (Fig. 11). Pancreatic body and tail lesions are sampled transgastrically. Endoscopic ultrasound-guided FNA is most commonly performed following EUS staging examination using the radial scanning echoendoscope.

The availability of Doppler flow analysis allows the assessment of vascular structures that may then be avoided with the course of the needle. This is an advantage over percutaneous aspiration techniques. Another advantage is the avoidance of the potential for malignant seeding, which most commonly occurs cutaneously. In patients with pancreatic head lesions, sampled through the duodenum, the duodenum is typically removed during surgery.

Table 7 lists the data on ultrasound-guided real-time FNA for pancreatic lesions. These data were derived from the evaluation of lesions not seen by or inaccessible to CT-guided percutaneous FNA. In our series of 23 patients, all lesions were either inaccessible or had failed attempted tissue sampling by CT guidance (45). Peripancreatic lymph nodes and celiac nodes may also be successfully aspirated to confirm suspected metastasis.

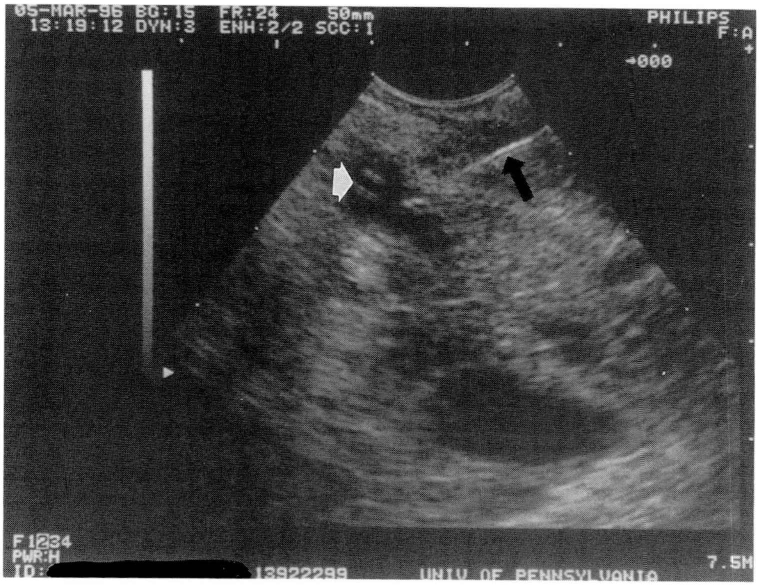

Figure 11. EUS-guided fine needle aspiration. The needle (black arrow) is seen impaled within a pancreatic head mass that had resulted in biliary obstruction. A previously placed plastic stent is seen within the CBD (white arrow).

The ability to perform EUS-guided FNA during the same session as a diagnostic or staging EUS exam, coupled with its high sensitivity, enhances its cost effectiveness. Employing this technique will (1) likely reduce the time to establish a definitive diagnosis, (2) avoid other less accurate tissue sampling techniques, and (3) decrease reliance on laparotomy for achieving tissue diagnosis.

CYSTIC NEOPLASMS OF THE PANCREAS

The ability to differentiate cystic tumors from pseudocysts has improved. However, this remains a troublesome clinical situation. The clinical history is of great signifi-

Table 7. Sensitivity and specificity of EUS-guided FNA cytology in the diagnosis of pancreatic carcinoma[a]

Authors	No. Patients	Sensitivity (%)	Specificity (%)
Giovanini et al. (102)	43	75	100
Wiersema et al. (103)	11	82	100
Bhutani et al. (104)	11	91	100
Chang et al. (105)	10	90	100
Faigle et al. (106)	20	88	100
Change et al. (107)	155	88	100
Total	250	86	100

[a]Modified from Reference 101 with permission of Thomas Rösch.

cance. Most patients undergo a cross-sectional imaging study. Endoscopic retrograde cholangiopancreatography and EUS play a role that continues to evolve.

The utility of ERCP and CT scanning in the preoperative assessment of patients with pancreatic cysts and pancreatic neoplasms associated with cysts was evaluated in 11 patients with proven pancreatic neoplasms associated with cysts (46). Four patients had adenomas, two had mucinous cystadenomas, one had a mucinous cyst adenocarcinoma, and four had adenocarcinomas associated with cysts. Computed tomography identified pancreatic cystic lesions in all 11 cases. Endoscopic retrograde cholangiopancreatography showed focal irregular narrowing, occlusion, or displacement of the main pancreatic duct at the corresponding location without ductal changes associated with the chronic pancreatitis. The authors concluded that ERCP is helpful in distinguishing preoperatively cystic neoplasms from pseudocysts associated with chronic pancreatitis.

Similarly, cystic tumors can be identified with regularity by EUS. However, distinguishing neoplastic from non-neoplastic cystic lesions based on endosonograpic criteria alone may be difficult. We evaluated the role of EUS for the evaluation of complex cystic pancreatic lesions. There were 25 complex cystic lesions identified among 231 EUS exams performed to evaluate pancreatic disease, and 72% were neoplastic with clinicopathological correlation (47) (Fig. 12). Although we describe features suggestive of a definitive diagnosis these criteria have not been tested prospectively. Endosonographically guided aspiration of solid and cystic components contributes to this distinction.

Differentiation of cystic tumors and pseudocysts has been aided by the use of cystic fluid analysis for tumor markers (48). In another study diagnostic accuracy was evaluated in 26 patients whose cystic fluid was examined for cytology, cystic fluid viscosity, and carcinoembryonic antigen (CEA), CA 19-9, CA 125, amylase, lipase, and amylase isoenzyme levels (49). Among the analyses performed, the CEA was the most reliable for distinguishing mucinous neoplasms from serocyst adenomas or pseudocyst. Amylase is expected to be elevated in fluid obtained from pseudocysts correlating with pseudocyst–pancreatic duct communication (50). The applicability of cyst aspiration via EUS-guided FNA has yet to be determined.

PANCREATIC NEUROENDOCRINE TUMORS

The diagnosis of a pancreatic neuroendocrine tumor is established by clinical signs and laboratory tests. However, noninvasive imaging tests such as transabdominal ultrasound and CT fail in the preoperative localization of these tumors in a considerable number of cases. Approximately 20% of insulinomas and up to 40% of gastrinomas are not visualized by radiological imaging. Gastrinomas are particularly challenging because they have a high frequency of extrapancreatic foci. Although the use of intraoperative palpation and intraoperative ultrasound and duodenal transillumination identify additional tumors, preoperative localization greatly facilitates the operative approach. Rösch et al. in a multicenter study detected 82% of 39 pancreatic endocrine tumors not localized on CT scan by EUS (51). These were small tumors (mean size 1.4 cm), with 95% measuring less than 2.0 cm in diameter. These lesions included 31 insulinomas, seven gastrinomas, and one glucagonoma. In 22 patients who had both EUS and angiography, EUS was significantly more

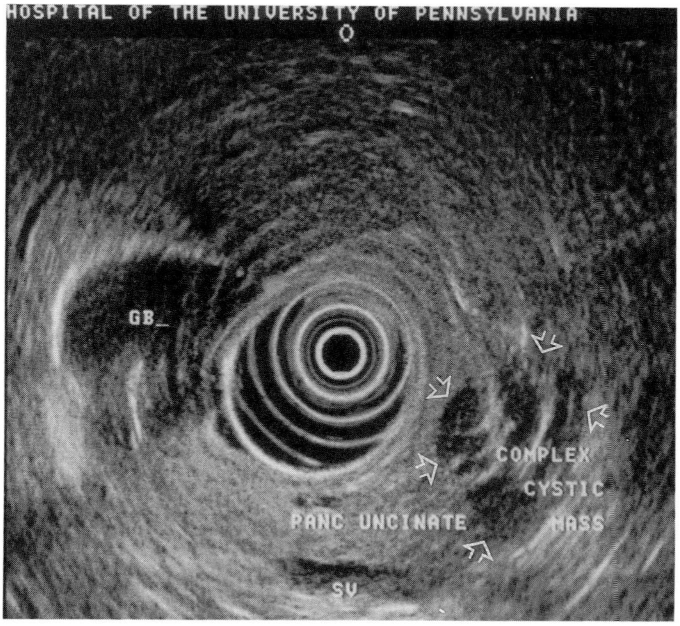

(A)

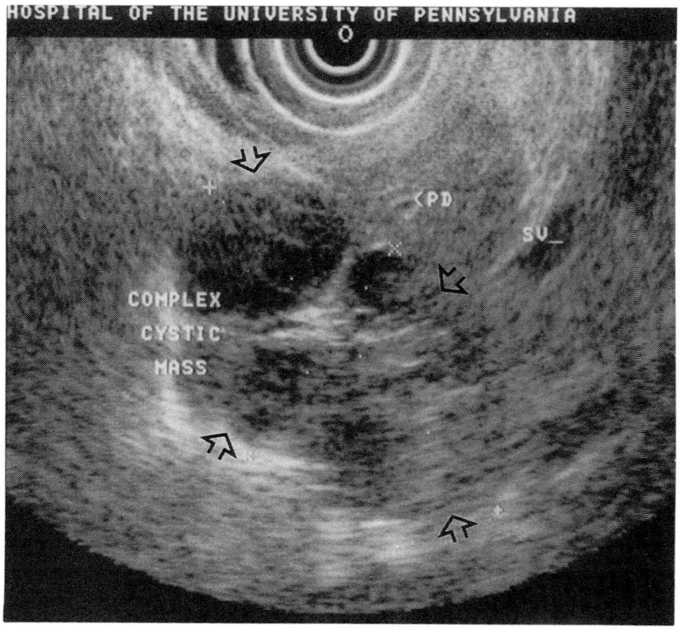

(B)

Figure 12. Two complex cystic lesions of the pancreas. Lesion (A), a microcystic or serous cystadenoma, has multiple fine septations and scant associated solid material (arrows, A). Lesion (B), a mucinous cystadenocarcinoma, has larger and fewer cyst cavities with greater associated solid component and indistinct margins suggesting infiltration (arrows, B).

Table 8. Comparison of EUS with TAUS, CT, MRI, SRS in localizing pancreatic endocrine tumors[a]

	EUS	TAUS[b]	CT	MRI	SRS[c]
Sensitivity (%)	84	30	2	24	52
No. Patients	176	111	126	25	25

[a]Data from References 109–118.
[b]TAUS = transabdominal ultrasonography.
[c]SRS = somatostatin receptor scintigraphy.

sensitive in detecting and localizing pancreatic endocrine tumors (82 versus 27%, $p < .05$). Table 8 compares the sensitivity of EUS with other modalities in the localization of pancreatic endocrine tumors. These authors also reported that in 19 patients thought to have endocrine tumors on initial work-up, but later found to have no such lesion, EUS was truly negative in 18 for a specificity of 95%. Based on these data, EUS is now solidly indicated for the preoperative localization of pancreatic neuroendocrine tumors when the clinical diagnosis is suggestive and other imaging modalities are negative or inconclusive.

Typically a pancreatic endocrine tumor appears as a homogeneous, echo-rich, well-demarcated lesion (Fig. 13). Because the majority of neuroendocrine tumors arises within the pancreatic parenchyma, not as ductal lesions, there is no defined

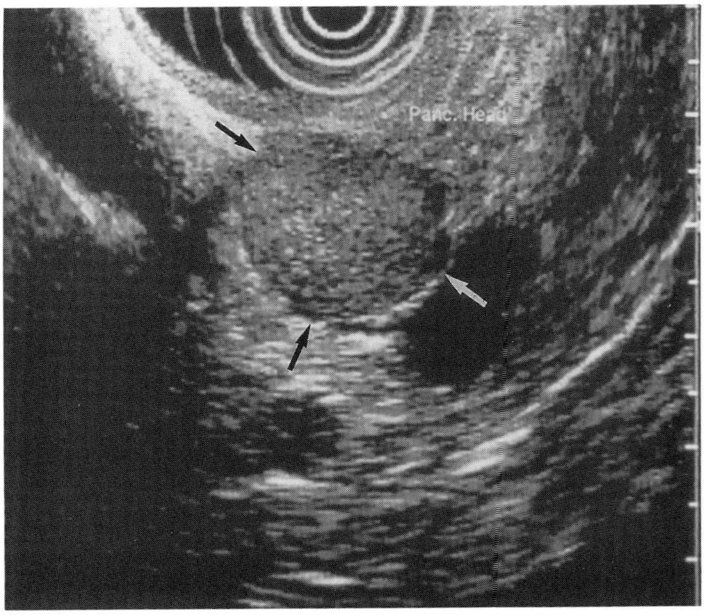

Figure 13. This 1.5-cm insulinoma was clinically suspected; however, it was not seen on CT or MRI scan. The presence of sharply demarcated borders on EUS exam (arrows) correctly predicted local resectability.

role for ERCP in their diagnosis or preoperative localization. Furthermore, EUS is an effective means of localizing duodenal wall tumors and lymph node metastasis. The duodenal wall lesions appear as submucosal, well-circumscribed lesions. Peri-pancreatic, mesenteric, and celiac adenopathy may also be identified.

AMPULLARY TUMORS

Adenocarcinomas and adenomas arising from the major papilla constitute a distinct pathological entity. Biliary obstruction is the most common presentation. Patients may also present with pancreatitis and/or anemia. Generally these tumors are uncommon, but there is an increased incidence of ampullary adenomas and carcinoma in patients with familial polyposis syndromes (52).

The diagnosis is usually made endoscopically with a side-viewing duodenoscope. Forceps biopsies of the suspect papilla occasionally achieve sufficient tissue for diagnosis. Biopsies obtained after sphincterotomy may increase the yield (53). In nonoperative candidates, endoscopic stenting is an effective palliative therapy either alone or with adjunctive endoscopic tumor ablation therapy.

Surgical excision is the preferred mode of treatment and prognosis depends on stage. Endosonography has been demonstrated to be an effective means of staging ampullary tumors (54). Ampullary tumors appear as a hypoechoic thickening. The presence of dilated pancreatic and/or common bile duct in the majority of patients with ampullary tumors aids in the identification by EUS. Small tumors may be seen by EUS that are below the resolution of CT or transabdominal ultrasound. However, in larger tumors, it may not be possible to distinguish primary carcinoma of the head of the pancreas from ampullary carcinoma. Papillary inflammation attributed to pancreatitis or following passage of gallstones may not be accurately distinguished from neoplasia.

In the AJCC classification system, T1 tumors are limited to the ampulla with intact duodenal wall layers; T2 tumors invade into the muscularis propria; T3 tumors invade into the pancreas less than 2 cm; T4 lesions invade into the pancreas more than 2 cm or into adjacent organs or vessels. Tio described a high accuracy of EUS in staging ampullary carcinomas, with a T stage accuracy of 80% and an overall accuracy of 77% (54). Bansal et al. reported the accuracy of T and N staging by EUS compared to that of CT and/or MRI in 14 patients with ampullary carcinoma (55). Endosonography had a T stage accuracy of 71% versus 0 and 40% for CT and MRI, respectively. N-stage accuracy was also 71% for EUS versus 9 and 60% for CT and MRI, respectively. Furthermore, EUS accurately confirmed absence of vascular invasion in all 14 cases, whereas angiography reported one false positive result.

The majority of ampullary carcinomas are resectable. Precise staging is most important in patients at increased surgical risk; endoscopic palliation versus surgical resection or possibly local regional resection is based on staging information. Computed tomography or MRI is generally required to exclude distal metastasis and ERCP is necessary for palliation of biliary obstruction. Endoscopic ultrasound should be performed for tumor and nodal staging to rule out unresectability and to assess the potential for local excision in patients otherwise deemed poor operative candidates.

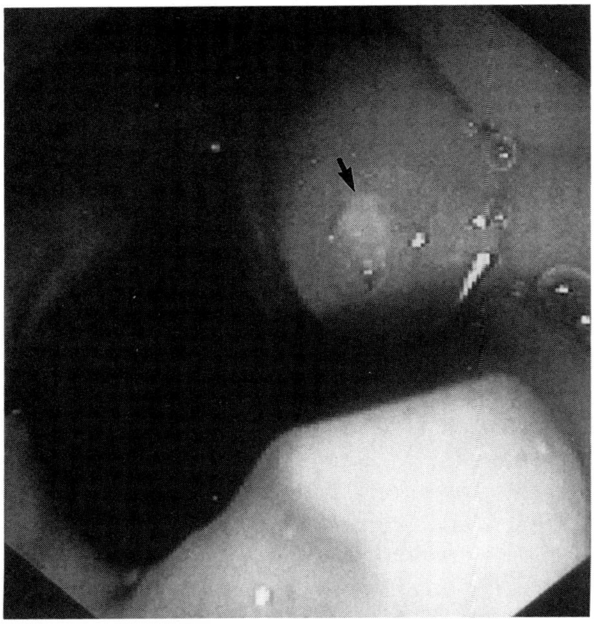

Figure 14. Impacted common bile duct stone (arrow) was seen on ERCP in a patient with severe acute gallstone pancreatitis and cholangitis. Endoscopic sphincterotomy and stone extraction were performed, leading to full recovery.

PANCREATITIS

Acute Pancreatitis

The diagnosis of acute pancreatitis is based on the clinical presentation, laboratory features, and in some instances, correlation with radiological imaging. Transabdominal ultrasound, CT, or MRI may show a large edematous gland with stranding in the peripancreatic fat due to inflammation. There is no defined role for EUS in the diagnosis and management of acute pancreatitis.

Endoscopic retrograde cholangiopancreatography is indicated in patients with severe pancreatitis attributed to gallstones early in its course. In a randomized study of 121 patients, Neoptolemos et al. reported that the removal of gallstones within 24 hr of presentation via ERCP and endoscopic sphincterotomy in patients with acute gallstone-induced pancreatitis led to a lower morbidity rate than conventional medical treatment alone (24 versus 61%) (56). Similarly, Fan et al. reported that the use of ERCP and endoscopic sphincterotomy within 24 hr of admission reduced the incidence of biliary sepsis and demonstrated a trend toward reduction of mortality in patients treated endoscopically rather than conservatively or with urgent laparotomy (57) (Fig. 14).

Idiopathic Recurrent Pancreatitis

Endoscopic retrograde cholangiopancreatography plays a role in the diagnosis of patients in whom no apparent etiology for the pancreatitis is identified. Diagnostic

ERCP with the addition of sphincter of Oddi manometry and biliary crystal analysis can provide information about the cause of pancreatitis in the majority of such patients (58). Abnormalities revealed by these studies may include small pancreatic tumors, pancreatic ductal lesions, biliary lithiasis, pancreas divisum, choledochocele, and hypertensive sphincter of Oddi (59). Venu et al. evaluated 116 patients initially diagnosed with idiopathic recurrent pancreatitis with ERCP (60). Seventeen patients had findings suggestive of sphincter of Oddi dysfunction. An additional 27 patients had the following abnormalities: pancreas divisum (11 patients), choledochocele (four patients), cholelithiasis (eight patients), papillary tumors (three patients), and malignant stricture of the pancreatic duct (one patient). In their series, ERCP with sphincter of Oddi manometry revealed the possible etiology of recurrent pancreatitis in 38% of patients categorized as idiopathic recurrent pancreatitis by conventional criteria. They reported that appropriate therapeutic intervention was carried out in 43 of the 44 patients with a favorable outcome in the majority of patients during long-term follow-up.

Lee et al. prospectively evaluated 86 patients who had acute pancreatitis with no known cause and no ultrasonographic evidence of gallstones or dilatation of the biliary ducts (61). As a potential etiology, they examined for the presence or absence of biliary sludge (a suspension of cholesterol monohydrate crystals or calcium bilirubinate granules typically found in the gallbladder). Patients with biliary sludge were treated with cholecystectomy or endoscopic papillotomy and their outcomes compared with those of untreated patients. Pancreatitis was considered idiopathic in 31 of 86 patients (36%), of whom 23 had microscopic evidence of biliary sludge aspirated during biliary endoscopy. Biliary sludge was detected by transabdominal ultrasonography in only 11 of the 23 patients (43%). Approximately half the patients with biliary sludge were treated with cholecystectomy ($n = 6$) or papillotomy ($n = 4$). These patients had fewer recurrences of acute pancreatitis during follow-up (up to 7 years) than 11 untreated patients ($p = .011$). The presence of biliary sludge was associated with an increased likelihood of recurrent attacks of pancreatitis ($p = .02$). This study supports the notion that biliary sludge is an underestimated cause of acute recurrent idiopathic pancreatitis. It also supports therapy with endoscopic sphincterotomy and/or cholecystectomy.

Chronic Abdominal Pain of Suspected Pancreatic Origin

The diagnosis of early chronic pancreatitis remains problematic owing to limited correlation between symptoms, imaging studies, and laboratory assessment. The diagnosis is commonly established using pancreatic function secretory tests and imaging combining conventional abdominal ultrasound, CT, and ERCP. Two studies have evaluated the role of endoscopic ultrasonography in the diagnosis of chronic pancreatitis. Wiersema et al. identified EUS features that were found to indicate chronic pancreatitis (62). Sensitivity and specificity were high when a combination of abnormal parenchymal or ductal features were found. In patients with early disease, the sensitivity of EUS was significantly greater than that of ERCP (Fig. 15).

Buscail et al. evaluated the usefulness and accuracy of endosonography in the diagnosis of chronic pancreatitis prospectively in 81 patients with suspected pancreatic disease (63). All patients underwent EUS, abdominal ultrasound, and CT. Endoscopic retrograde cholangiopancreatography was performed in 55 patients.

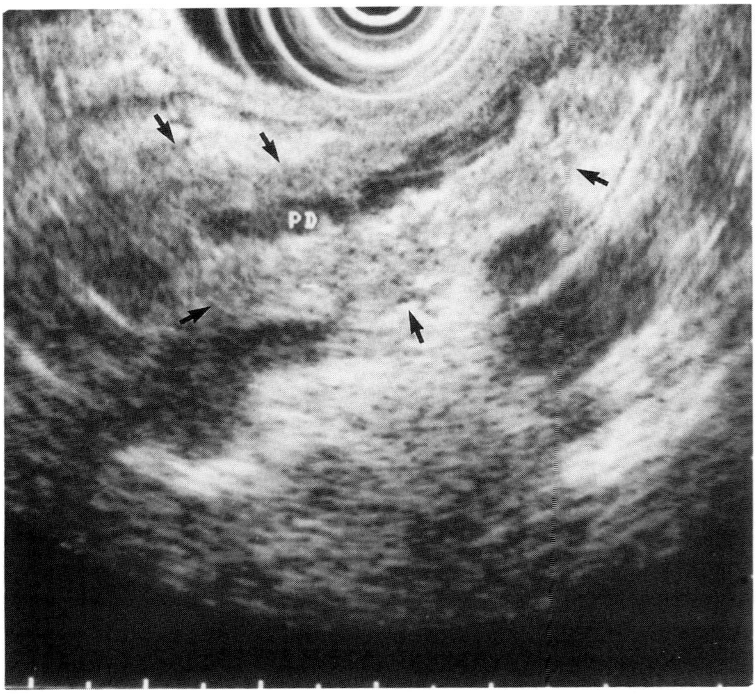

Figure 15. EUS image of pancreas in patient with chronic pancreatitis. The dorsal pancreatic duct is dilated. The surrounding pancreatic parenchyma is atrophic, inhomogeneous, and has increased echogenicity (arrows).

The diagnosis of chronic pancreatitis was ultimately established in 44 patients including 24 with calcifications. No pancreatic disease was observed in 18 patients who served as a control group, and 19 patients had pancreatic carcinoma. In the chronic pancreatitis group, EUS and CT scanning performed identically and were superior to abdominal ultrasound. Endosonographic findings that correlated with chronic pancreatitis were dilatation of the main pancreatic duct, heterogeneous echogenicity of the pancreatic parenchyma, and small cysts. The sensitivity of EUS for the diagnosis of pancreatitis was 88% compared to 58% for abdominal ultrasound, 74% for ERCP, and 75% for CT scanning; the specificity was 100% for ERCP and EUS, 95% for CT scanning, and 75% for abdominal ultrasound. Endosonography identified tumor in all patients within this category.

Pancreatic Duct Strictures

Isolated strictures of the pancreatic duct may be due to neoplasm, chronic pancreatitis, or previous trauma. Other pancreatographic findings are generally helpful in distinguishing these features. However, because pancreatic carcinoma may arise in the presence of chronic pancreatitis, reliable distinction is critical. Brush cytology should be obtained. Correlation with CT and EUS findings are likely to be indicated. The most common cause of benign pancreatic duct strictures is that associated with chronic alcoholic pancreatitis. Patients who have proximal pancreatic duct strictures with dilatation of the distal pancreatic duct are most apt to respond to therapy, endoscopic or surgical. The Puestow procedure is a time-honored, successful means of achieving pain relief in patients with these anatomic features. In patients who are nonoperative candidates and those patients preferring an alternative to surgical therapy, endoscopic balloon dilation and temporary stent placement may be attempted. However, these strictures tend to recur after endoscopic dilation and because long-term pancreatic duct stenting is undesirable, one short-term goal of this therapy is to allow prediction of which patients may benefit from surgery (64–68 (Fig. 16).

Endoscopic Treatment for Chronic Pancreatitis

Before one considers endoscopic therapy for chronic pancreatitis it is axiomatic that a surgical decision regarding treatment must be made, for a failed endoscopic procedure might necessarily lead to its surgical counterpart. This is particularly true when performing ERCP in the evaluation or management of pancreatic pseudocysts because injection of contrast into the pseudocyst may be complicated by bacterial contamination. Therefore, the decision to employ endoscopic therapy should be made by the consulting gastroenterologist and surgeon together. Techniques for endoscopic management of chronic pancreatitis include sphincterotomy of the major or the minor papilla, transpapillary stenting, and removal of duct calculi. Stones identified on pancreatography may be fragmented by laser or by contact or extracorporeal shock wave lithotripsy or extracted by a basket (69).

Pancreatic Pseudocyst

Pseudocyts can complicate chronic pancreatitis in up to 20% of patients. The majority of pancreatic pseudocysts resolve with conservative management. Even persistent, large pseudocysts may be followed expectantly (70); however, patients who have pseudocysts that continue to enlarge or who are symptomatic require therapy. Surgical therapy is generally applied. Preoperative pancreatography provides the surgeon with an anatomic road map that may be helpful intraoperatively.

Percutaneous aspiration is seldom successful as a definitive therapy, and external catheter drainage may be complicated by infection and persistent external fistula. Several studies have reported high success rates for endoscopic drainage of pseudocysts contiguous with the stomach or the duodenum with few complications (71, 72). Kozarek et al. also reported successful drainage of cysts by the transpapillary approach (73). Via the transgastric or transduodenal approach an electrocautery needle knife is used to perforate the gastric and the cyst walls under endoscopic and fluoroscopic guidance. Once access is achieved, a guide wire is placed into the cyst lumen and a double pigtail endoprosthesis is placed. Until recently, application of this methodology was limited to cysts that demonstrated an endoscopically visible bulge into the gastric or duodenal lumen. However, the evolution of endosonography has allowed endosonographic marking of the pseudocyst as well as accurate measurement of the depth between the bowel wall and the cyst lumen. Furthermore, EUS can identify large blood vessels in a proposed line of drainage, thereby reducing the risk of a bleeding catastrophe from a needle puncture (74, 75).

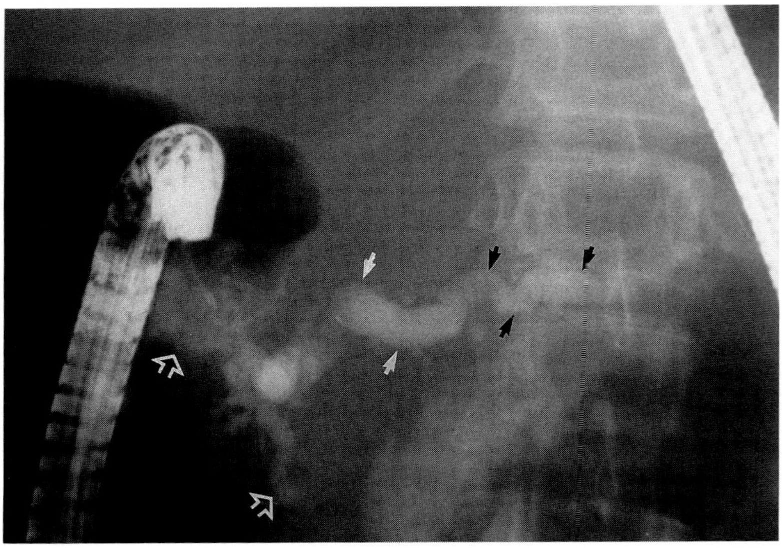

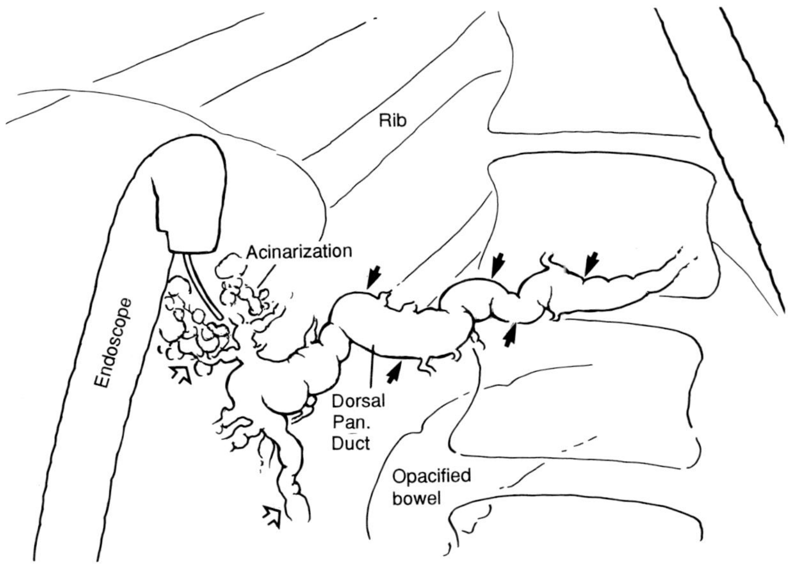

Figure 16. Pancreatogram obtained via minor (seen here) and major duct cannulation. There are focal strictures in the head region (open arrows) and gross ductal dilatation of the dorsal duct in the body and tail (solid arrows). These features, along with clubbing of the side branches and calcifications in the head region, suggest chronic pancreatitis. This impression was supported by the clinical history. The patient's chronic pain resolved following a Pustow procedure.

The largest reported series is an 11-year study in which 170 cysts and pseudocysts complicating chronic pancreatitis were managed in 143 patients (76). Among these, 78 endoscopic cyst enterostomies were performed in 71 patients, 66 transduodenal and 12 transgastric. There was a 72% cure rate among patients who underwent cyst enterostomy as initial therapy. However, there was a recurrence rate of 18%, and a complication rate of 15%, including one death due to uncontrolled hemorrhage. Other complications included infection, hemorrhage, and retroperitoneal perforation.

Another large series was reported by Cremer et al., which included 33 patients, 22 having transduodenal and 11 transgastric cyst enterostomies (71). In this series initial success was achieved in 32 of 33 patients. There were eight recurrences. Complications included three infections responsive to antibiotic therapy, percutaneous drainage in one case, and bleeding in one instance.

Transpapillary drainage of pseudocysts has been reported in several series (77). Combining data from several recent series shows that endoscopic transpapillary stent or nasopancreatic drain placement was successful in 97% of 93 patients, with successful resolution of cysts being achieved in 86% (78–81). Duration of treatment ranged from 3 weeks to 8 months, with the majority of patients responding within 3 to 5 months. The complication rate was 5.6% and generally minor, with no mortalities.

Pancreatic Fistula

Endoscopic retrograde cholangiopancreatography is the "gold standard" for diagnosing pancreatic fistulas. When the fistula tract or duct disruption communicates with the main pancreatic duct proximally, the pancreatography is highly sensitive. In instances where there is duct "blow-out" in the tail region, the presence of a mass or inflammation may preclude dorsal duct filling to the region of duct disruption. The majority of patients with pancreatic fistulas respond to conservative medical therapy or surgery. Two series have described successful resolution of pancreatic fistulas and duct disruptions with endoscopic transpapillary stent therapy. Kozarek et al. reported 18 patients with active pancreatic duct disruptions treated with transpapillary pancreatic stents (77). The majority of these patients had undergone previous attempts at percutaneous or surgical drainage procedures. Transpapillary stents were placed across the duct disruption or directly into fluid collection in each case. Resolution of the pancreatic duct disruption was observed in 16 of 18 patients, and fluid collection resolution in 12 of 14 patients. Complications were minor. However, at 16-month follow-up, seven of 18 patients required surgery for ongoing pancreatic pain or residual/recurrent fluid collection (Fig. 17).

Saeed et al. reported successful resolution of chronic pancreatic fistulas in five consecutive patients who had failed to respond to conservative management (82). There were no recurrences in 14–30 months follow-up. These two series demonstrate that transpapillary endoscopic management of pancreatic fistulas may be achieved in the majority of patients once conservative management has failed. Because this technique appears to be safe and well tolerated, it may avert surgery in some patients and change an urgent surgical procedure to an elective one in others.

Traumatic Pancreatitis

Traumatic injury is an uncommon but important etiology of acute pancreatitis and pancreatic duct disruption. This may occur following steering wheel injuries due to rapid deceleration during automobile accidents, bicycle accidents, knife and bullet wounds, and intraoperative trauma to the pancreas during other abdominal pro-

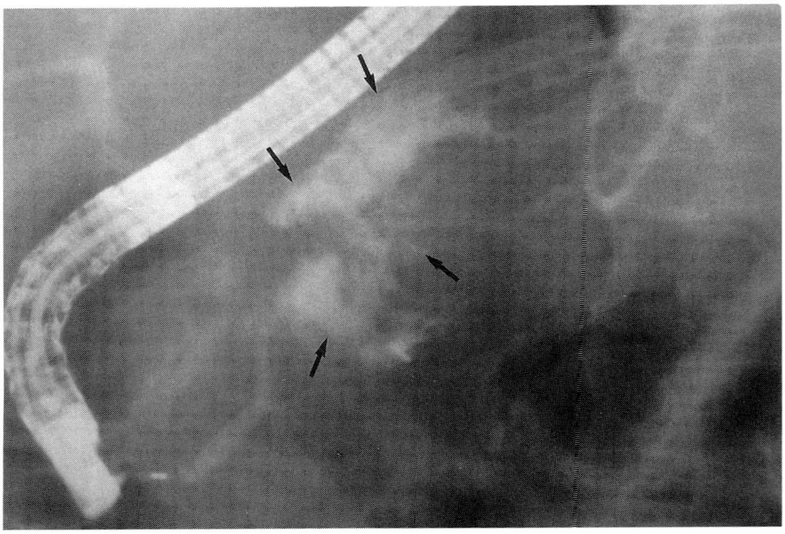

(A)

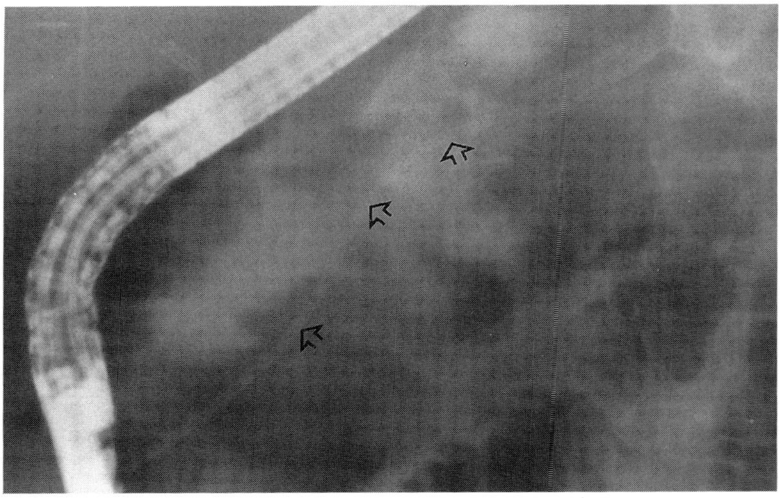

(B)

Figure 17. A postoperative pancreatic duct leak is observed on the pancreatogram (arrows, A). After a guide wire was passed across the leak, a 7-French endoprosthesis (arrows, B) was placed. Pancreatic ascites gradually resolved.

cedures. In the pediatric population blunt trauma due to physical abuse occurs with surprising frequency. The principal function of ERCP in the context of acute pancreatic trauma is to define the nature and extent of pancreatic duct disruption (83).

Localization of pancreatic duct disruption provides the important anatomic data for assessing operative and nonoperative management. The application of endoscopic transpapillary therapy for disruptive pancreatic duct may be considered.

SUMMARY

Endoscopic retrograde cholangiopancreatography and EUS are safe and effective imaging tools for the evaluation and management of pancreatic diseases. Endoscopic retrograde cholangiopancreatography contributes to the diagnosis of pancreatic adenocarcinoma and is the procedure of choice for initial palliation of obstructive jaundice. In many patients endoscopic palliation is the preferred management.

Endosonography is valuable in identifying small neoplasms that are more likely to benefit from attempted curative resection, in providing accurate staging information by which treatment selection can more logically be determined, and in accurately assessing response to neoadjuvant therapy. Precise staging of pancreatic tumor decreases the number of surgical interventions that do not benefit patients with advanced disease. The application of ultrasound-guided FNA appears to be a more accurate means of achieving tissue diagnosis and will reduce the number of patients requiring laparotomy for tissue diagnosis.

Given the poor outlook for the majority of patients who turn out to have unresectable locally advanced and metastatic disease, nonoperative approaches to palliation should be employed when possible to minimize procedure-associated complications and unrealistic therapeutic expectations while maximizing function and quality of life outside the hospital. Surgical exploration should be reserved for those patients in whom resection for cure is a realistic possibility and those who require palliation of gastroduodenal obstruction or in whom nonoperative biliary palliation cannot be achieved. The accompanying algorithm (Fig. 18) outlines the utilization of ERCP and EUS in the evaluation and management of patients with suspected pancreatic cancer.

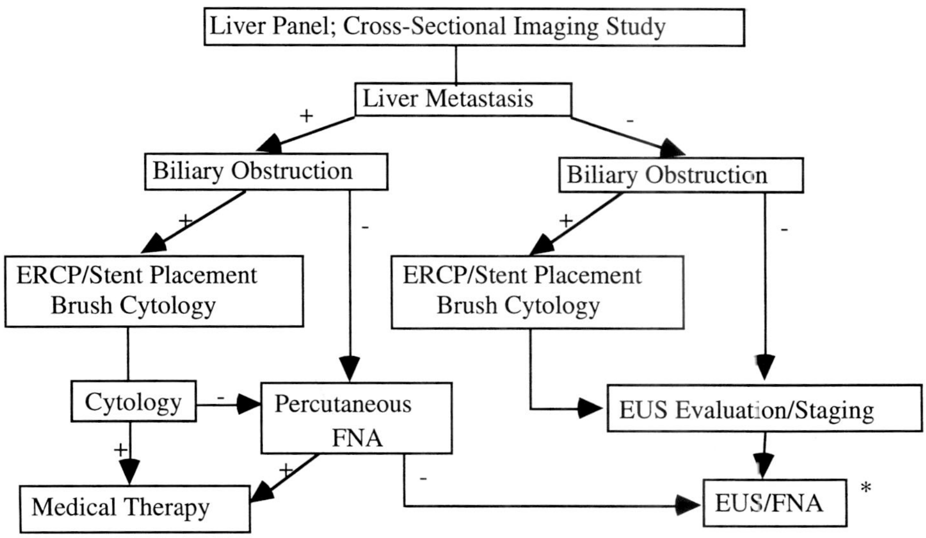

Figure 18. Suggested algorithm for the application of ERCP and EUS in the evaluation of patients with suspected pancreatic cancer. EUS/FNA = endoscopic ultrasound-guided real-time fine needle aspiration for cytology if (1) prior attempts at brush or percutaneous cytology are unsuccessful; (2) a malignant-appearing mass or lymph node is seen, the EUS staging of which confers unresectability; (3) the clinical history and EUS appearance require histology to distinguish an inflammatory versus neoplastic lesion.

Urgent ERCP is indicated in patients with severe gallstone pancreatitis early in the course of the illness. Patients who have recurrent episodes of pancreatitis should undergo ERCP evaluation to evaluate for treatable causes. Pancreatography contributes to the preoperative evaluation of patients with traumatic pancreatitis, or those with chronic pancreatitis complicated by stricture, fistula, or pseudocyst.

REFERENCES

1. Nebel OT, Silvis SE, Rogers G, et al. Complications associated with endoscopic retrograde cholangiopancreatography. Result of the 1974 ASGE Survey. *Gastrointest Endosc.* 1975;22:346.
2. Ruppin H, Aron R, Ett W, et al. Acute pancreatitis after endoscopic retrograde pancreatography. *Endoscopy.* 1974;6:94–98.
3. Kadish SL, Ginsberg GG, Faigel DO, Pollack BJ, Smith D, Kochman ML. Accuracy of celiac axis detection on endoscopic ultrasound. *Am J Gastroenterol.* 1995;9:A1162.
4. Soehendra N, Grimm H, Berger B, Nam VC. Malignant jaundice: results of diagnostic and therapeutic endoscopy. *World J Surg.* 1989;13:171–177.
5. Ogoshi K. Diseases of the pancreas and biliary system. Cancers of the pancreas. In: Takemoto T, Kasugai T, eds. *Endoscopic Retrograde Pancreatography.* Tokyo, New York: Igaku Shoin; 1979:159–176.
6. Sahel J. Pancreatic cancer: ERCP. In Kawai K, ed. *Early Diagnosis of Pancreatic Cancer.* Tokyo: Igaku Shoin; 1980:118–139.
7. Nakajima M, Yamaguchi K, Akasaka Y. Endoscopic retrograde cholangiopancreatography in the diagnosis of pancreatic cancer. In Kawai K, ed. *Early Diagnosis of Pancreatic Cancer.* Tokyo: Igaku Shoin; 1980:140–154.
8. Niederau C, Grendell JH. Diagnosis of pancreatic carcinoma: imaging techniques and tumor markers. *Pancreas.* 1992;7:66–68.
9. Cotton PB: ERCP. Progress report. *Gut.* 1977;18:316–341.
10. Aohto M, Ono T, Tsuchiya Y, et al. *Cholangiography and Pancreatography.* Tokyo, New York: Igaku Shoin, 1978:172–178.
11. Plumley TF, Rohrman CA, Freeny PC, Silverstein FE, Ball TJ. Double duct sign: reassessed the significance in ERCP. *Am J Radiol.* 1982;138:31–35.
12. Seligson U, Soderlund C. ERCP and serum alkalinephosphatates in pancreatic carcinoma. *ACTA Chir Scand.* 1986;152:309–312.
13. Frick NP, O'leary JF, Walker HC, Goodale RL. Accuracy of endoscopic retrograde cholangiopancreatography (ERCP) in differentiating benign and malignant disease. *Gastrointest Endosc.* 1982;7:241–244.
14. Shemesh E, Czerniak A, Nass S, Klein E. World with endoscopic retrograde cholangiopancreatography in differentiating pancreatic cancer coexisting with chronic pancreatitis. *Cancer.* 1990;65:893–896.
15. Foutch PG, Kerr DM, Harlan JR, Kummet TD. A prospective controlled analysis of endoscopic cyto techniques for diagnosis of malignant biliary structures. *Am J Gastroenterol.* 1991;86:577–580.
16. Howell DA, Beveridge PR, Bosco J, Jones M. Endoscopic needle aspiration biobsy at ERCP in the diagnosis of biliary strictures. *Gastrointest Endosc.* 1992;38:531–535.
17. Foutch PG, Kerr DM, Harlan JR, et al. Endoscopic retrograde wire-guided brush cytology for diagnosis of patients with malignant obstruction of the bile duct. *Am J Gastroenterol.* 1990;85:791–795.

18. Sawada Y, Gonda H, Hayashida Y. Combined use of brushing cytology in endoscopic retrograde pancreatography for the early detection of pancreatic cancer. *Acta Cytol.* 1989;33:870–874.

19. Ryan ME. Cytologic brushings of ductal lesions during ERCP. *Gastrointest Endosc.* 1991;37:139–142.

20. Berthelemy P, Bouisson M, Escourrou J, Vaysse N, Rumeau JL, Pradayrol L. Identification of K-ras mutations in pancreatic juice in the early diagnosis of pancreatic cancer. *Ann Intern Med* 1995;123:188–191.

21. Gentiloni N, Caradonna P, Costamagna G, et al. Pancreatic juice 90K and serum CA 19-9 combined determination can discriminate between pancreatic cancer and chronic pancreatitis. *Am J Gastroenterol.* 1995;90:1069–1072.

22. Speer AG, Cotton PB, Russell RCG, Mason RR, Hatfield ARW, et al. Randomized trial of endoscopic versus percutaneous stent insertion in malignant obstructive jaundice. *Lancet.* 1987;2:57–62.

23. Andersen JR, Sorensen SM, Kruse A, Rokkjaer M, Matzen P. Randomized trial of endoscopic endoprothesis versus operative bypass and malignant obstructive jaundice. *Gut.* 1989;30:1132–1135.

24. Shepherd HA, Diba A, Ross AP, Arthur M, Ryle G, Collin-Jones D. Endoscopic biliary prothesis and the palliation of malignant biliary obstruction-A randomized trial. *Gut.* 1986;27:A1284.

25. Smith AC, Dowsett JF, Russell RCG, Hatfield ARW, Cotton PB. Randomized trial of endoscopic stenting versus surgical bypass in malignant low bile duct obstruction. *Lancet.* 1194;344:1655–1660.

26. van den Bosch RP, van der Schelling GP, Klinkenbijl JHG, et al. Guidelines for the application of surgery and endoprostheses in the palliation of obstructive jaundice in advanced cancer of the pancreas. *Ann Surg.* 1994;219:18–24.

27. Brandabur JJ, Kozarec RA, Ball, et al. Nonoperative versus operative treatment of obstructive jaundice in pancreatic cancer: cost and survival analysis. *Am J Gastroenterol.* 1988;83:1132–1138.

28. Rösch T, Lorenz R, Braig C, et al. Endoscopic ultrasound and pancreatic tumor diagnosis. *Gastrointest Endosc.* 1991;37:347–352.

29. Lees WR. The Pancreas: differential diagnosis and pancreatitis. In: Lightdale CJ, ed. Endoscopic ultrasonography. *Gastrointest Endosc Clin North Am.* 1992;2:657–672.

30. Rösch T, Classen M. *Gastroenterologic Endosonography.* Stuttgart, New York: Thieme; 1992:114–167.

31. Palazzo L, Roseau G, Gayet B, et al. Endoscopic ultrasonography in diagnosis and staging of pancreatic adenocarcinoma: results of a prospective study with comparison to ultrasonography and CT scan. *Endoscopy.* 1993;25:143–150.

32. Rösch T, Neuhaus H, Gmeinweiser J, et al. Role of endoscopic ultrasonography in the evaluation of patients with suspected pancreatic disease. *Gastroenterology.* 1993; 104:21A.

33. Rösch T, Roder JR, Decassian T, et al. Indeterminant pancreatic tumors: still a problem evan with modern diagnostic methods. *Endoscopy.* 1995, in press.

34. Kadish SL, Kochman ML, Rosato EP, et al. Endosonography: the modality of choice for T staging and vascular involvement in patients with pancreatic carcinoma? *Gastroenterology.* 1995;108:A486.

35. Gress F, Savides R, Zaidi S, et al. Endoscopic ultrasound (EUS) staging of pancreatic cancer (PCa) accuratly predicts patient outcome and survival. *Gasrtointest Endosc.* 1996;43(suppl):A8.

36. Snady H. Pancreatic cancer: influence of endoscopic ultrasonography on management and outcomes. *Gastrointest Endosc Clin North Am.* 1995;5:755–762.
37. Cooperman A. When is surgery indicated as the initial treatment for pancreatic neoplasm? In: Snady H, Lambroza A, Falkenstein D, eds.: *Clinical Endoscopy: Practice and Opinions* (postgraduate course). New York: New York Society for Gastrointestinal Endoscopy; 1994:37.
38. Warshaw AL, Fernandez-Del Castillo. Medical progress: pancreatic carcinoma. *N Engl J Med.* 1992;326:455–465.
39. Snady H, Bruckner H, Siegel J, et al. Influence of combined chemotherapy, radiotherapy and surgery on survival of patients with unresectable pancreatic carcinoma using computed tomography and endoscopic ultrasound to select treatment. *Gastroenterology.* 1994;106:A28.
40. Niederau, Grendell, Hall-Craggs MA, Lees WR. Fine needle aspiration biopsy: pancreatic and biliary tumors. *Am J Radiol.* 1986;147:359–403.
41. Al-Kaisi N, Siegler EE. Fine needle cytology of the pancreas. *Acta Cytol.* 1989; 33:145–152.
42. Phillips VM, Hersh T, Erwin BC, et al. Percutaneous biopsy of pancreatic masses. *J Clin Gastroenterol.* 1985;7:506–510.
43. Warshaw AL. Implications of peritoneal cytology for staging of early pancreatic cancer. *Am J Surg.* 1991;161:26–30.
44. Staley CA, Lee JE, Cleary KR, et al. Preoperative chemoradiation, pancreaticoduodenectomy, and intraoperative radiation therapy for adenocarcinoma of the pancreatic head. *Am J Surg.* 1996;171:118–125.
45. Faigel DO, Ginsberg GG, Smith D, Kadish SL, Kochman ML. Endoscopic ultrasound (EUS) guided fine needle aspiration (FNA) of pancreatic tumors. *J Clin Oncol.* 1996;15:A224.
46. Pinson CW, Munson JL, Deveney CW. Endoscopic retrograde cholangiopancreatography in the preoperative diagnosis of pancreatic neoplasms associated with cyst. *Am J Surg.* 1990;159:510–513.
47. Faigle DO, Kochman ML, Kadish SL, Smith D, Ginsberg GG. Endosonography of complex cystic masses of the pancreas with clinicopathologic correlation. *Gastrointest Endosc.* 1996;43:A513.
48. Hammel P, Levy P, Voitot H, et al. Preoperative cyst fluid analysis useful for differential diagnosis of cystic lesions of the pancreas. *Gastroenterology.* 1995;108:1230–1235.
49. Leawandrowski KB, Southern JF, Pins MR, et al. Cyst fluid analysis in the differential diagnosis of pancreatic cysts. A comparison of pseudocysts, serocyst adenomas, mucinous cystic neoplasms, and mucinous cyst adenocarcinoma. *Ann Surg.* 1993;217:41–47.
50. Duvenjak M, Rotvic I, Vucelic B, et al. The value of pancreatic pseudocyst amylase concentration in the detection of pseudocyst communication with the pancreatic duct. *Am J Gastroenterol.* 1991;86:595–598.
51. Rösch T, Lightdale CT, Botet JF, et al. Endosonographic localization of pancreatic endocrine tumors. *New Engl J Med.* 1992;326:1721–1726.
52. van Stolke R, Sivak MV, Petrini JL, et al. Endoscopic management of upper gastrointestinal polyps and periampullary lesions in familial adenomatous polyposis and Gardner's syndrome. *Endoscopy.* 1987;19:19–22.
53. Nakao NL, Seigle JH, Stenger R, et al. Tumors of the ampulla of Vater: early diagnosis by intraampullary biopsy during endoscopic cannulation. *Gastroenterology.* 1982; 83:459–464.

54. Tio TL. Endosonography in diagnosis and staging of pancreatic ampullary tumors. In: Lightdale CJ, ed. Endoscopic ultrasonography. *Gastrointest Endosc Clin North Am.* 1992;2:673–684.

55. Bansal R, Kadish S, Carpenter S, et al. Accuracy of endoscopic ultrasound vs. CT scan, MRI, and angiography for the staging of adenocarcinoma of the ampulla of Vater. *Gastrointest Endosc.* 1995;41:A296.

56. Neoptolemos JP, Carr-Locke DL, London NJ, Bailey IA, James D, Fossard DP. Controlled trial of urgent endoscopic retrograde pancreatography and endoscopic sphincterotomy versus conservative treatment for acute pancreatitis due to gallstones. *Lancet.* 1988;2:979–983.

57. Fan ST, Lai ECS, Mok PFT, Lo CM, Zheng SS, Wang J. Early treatment of acute biliary pancreatitis by endoscopic papillotomy. *New Engl J Med.* 1993;328:228–232.

58. Steinberg W, Tenner S. Acute pancreatitis. *New Engl J Med.* 1994;330:1198–1210.

59. Feller ER. Endoscopic retrograde cholangiopancreatography in the diagnosis of unexplained pancreatitis. *Arch Intern Med.* 1984;144:1797–1799.

60. Venu RP, Geenen JE, Hogan W, Stone J, Johnson GK, Soergel K. Idiopathic recurrent pancreatitis: An approach to diagnosis and treatment. *Dig Dis Sci.* 1989;34:56–60.

61. Lee SP, Nicholls JF, Park HZ. Biliary sludge as a cause of acute pancreatitis. *New Engl J Med.* 1992;326:589–593.

62. Wiersema MJ, Hawes RH, Lehman GA, Kochman ML, Sherman S, Kopecky KK. A prospective evaluation of endoscopic ultrasonography and endoscopic retrograde cholangiopancreatography in patient with chronic abdominal pain of suspected pancreatic origin. *Endoscopy.* 1993;25:555–565.

63. Buscail L, Escourrou J, Moreau J, et al. Endoscopic ultrasonography and chronic pancreatitis comparative prospective study with conventional ultrasonography, computed tomography, and ERCP. *Pancreas.* 1995;10:251–257.

64. Huibregtse K, Schneider B, Brij A, Titgat GNJ. Endoscopic pancreatic drainage in chronic pancreatitis. *Gastrointest Endosc.* 1988;34:9–15.

65. Kozarek RA, Patterson DJ, Ball TJ, Traverso LW. Endoscopic placement of endoscopic drains in the management of pancreatitis. *Ann Surg.* 1989;209:261–256.

66. Cremer M, Deviere J, Delahay M, Baize M, Vandermeeren A. Stenting in severe chronic pancreatitis, results of median term follow-up in 76 patients. *Endoscopy.* 1991;23:171–176.

67. Carr-Locke DL. Endoscopic procedures in the treatment of pancreatic pain. *Acta Chir Scand.* 1990;156:293–298.

68. Geenen JE, Rolny P. Endoscopic therapy of acute and chronic pancreatitis. *Gastrointest Endosc.* 1991;37:377–382.

69. Bornman PC, Russell RCG. *Br J Surg.* 1992;79:1260–1261.

70. Yeo CJ, Bastidas JA, Lynch-Nyhan A, et al. The natural history of pseudocysts documented by computed tomography. *Surg Gynecol Obstet.* 1990;170:411–417.

71. Cremer M, Deviere J, Engelholm L. Endoscopic management of cysts and pseudocysts in chronic pancreatitis: Long-term follow-up after seven years experience. *Gastrointest Endosc.* 1989;35:1–9.

72. Zahel J. Endoscopic drainage of pancreatic cysts. *Endoscopy.* 1991;23:181–184.

73. Kozarek RA, Brayko CM, Harlin J, Samowski RA, Cintoria I, Koval A. Endoscopic drainage of pancreatic pseudocysts. *Gastrointest Endosc.* 1990;36:96–100.

74. Grimm H, Binmoellr KF, Soehindra N. Endosonography pseudocysts. *Gastrointest Endosc.* 1992;38:170–171.

75. Ginsberg GG, Al-Kawas FH, Tio TL, et al. Endoscopic ultrasound evaluation of vascular involvement in pancreatic lesions: a comparison with computed tomography. *Gastrointest Endosc.* 1993;39:A251.

76. Barthet M, Bugallo M, Moreira LS, et al. Management of cysts and pseudocysts complicating chronic pancreatitis. A retrospective study of 143 patients. *Gastroenterol Clin Biol.* 1993;17:270–280.

77. Kozarek RA, Ball TJ, Patterson DJ, Freeny PC, Ryan JA, Traverso LW. Endoscopic trans-papillary therapy for disrupted pancreatic duct and peri-pancreatic fluid collections. *Gastroenterology.* 1991;100:1362–1370.

78. Catalano MF, Geenen JE, Schmalz MJ, Johnson GK, Dean RS, Hogan WJ. Treatment of pancreatic pseudocysts with ductal communication by trans-papillary pancreatic duct endoprosthesis. *Gastrointest Endosc.* 1995;42:214–218.

79. Smits ME, Rauws EAJ, Tytgat GNJ, Huibregtse K. The efficacy of Endoscopic Treatment of Pancreatic Pseudocysts. *Gastrointest Endosc.* 1995;42:202–207.

80. Barthet M, Sahel J, Bodiou-Bertei C, Bernard JP. Endoscopic transpapillary drainage of pancreatic pseudocysts. *Gastrointest Endosc.* 1995;42:208–213.

81. Binmowller KF, Seifert H, Walter A, Soehendra N. Transpapillary and transmural drainage of pancreatic pseudocysts. *Gastrointest Endosc.* 1995;42:219–224.

82. Saeed ZA, Ramirez FC, Hepps KS. Endoscopic stent placement for internal and external pancreatic fistulas. *Gastroenterology.* 1993;105:1213–1217.

83. Barkin KS, Ferstenberg RM, Panullo W, et al. Endoscopic retrograde cholangiopancreatography and pancreatic trauma. *Gastrointest Endosc.* 1988;34:102–105.

84. Muller MF, Meyenberger C, Bertschinger P, et al. Pancreatic tumors: Evaluation with endoscopic US, CT, and MR imaging. *Radiology.* 1994;190:745–751.

85. Forsmark CE, Allbert CA, Lambiase L, et al. Diagnostic tests for pancreatic cancer. *Gastrointest Endosc.* 1993;39:A314 (abstract).

86. Giovannini M, Seitz JF. Endoscopic ultrasonography with a linear type echoendoscope in the evaluation of 94 patients with pancreatobiliary disease. *Endoscopy.* 1994;26: 579–585.

87. Kallimanis G, Axiotis E, Papantoniou P, et al. EUS, ERCP, US, CT in the diagnosis of pancreatic cancer. *Endoscopy.* 1992;24:656 (abstract).

88. Akahoshi K, Chijiiwa Y, Nakano I, et al. Role of endosonography in diagnosis and staging of pancreatic cancer. Unpublished data.

89. Nakaizumi A, Uehara H, Lishi H, et al. Endoscopic ultrasonography in diagnosis and staging of pancreatic cancer. *Dig Dis Sci.* 1995;40:696–700.

90. Yasuda K, Mukai H, Fujimoto S, et al. The diagnosis of pancreatic cancer by endoscopic ultrasonography. *Gastrointest Endosc.* 1988;34:1–8.

91. Grimm H, Maydeo A, Soehendra N. Endo-luminal ultrasound for the diagnosis and staging of pancreatic cancer. *Baillieres Clin Gastroenterol.* 1990;4:869–887.

92. Tio TL, Tytgat GNJ, Cikot RJLM, et al. Ampullopancreatic carcinoma: Preoperative TNM classification with endosonography. *Radiology.* 1990;175:455–461.

93. Kallimanis G, Axiotis E, Papantoniou P, et al. Endoscopic ultrasonography in preoperative TNM classification of pancreatic cancer. *Endoscopy.* 1992;24:656 (abstract).

94. Rösch T, Dittler HJ, Lorenz R, et al. Endosonographisches staging des pankreaskarzinoms. *Dtsch Med Wochenschr.* 1992;117:563–569.

95. Wiersema MJ, Chak A, Hawes RH, Kopecky KK. Evaluation of endosonography in distinguishing malignant from inflammatory pancratic masses. *Gastrointest Endosc* 1993;39:A336 (abstract).

96. Rösch T, Dittler HJ, Strobel K, et al. Local staging of pancreatic head cancer by endoscopic ultrasonography: A re-evaluation using blind videotape assessment. *Endoscopy* 1995;27(abstract) (in press).

97. Yasuda K, Mukai H, Nakajima M, Kawai K. Staging of pancreatic carcinoma by endoscopic ultrasonography. *Endoscopy.* 1993;25:151–155.

98. Kadish SL, Kochman ML, Rosato EP, et al. Endosonography: the modality of choice for T staging and vascular involvement in patients with pancreatic carcinoma? *Gastroenterology.* 1995;108:A486 (abstract).

99. Kadish SL, Kochman ML, Rosato EP, et al. Endosonography for pancreatic cancer staging: superiority vs. angiography for assessing vascular invasion *Am J Gastroenterol.* 1995;90:A211.

100. Snady H, Cooperman A, Siegel JH. Assessment of vascular involvement by pancreatic disease—a comparison endoscopic ultrasonography to computerized tomography and angiography. *Gastrointest Endosc.* 1990;36:197 (abstract).

101. Rösch T, Braig C, Gain T, et al. Staging of pancreatic and ampullary carcinoma by endoscopic ultrasonography. *Gastroenterology.* 1992;102:188–199.

102. Giovannini M, Seitz JF, Monges G, et al. Fine-needle aspiration biopsy guided by endoscopic ultrasonography. Results in 141 patients. *Endoscopy.* 1995;27:171–177.

103. Wiersema MJ, Kochman ML, Cramer HM, et al. Endosonography-guided real-time fine-needle aspiration biopsy. *Gastrointest Endosc.* 1994;40:700–770.

104. Bhutani M, Hoffman B, van Velse A, et al. Endoscopic ultrasound (EUS) guided fine needle aspiration (FNA) of malignant prancreatic lesions: Accuracy, safety and clinical utility. *Gastrointest Endosc.* 1995;41:298 (abstract).

105. Chang K, Nguyen P, Durbin T, et al. Endoscopic ultrasound (EUS) guided fine needle aspiration (FNA) in the diagnosis and staging of pancreatic carcinoma. *Gastrointest Endosc.* 1994;40:A62.

106. Faigel DO, Ginsberg GG, Kadish SL, et al. Endoscopic ultrasound (EUS) guided fine needle aspiration (FNA) of extraluminal masses. *Gastroenterology.* 1996:110(4):A511.

107. Chang K, Wiersema MJ, Giovannini M, Villmann P, Erickson RA. Multi-centerexperience with endoscopic ultrasound guided fine needle aspiration of the pancreas. *Gastrointest Endosc.* 1996;43(suppl):A1.

108. Schumacher B, Lubke HJ, Frieling T, et al. Prospective detection of insulinomas by endoscopic ultrasonography. *Endoscopy* 1996;28:310–1.

109. Bansal R, Nostrant TT, Elta GH, et al. Comparison of radial and sector array endoscopic ultrasound for localization of pancreatic endocrine tumors. *Gastrointest Endosc.* 1995;41:296A.

110. Thompson NW, Czako PF, Fritts LL, et al. The role of endoscopic ultrasonography in the localization of insulinomas and gastrinomas. *Surgery.* 1994;116:1131–1138.

111. Lightdale CJ, Botet JP, Woodruff JM, Brennan MF. Localization of endocrine tumors of the pancreas with endoscopic ultrasound. *Cancer.* 1991;68:1815–1820.

112. Rösch T, Lorenz R, Braig C, et al. Preoperative localization of endocrine tumors of the pancreas: Endoscopic ultrasound is superior to trans-abdominal sonography and computed tomography. *Gastrointest Endosc.* 1990;36:199–200A.

113. Yamada N, Komoto E, Naito Y, et al. Endoscopic ultrasonography in the diagnosis of pancreatic islet cell tumors. *J Ultrasound Med.* 1991;23:85–87.

114. Ruszniewski P, Amouyal P, Amouyal G, et al. Diagnostic value of endoscopic ultrasonography for the localization of gastrinomas. *Gastroenterology.* 1993;104:A331.

115. Glover JR, Shover PJ, Lees WR. Endoscopic ultrasound for localization of islet cell tumors. *Gut.* 1992;33:108–110.

116. Ruszniewski P, Amouyal P, Amouyal G, et al. Endoscopic ultrasonography in the localization of insulinomas: Results of a multicenter prospective study. *Gastroenterology.* 1993;104:A332.

117. Palazzo L, Roseau G, Salmeron M. Endoscopic ultrasonography in the preoperative localization of pancreatic endocrine tumors. *Endoscopy.* 1992;24:350–353.

118. Zimmer T, Zeigler K, Bader N, et al. Localization of neuro-endocrine tumors of the upper gastrointestinal tract. *Gut.* 1994;35:471–475.

26

SURGICAL SUMMARY: PANCREATIC DISEASE

Keith D. Lillemoe, M.D.
The Johns Hopkins Medical Institutions
Baltimore, Maryland

The preceding chapters have discussed the diagnostic modalities available for investigating pancreatic pathology. Each of the techniques described has the potential to provide useful information to the clinician in the diagnosis and management of pancreatic disease. In many situations, one diagnostic study may complement another and more than one technique may be indicated. In other scenarios, the information provided by different examinations may be redundant and therefore the clinician must base his or her choice of studies on the benefits of each test in that specific clinical presentation while reflecting on the relative risks and costs of the procedure.

In this chapter, a general overview of the clinical presentation of pancreatic disease including both acute and chronic, benign and malignant pancreatic conditions is first provided. Finally, a number of specific pancreatic conditions are reviewed, and the role of various diagnostic studies are discussed with respect to each specific diagnosis.

CLINICAL PRESENTATION OF PANCREATIC DISEASE

The most common presenting complaints in patients with pancreatic disease are pain and jaundice. Pain can be located either in the abdomen—usually in the epigastrium or left upper quadrant—or radiating into the back. The pain may be of acute onset or of a chronic nature. Severe pain of an acute onset usually represents a benign process—acute pancreatitis. Chronic pain, however may be seen with either a benign or malignant process. Jaundice associated with pancreatic disease is the result of obstruction of the distal common bile duct as it passes through the pancreatic head en route to the ampulla of Vater. Pancreatic carcinoma is by far the most common form of pancreatic pathology presenting with obstructive jaundice. Chronic pancreatitis with parenchymal fibrosis, a pancreatic pseudocyst, or benign pancreatic neoplasms are uncommon causes of biliary obstruction. The final symptoms suggesting pancreatic disease are those of pancreatic exocrine and endocrine insufficiency. These symptoms are much less common and are seen only in advanced stages of chronic pancreatitis. Patients with pancreatic exocrine insufficiency manifest symptoms of malabsorption with diarrhea and steatorrhea. Endocrine insufficiency may be asymptomatic with only laboratory evidence of glucose intolerance, or frank symptoms of diabetes may be present.

The physical findings associated with pancreatic disease are generally not specific. Patients with acute pancreatitis show signs of abdominal tenderness as well as evidence of systemic manifestations of the disease such as fever, tachycardia, and in severe cases, associated pulmonary findings. Patients with severe pancreatitis may develop either a pancreatic phlegmon or a peripancreatic fluid collection during the course of their disease, and an abdominal mass may be palpable. Patients with chronic pancreatitis usually lack physical findings. Patients with periampullary pancreatic carcinoma show evidence of jaundice and, with advanced disease, signs of cachexia and weight loss. A palpable mass is uncommon with any pancreatic neoplasm.

Laboratory tests for pancreatic disease, in general, lack specificity with the exception of serum amylase or lipase elevations associated with acute pancreatitis. A number of other abnormal laboratory values may also be present in patients with acute pancreatitis including an increased white blood cell count, a fall in hematocrit and serum calcium, a rise in serum urea nitrogen and creatinine, increased serum glucose, and metabolic acidosis. These abnormalities reflect the severity of the disease and may predict prognosis (1) but are not specific for the diagnosis of pancreatic disease. Patients with chronic pancreatitis may have totally normal laboratory values. Patients with a periampullary pancreatic carcinoma have evidence of biliary obstruction with elevated serum bilirubin and other liver function tests. Recently attention has focused on the serum tumor marker, CA 19-9, which has been reported to have a sensitivity and specificity approaching 90% for pancreatic carcinoma (2). Unfortunately, CA 19-9 is frequently normal in the early stages of disease and can not be used as a screening test.

The lack of specific symptoms, signs, and laboratory tests associated with most pancreatic disease emphasizes the importance of diagnostic radiological studies in the diagnosis and management of patients with these disorders.

BENIGN PANCREATIC DISORDERS

Acute Pancreatitis

Acute pancreatitis includes a broad spectrum of pancreatic pathology, varying from mild interstitial edema to severe hemorrhagic necrosis. The clinical presentation can vary, ranging from mild self-limited episodes of abdominal discomfort to a severe systemic illness associated with fluid sequestration, metabolic derangements, hypotension, and death. The great majority of patients with acute pancreatitis have only mild to moderate symptoms, follow a self-limited course, and respond to supportive care alone. However, approximately 10% of the patients develop a severe illness that may be life-threatening, associated with pancreatic hemorrhage or necrosis, and that is often attended by significant morbidity and mortality despite maximal supportive care. The early recognition of those patients with severe disease who at are increased risk for complications is a challenge of the management of acute pancreatitis. It is in these patients that the role of diagnostic radiologic imaging is most significant.

Although a number of causes of pancreatitis have been defined, more than 90% of cases are related to biliary tract disease or excessive alcohol intake. The relative frequency of these two principal causes of acute pancreatitis varies, depending upon the patient population. Although not a common cause, pancreatitis occurring in a postoperative period is often particularly severe and associated with a significantly increased risk of pancreatic sepsis and associated mortality. In many cases, a secure diagnosis of acute pancreatitis is possible based on the clinical presentation. In more than 90% of patients, the predominant feature is abdominal pain. Pain begins as a gradually increasing mid-epigastric pain reaching its maximal intensity several hours after the onset of the illness. Nausea and vomiting usually accompany the abdominal pain. Physical findings can be quite variable and include fever, tachycardia, epigastric tenderness, and abdominal distension. In patients with severe pancreatitis, major systemic manifestations may be present. These include hypotension, hypovolemia, hypoperfusion, and obtundation. Evidence of pulmonary complications including tachypnea, dyspnea, and cyanosis may be present in patients with severe disease.

The diagnosis of pancreatitis in the face of a typical clinical presentation can usually be confirmed by determination of serum amylase. Hyperamylasemia is observed generally within 24 hr of onset of symptoms. The degree of initial hyperamylasemia does not reliably predict the severity of the pancreatic injury.

Radiological Studies in Patients with Acute Pancreatitis. The indication for various radiological studies in patients with acute pancreatitis includes confirmation of the diagnosis, identification of the etiology, and detection of associated complications (Fig. 1). In patients with a typical presentation and a self-limited attack, there is little role for extensive radiological work-up. In contrast, in patients with severe acute pancreatitis with associated pancreatic necrosis, multiple diagnosis studies with frequent repetition may be indicated during the course of management.

Confirmation of the Diagnosis of Acute Pancreatitis. At the time of initial presentation of an acute abdomen, a standard chest X-ray and abdominal series should be obtained. The indications for these examinations are often to rule out other conditions such as a perforated viscus with free air, bowel obstruction, or a pulmonary process such as pneumonia. Findings that may be seen in patients with acute pancreatitis include nonspecific abnormalities such as a "sentinal loop" or a "colon cutoff" sign, a nonspecific ileus pattern, or in patients with previous episodes of pancreatitis, the presence of pancreatic calcifications. The findings on chest X-ray may include a left pleural effusion or left basilar atelectasis. If a diagnostic study is indicated to confirm the diagnosis of acute pancreatitis, a dynamic contrast-enhanced abdominal computed tomography (CT) scan is currently the most sensitive, noninvasive imaging method widely available to confirm the diagnosis. The

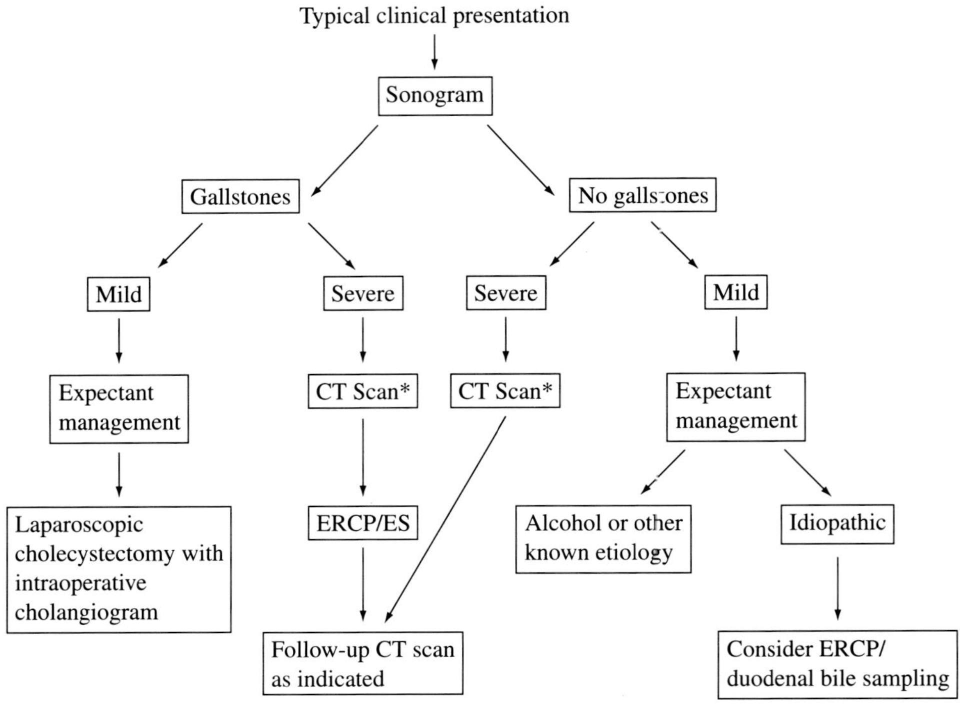

Figure 1. Radiologic studies in the evaluation of acute pancreatitis.

findings in acute pancreatitis may be divided into pancreatic and peripancreatic changes (Table 1). The use of intravenous contrast is particularly important in both the diagnosis and the detection of the complication of necrosis. In acute pancreatitis, hyperemia of the gland is common. Areas devoid of enhancement may indicate the presence of necrosis. Although ultrasound may demonstrate findings of decreased echogenicity and enlargement of the gland, the gland may appear normal during the first 24 hr after the onset of pain. Furthermore, the examination may be difficult in the acute phase owing to abdominal pain and ileus. Although magnetic resonance imaging (MRI) may provide similar morphological changes as CT scan, there is no real clinical advantage save for patients with an allergy to iodinated contrast and/ or impaired renal function.

Identification of the Etiology of Pancreatitis. The etiology of acute pancreatitis is either gallstones or alcohol abuse in over 90% of patients. In many cases, a history of heavy alcohol intake may strongly suggest that diagnosis. However, in all patients, even those likely to have pancreatitis on the basis of alcohol abuse, ultrasound examination is indicated to rule out gallbladder and common bile duct stones. Although highly accurate in the detection of gallstones, the accuracy and identification of common bile duct stones is significantly less, usually in the range of 70–80%

(3). The widespread use of MR cholangiography may in the future provide a more accurate noninvasive technique for demonstrating the presence of common duct calculi. If gallstone pancreatitis is expected, the performance of endoscopic retrograde cholangiopancreatography (ERCP) should be considered in selected patients with severe disease. Two randomized studies have been reported, suggesting that early ERCP with sphincterotomy is associated with a decrease in the complication rate in selected patients with severe gallstone pancreatitis (4, 5). Furthermore, endoscopic intervention was shown to be safe in the setting of acute pancreatitis. There appears to be no role for ERCP or sphincterotomy in patients with alcohol-induced pancreatitis or pancreatitis secondary to other processes.

Historically, in a significant percentage of patients with acute pancreatitis, no etiology can be identified, and the etiology is classified as "idiopathic." In such patients, routine abdominal ultrasound has failed to show evidence of gallstones and no other risk factors could be identified. Recent studies have demonstrated, however, that more than two-thirds of these patients may be found to have biliary gravel or sludge, termed microlithiasis, based on evaluation of duodenal bile collected during endoscopic aspiration (6). In a number of patients, ERCP may identify anomalies of the pancreatic and biliary tree that may contribute to the development of pancreatitis (7). Therefore a thorough evaluation for the cause of acute pancreatitis should be completed in all patients to identify a treatable cause.

Detection of Complications of Pancreatitis. A correlation exists between the degree of CT abnormality and the clinical course and severity of acute pancreatitis. In this system described by Ranson and colleagues (8) (known as Balthazar stage) an excellent correlation has been seen between CT changes, the incidence of peri-

Table 1. Computed tomographic findings in acute pancreatitis

Pancreatic Changes
Parenchymal enlargement
Diffuse
Focal
Parenchymal edema
Parenchymal vascular enhancement
Necrosis
Peripancreatic Changes
Blurring of fat planes
Thickening of fascial planes
Presence of fluid collections
Nonspecific Findings
Bowel distension
Pleural effusion
Mesenteric edema

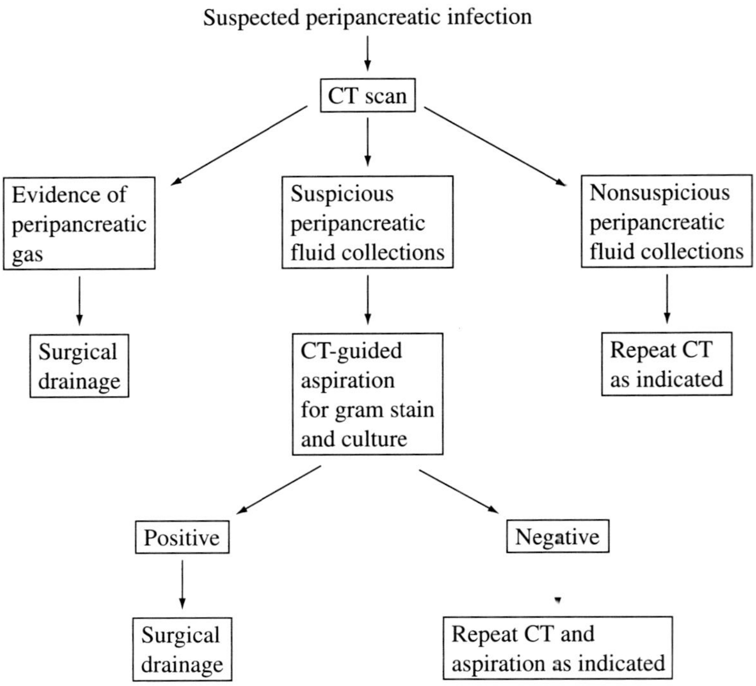

Figure 2. Radiologic studies in the evaluation of secondary peripancreatic infection.

pancreatic infection, and overall prognosis. The incidence of abscess formation in patients with Balthazar E class changes (two or more collections of peripancreatic fluid) approaches 60%. If indeed such findings are detected, a CT scan should be repeated at regular intervals (approximately 1 week) to monitor for further development of changes or progression to signs of peripancreatic infection. Although ultrasound examination can also detect fluid collections or phlegmon involving the lesser sac, the CT scan remains the study of choice. Similarly, MRI can be useful for detection of such changes.

Complications of Acute Pancreatitis

Secondary pancreatic infections account for more than 80% of the late deaths in patients with acute pancreatitis. These entities occur with increasing frequency in direct proportion to the severity of acute pancreatitis. Secondary pancreatic infections occur as the result of infection of necrotic pancreatic and peripancreatic tissue. Patients with significant pancreatitis and resultant extensive pancreatic and peripancreatic necrosis are therefore at significant risk for the development of this complication. Radiographic investigation is particularly helpful in the diagnosis of secondary pancreatic infection (Fig. 2). Extraluminal retroperitoneal air on abdominal X-ray can be pathognomonic when present, but is seen in only a minority of patients. At present, CT scanning with percutaneous aspiration as needed is the most accurate procedure for evaluating for potential secondary pancreatic infections. The

CT finding of air bubbles in the peripancreatic fluid collection is diagnostic of a secondary pancreatic infection but is not present in all cases. Focal or diffuse, well-marginated zones of nonenhanced pancreatic parenchyma that are larger than 3 cm or involve more than 30% of the area of the pancreas are typical criteria for the diagnosis of pancreatic necrosis. The combination of imaging via CT scan and guided percutaneous needle aspiration appears to be highly reliable in differentiating a secondary pancreatic infection from sterile peripancreatic necrosis. The sample obtained by percutaneous aspiration is gram stained and cultured, and the aspiration is considered to be positive for infection if either the gram stain or the culture reveals organisms. The treatment of secondary peripancreatic infection involves appropriate antibiotic therapy and prompt surgical drainage. Percutaneous or endoscopic techniques have a limited role in the drainage of these infections in that treatment requires extensive surgical debridement of necrotic tissue and either open packing or wide sump drainage of the cavity.

Extensive pancreatic necrosis and peripancreatic infection can be associated with complications involving the peripancreatic vessels. Massive hemorrhage can occur either in patients with peripancreatic infection or with erosion from an enlarging pancreatic pseudocyst. In some patients a pseudoaneurysm will form as the bleeding site is initially contained. Hemorrhage from peripancreatic vessels is associated with significant mortality, and therefore an aggressive approach to diagnosis should be instituted at the first clinical suggestion of bleeding. Although real-time ultrasound with pulse and color Doppler may identify vascular complications, visceral angiography is usually required to confirm the diagnosis. Angiographic embolotherapy has gained increasing acceptance and utility in the management of many arterial bleeding sources associated with pancreatitis. Angiography followed by the selective administration of surgical sponge pledgets or wire coils into the artery serving as the source of hemorrhage has been successful as definitive therapy. This technique is the treatment of choice for most patients with the exception of individuals with unstable vital signs associated with massive hemorrhage. In these patients a direct surgical approach is indicated.

Splenic or portal vein thrombosis can occur with either acute or chronic pancreatitis (as well as pancreatic neoplasms). Real-time ultrasound with color flow Doppler, or spiral CT or MRI with intravenous contrast demonstrates not only evidence of the absence of venous flow but also associated collateral vessels or varices. Angiography is usually not indicated for either diagnosis or treatment.

Pancreatic Pseudocysts

A pancreatic pseudocyst is a localized collection of pancreatic juice enclosed by a wall of fibrous or granulation tissue, arising as a consequence of pancreatitis, pancreatic trauma, or a neoplastic obstruction of the pancreatic duct. Pseudocysts account for more than 75% of all cystic lesions of the pancreas, contain a high concentration of pancreatic enzymes, and lack an epithelial lining. Pancreatic pseudocysts may develop following an attack of acute pancreatitis or may occur without a specific attack in patients with recurrent chronic pancreatitis. Pseudocysts typically are present as long as there is a communication with the pancreatic duct. When the communication between the pancreatic duct and pseudocyst closes secondarily to syccytrization, the intracystic fluid is reabsorbed by the body and the pseudocyst

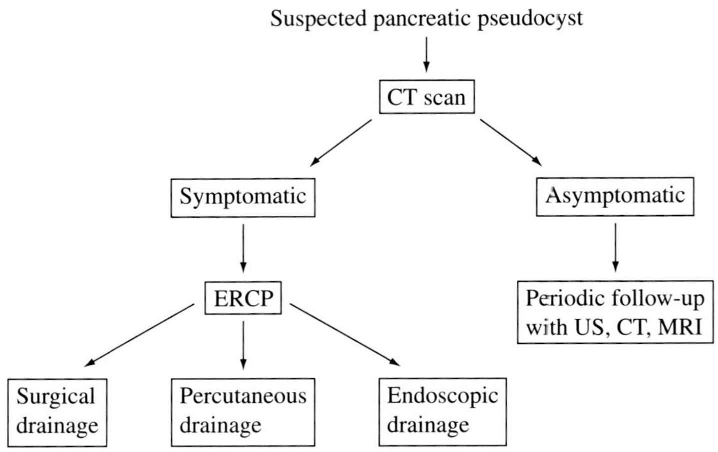

Figure 3. Radiologic studies in the evaluation and management of suspected pancreatic pseudocysts.

resolves. Persistence of a pseudocyst implies an ongoing communication with the pancreatic ductal system whether or not the ductal system can be demonstrated radiographically or pathologically. It is important to differentiate pseudocysts from acute fluid collections (pseudo-pseudocysts), which may arise early in the course of an attack of acute pancreatitis and lack the wall of fibrous or granulation tissue. Such fluid collections are common in patients with severe pancreatitis, but most regress spontaneously and do not require specifically directed treatment. Pseudocysts must also be differentiated from cystic neoplasms of the pancreas.

Alcohol is the most common causative factor for pancreatitis-related pseudocysts, being a cause in 65% of all cases. The clinical presentation of patients who develop pseudocysts following an episode of acute pancreatitis involves the persistence or recurrence of upper abdominal pain for a period of time that is longer than when uncomplicated pancreatitis occurs. Other symptoms include nausea and vomiting, weight loss, and jaundice. Patients have upper abdominal tenderness on physical examination and a palpable mass may be present. Symptoms of early satiety, nausea, and vomiting may be the result of gastroduodenal obstruction from the mass effect of the pseudocyst. Less common modes of presentation in patients with pancreatic pseudocysts include evidence of sepsis secondary to pseudocyst infection, evidence of hypovolemia related to pseudocyst-associated intraabdominal hemorrhage, pruritus and jaundice secondary to common bile duct obstruction, and rarely, severe acute abdominal pain secondary to free rupture of the pseudocyst.

There is no definitive laboratory test for the diagnosis of a pancreatic pseudocyst. Patients may have elevations of serum amylase and lipase; however, this is not the case in many patients. Radiologic examination remains the hallmark for the identification and diagnosis as well as the follow-up in patients with pseudocysts (Fig. 3). A CT scan of the abdomen is currently the favored study for demonstrating a pancreatic pseudocyst. Ultrasound evaluation is nearly as accurate as CT scanning and may be used as an efficient means for following fluid collections to ensure resolution. Magnetic resonance imaging provides parenchymal information similar to CT scan as well as cholangiographic information, which may have therapeutic significance.

Endoscopic retrograde cholangiopancreatography is important in the diagnosis and management of many patients with pancreatic pseudocysts. Patients with pseudocysts have nearly universal abnormalities in their pancreatograms, with between 20 and 50% having demonstrable abnormalities of their cholangiogram as well (9, 10). Endoscopic retrograde cholangiopancreatography may be important in dictating management in that if a major duct disruption or communication exists or a bile duct stricture is present, surgical drainage may be indicated.

The appropriate management of pancreatic pseudocysts requires knowledge of their natural history. Traditionally, it was considered that any pseudocyst that persisted over a 6-week period should undergo operation to avoid the development of complications. More recent data would suggest that asymptomatic pseudocysts can be preferentially managed nonoperatively independent of pseudocyst size (11). If they are asymptomatic, routine follow-up with ultrasound, CT scan, or MRI is appropriate. The options for management of symptomatic pancreatic pseudocysts include internal surgical drainage or surgical excision. In recent years there has also been significant enthusiasm for nonsurgical drainage of pancreatic pseudocysts by percutaneous aspiration with or without catheter drainage, using either ultrasound or CT guidance. Endoscopic approaches involving localization, aspiration, and drainage of pseudocysts into the adjacent stomach or duodenum have also been developed. Endoscopic ultrasound is particularly helpful in this technique, which involves placement of an endoprosthesis to create a fistula between the gastric or duodenal lumen and the pseudocyst. Although the initial experience with these techniques appears favorable, long-term follow-up and more widespread application are necessary prior to the conclusion that these techniques are favorable to traditional surgical drainage.

Chronic Pancreatitis

Chronic pancreatitis is characterized clinically by recurrent or persistent episodes of abdominal pain. Evidence of functional pancreatic insufficiency such as steatorrhea or diabetes is often, but not invariably seen. The morphological changes of chronic pancreatitis include sclerosis with destruction and permanent loss of exocrine elements. These changes may be focal, segmental, or diffuse, and may be associated with various degrees of dilatation of the pancreatic ductal system. Ductal dilatation is most often associated with strictures of the ducts and/or intraductal protein plugs or calculi.

Alcoholism is the cause of 75% of cases of chronic pancreatitis in the United States and in other developed countries. Biliary tract disease is seldom associated with the development of chronic pancreatitis.

Abnormal physical findings are rare in patients with chronic pancreatitis. There may be some epigastric tenderness and evidence of weight loss. Routine laboratory studies are rarely of benefit in the diagnosis of chronic pancreatitis.

Radiological Examination in Patients with Chronic Pancreatitis. The findings of diffuse speckled calcifications within the pancreas on plain abdominal radiographs is pathognomonic for chronic pancreatitis and is seen in approximately 30–50% of

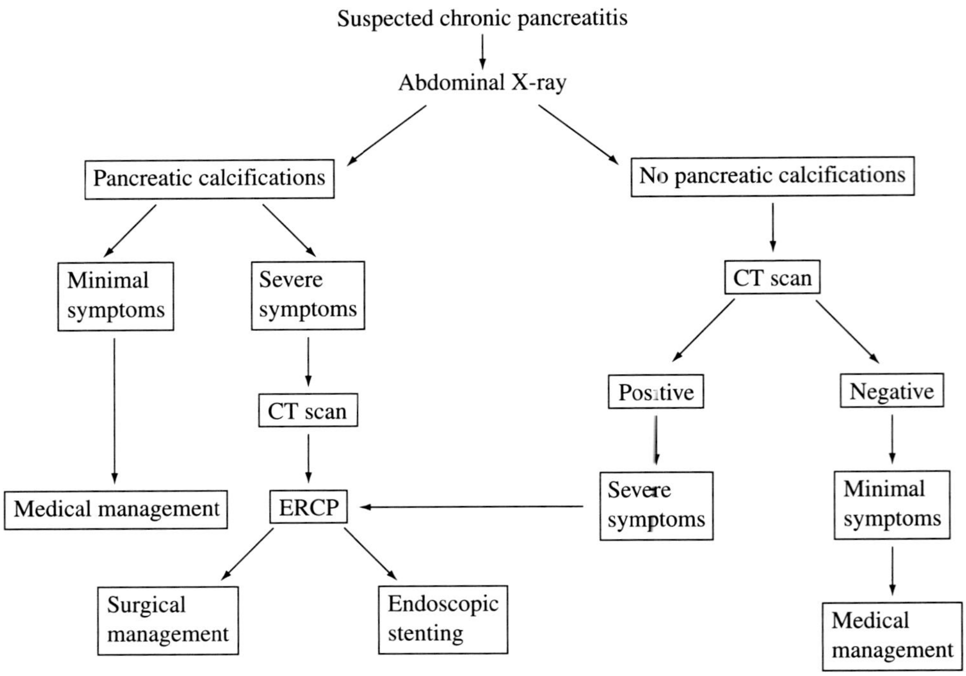

Figure 4. Radiologic studies in the evaluation and treatment of chronic pancreatitis.

patients (Fig. 4). Computed tomographic scanning is probably the most sensitive radiological imaging examination for diagnosing chronic pancreatitis. The most common CT findings in chronic pancreatitis include pancreatic ductal dilatation, pancreatic calcifications, and cystic lesions in or near the pancreas. Less commonly, pancreatic enlargement or atrophy, heterogeneous pancreatic density, and splenic vein thrombosis may be seen. Endoscopic retrograde cholangiopancreatography is the invasive radiological procedure of choice in the diagnosis and management of chronic pancreatitis. The accuracy of ERCP in making the diagnosis increases with the duration of the disease, reaching 92% of patients who have been affected for more than 5 years (12). The radiologic appearance on ERCP of the pancreatic ductal system may show caliber variation, stricture, obstruction, ductal filling defects (stones), or filling of pseudocysts. Despite the usefulness of ERCP, this invasive and costly procedure should be performed only in those patients who are being evaluated for operation or other modes of treatment. The role of MRCP is currently under investigation.

Surgical treatment of chronic pancreatitis includes either ductal drainage procedures or ablative procedures. Endoscopic retrograde cholangiopancreatography is critical in defining the anatomy of the pancreatic and biliary ductal system in dictating surgical management. Recently the role of therapeutic endoscopic interventions such as stenting of the major or minor pancreatic ducts has been reported (13, 14). These interventions at this time remain preliminary, reporting only small numbers of patients with long-term follow-up.

PANCREATIC NEOPLASMS

There are three common types of pancreatic neoplasms: pancreatic adenocarcinoma, cystic neoplasms of the pancreas, and islet cell tumors of the pancreas. Ductal adenocarcinoma of the pancreas is by far the most common of these neoplasms. Two-thirds of these tumors arise in the periampullary region and are difficult to distinguish from other periampullary carcinomas arising in the ampulla of Vater, distal common bile duct, and duodenum. Frequently, the clinical presentation with obstructive jaundice, preoperative imaging studies, and findings at laparotomy do not allow differentiation of the specific site of origin. Pathological examination of resected specimens shows that adenocarcinoma of the pancreas accounts for 50–60% of these tumors; however, because these data arise from resected specimens, the incidence of ampullary, distal bile duct, and duodenal carcinomas is probably somewhat higher owing to the fact that these tumors have a greater rate of resectability than tumors arising in the head of the pancreas. Therefore carcinoma of the pancreas is the likely site of origin in up to 90% of periampullary carcinomas. Islet cell tumors or neuroendocrine tumors may be either histologically benign or malignant and may be functional with excessive hormone production resulting in clinical manifestations. Nonfunctional islet cell tumors produce no recognizable hormonal manifestations and are usually detected owing to their space-occupying characteristics. Cystic neoplasms of the pancreas arise from the exocrine pancreas and are classified as either benign serous cystadenomas, potentially malignant mucinous cystadenomas, or malignant mucinous cystadenocarcinomas. Cystic neoplasms are much less common than ductal adenocarcinoma, tend to occur in women, and can be found throughout the entire gland. Although malignant cystic neoplasms of the pancreas can produce obstructive jaundice, this presentation is much less common than is seen with ductal carcinoma.

Pancreatic Carcinoma

The early symptoms of pancreatic carcinoma are usually vague and include anorexia, weight loss, abdominal discomfort, and nausea. Specific symptoms usually develop only after invasion or obstruction of a nearby structure, usually the common bile duct. In this case, jaundice is progressive and is often associated with pruritus. Pain of moderate intensity may be present as the result of obstruction of either the biliary or pancreatic ducts. This pain, often described as dull and located in the epigastrium, may be accompanied by back pain and is often worse in the supine position and relieved by sitting forward. In patients with carcinoma of the head of the pancreas, more intense pain can be caused by invasion of the tumor into the splanchnic plexus of the retroperitoneum as well as obstruction of the pancreatic duct. Pain is generally the only symptom in patients with tumors arising in the body and tail of the pancreas. The pain is again subtle, vague, and nondescript initially but can become intense as the tumor progresses and retroperitoneal and splanchnic nerve invasion occurs.

There are no specific laboratory tests for pancreatic neoplasms. Virtually all patients with lesions in the head of the pancreas present with liver function test abnormalities including increased levels of total bilirubin, alkaline phosphatase, and transaminases. The tumor antigen CA 19-9 may be elevated in patients with

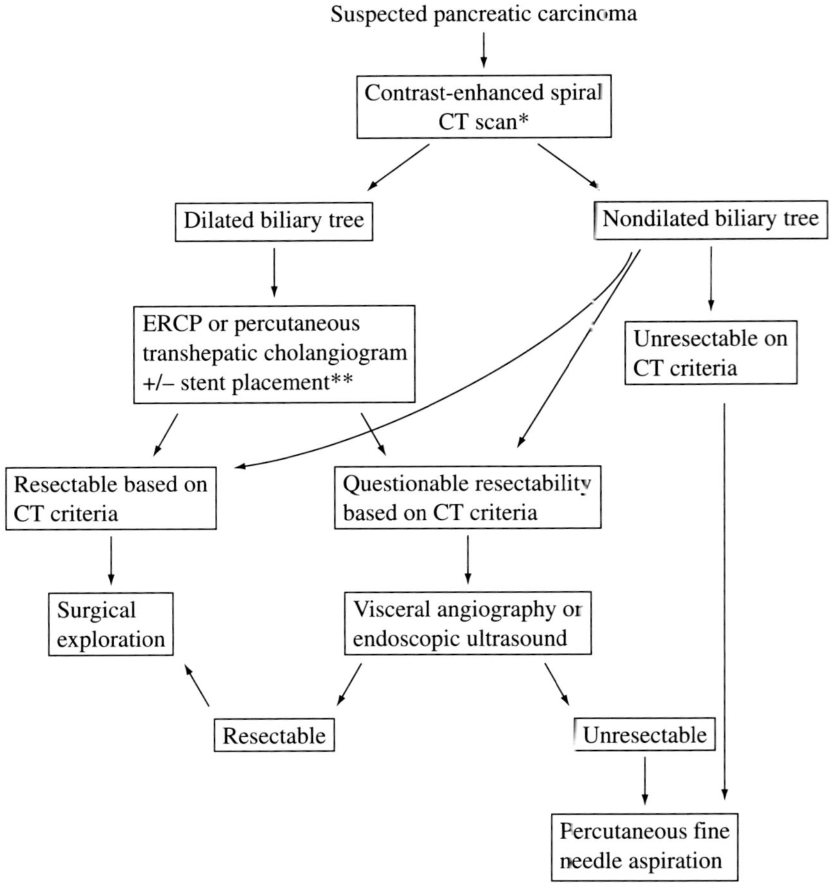

*MRI if contraindications to contrast-enhanced CT or equivocal CT examination.
**MRCP may have a role to play.

Figure 5. Radiologic studies in the evaluation and treatment of suspected pancreatic carcinoma.

pancreatic carcinoma although it is not sensitive in the early stages of disease and therefore is not valuable as a screening test.

Radiologic Studies in Patients with Pancreatic Carcinoma. Radiologic studies play two primary roles in patients with pancreatic carcinoma. First, radiologic studies are essential in making the preoperative diagnosis. Secondly, radiologic studies are important in the preoperative staging of pancreatic cancer and assisting in determining the role for either surgical management or nonoperative palliation (Fig. 5). Finally, radiologic techniques are essential in the performance of nonoperative palliation of pancreatic carcinoma.

Diagnosis of Pancreatic Carcinoma. The early diagnosis of pancreatic carcinoma requires a high index of suspicion and appropriate aggressiveness in proving the diagnosis. The prompt evaluation of patients with jaundice, however, offers the opportunity for early diagnosis. Any patient with jaundice should undergo prompt diagnostic imaging with either ultrasound or CT. Both tests confirm the obstructive nature of jaundice by demonstrating dilated intra- and extrahepatic bile ducts. Conventional ultrasonography is a safe and easy examination, does not entail radiation exposure, and is relatively inexpensive. This technique is more sensitive for detecting gallstones than other modalities, but suffers from being technically suboptimal in a significant percentage of patients. Currently the use of intravenous and oral contrast-enhanced spiral CT offers the best form of imaging of the pancreas because it can determine the level of obstruction, demonstrate the presence of a pancreatic mass (as small as 1 cm in size), and detect liver metastases or local vascular invasion. Magnetic resonance imaging is comparable to CT in the work-up of suspected neoplasm. Recently MRI has been shown to be useful in cases with indeterminate pancreatic head enlargement or spiral CT (15).

Once biliary obstruction has been confirmed by imaging studies, the next step in the evaluation of the jaundiced patient is cholangiography. Either the endoscopic or percutaneous approach is appropriate, with the choice of technique depending on the local expertise. Using the endoscopic approach, ampullary and duodenal carcinomas can be visualized and biopsied. In addition, a pancreatogram may be obtained that may be important if the differential diagnosis includes chronic pancreatitis. In most cases of pancreatic cancer, the ductal system is obstructed with no distal filling of the duct. The percutaneous approach is technically easier with a dilated biliary tree and offers the advantage of defining the proximal biliary system that will be used in reconstruction. A biliary stent can be placed through the obstructing lesion in the bile duct by other endoscopic or percutaneous approach to alleviate jaundice. The use of biliary stents preoperatively in an attempt to improve the overall operative risk has been addressed by a number of prospective, randomized studies with mixed results (16, 17). It appears likely, although not routinely indicated, that in selected patients with advanced malnutrition, sepsis, and/or correctable medical conditions, or those in which a significant delay will ensue between diagnosis and definitive surgery, preoperative biliary drainage is useful

A preoperative attempt to obtain a histological diagnosis is not routinely indicated in patients who are considered operative candidates to attempt resection or for palliation. However, if preoperative staging precludes surgical resection for cure, unresectable pancreatic carcinoma may respond to radiation or chemotherapy with both a benefit with respect to survival and palliation of symptoms. Either CT- or ultrasound-guided fine needle aspiration for cytological diagnosis is indicated in this setting with diagnostic results in up to 90% of patients.

Preoperative Staging of Pancreatic Carcinoma. The goal of preoperative staging of pancreatic carcinoma is to determine the role of surgery and the optimal treatment for each individual patient. In general, preoperative staging is more useful for pancreatic tumors than any other form of periampullary cancer, because resectability for the latter lesions is usually significantly higher at the time of presentation than for pancreatic cancer. In many patients, dynamic abdominal spiral CT with oral and intravenous contrast provides all the information necessary by demonstrating liver metastases and/or major vascular invasion. The extent of further staging to be performed depends on the individual patient and the preference of the surgeon. If the surgeon's philosophy is to pursue surgical treatment of all patients, in order either to attempt resection or to provide palliation, further staging is unnecessary. However, if findings at staging could preclude an operation and lead to nonoperative palliation, these efforts are worthwhile.

Local invasion of adjacent visceral vessels preclude resection in a significant number of patients explored for periampullary carcinoma. Of the periampullary malignancies, major vessel involvement is far more common in tumors originating in the head of the pancreas. Preoperative visceral angiography with arterial injection of the celiac and superior mesenteric arteries with venous phase studies provides the best demonstration of vascular anatomy and major vessel encasement or occlusion. In a review of this technique in patients with periampullary carcinoma identified by CT scan at The Johns Hopkins Hospital, 77% of patients without evidence of major visceral vessel occlusion or encasement were resectable (18). Major vessel encasement indicated a lower resectability rate (35%). Furthermore, in all patients with major vessel occlusion, the tumor was found to be unresectable at operation. Finally, visceral angiography will also detect anatomy variations such as replaced right hepatic artery or atherosclerotic stenosis or occlusion of the celiac axis that may alter operative management. In patients with tumors of the body or tail of the pancreas, encasement or occlusion of the splenic artery or vein is common. Although this finding alone does not preclude resection, angiography is indicated to rule out involvement of superior mesenteric and portal vein and/or the celiac axis.

Recently experience has been gained with less invasive techniques to evaluate the status of peripancreatic vessels in patients with pancreatic carcinoma. Contrast-enhanced spiral CT is a sensitive technique with results comparable to those seen with angiography. Similarly MRI can provide comparable information. Additionally its volumetric data acquisition affords "angiographic display" in multiple imaging planes. Magnetic resonance imaging is also indicated in patients with contrast allergy. Transabdominal ultrasound may reliably detect major vessel occlusion but lacks the sensitivity of the other examinations.

Endoscopic ultrasonography is a minimally invasive technique in which a high-frequency transducer is placed in the gastric and duodenal lumen in close proximity to the pancreas and adjacent organs. The main usefulness of this technique is to detect small pancreatic lesions (less than 2 cm) and also lymph node and vascular involvement. This technique is also particularly useful in evaluation of ampullary tumors with respect to invasion of the duodenal wall and pancreas. Recent data would suggest that endoscopic ultrasound examination is superior to conventional sonography, CT, and angiography in assessing resectability (19). Experience with this technique, which is operator dependent, is still limited, precluding its widespread use.

The information gained from preoperative staging provides a basis for planning for each individual patient. If preoperative staging with CT scan and angiography is completed, resectability rates may approach 90% of tumors of the head of the pancreas (20). Preoperative staging therefore results in considerable improvement from previous resectability rates of 25%, thus eliminating the need for unnecessary operation in a number of patients.

Nonoperative Palliation of Pancreatic Carcinoma. Patients in whom preoperative staging detects disease precluding surgical resection may be candidates for

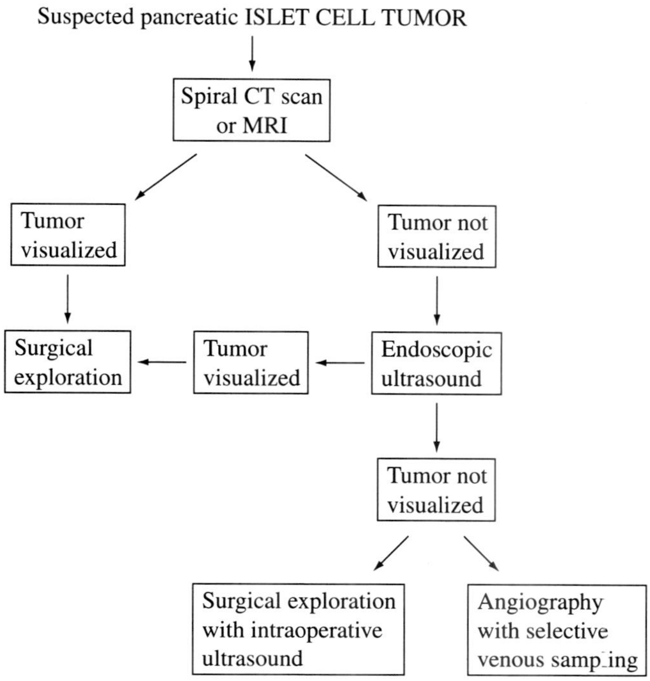

Figure 6. Radiologic studies in the evaluation and detection of pancreatic suspected islet cell tumor.

nonoperative palliation. Nonoperative palliation in patients with carcinoma of the head of the pancreas is primarily directed at relief of obstructive jaundice and can be accomplished either by an endoscopic or percutaneous route. A number of studies have demonstrated that nonoperative biliary stenting is as effective as surgical palliation in the short term and associated with lower procedure-related morbidity and mortality (21, 22). Recently, the use of metallic endoprostheses has been shown to be associated with a longer stent patency and therefore a decreased need for reintervention (23).

Islet Cell Neoplasms

Islet cell tumors are neoplasms that form from the neuroendocrine elements of the pancreas known as the islets of Langerhans, which are responsible for pancreatic hormone production. Therefore, many of these tumors present with symptoms due to excess hormone secretion. The most common islet cell tumors are gastrinomas resulting in excessive gastric acid secretion presenting with complications with either intractable symptoms or complications of duodenal ulcer disease. The next most common islet cell tumors are insulinomas, which present with excessive production of insulin and episodes of hypoglycemia. Nonfunctional islet cell tumors are either symptomatic secondary to a space-occupying nature or detected incidentally.

The role of radiology in the diagnosis and evaluation of islet cell tumors consists of both identifying the primary tumor and determining the extent of disease (Fig. 6). The localization of functional endocrine tumors can be very challenging. Approximately 20% of insulinomas and up to 40% of gastrinomas may not be visualized by radiologic imaging. Gastrinomas are particularly challenging because they have a high frequency of extrapancreatic foci. The initial study to be obtained in an attempt to identify the location of a functional islet cell tumor is usually a spiral CT scan. Islet cell tumors are known for their hypervascularity. Therefore, the use of helical scanning can be more sensitive in detecting these tumors. Similarly, MRI techniques that utilize dynamic contrast enhancement can also be valuable in their detection. Recently favorable results have been reported with the use of endoscopic ultrasound in detection of these tumors. In one report 82% of pancreatic endocrine tumors not detected by traditional CT assessment were seen by endoscopic ultrasound (24). Therefore, owing to its effectiveness and minimally invasive nature, endoscopic ultrasound has become the primary technique for preoperative localization of functional pancreatic islet cell tumors.

The hypervascular nature of these tumors has traditionally made angiography useful in the detection of islet cell tumors. Although endoscopic ultrasound has replaced angiography at the early stages of evaluation, in those patients in which all imaging techniques prove unsuccessful, angiography with visceral venous sampling may help identify an area of increased hormone production to aid the surgeon in localizing the tumor at the time of surgery. This technique is, quite complex, tedious, and expensive, however. Whether this technique should be considered prior to initial surgical exploration in patients with suspected but undetected islet cell tumors is unclear. Finally, the use of intraoperative ultrasound to detect the primary lesion or other synchronous lesions is also recommended.

The treatment of an islet cell tumor is surgical resection. In a significant percentage of patients, liver metastasis may be present at the time of presentation. In selected patients, resection of the primary tumor and metastasis may prove useful in alleviating the symptoms of excess hormone production. Contrast-enhanced CT or MRI scans are both useful in the detection of liver metastasis and should be obtained preoperatively in all patients in which surgical intervention for an islet cell tumor is considered.

In nonfunctional islet cell tumors, detection of the tumor mass is seldom a significant problem in that the diagnosis is made only because of the space-occupying nature of the lesion or because it is detected on an imaging study. In these patients, a significant percentage of the tumors are malignant and therefore surgical resection should be considered unless metastatic disease is detected. There is a very low incidence of visceral vessel involvement with islet cell tumors; therefore staging with spiral CT scan alone is sufficient in most cases.

Cystic Neoplasms of the Pancreas

Cystic neoplasms of the pancreas may cause symptoms of abdominal pain or discomfort and are frequently seen in middle-aged women. The tumors can be found throughout the entire gland and may present with obstructive jaundice as the result of bile duct obstruction. Cystic neoplasms of the pancreas can be benign (serous cystadenomas), potentially malignant (mucinous cystadenomas), or malignant (cystadenocarcinoma).

The role of radiologic studies in the management of cystic neoplasms involves distinguishing a neoplastic cystic lesion from a benign inflammatory pancreatic

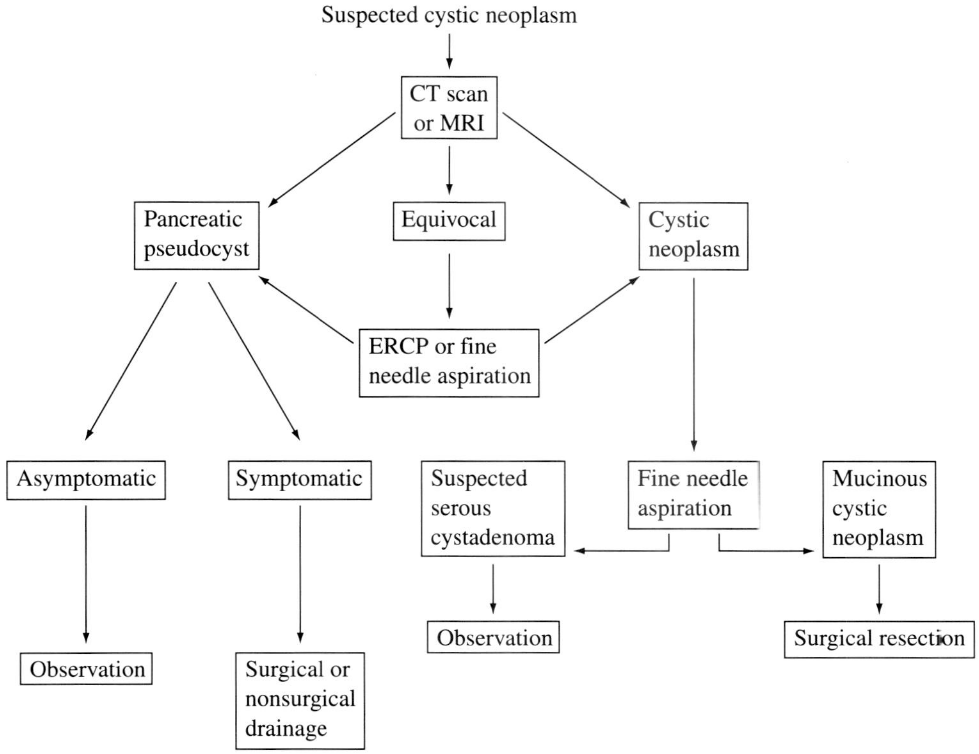

Figure 7. Radiologic studies in the evaluation of suspected cystic neoplasms.

pseudocyst (Fig. 7). Furthermore, if a lesion can be defined preoperatively as a serous cystadenoma, a conservative approach with prolonged observation rather than surgery may be indicated. Although both ultrasonography and CT or MRI may detect the presence of a cystic neoplasm, CT or MRI scan appears to be more valuable in distinguishing a neoplastic growth from an inflammatory pseudocyst. A pancreatic pseudocyst generally has a single cyst with evidence of pancreatic and peripancreatic inflammation, whereas a cystic neoplasm has multiple cysts with no adjacent inflammation. The presence of an eccentric solid component within the wall of the cyst and the lack of calcification also helps differentiate neoplasms from pseudocysts.

Serous cystadenomas usually demonstrate multiple small cysts with a calcified sunburst appearance on CT scan, whereas with mucinous lesions, one or more dominant cysts up to several centimeters in size may be seen. Overall size is of no discriminant value. Distinguishing a benign from a malignant mucinous lesion can be difficult in the absence of distant metastasis. However, local changes such as evidence of biliary obstruction, portal or splenic vein occlusion, or duodenal obstruction strongly suggest cystadenocarcinoma. Magnetic resonance imaging provides similar information. Angiography offers no advantage compared to CT scan in distinguishing the type of cystic neoplasm.

Endoscopic retrograde cholangiopancreatography alone has little to offer in evaluating a presumed cystic neoplasm, although ductal changes of chronic pancreatitis or direct communication with the cystic mass may be strong evidence in support of a diagnosis of pancreatic inflammatory disease from a cystic neoplasm. Cystic neoplasms may, but do not normally, communicate with the ductal system and usually only create an extrinsic mass effect on pancreatogram. Endoscopic ultrasound also adds little in differentiating neoplasms versus pseudocysts.

Percutaneous cytological sampling and biopsy and cystic fluid markers have been advocated in the diagnosis of cystic neoplasms (25). The fluid should be analyzed for amylase; an increased level is highly suggestive of a pseudocyst. However, if fluid amylase is normal and the lesion returns cells for analysis, the diagnosis of a neoplasm, either benign or malignant, may be obtained by standard cytological techniques. Evaluation for mucin, increased viscosity, and tumor markers such as carcinoembryonic antigens and CA 19-9 have been suggested to be highly specific for mucinous versus serous cystadenomas and especially for mucinous cystadenocarcinomas. Finally, despite efforts to distinguish inflammatory cysts from neoplastic cysts or to identify the specific type of cystic neoplasm, a high index of suspicion should be maintained. Only surgical resection can ultimately prove the true nature of a pancreatic cystic lesion and should be strongly considered unless the clinical evidence of the inflammatory nature of the lesion is overwhelming.

REFERENCES

1. Ranson JHC, Rifkind KM, Roses TF, et al. Prognostic signs and the role of operative management in acute pancreatitis. *Surg Gynecol Obstet.* 1974;139:69–81.
2. Steinberg W. The clinical utility of CA 19-9 tumor-associated antigen. *Am J Gastroenterol.* 1990;85:350–355.
3. Dong B, Chen M. Improved sonographic visualization of choledocholithiasis. *J Clin Ultrasound.* 1987;15:185–190.
4. Neoptolemos JP, London NJ, James D, Carr-Locke DL, Bailey IA, Fossard DP. Controlled trial of urgent endoscopic retrograde cholangiopancreatography and endoscopic sphincterotomy versus conservative treatment for acute pancreatitis due to gallstones. *Lancet.* 1988;979–983.
5. Fan ST, Lai ECS, Mok FPT, Lo CM, Zheng SS, Wong J. Early treatment of acute biliary pancreatitis from endoscopic pappilotomy. *New Engl J Med.* 1993;328:228–232.
6. Lee SP, Nicholls JF, Park HC. Biliary sludge is a cause of acute pancreatitis. *New Engl J Med.* 1992;326:589–593.
7. Feller ER. Endoscopic retrograde cholangiopancreatography in the diagnosis of unexplained pancreatitis. *Arch Intern Med.* 1984;144:1797–1799.
8. Ranson JHC, Balthazar E, Caccaual ER, et al. Computed tomography and the prediction of pancreatic abscess in acute pancreatitis. *Ann Surg.* 1985;201:656–663.
9. Laxson LC, Fromkes JJ, Cooperman M. Endoscopic retrograde cholangiopancreatography in the management of pancreatic pseudocysts. *Am J Surg.* 1985;150:683–686.
10. Nealon WH, Townsend CM, Thompson JC. Preoperative endoscopic retrograde cholangiopancreatography (ERCP) in patients with pancreatic pseudocysts associated with resolving acute and chronic pancreatitis. *Ann Surg.* 1989;209:532–540.
11. Yeo CJ, Bastidas JA, Lynch-Nyhan A, et al. The natural history of pancreatic pseudocysts documented by computed tomography. *Surg Gynecol Obstet.* 1990;170:411–417.
12. Caletti G, Brocchi E, Agostini D, et al. Sensitivity of endoscopic retrograde pancreatography in chronic pancreatitis. *Br J Surg.* 1982;69:507–509.

13. Kozarek RA, Ball TJ, Patterson DJ, et al. Endoscopic pancreatic duct sphincterotomy: Indications, technique, and analysis of results. *Gastrointest Endosc.* 1994;40:592–598.

14. Cremer M, Duviere J, Delhay EM, et al. Endoscopic management of chronic pancreatitis. *Acta Gastroenterol Belg.* 1993;56:192–200.

15. Semecka KC, Kelekis NL, Molina PL, et al. Pancreatic masses with inconclusive findings on spiral CT: Is there a role for MRI? *JMRI.* 1996;6:585–588.

16. Pitt HA, Gomes AS, Lois JF, et al. Does preoperative percutaneous biliary drainage reduce operative risk or increase hospital costs? *Ann Surg.* 1985;201:545–553.

17. Lygidakis NJ, VanDerHeyde M, and Lubler MJ. An evaluation of preoperative biliary drainage in the surgical management of pancreatic head carcinoma. *Acta Chir Scand.* 1987;153:665–668.

18. Dooley WC, Cameron JL, Pitt HA, et al. Is preoperative angiography useful in patients with periampullary tumors? *Ann Surg.* 1990;211:649–655.

19. Rosch T, Braig C, Gain T, et al. Staging of pancreatic and ampullary carcinoma by endoscopic ultrasonography: Comparison with conventional sonography, computed tomography, and angiography. *Gastroenterology.* 1992;102:188–199.

20. Warshaw AL, Gu ZY, Wittenberg J, and Waltman AC. Preoperative staging and assessment of resectability in pancreatic cancer. *Arch Surg.* 1990;125:230–233.

21. Anderson JR, Sorensen SM, Kruse A, et al. Randomized trial of endoscopic endoprosthesis versus operative bypass in malignant obstructive jaundice. *Gut.* 1989;30:1132–1135.

22. Smith AC, Dowsett JF, Russell RCJ, et al. A randomized trial of endoscopic stenting versus surgical bypass and malignant low bile duct obstruction. *Lancet.* 1994;344:1655–1657.

23. Carr-Locke DL, Ball TJ, Connors PJ, et al. Multicenter randomized trial of Wallstent biliary endoprosthesis versus plastic stents. *Gastrointest Endosc.* 1993;39:310–314.

24. Rosch T, Lightdale CT, Botet JF, et al. Endosonographic location of pancreatic endocrine tumors. *New Engl J Med.* 1992;326:1721–1726.

25. Lewandrowski KB, Southern JF, Pins MR, et al. Cyst fluid analysis in the differential diagnosis of pancreatic cysts: a comparison of pseudocysts, serous cystadenomas, mucinous cystic neoplasms, and mucinous cystadenocarcinoma. *Ann Surg.* 1993;217:41–47.

INDEX